INTRODUCTION TO
Radiologic Sciences
and
Patient Care

Fourth Edition

INTRODUCTION TO
Radiologic Sciences
and
Patient Care

Arlene M. Adler, MEd, RT(R), FAERS
Professor and Director
Radiologic Sciences Programs
Indiana University Northwest
Gary, Indiana

Richard R. Carlton, MS, RT(R)(CV), FAERS
Director and Associate Professor of Radiologic and Imaging Sciences
Grand Valley State University
Grand Rapids, Michigan

with 348 illustrations

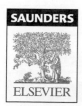
SAUNDERS

ELSEVIER

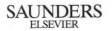

11830 Westline Industrial Drive
St. Louis, Missouri 63146

INTRODUCTION TO RADIOLOGIC SCIENCES AND PATIENT CARE, ED 4   ISBN-13: 978-1-4160-3194-9
ISBN-10: 1-4160-3194-4

Copyright © 2007, 2003, 1999, 1994 by Saunders, an imprint of Elsevier Inc.

ISBN-13: 978-1-4160-3194-9
ISBN-10: 1-4160-3194-4

Acquisitions Editor: Jeanne Wilke
Developmental Editor: Becky Swisher
Publishing Services Manager: Julie Eddy
Project Manager: Andrea Campbell
Design Direction: Andrea Lutes

Printed in the United States of America

Last digit is the print number: 9 8 7 6 5 4 3 2

To Don, Meredith, and Katie Adler
and to D. Raleigh and Hazel Carlton

Contributors

Arlene M. Adler, MEd, RT(R), FAERS
Professor and Director
Radiologic Sciences Programs
Indiana University Northwest
Gary, Indiana

Angie Arnold, MEd,RT(R)
Assistant Professor and Radiologic Technology Program
    Director
University of Cincinnati
Raymond Walters College
Cincinnati, Ohio

Sarah S. Baker, EdD,RT(R), FASRT
Associate Professor
Indiana University School of Medicine
Radiologic Sciences Programs
Indianapolis, Indiana

Norman E. Bolus, MPH,CNMT
Assistant Professor and Clinical Coordinator
Nuclear Medicine Program
University of Alabama at Birmingham
Birmingham, Alabama

Jan Bruckner, PhD, PT
Physical Therapist
Penn Care at Home
University of Pennsylvania Health Care System
Bala Cynwyd, Pennsylvania

Robert A. Buerki, PhD, RPh
Professor
Division of Pharmacy Practice and Administration
The Ohio State University College of Pharmacy
Columbus, Ohio

Richard R. Carlton, MS, RT(R)(CV), FAERS
Director and Associate Professor of Radiologic and
    Imaging Sciences
Grand Valley State University
Grand Rapids, Michigan

Steven B. Dowd, EdD, RT(R),(QM), (MR),(M)(CT)
Associate Professor, Radiography Program
University of Alabama at Birmingham
Birmingham, Alabama

Jody L. Ellis, MMS, PA-C, RT(R)
Physician Assistant
Radiology Department
Community Hospital
Munster, Indiana

Larry A. Genzink, MBA, RT(R)
Administrative Director
Spectrum Health
Grand Rapids, Michigan

Joanne S. Greathouse, EdS, RT(R), FASRT, FAERS
Chief Executive Officer
Joint Review Committee on Education in Radiologic
    Technology
Chicago, Illinois

Samuel L. Gurevitz, RPh, PharmD
Consultant Pharmacist
Care Pharmaceutical Service, Inc.
Griffith, Indiana

Audrey Harris, MAEd,RT(R)(CT)(M)(QM)
Director/Assistant Professor, Radiography Program
University of Alabama at Birmingham
Birmingham, Alabama

Tracy Herrmann MEd,RT(R)
Associate Professor and Chairperson of Allied Health
University of Cincinnati
Raymond Walters College
Cincinnati, Ohio

Lyn Hubbard, MSE, RT(R)(M)
Assistant Professor and Clinical Coordinator
Radiologic Sciences
Arkansas State University
State University, Arkansas

Robin Jones, MS, RT(R)
Clinical Assistant Professor and Clinical Coordinator
Radiologic Sciences Programs
Indiana University Northwest
Gary, Indiana

Denise E. Moore, MS, RT(R)
Professor, Radiologic Technology
Online CE Program Director
Sinclair Community College
Dayton, Ohio

Marcia S. Mulcahey, MSN, RN, NP
Lecturer
School of Nursing
Indiana University Northwest
Gary, Indiana

Ann M. Obergfell, JD, RT(R)
Dean of Health Sciences
St. Catharine College
St. Catharine, Kentucky

Sandy L. Piehl, MPA, RT(R)(T)
Director, Radiation Therapy Program
Indiana University Northwest
Gary, Indiana

Margaret A. Skurka, MS, RHIA, CCS
Professor and Director
Health Information Management Programs
Indiana University Northwest
Gary, Indiana

Tracy B. White, MS, RT(R)(T)
Associate Professor and Coordinator
Radiation Therapy Program
Arkansas State University
State University, Arkansas

Bettye G. Wilson, MAEd,RT(R)(CT),ARRT, RDMS, FASRT
Associate Professor, Radiography Program
University of Alabama at Birmingham
Birmingham, Alabama

Thomas Wolfe, MSRS, RT(R)
Program Director, Radiologic Technology
Southwest Tennessee Community College
Memphis, Tennessee

Louis D. Vottero, MS, RPh
Emeritus Professor of Pharmacy
Ohio Northern University
Ada, Ohio

Preface

It has now been 12 years since we first published *Introduction to Radiologic Sciences and Patient Care*. We continue to be pleased with the success of the book as it was quickly adopted in radiologic and imaging science classrooms, and we continue to receive comments and suggestions from our colleagues as they make it part of their teaching. We have been delighted with the success of many of our contributing authors over the years and we think you will find this new edition to be no exception in the quality and relevance of their coverage of the critical issues for beginning clinical practice in our field.

We are always pleased when we are contacted by a teacher, and even more pleased when we are contacted by a student, in regard to this book. We encourage you to email, phone, write, or simply come up and talk to us at one of our professional meetings. We consider dialogue with you to be absolutely critical to improving our profession, and we do value each and every comment, suggestion, correction, or improvement that you can provide. As with any new book, there are numerous updates, clarifications, expanded coverage, and new topics that we added as a result of the commentary we received from students and faculty.

We remain committed to providing a reasonably priced but comprehensive introduction to our profession. We continue to strive to provide the breadth necessary to permit well-informed and properly orientated students their first real clinical practice. We attempt to sufficiently pry open the doors to technical areas so that students will respect not only what they know but how much they don't know as well. We have found that the most dangerous person in a school may well be the first-year student who has had an introduction to psychology but has not yet glimpsed the vast depth of knowledge in this field. He or she runs around trying to apply elementary concepts in interpersonal relationships just enough to thoroughly damage the friendships of anyone foolish enough to take their advice. The danger, of course, is not in what the student knows, but in the failure to appreciate what they do not know. We hope we have avoided setting anyone up for this error by treating our readers as serious new professionals, who are perfectly capable of deducting the potential dangers of the clinical environment while at the same time beginning to learn how to function competently in a manner that begins to make a contribution to our field.

The major changes you will find in the fouth edition include:

- a new chapter on Critical Thinking and Problem Solving that provides the steps involved in the process along with clinical applications of the concepts
- a new chapter on the important topic of Human Diversity which explores the various characteristics of human diversity and the development of cultural competency
- a table of common commands and questions in six different languages
- ancillary support for teachers that includes a test bank as well as all artwork for cut and paste use by faculty members—this is available both on the CD-ROM and on the accompanying *Evolve* site online at http://evolve.elsevier.com/Adler
- patient care laboratories that can be removed from the text without damaging the rest of the book

We continue to assume full responsibility for any errors, including those that may be construed as having arisen from quoting others out of context. We have made every effort to ensure the accuracy of the information. We ask that you remember that it is the responsibility of every practitioner to evaluate the appropriateness of a particular procedure in the context of an actual clinical situation. Consequently, neither the authors nor the publishers take responsibility or accept any liability for the actions of persons applying the information contained herein in an unprofessional manner.

We highly value your point of view. We have learned that the most precious commodity to an author is criticism. As the reader, your perceptions are very important to us and we always appreciate that you communicate with us regarding any aspect of the book you like, dislike, or would like to see changed. As in all our books, we point out that a book such as this is never finished but merely abandoned until the next edition.

Arlene M. Adler, Indiana University Northwest

3400 Broadway, Gary, IN 46408
219-980-6540
aadler@iun.edu

Rick Carlton, Grand Valley State University

Suite 200, Center for Health Sciences, 301 Michigan St. NE, Grand Rapids, MI 49503
616-331-5953
carltonr@gvsu.edu

Acknowledgements

Students are always the best teachers, and we have had some of the very greatest at Indiana University Northwest, Michael Reese Hospital in Chicago, Grand Valley State University, Wilbur Wright College in Chicago, Lima Technical College in Lima, Ohio; City College of San Francisco; Mills-Peninsula School of Radiologic Technology, Burlingame, California; Memphis' Methodist School of Radiologic Technology; and Arkansas State University. We thank you all for listening and valuing what we have tried to teach you.

Rick offers many thanks for the constant and solid support of Bonita Pawloski, Susan Raaymakers, and Lynn Carlton at Grand Valley State University. Finally, and nowhere near last, he must confess to his Dean, Dr. Jane Toot, that he is at a loss to express his thanks for bringing him to Grand Valley State and giving him a role in the new wave of radiologic sciences education.

Arlene would like to thank her professional colleagues: Robin Jones, MS,RT(R); Sandy Piehl, MPA, RT(T)(R); Sharon Lakia, RDMS, BS,RT(R); Bradley Johnson, BS,RT(R); Becky Bilyak, AS,RT(R); Jan Borden BS,RT(R); Helen Campbell, RT(R); Carol Collins, RT(R); Martha Foreman, RT(R); Char Gilpin, RT(R); Patricia Lewis, RT(R), Tiffany Long, BS,RT(R); Becky Wantland RT(R); Sue Wilson, AS, RT(R); Jane Wuchenich, AS,RT(R); Sue Woods, AS, RT(R); and Laura Zlamal,

RT(R), all with the Radiologic Sciences Programs at Indiana University Northwest.

Steve Dowd wishes to acknowledge the support of Mark Harbaugh, PhD, Joan Lewis, MSN, and the Radiography Program Class of 1992, all of Lincoln Land Community College; Mike Drafke, MS, RT(R); and Bettye Wilson, MAEd, RT(R), of the University of Alabama Radiography Program.

Special thanks are owed to the Radiology Department at St. Rita's Medical Center in Lima, Ohio, Edyta Postolowicz, Dennis Stryker, Brian Nye, John Jacobs, Jill Steinbrenner, and Sally Singer, and Jeff Lloyd and Kay Williams at Spectrum Health in Grand Rapids, Michigan. Appreciation is also extended to our photographers, Jenny Torbett from the Biomedical Communications Department at the Ohio State University, George D. Greathouse of Downers Grove, Illinois, and Curt Steele of Arkansas State University. Many of our photographs were great because of the spectacular performance of the best pediatric model ever, Meredith Adler.

Arlene M. Adler, MEd, RT(R), FAERS

Richard R. Carlton, MS, RT(R)(CV), FAERS

Contents

The Profession of Radiologic Technology

1

Introduction to Radiologic Technology

Arlene M. Adler, MEd, RT(R), FAERS
Richard R. Carlton, MS, RT(R)(CV), FAERS

During World War I, the demand for x-ray technicians in military hospitals was so great that a shortage of technical workers became acute at home. The value of the well-trained technician was emphasized, and the radiologist was no longer satisfied with someone who knew only how to throw the switch and develop films.

Margaret Hoing, The First Lady of Radiologic Technology
A History of the American Society of X-Ray Technicians, *1952*

OBJECTIVES

On completion of this chapter, the student will be able to:

1. Explain the use of radiation in medicine.

2. Describe the discovery of x-rays.

3. Define terms related to radiologic technology.

4. Explain the career opportunities within the profession of radiologic technology.

5. Identify the various specialties within a radiology department.

6. Describe the typical responsibilities of the members of the radiology team.

7. Explain the career-ladder opportunities within a radiology department.

8. Discuss the roles of other members of the health care team.

GLOSSARY

Bone Densitometry (BD): the measurement of bone density using dual-energy x-ray absorptiometry (DXA or DEXA) to detect osteoporosis

Cardiovascular Interventional Technology (CVIT): radiologic procedures for the diagnosis and treatment of diseases of the cardiovascular system

Computed Tomography (CT): recording of a predetermined plane in the body using an x-ray beam that is measured, recorded, and then processed by a computer for display on a monitor

Diagnostic Medical Sonography: visualization of deep structures of the body by recording the reflections of pulses of ultrasonic waves directed into the tissue

Energy: capacity to operate or work

Ionization: any process by which a neutral atom gains or loses an electron, thus acquiring a net charge

Magnetic Resonance Imaging (MRI): process of using a magnetic field and radiofrequencies to create sectional images of the body

Mammography: radiography of the breast

Nuclear Medicine Technology: branch of radiology that involves the introduction of radioactive substances into the body for both diagnostic and therapeutic purposes

Radiation: energy transmitted by waves through space or through a medium

Radiation Therapy: branch of radiology involved in the treatment of disease by means of x-rays or radioactive substances

Radiography: making of records (radiographs) of internal structures of the body by passing x-rays or gamma rays through the body to act on specially sensitized film or imaging plate or system

Radiologic Technologist: general term applied to an individual who performs radiography, radiation therapy, or nuclear medicine technology

Radiologist: physician who specializes in the use of roentgen rays and other forms of radiation in the diagnosis and treatment of disease

Radiologist Assistant: an advanced-level radiographer who extends the capacity of the radiologist in the diagnostic imaging environment, thereby enhancing patient care

Radiology: branch of the health sciences dealing with radioactive substances and radiant energy and with the diagnosis and treatment of disease by means of both ionizing (e.g., roentgen rays) and nonionizing (e.g., ultrasound) radiation

Roentgen Ray: synonym for x-ray

X-ray: electromagnetic radiation of short wavelength that is produced when electrons moving at high velocity are suddenly stopped

MEDICAL RADIATION SCIENCES

When the term *radiation* is used, it generally evokes concern and a sense of danger. This circumstance is unfortunate because radiation is not only helpful, it is also essential to life. **Radiation** is energy that is transmitted by waves through space or through a medium (matter); it has permeated the universe since the beginning of time and is a natural part of all of our lives. For example, the sun radiates light energy, and a stove radiates heat energy.

Energy is the capacity to operate or work. The many different forms of energy include mechanical, electrical, heat, nuclear, and electromagnetic. Many forms of energy are used in medicine to create images of anatomic structures or physiologic actions. These images are essential for the proper diagnosis of disease and treatment of the patient. All these energy forms can be described as radiation because they can be, and in many instances must be, transmitted through matter.

Some higher-energy forms, including x-rays, have the ability to ionize atoms in matter. **Ionization** is any process by which a neutral atom gains or loses an electron, thus acquiring a net charge. This process has the ability to disrupt the composition of the matter and, as a result, is capable of disrupting life processes. Special protection should be provided to prevent excessive exposure to ionizing radiation.

Sound is a form of mechanical energy. It is transmitted through matter, and images of the returning sound waves can be created. Diagnostic medical sonography is the field of study that creates anatomic images by recording reflected sound waves. Sound waves are a form of nonionizing radiation.

Electrocardiography and *electroencephalography* are methods of imaging the electrical activities of the heart and of the brain, respectively. The graphs they produce provide useful information about the physiologic activities of these organs.

The body's naturally emitted heat energy can produce images for diagnostic purposes as well. These images are called *thermograms,* and they can be useful in demon-

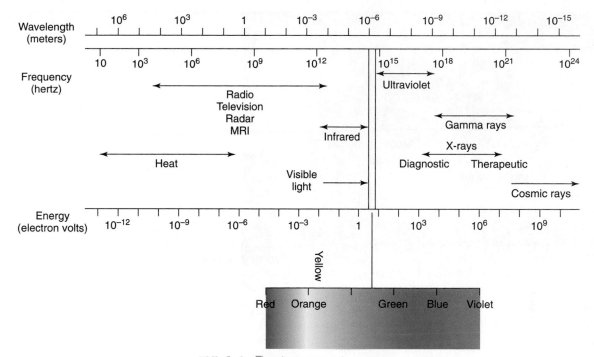

FIG. 1–1 The electromagnetic spectrum.

strating conditions such as changes in the body's circulation.

Nuclear energy is emitted by the nucleus of an atom. Nuclear medicine technology uses this type of energy to create images of both anatomic structures and physiologic actions. It involves the introduction of a radioactive substance into the body for diagnostic and therapeutic purposes. These substances emit gamma radiation from their nuclei. *Gamma radiation* is a form of electromagnetic energy that has the ability to ionize atoms. As a result, proper radiation protection is important in the nuclear medicine department.

Electromagnetic energy has many forms (Fig. 1–1). Many of these forms are used in medicine to deliver high-quality patient care. For example, light is an essential energy form in many of the scopes used by physicians to view inside the body. In addition, **x-rays** are a man-made form of electromagnetic energy. They are created when electrons moving at high speed are suddenly stopped. X-rays, also called **roentgen rays,** named after their discoverer, Wilhelm Röntgen, allow physicians to visualize many of the anatomic structures that were once visible only at surgery.

Radiography is the making of records, known as *radiographs,* of internal structures of the body by passage of x-rays or gamma rays through the body to act on specially sensitized film or imaging plate or system. In the diagnostic radiography department, images are created using x-rays that pass through the body (Fig. 1–2). In addition, very-high-energy x-rays are used in the radiation therapy department for the treatment of many forms of cancer. In both of these departments, proper radiation protection is essential.

Radio waves are another form of electromagnetic radiation. They are a nonionizing form of radiation and are important in the creation of **magnetic resonance images (MRI)** (Fig. 1–3).

Medical radiation science involves the study of the use of radiation throughout medicine. The fact that many forms of radiation are used in all branches of medicine should be apparent.

AN OVERVIEW OF THE HISTORY OF MEDICINE

Humankind's attempt to treat and cure diseases can be dated back almost 5000 years to Egypt and Mesopotamia, where evidence exists that medicine was being practiced in combination with religious beliefs. Prehistoric skulls found in Europe and South America also demonstrate that early humans deliberately removed bone from the skull successfully. Whether this action was performed as a surgical treatment or as a religious attempt to release evil spirits is unknown. In addition, evidence exists that

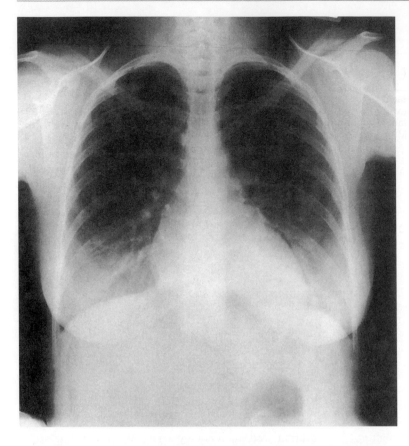

FIG. 1–2   Radiograph of the chest. (Courtesy Robin Jones, MS, RT[R], Methodist Hospital Southlake Campus, Merrillville, Indiana.)

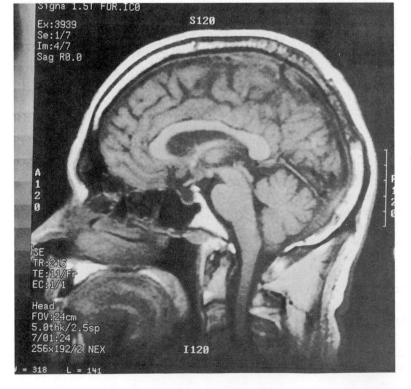

FIG. 1–3   Sagittal image of the brain created using magnetic resonance imaging. (Courtesy Robin Jones, MS, RT[R], Methodist Hospital Southlake Campus, Merrillville, Indiana.)

many potent drugs still in use today, such as castor oil and opium, were used in ancient Egypt for medicinal purposes. The Egyptians demonstrated little knowledge of anatomy, however, despite their sophisticated embalming skills.

The understanding of human anatomy and physiology by the early Greek philosophers was of such high quality that it was not equaled for hundreds of years. Hippocrates (c. 460-370 BC) was a Greek physician who is considered the father of Western medicine. Little is really known about him, but the fact that he was a contemporary of Socrates and was one of the most famous physicians and teachers of medicine of his time is generally accepted. More than 60 medical treatises, called the *Hippocratic Corpus,* traditionally have been attributed to him; however, Hippocrates did not write most of them himself. The writings are similar in that they emphasize rational and natural explanations for the treatment of disease and reject sorcery and magic. Hippocrates emphasized the importance of carefully observing the patient. He believed in the powers of nature to heal over time and taught the prevention of disease through a regimen of diet and exercise. He is also attributed with developing a high standard of ethical conduct, as incorporated in the Hippocratic oath, which provided guidelines for physician-patient relationships, for the rights of patient privacy, and for the use of treatment for curative purposes only. The Hippocratic oath still governs the ethical conduct of physicians today.

The Romans recognized the importance of proper sanitation for good public health through their construction of aqueducts, baths, sewers, and hospitals. Unfortunately, during the Middle Ages, the destruction or neglect of the Roman sanitary facilities resulted in many local epidemics that eventually led to the great plague, known as the Black Death, during the fourteenth century. Medicine was strongly controlled by religious groups during this period, and it was not until the early 1500s that a physician in England had to be licensed to practice.

By the seventeenth century, medicine began to develop an increasingly scientific experimental approach. William Harvey (1578-1657), an English physician, is considered by many scholars to have laid the foundation of modern medicine. Harvey was first to demonstrate the function of the heart and the circulation of the blood. This feat is especially remarkable because it was accomplished without the aid of a microscope. By the end of the seventeenth century, bacteria had been described by Anton Van Leeuwenhoek (1632-1723), a Dutch zoologist, who isolated the microorganism with a microscope he made. With the development of improved microscopes, the dis-covery of the capillary system of the blood helped complete Harvey's explanation of blood circulation.

During the eighteenth century, a significant number of developments in medicine occurred. Surgery was becoming an experimental science, a large number of reforms were taking place in the area of mental health, and the heart drug digitalis was introduced. In 1796, Edward Jenner (1749-1823), an English physician, introduced a vaccine to prevent smallpox when he inoculated an 8-year-old boy, which proved that cowpox provided immunity against smallpox. This discovery served as the foundation for the field of immunology.

In the nineteenth century, the theory that germs cause disease was established. Louis Pasteur (1822-1895), a French chemist, worked with bacteria to prove the germ theory of infection. Through his work, the process of pasteurization was developed. Robert Koch (1843-1910), a German bacteriologist, established the bacterial cause for many infections, such as anthrax, tuberculosis, and cholera. In 1905, Koch received a Nobel Prize for his work in developing tuberculin as a test for tuberculosis. During the mid-1800s, Florence Nightingale (1820-1910), an English nurse, developed the foundations for modern nursing. In 1895, Wilhelm Röntgen discovered x-rays, and the radiologic imaging sciences had their start.

The twentieth century saw development of the use of the scientific method throughout medicine. The early part of the century welcomed discovery of the first antibiotics. Sir Alexander Fleming (1881-1955), a Scottish bacteriologist, discovered penicillin in 1928. Further medical advances included the increased use of chemotherapy and a better understanding of the immune system, which resulted in the increased prophylactic use of vaccines such as the Salk vaccine, discovered by Jonas Salk (1914-1995), which helped control and prevent poliomyelitis. Increased knowledge of the endocrine system has helped treat diseases resulting from hormone imbalance, including the use of insulin to treat diabetes.

In 1953, at Cambridge University in England, Francis Crick (1916-2004), an English scientist, and James Watson (1928-), an American biologist, announced that they had discovered the *secret of life.* Through their work, they identified the molecular structure of deoxyribonucleic acid (DNA), a key to heredity and genetics. Today, much research is being devoted to the field of genetics. Completed in 2003, the Human Genome Project (HGP) was a 13-year project coordinated by the U.S. Department of Energy and the National Institutes of Health. During the early years of the HGP, the Wellcome Trust (United Kingdom) became a major partner; additional partners came from Japan, France, Germany, China, and others. The project goals were to:

- *Identify* all of the approximately 20,000 to 25,000 genes in human DNA
- *Determine* the sequences of the 3 billion chemical base pairs that make up human DNA
- *Store* this information in databases
- *Improve* tools for data analysis
- *Transfer* related technologies to the private sector
- *Address* the ethical, legal, and social issues (ELSI) that may arise from the project

Though the HGP is finished, analyses of the data will continue for many years. The replacement of faulty genes through gene therapy offers promises of cures for a variety of hereditary diseases, and, through genetic engineering, important pharmaceuticals have been developed.

HISTORY OF RADIOLOGIC TECHNOLOGY

The field of radiologic technology began on November 8, 1895, when Wilhelm Conrad Röntgen, a German physicist, was working in his laboratory at the University of Wurzburg. Röntgen had been experimenting with cathode rays and was exploring their properties outside glass tubes. He had covered the glass tube to prevent any visible light from escaping. During this work, Röntgen observed that a screen that had been painted with barium platinocyanide was emitting light *(fluorescing)*. This effect had to be caused by invisible rays being emitted from the tube. During the next several weeks, Röntgen investigated these invisible rays. During his investigation, he saw the very first radiographic image, his own skeleton. Röntgen became the first radiographer when he produced a series of photographs of radiographic images, most notably the image of his wife's hand (Fig. 1–4). He termed these invisible rays *x-rays* because *x* is the symbol for an unknown variable.

Wilhelm Conrad Röntgen was born in Lennep, Germany, on March 27, 1845. In 1872, he married Anna Bertha Ludwig (1839-1919), and they had one adopted daughter. In 1888, Röntgen began working at the University of Wurzburg in the physics department. During the 1870s and 1880s, many physics departments were experimenting with cathode rays, electrons emanating from the negative (cathode) terminal of a tube. During his discovery, Röntgen worked with a Crookes tube. Sir William Crookes (1832-1919) used a large, partially evacuated glass tube that encompassed a cathode and an

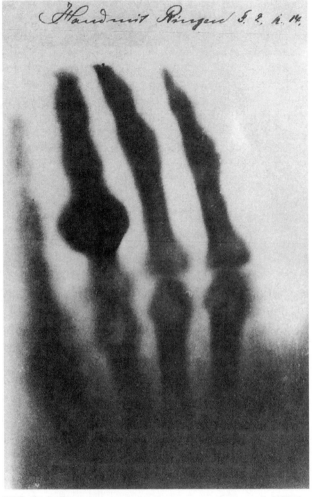

FIG. 1–4 The first radiograph was an image of Wilhelm Röntgen's wife's hand.

anode attached to an electrical supply. His tube was the early version of the modern fluorescent light. Crookes actually produced x-rays during his experimentation in the 1870s but failed to grasp the significance of his finding. He often found that photographic plates stored near his worktable were fogged. He even returned fogged photographic plates to the manufacturer, claiming they were defective. Many physicists created x-rays during the course of their work with cathode rays, but Röntgen was the first to appreciate the significance of the penetrating rays.

The actual day that the significance of Röntgen's finding became clear to him is the subject of much debate. However, Friday, November 8, 1895, is believed by historians to be the day that Röntgen created the famous image of his wife's hand (see Fig. 1–4). On Saturday, December 28, 1895, Röntgen submitted his

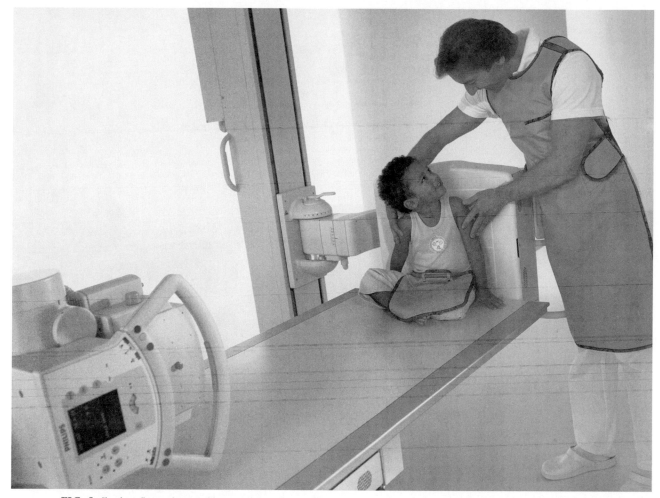

FIG. 1–5 A radiographer positions a patient for a radiographic examination. (Courtesy of Philips Medical Systems.)

first report, titled *On a New Kind of Rays,* to the Wurzburg Physico-Medical Society. Through his investigative methods, Röntgen identified the properties of x-rays. His methods were so thorough that no significant additions have been made to his work.

For his efforts, W. C. Röntgen was honored, in 1901, with the first Nobel Prize in physics. He refused to patent any part of his discovery and rejected many commercial company offers. As a result, he saw little financial reward for his work. He died on February 10, 1923, of colon cancer.

OPPORTUNITIES IN RADIOLOGIC TECHNOLOGY

Radiologic technology is the technical science that deals with the use of x-rays or radioactive substances for diagnostic or therapeutic purposes in medicine. **Radiologic**

technologist is a general term applied to persons qualified to use x-rays *(radiography)* or radioactive substances *(nuclear medicine)* to produce images of the internal parts of the body for interpretation by a physician known as a **radiologist.** Radiologic technology also involves the use of x-rays or radioactive substances in the treatment of disease *(radiation therapy)*.

In addition to the use of x-rays and radioactive substances, radiologic technologists have become involved in using high-frequency sound waves (diagnostic medical sonography) and magnetic fields and radio waves (MRI) to create images of the internal anatomy of the body.

Radiography

A radiologic technologist specializing in the use of x-rays to create images of the body is known as a *radiographer* (Fig. 1–5). Radiographers perform a wide variety of

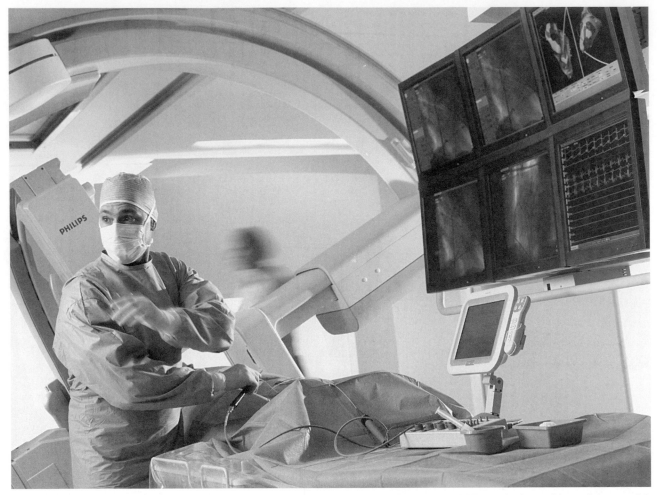

FIG. 1–6   A physician performs a cardiovascular interventional procedure in a vascular suite, which may be located in cardiology, radiology, or surgery. (Courtesy of Philips Medical Systems.)

diagnostic x-ray procedures, including examinations of the skeletal system, the chest, and the abdomen. They administer contrast media to visualize the gastrointestinal tract and the genitourinary system. They also assist the radiologist during more specialized contrast media procedures, such as those used to visualize the spinal cord (*myelography*) and the joint spaces (*arthrography*).

To become a registered radiographer, an accredited radiography program must be completed. Programs are most commonly sponsored by hospitals, community colleges, and universities. Approximately 600 radiography programs are available in the United States. On successful completion of an accredited program, individuals are awarded a certificate, an associate degree, or a baccalaureate degree and are eligible to take the national examination in radiography offered by the American Registry of Radiologic Technologists (ARRT). A registered radiogra-

pher uses the initials *RT(R)* after his or her name. This abbreviation means *registered technologist (radiography)*.

Appendix A contains Clinical Practice Standards for Radiography, developed by the American Society of Radiologic Technologists (ASRT). These practice standards help define the role of the radiographer and establish criteria used to judge performance.

CARDIOVASCULAR INTERVENTIONAL TECHNOLOGY. Radiographers can specialize in performing radiologic examinations of the cardiovascular system, a discipline called **cardiovascular interventional technology (CVIT)** (Fig. 1–6). These procedures involve the injection of iodinated contrast media for diagnosing diseases of the heart and blood vessels. *Angiography* is the term for radiologic examination of the blood vessels after injection of a contrast medium. Most often, the contrast material is injected through a catheter, which can be directed to a variety of major arteries or veins for visualization of these structures. By way of a catheter, injecting contrast media into structures such as the carotid arteries leading to the brain, the renal arteries leading to the kidneys, the femoral artery of the leg, and many other sites is relatively easy.

Placing a catheter into one of the chambers of the heart is termed *cardiac catheterization*. This catheter then can be directed into one or both of the two main arteries that supply blood to the heart itself. These arteries are called the *coronary arteries*.

Coronary arteriography is an extremely valuable tool in diagnosing atherosclerosis, which can block the coronary arteries and cause a heart attack (*myocardial infarction*). By way of a special catheter with a balloon tip, effective treatment of atherosclerosis is possible. This treatment of a blocked blood vessel is termed *angioplasty*. Angioplasty is used to treat patients without the need for invasive open-heart surgery. In addition to angioplasty, blocked vessels are also treated by placing a stent in the vessel to physically keep it open.

CVIT involves the use of highly specialized equipment and complex procedures. This specialization of equipment and supplies has resulted in a need for radiographers to be specially trained in this advanced technology. Most of this advanced education and training occurs through continuing education classes and on-the-job training. In 1991 the ARRT began offering a postprimary examination in CVIT. This examination is no longer offered but has been split into two separate examinations, one for cardiac interventional (CI) technology and another for vascular interventional (VI) technology. To qualify to take either examination, individuals must be ARRT certified in radiography and meet clinical requirements.

MAMMOGRAPHY. Radiographers can specialize in performing radiologic examination of the breast, a procedure called **mammography.** Mammography is a valuable diagnostic tool for the early detection of breast disease, especially breast cancer. Current statistics indicate that one of every eight or nine women in the United States will develop breast cancer. Men are not excluded from this disease; approximately 1% of breast cancers are found in men. Early detection of breast cancer is important to successful treatment and cure. As a result, the American Cancer Society has recommended regular mammography screening for all women over 40 years of age.

This emphasis on screening mammography has resulted in an increase in the number of mammographic examinations being performed across the country. Special breast imaging centers have been built to accommodate the demand for these procedures. Equipment and supplies, such as film and screens, have been specially designed to create high-quality breast images. This specialization of equipment and supplies has resulted in a need for radiographers to be specially trained in this advanced technology. Most of this advanced education and training occurs through continuing education classes and on-the-job training. In 1992 the ARRT began offering a postprimary examination in mammography. To qualify to take the examination, individuals need to be ARRT certified in radiography and meet educational and clinical requirements.

RADIOLOGIST ASSISTANT. A **radiologist assistant** is an advanced-level radiographer who extends the capacity of the radiologist in the diagnostic imaging environment, thereby enhancing patient care. The radiologist assistant is an ARRT-certified radiographer who has completed an advanced academic program encompassing a nationally recognized radiologist assistant curriculum and a radiologist-directed clinical preceptorship.

The concept of a radiologist assistant has moved in and out of popularity in the United States. Pilot programs at the University of Kentucky and Duke University were launched in the mid-1970s to educate technologists who can carry out certain tasks traditionally performed by radiologists. The programs produced a small number of graduates before they were forced to close when federal funding was cut in the late 1970s. The American College of Radiology was not in support of the concept, and the programs slowly died over the next 20 years. A new era of radiologist assistant programs began in 1995 when Weber State University in Utah started a 2-year educational program for registered radiologic technologists who had at least 5 years of experience and wanted to work in an advanced clinical role. Although this program has also been somewhat controversial, in 2003 it was joined by a Bachelor of Science program at Loma Linda University in California and in 2004 by several other undergraduate programs around the country. This number is expected to increase and may even be joined by new graduate programs in conjunction with physician assistant programs already in existence. In 2005 the ARRT began offering a postprimary examination for radiologist assistants (RAs). To qualify to take the examination, individuals need to be ARRT certified in radiography and meet the educational, ethics, and examinations standards established by the ARRT.

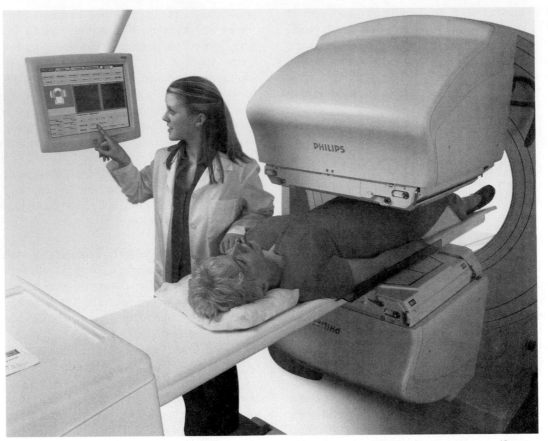

FIG. 1–7   A nuclear medicine technologist performs procedures requiring the use of radioactive substances. (Courtesy of Philips Medical Systems.)

Nuclear Medicine

The branch of radiologic technology that involves procedures that require the use of radioactive materials for diagnostic or therapeutic purposes is **nuclear medicine technology** (Fig. 1–7). Nuclear medicine procedures usually involve the imaging of a patient's organs—such as the liver, heart, or brain—after the introduction of a radioactive material known as a *radiopharmaceutical.* Radiopharmaceuticals are usually administered intravenously but can be administered orally or by inhalation. Procedures also can be performed on specimens such as blood or urine. Samples from a patient can be combined with a radioactive substance to measure various constituents in the sample. Radiopharmaceuticals are also used to perform positron emission tomography (PET) procedures. PET scans create sectional images of the body that demonstrate the physiologic function of various organs and systems.

To become a registered nuclear medicine technologist, completing an accredited nuclear medicine technology program is necessary. Approximately 100 programs are available in the United States. Most commonly sponsored by hospitals, community colleges, or universities, these programs vary in length from 1 year to a 4-year baccalaureate program. One-year programs are usually designed for persons who already hold credentials in radiography, medical technology, or nursing or who possess a bachelor's degree in one of the basic sciences. Graduates of an accredited program are eligible to take the national examination in nuclear medicine technology offered by either the ARRT or the Nuclear Medicine Technology Certification Board (NMTCB). Successful completion of one of these two examinations is usually required for employment. An ARRT-certified person uses the initials *RT(N)* after his or her name, meaning *registered technologist (nuclear medicine technology).* An

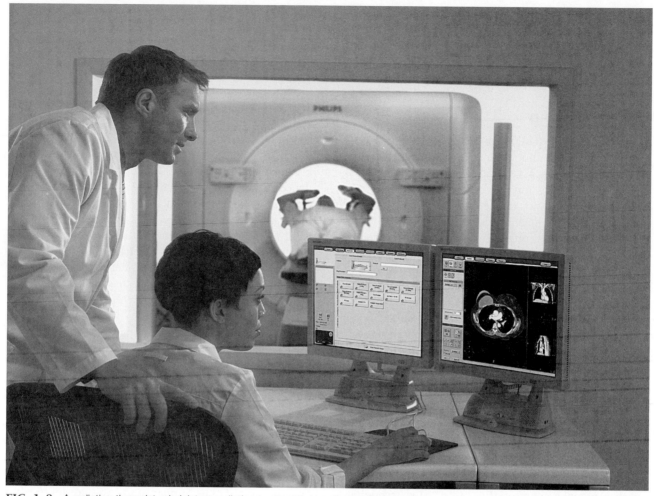

FIG. 1–8 A radiation therapist administers radiation treatments to patients with lesions. A radiation therapist is using a specialized oncology computed tomography unit to perform initial treatment planning studies on a patient. (Courtesy of Philips Medical Systems.)

NMTCB-certified individual uses the initials *CNMT* after his or her name, signifying *certified nuclear medicine technologist.*

Radiation Therapy

A **radiation therapy** technologist, or *radiation therapist,* is a person who administers radiation treatments to patients according to the prescription and instructions of a physician, known as a *radiation oncologist* (Fig. 1–8). *Radiation oncology* involves the use of high-energy ionizing radiation to treat primarily malignant tumors (*cancer*). Therapists are responsible for administering a planned course of prescribed radiation treatments using high-technology therapeutic equipment and accessories. They provide specialized patient care and observe the clinical progress of their patients. Radiation therapists can specialize in the area of medical dosimetry. *Medical dosimetrists* are involved in treatment planning and dose calculations. This specialized area usually requires advanced education and certification.

To become a registered radiation therapy technologist, completing an accredited radiation therapy technology program is necessary, of which approximately 80 are available in the United States. Programs are most commonly sponsored by hospitals, community colleges, or universities and vary in length from 1 year to 4-year baccalaureate programs. One-year programs usually are designed for persons who already have credentials in radiography or who can demonstrate competence in the areas identified in the essentials for a radiation therapy technology program. Graduates of an accredited program are eligible to take the national examination in radiation therapy technology offered by the ARRT. An ARRT-certified individual uses the initials *RT(T)* after his or her name. This abbreviation means *registered technologist (radiation therapy technology)*.

Bone Densitometry

Bone densitometry (BD) is most often used to diagnose osteoporosis, a condition that is often recognized in menopausal women but can also occur in men. Osteoporosis involves a gradual loss of calcium, causing the bones to become thin, fragile, and prone to fractures. Routine x-rays can diagnose bone fractures but are not the best way to assess bone density. To detect osteoporosis accurately, dual-energy x-ray absorptiometry (DXA or DEXA) is used. DEXA BD is the current standard for measuring bone mineral density (BMD). Measurement of the lower spine and hips is most often performed. In 2001 the ARRT began offering a postprimary examination in BD. To qualify to take the examination, individuals need to be ARRT certified in radiography, nuclear medicine technology (or NMTCB certified), or radiation therapy and meet clinical requirements.

Computed Tomography

Computed tomography (CT) is the recording of a predetermined plane in the body using an x-ray beam that is measured, recorded, and then processed by a computer for display on a monitor (Fig. 1–9). This technology allows physicians to visualize patient anatomy from various sectional planes.

CT involves the use of highly specialized equipment and complex procedures, which has resulted in a need for radiographers to be specially trained in this advanced technology. Most of this advanced education and training occurs through continuing education courses and on-the-job training. In 1995 the ARRT began offering a postprimary examination in CT. To qualify to take the examination, individuals need to be ARRT certified in radiography, nuclear medicine technology (or NMTCB certified), or radiation therapy technology and meet clinical requirements.

Diagnostic Medical Sonography

Diagnostic medical sonography is the visualization of structures of the body by recording the reflections of pulses of high-frequency sound (*ultrasound*) waves directed into the tissue. A person who specializes in this field is known as a *diagnostic medical sonographer* (Fig. 1–10).

Sonographers often have previous experience as radiographers, but this experience is not required. To become a sonographer, the candidate can either complete an accredited diagnostic medical sonography program or be trained on the job. Approximately 140 programs are available in the United States. On-the-job training is typically provided only to persons who have previous experience in another allied health specialty, such as radiography. Graduates of accredited programs or experienced sonographers are eligible to take a national examination offered by the American Registry of Diagnostic Medical Sonographers (ARDMS). A *registered diagnostic medical sonographer* uses the initials *RDMS* after his or her name. A *registered diagnostic cardiac sonographer* uses the initials *RDCS* after his or her name. In addition, a *cardiovascular credentialing international* organization provides cardiac sonographers with a credential that allows them to use the initials *CCI* after their names.

In 1999 the ARRT began offering a postprimary examination in sonography. To qualify to take the examination, individuals need to be ARRT certified in radiography, nuclear medicine technology (or NMTCB certified), or radiation therapy and meet clinical requirements.

Magnetic Resonance Imaging

MRI uses a strong magnetic field and radio waves along with a computer to generate sectional images of patient anatomy (Fig. 1–11). Similar to CT, this advanced technology uses highly specialized equipment and requires specialized education. Although many MRI technologists have obtained their education through continuing education courses and on-the-job training, more and more formal educational programs now exist with baccalaureate, associate, or certificate credentials. For the most part, MRI technologists have credentials in radiography, and many are also experienced CT technologists. In 1995 the ARRT began offering a postprimary certification examination in MRI. To qualify to take the examination, individuals need to be ARRT-certified in radiography, nuclear medicine technology (or NMTCB certified), or radiation therapy technology and meet clinical requirements.

Additional Opportunities

Regardless of the area in which an individual chooses to specialize within the profession of radiologic technology, additional opportunities exist in education, management, and commercial firms.

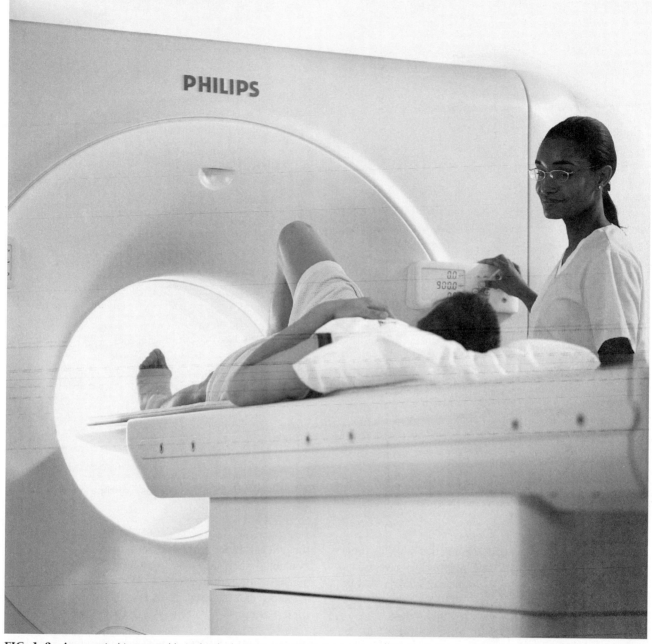

FIG. 1–9 A computed tomographic technologist uses a computerized x-ray system to produce sectional anatomic images of the body. (Courtesy of Philips Medical Systems.)

EDUCATION. Individuals who have an interest in teaching any of the specific disciplines can find opportunities in hospitals, colleges, and universities. Careers include clinical instructor, didactic faculty member, clinical coordinator, and program director.

A *clinical instructor* teaches students primarily on a one-on-one basis in the clinical setting. A *didactic faculty member* teaches students typically through classroom lectures and laboratory activities. A *clinical coordinator* has teaching responsibilities along with administrative duties in overseeing clinical education, most often in programs using many clinical education centers. A *program director* has teaching responsibilities, as well as overall administrative responsibility, for the entire educational program.

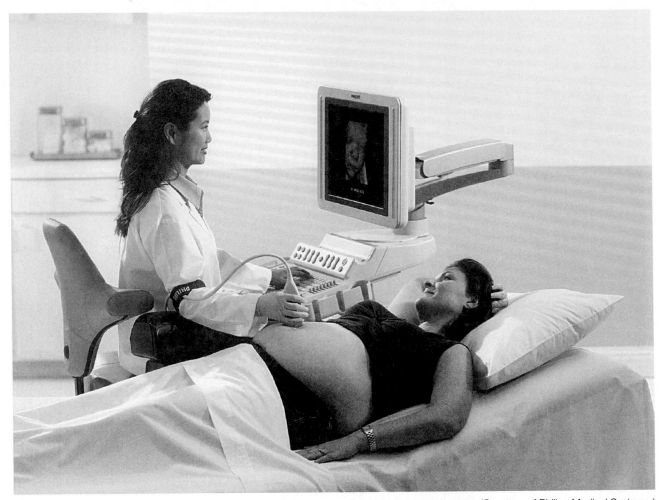

FIG. 1–10 A diagnostic medical sonographer uses high-frequency sound waves to create images. (Courtesy of Philips Medical Systems.)

Advanced coursework in education is desirable for these positions. Program directors are required to have a baccalaureate degree, and by 2009 a master's degree will be required.

ADMINISTRATION. Persons who have an interest in the management of the radiology services in a given facility can specialize for a wide spectrum of supervisory and administrative positions. Many departments have supervisory positions in areas such as CT, MRI, CVIT, sonography, and quality management. In 1997 the ARRT began offering a postprimary examination in quality management. To be eligible to take the examination, individuals need to be ARRT certified in radiography, nuclear medicine technology (or NMTCB certified), or radiation therapy technology and meet clinical requirements. In addition, depending on the size of

the department, upper-management positions are available, such as chief technologist and radiology manager or administrator. Along with experience, advanced coursework in management is desirable for these positions.

COMMERCIAL FIRMS. Opportunities for radiologic technologists and sonographers exist in a variety of areas within commercial companies involved in the selling of x-ray equipment, film, processing chemicals, and related x-ray supplies. These companies need sales representatives with technical knowledge of the radiologic procedures and equipment, as well as the ability to sell. In addition, companies hire technical specialists who are not directly involved in sales but who are involved with the education and training of the staff at the sites where the equipment is installed. Sales representatives and

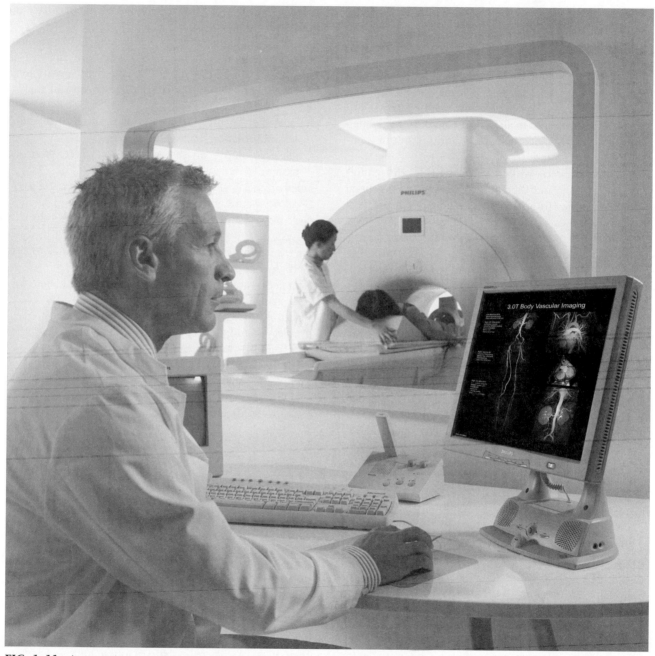

FIG. 1–11 A magnetic resonance imaging technologist uses electromagnetics, specifically radio waves and magnetism, to create diagnostic sectional images of the body. (Courtesy of Philips Medical Systems.)

technical specialists generally have some travel requirements as part of their responsibilities.

HEALTH CARE TEAM

A wide array of specialists makes up the health care team. More than 200 different health careers have been identified. Most of these careers have been grouped into the large category known as allied health. *Allied health* is a term that includes all the health-related disciplines with the exception of nursing and the MODVOPP careers. *MODVOPP* is an acronym that stands for *m*edicine, *o*steopathy, *d*entistry, *v*eterinary medicine, *o*ptometry, *p*harmacy, and *p*odiatry.

Although not all of the various disciplines can be detailed here, some health care services that a radiologic technologist encounters on a regular basis are highlighted. These services include medicine and osteopathy, nursing, and the allied health careers that encompass many of the diagnostic services, therapeutic services, and health information services. Persons employed in health care find opportunities in all kinds of environments, such as hospitals, clinics, doctors' offices, long-term care facilities, schools, and industry.

Many health care workers share the titles of technologist, technician, and therapist. *Technologist* is a general term that applies to an individual skilled in a practical art. This health care provider applies knowledge to practical and theoretical problems in the field. *Technician* is a term that applies to a person who performs procedures that require attention to technical detail. Technicians work under the direction of another health care provider. The terms *technologist* and *technician* are often used interchangeably, which can create problems in disciplines in which the terms are used to denote differing levels of education. In the clinical laboratory sciences, a medical technologist (MT) has earned a 4-year degree, and a medical laboratory technician (MLT) has completed a 2-year program. In general, technologists are involved in higher-level problem-solving skills and have more extensive educational preparation than do technicians. Technologists and technicians work throughout all areas of health care; many provide direct patient care, whereas others serve in support roles.

Therapists specialize in carrying out treatments designed to correct or improve the function of a particular body part or system. Therapists possess varied levels of educational experiences. Most therapists have either a 2-year or a 4-year college degree.

Medicine and Osteopathy

Physicians are primary care providers who promote the optimal health of their patients and who provide for patients' care during an illness. Two principal types of physicians are the medical doctor (MD) and the doctor of osteopathy (DO). MDs generally complete a baccalaureate degree program with a science major such as biology or chemistry and then complete 4 years of medical school. DOs have educations similar to those of MDs. The philosophy of osteopathic medicine differs from that of traditional medicine. In addition to learning the important concepts of medicine, DOs are trained to do manipulations of muscles and bones as a part of the healing process. Both MDs and DOs must be state licensed to practice.

After medical school, most MDs and DOs complete additional training, known as a *residency,* in an area of specialization. Residencies are usually 3 or 4 years long and may include the following branches of medicine:

Anesthesiology—study of the use of medication to cause loss of sensation during surgery
Cardiology—study of diseases of the cardiovascular system
Family practice—study of diseases in patients of all ages
Geriatrics—study of diseases of older adults
Gynecology—study of diseases of the female reproductive system
Internal medicine—study of diseases of the internal organs of the chest and abdomen
Neurology—study of diseases of the brain and nervous system
Obstetrics—study of pregnancy and childbirth
Oncology—study of the treatment of tumors
Orthopedics—study of diseases of muscles and bones
Pediatrics—study of diseases in children
Radiology—study of the use of x-rays and radioactive substances to diagnose and treat diseases
Surgery—study of the use of operative procedures to treat diseases
Urology—study of diseases of the urinary system

In addition, many physicians choose a subspecialty; for example, the primary duties of a pediatric cardiovascular surgeon include performing surgery on the heart and blood vessels of children.

Nursing

A *nurse* provides direct patient care, typically under the direction of physicians. Nurses are classified as nursing assistants, licensed practical nurses (LPNs), or registered nurses (RNs). RNs have a variety of duties, depending on their area of expertise. Nurses often choose to work exclusively in one specialty area (e.g., pediatrics, orthopedics, intensive care) or the emergency department. To become an RN, the candidate must pass a state licensing examination after completion of a 2-, 3-, or 4-year program of study.

Advanced education for the nurse can lead to work as a nurse practitioner, a nurse midwife, or a nurse anesthetist. A *nurse practitioner* performs physical examinations, orders and interprets some tests, and, in some states, prescribes medications. A *nurse midwife* provides perinatal care and can deliver infants under the supervision of an obstetrician. A *nurse anesthetist* provides anesthesia under the supervision of an anesthesiologist.

Nursing assistants and LPNs generally work under the direction of an RN or a physician to provide basic care to patients. Nursing assistants generally have limited training, most of which is done on the job. LPNs complete a 1-year program and can legally administer drugs except by the intravenous route.

Diagnostic Services

Health care workers in diagnostic service areas perform tests or evaluations that aid the physician in determining the presence or absence of a disease or condition. Many health care specialists perform diagnostic procedures. *Electrocardiographic technicians* operate equipment that records the electrical impulses of the heart. *Electroencephalographic technologists* operate equipment to record the electrical impulses of the brain.

The clinical laboratory sciences involve a wide variety of careers in health care. An MT works in the laboratory performing tests and analyzing results. Several areas of specialization exist in the laboratory, including hematology, microbiology, clinical chemistry, immunology, and blood banking. MLTs generally work under the supervision of an MT or physician to perform basic laboratory tests in all the various departments of the laboratory. Other laboratory personnel include the cytotechnologist, who specializes in the preparation and screening of cells, and the histologic technologist, who specializes in the preparation of tissues.

Radiology is predominantly a diagnostic service. These careers have already been detailed. Educational requirements for careers in the diagnostic services vary considerably across the disciplines, but most require 2 to 4 years of education beyond high school.

Therapeutic Services

Therapists provide services designed to help patients overcome some form of physical or psychological disability. Examples include *occupational therapists,* who teach useful skills to patients with physical or emotional illnesses; *physical therapists,* who help restore muscle strength and coordination through exercise and the use of special devices such as braces or crutches; *radiation therapists,* who treat cancer patients using high-energy x-rays and gamma rays; and *respiratory therapists*, who help treat patients with breathing difficulties. Educational requirements vary considerably across the disciplines,

but most require 2 to 6 years of education beyond high school.

Health Information Services

Health information services involve careers that are responsible for the management of health information, such as that contained in the patient's health record. These careers do not involve direct patient contact but are essential to the efficient operation of any health care facility. For example, health information technologists are involved in the coding of patient conditions, and these codes are used to determine the amount of money a facility is reimbursed for providing care to a patient. Educational requirements for careers in health information management vary considerably across disciplines, but most require 2 to 4 years of education beyond high school.

Other Health Services

A vast number of other careers exist within the health care environment. Other health services include such disciplines as dental health, dietetics, psychosocial health care, and emergency care.

SUMMARY

Radiation is energy transmitted by waves through space or through a medium (matter). It is both helpful and essential for life. *Energy* is the capacity to operate or work. One form of energy is electromagnetic energy, which includes radio waves, light, and x-rays. Many forms of energy are used in medicine to help diagnose and treat patients. Some higher-energy forms, such as x-rays, are capable of causing ionization. This process is capable of causing biologic damage, and caution should be exercised to prevent unnecessary exposure to ionizing radiation.

X-rays were discovered by Wilhelm Conrad Röntgen on November 8, 1895. For his discovery, Röntgen was awarded the first Nobel Prize in physics in 1901.

Radiologic technology is the technical science that deals with the use of x-rays or radioactive substances for diagnostic or therapeutic purposes in medicine. *RT* is a general term applied to an individual qualified to use x-rays (radiography) or radioactive substances (nuclear medicine) to produce images of the internal parts of the body for interpretation by a physician known as a *radiologist*. RTs also use x-rays or radioactive substances in the treatment of disease (radiation therapy).

In addition to using x-rays and radioactive substances, RTs have become involved in using high-frequency sound waves (diagnostic medical sonography) and magnetic fields and radio waves (MRI) to create images of the internal anatomy of the body. Additional opportunities also exist for RTs in education, management, and commercial firms.

The health care team comprises a wide array of specialists. More than 200 different health careers have been identified, most of which have been grouped into the large category known as allied health. *Allied health* is a term that includes all health-related disciplines with the exception of nursing and the MODVOPP (*m*edicine, *o*steopathy, *d*entistry, *v*eterinary medicine, *o*ptometry, *p*harmacy, and *p*odiatry) careers.

Radiologic technologists work as a part of the health care team and interact with many of the other health care members on a regular basis. These other members are employed in such health services as medicine and osteopathy, nursing, and the allied health careers that encompass many of the diagnostic services, therapeutic services, and health information services.

Individuals employed in health care find opportunities in all kinds of environments, such as hospitals, clinics, doctors' offices, long-term care facilities, schools, and industry.

BIBLIOGRAPHY

American Medical Association: *Health professions career and education directory,* ed 33, Chicago, 2005, The Association.

Carlton R, Adler AM: *Principles of radiographic imaging: an art and a science,* ed 4, Albany, NY, 2006, Thomson Delmar Publishers.

Curry TS, Dowdey JE, Murry RC: *Christensen's physics of diagnostic radiology,* ed 44, Philadelphia, 1990, Lea & Febiger.

Eisenberg RL: *Radiology: an illustrated history,* 1992, St Louis, Mosby–Year Book.

Gerdin JA: *Health careers today,* ed 2, St Louis, 2003, Mosby.

Grigg ERN: *The trail of the invisible light,* 1965, Springfield, Ill, Charles C. Thomas.

Gurley LT, Calloway WJ: *Introduction to radiologic technology,* ed 5, St Louis, 2002, Mosby.

Papp J: *Quality management in the imaging sciences,* ed 2, St Louis, 2002, Mosby.

Röntgen WC: On a new kind of rays, *Nature* 53:1369, 1896.

Simmers L: *Diversified health occupations,* ed 6, Albany, NY, 2004, Thomson Delmar Publishers.

Professional Organizations

Richard R. Carlton, MS, RT(R)(CV), FAERS
Arlene M. Adler, MEd, RT(R), FAERS

Be active in your local, state and national organizations; never be satisfied until the highest goal has been attained.

Professor Ed C. Jerman
The Father of Radiologic Technology, Circa 1920

OBJECTIVES

On completion of this chapter, the student will be able to:

1. Differentiate accreditation, certification, and representation functions of various professional organizations.

2. Describe the organizations that carry out the professional aspects of a specific radiologic technology area of specialization.

3. Describe the relationship of various radiologist and physicist organizations with radiologic technology.

ACCREDITATION OF SCHOOLS

Accreditation of schools sets the conditions under which new members qualify for entry into the profession. Accredited programs have satisfactorily demonstrated compliance with educational standards developed by and for the profession. These standards are set by the organizations that sponsor the accrediting agency. Each **sponsoring organization** appoints one or more members to the board of directors known as a **joint review committee** (JRC). This board is the governing body of the organization, and its members make recommendations on the accreditation status of schools. The sponsoring organizations of the JRCs approve a document formerly known as the *Essentials* and now known as the *Standards,* which details exactly how an accredited program must operate. These documents typically require a program to demonstrate its purposes, resources, effectiveness of its outcomes, and other elements deemed important by the sponsoring organizations.

The process of accreditation begins with an application from the program. On approval of the application, a comprehensive document known as a *self-study* must be compiled by the program according to guidelines set by the accrediting agency. On submission of this document, a team of site visitors is sent to verify the information provided in the self-study. Site visitors are volunteers from the profession who serve without pay, although the program being visited pays their expenses. The site-visiting team submits a report to the accrediting agency, and the agency staff reviews this report and presents it to the board for a vote on recommended accreditation status. Typical accreditation award classifications include provisional, probationary, and up to 8-year status. Fees are collected for the application and the site-visit expenses, as is an annual fee from the sponsor of the program and from each clinical education site.

Accreditation is a voluntary peer-review process. Although accreditation is voluntary, few programs choose not to undergo the accreditation process. Nearly all schools value their accreditation status highly and work hard to maintain standards that meet all the accreditation recommendations. A program may choose not to pursue programmatic accreditation and rely on the accreditation awarded to the college or university under a regional institutional accrediting agency. A list of accrediting agencies, certification agencies, and professional societies with addresses and telephone numbers is supplied in Appendix B.

Joint Review Committee on Education in Diagnostic Medical Sonography

The Joint Review Committee on Education in Diagnostic Medical Sonography (JRCDMS) was established in 1979 and is currently sponsored by nine organizations: the American College of Cardiology, the American College of Obstetrics and Gynecology (OB/GYN), the American College of Radiology, the American Institute of Ultrasound in Medicine, the American Medical Association (AMA), the American Society of Echocardiography, the American Society of Radiologic Technologists, the Society of Diagnostic Medical Sonographers, and the Society of Vascular Technologies. The JRCDMS accredits approximately 140 diagnostic medical sonography programs (web site: *http://www.jrcdms.org*).

Joint Review Committee on Education in Nuclear Medicine Technology

The Joint Review Committee on Education in Nuclear Medicine Technology (JRCNMT) was established in 1970 and is currently sponsored by four organizations: the American College of Radiology, the American Society of Radiologic Technologists, the Society of Nuclear Medicine, and the Society of Nuclear Medicine—Technologist Section. The JRCNMT accredits approximately 100 nuclear medicine technology programs (web site: *http://www.jrcnmt.org*).

Joint Review Committee on Education in Radiologic Technology

Radiography is considered to be the fifth oldest allied health profession because the first *Essentials* document was established in 1944, after occupational therapy, medical technology, physical therapy, and medical records administration. Not until 1969 was the Joint Review Committee on Education in Radiologic Technology (JRCERT) established. The JRCERT board is currently nominated by the American College of Radiology, the American Society of Radiologic Technologists, the Association of Educators in Radiological Sciences, and the American Healthcare Radiology Administrators. The JRCERT accredits approximately 600 radiography programs (more than any other allied health profession), as well as approximately 80 radiation therapy technology programs (web site: *http://wwwjrcert.org*).

CERTIFICATION OF INDIVIDUALS

Professional **certification** is a process through which an agency grants recognition to an individual on demonstration, usually by examination, of specialized professional skills. It is a voluntary process and is the responsibility of the person, not of the person's school or employer. Each certification organization sets requirements for the recognition of professionals through registration, certification, or other recognition of skills by examination. Fees are charged for these services. Especially important are the annual fees for continued recognition. Failure to pay these fees or meet other requirements, such as verification of continuing education activities, results in the removal of an individual from the registration lists of the profession. Reinstatement

usually does not involve retaking an examination, but a special fee is often charged.

Actually, a **registry** is simply a listing of individuals holding a particular certification. The term *registry* is commonly applied to the agency that carries out the certification function and maintains the registry list. Each registry is sponsored by appropriate professional organizations. The sponsoring organizations appoint the members of the board, and this board then determines the standards for the registry, such as eligibility requirements, examination questions, fees, and ethical standards.

Nearly all hospitals in the United States require appropriate professional certification as a condition of employment. Physicians who desire quality imaging also insist on appropriate professional certification for the technologists who perform radiography, ultrasonography, and mammography in their offices and clinics.

American Registry of Diagnostic Medical Sonographers

The American Registry of Diagnostic Medical Sonographers (ARDMS) offers voluntary certification through examination to eligible sonographers and vascular technologists. Since its inception in 1975, the ARDMS has certified approximately 45,000 persons. The ARDMS offers three credentials: registered diagnostic medical sonographer (RDMS), registered diagnostic cardiac sonographer (RDCS), and registered vascular technologist (RVT).

American Registry of Radiologic Technologists

The American Registry of Radiologic Technologists (ARRT) was founded in 1922 by the Radiological Society of North America (RSNA), with the support of the American Roentgen Ray Society (ARRS) and the cooperation of the Canadian Association of Radiologists and the American Society of X-Ray Technicians (now known as the American Society of Radiologic Technologists [ASRT]). In 1936 the ARRT was incorporated, and in 1944 the American College of Radiology and the ASRT became co-sponsors of the ARRT. Currently, the ASRT appoints five members to the ARRT board, and the ACR appoints four members.

The purposes of the ARRT include encouraging the study and elevating the standards of radiologic technology, examining and certifying eligible candidates, and periodically publishing a listing of registrants. This mission is accomplished through voluntary certification by examination. Once an individual has passed the appropriate examination, he or she is listed in the registry and granted the right to use an appropriate professional title. These designations are registered technologist (RT), with a specialty designation for radiographer (R), radiation therapy (T), nuclear medicine (N), cardiac interventional technology (CI), vascular interventional technology (VI), mammography (M), computed tomography (CT), magnetic resonance imaging (MR), or quality management (QM). In addition, the ARRT has added sonography (S), vascular sonography (VS), breast sonography (BS), and bone densitometry (BD) examinations. For example, a registered radiographer is designated as RT(R) (ARRT). This designation is a registered trademark, and its use by non–ARRT-registered individuals is illegal.

Individuals must pay an annual fee to maintain active status with the ARRT and must adhere to the ARRT code of ethics. Members of the profession who violate the code of ethics, usually through criminal activity, may have their registration revoked. For example, former registered technologists who have been convicted of stealing from their employers often have their registration revoked. ARRT registrants also must certify that they have attended 24 hours of continuing education during the previous 2 years to maintain their registration status. Continuing education became mandatory for ARRT registrants in 1995.

The ARRT began offering registration in nuclear medicine technology and radiation therapy in 1962 and started postprimary examinations in 1991. Currently, the ARRT listed more than 250,000 registered technologists, thousands of whom were certified in more than one professional specialty. Registered technologists hold more than 235,000 certifications in radiography, 15,000 certifications in radiation therapy, more than 11,000 in nuclear medicine, more than 4200 in cardiovascular interventional technology, more than 46,000 in mammography, more than 24,000 in computed tomography (CT), more than 15,000 in magnetic resonance imaging (MRI), and more than 1300 in quality management.

Nuclear Medicine Technology Certification Board

The Nuclear Medicine Technology Certification Board (NMTCB) was founded in 1977. Current sponsors include the Society of Nuclear Medicine, the Society of Nuclear Medicine—Technologist Section, the American Society of Clinical Pathologists, the College of Physicists, the American Society of Medical Technology, and the Association of Physicists in Medicine. The NMTCB consists of 15 persons plus an advisory council, whose chair also sits on the board.

The purposes of the NMTCB include examining and certifying eligible candidates and periodically publishing a listing of registrants. This mission is accomplished through voluntary certification by examination. Once an individual has passed the appropriate examination, he or she becomes registered and is granted the right to use the title certified nuclear medicine technologist. The NMTCB has approximately 15,000 registrants. The NMTCB also offers two specialty examinations for nuclear medicine technologists, the nuclear cardiology (NCT) and positron emission tomography (PET) examinations.

State Licensing Agencies

Requirements to practice the radiologic professions vary from state to state. More than 35 states and territories require a license, which can usually be obtained on providing proof of certification from the appropriate national certification organization (a process known as **licensure**). The laws in effect vary tremendously from one state to another and can vary from year to year within a state as a result of new legislation. Most radiologic professionals do not experience difficulty in moving employment from one state to another because proper licensing is usually a matter of submitting the appropriate paperwork and fees. Verifying current licensing requirements is important before practicing in a new state because penalties may be assessed for practicing without a license. A list of state licensing bodies and their addresses and telephone numbers is supplied in Appendix C.

PROFESSIONAL SOCIETIES

Professional societies represent the interests of various groups to the public and to governmental bodies. The radiologic sciences have many such organizations, with new ones forming and others combining or ceasing operations from time to time. These organizations usually publish professional journals, conduct educational meetings, and represent their members to governmental bodies. They also often provide continuing education verification, scholarships, special reports, information networking, recruitment and promotional materials, malpractice insurance, and other services for their members. Some of the most important professional societies are described here. Contact information, including Internet web sites, can be found in Appendix B.

American Healthcare Radiology Administrators

The American Healthcare Radiology Administrators (AHRA) was organized to promote management practice in the administration of imaging services. Membership is open to professionals engaged in the practice of radiology administration in both hospital and nonhospital settings, as well as to others in service or education who have limited management responsibilities.

The AHRA provides a broad range of services for its members, including the journal *Radiology Management,* a newsletter, and monographs. The association holds regular educational meetings and an annual conference. They recently began offering an examination for radiology administrators. Persons who successfully complete the examination are given the title certified radiology administrator (CRA). The AHRA has strong cooperative ties with other professional associations and has spearheaded the Summit on Manpower, a consortium of radiology and health care organizations concerned with labor shortages in radiology.

American Society of Radiologic Technologists

The ASRT was founded in 1920. As the most prominent national professional voice for radiologic technologists, the ASRT represents individual practitioners, educators, managers and administrators, and students in radiography, radiation therapy, and nuclear medicine, as well as the many specialties within each modality. The ASRT has approximately 115,000 members (nearly one half of the registered technologists in the United States).

The goals of the ASRT are to advance the professions of radiologic technology and imaging specialties, to maintain high standards of education, to enhance the quality of patient care, and to further the welfare and socioeconomics of radiologic technologists. The ASRT publishes a peer-reviewed, refereed journal (*Radiologic Technology*), conducts regional and national conferences, and produces educational programs of all types.

Association of Educators in Imaging and Radiologic Sciences, Inc.

The Association of Educators in Imaging and Radiological Sciences (AEIRS), Inc., was founded in 1967. Its primary purposes are to encourage the exchange of teaching concepts, to help establish minimum standards for teaching radiologic technologies, and to advance radiologic education by encouraging educational research and technical writing by its members. The AEIRS is a national association of educators. The association holds meetings and publishes *Radiologic Science and Education, AEIRS Quarterly,* and other educational data.

Association of Vascular and Interventional Radiographers

The Association of Vascular and Interventional Radiographers (AVIR) was organized to represent radiographers and allied health care professionals specializing in cardiovascular and interventional radiology. AVIR offers members a quarterly newsletter and a national conference in conjunction with the Society of Cardiovascular and Interventional Radiology and the American Radiological Nurses Association.

International Society of Radiographers and Radiologic Technologists

The International Society of Radiographers and Radiologic Technologists (ISRRT) was founded in 1959 as an organization of national societies of radiologic technologists. The ISRRT is an international nongovernmental organization with official relations with the World Health Organization.

The primary objectives of the ISRRT are to facilitate communication among radiologic technologists worldwide, to advance the science and practice of radiologic technology, and to identify and help meet the needs of radiologic technologists in developing nations. The ISRRT sponsors three types of international meetings: world congresses, regional meetings, and teachers' seminars. These meetings are held on a 4-year cycle, with one type of meeting scheduled each year and the fourth year off. Three regions hold meetings: Europe and Africa, Asia and Australasia, and the Americas. The world congresses and the teachers' seminars rotate among the regions of the world. The ISRRT publishes a semiannual newsletter, proceedings of meetings, and translations of various documents of interest to the profession.

More than 65 member countries are represented by the ISRRT. Each member country appoints a representative to the ISRRT World Council, which serves as the governing body. The secretary-general of the organization serves as the liaison for the council, as well as the office. The ISRRT offers associate membership to individuals wishing to support the organization.

Society of Diagnostic Medical Sonographers

The Society of Diagnostic Medical Sonographers (SDMS) is the largest professional society for sonographers, representing every specialty and level of expertise. The SDMS was founded in 1970 to answer the needs of nonphysicians who were performing diagnostic sonographic procedures. Its goals are to promote, advance, and educate its members and the medical community in the science of diagnostic medical sonography and thereby to contribute to the enhancement of patient care. This goal is accomplished through educational programs, scientific and professional publications, and representation and collaboration with other organizations.

Society of Magnetic Resonance in Medicine/Society for Magnetic Resonance Imaging

The Society of Magnetic Resonance in Medicine (SMRM) was founded in 1981. Its major purpose is to further the development and application of magnetic resonance techniques in medicine and biology by promoting communications, research development applications, and the availability of information in the fields of MRI and spectroscopy. To accomplish this purpose, the society holds meetings and workshops, publishes journals and other documents, provides information and advice on aspects of public policy concerned with magnetic resonance in medicine, and otherwise performs charitable, scientific, and educational functions with respect to magnetic resonance in medicine and biology. SMRM's periodicals include a newsletter called *Resonance* and a journal titled *Magnetic Resonance in Medicine.*

The SMRM and the Society for Magnetic Resonance Imaging (SMRI) also support a joint Section for Magnetic Resonance Technologists (SMRT). SMRI publishes a journal, *Magnetic Resonance Imaging Technology.*

Society of Nuclear Medicine— Technologist Section

The Society of Nuclear Medicine (SNM) is a multidisciplinary organization of physicians, physicists, chemists, radiopharmacists, technologists, and others interested in the diagnostic, therapeutic, and investigational use of radiopharmaceuticals. Founded in Seattle in 1954, the SNM is the largest scientific organization dedicated to nuclear medicine.

The Technologist Section of SNM was formed in 1970 to meet the needs of the nuclear medicine technologist.

It is a scientific organization formed with, but operating autonomously from, the SNM to promote the continued development and improvement of the art and science of nuclear medicine technology. Its ongoing objectives are to enhance the development of nuclear medicine technology, to stimulate continuing education activities, and to develop a forum for the exchange of ideas and information. The Technologist Section provides nuclear medicine technologists with a mechanism to deal directly with issues that concern them, such as continuing education, academic affairs, and socioeconomic issues. The organization publishes a journal called *Journal of Nuclear Medicine Technology,* or *JNMT.*

State and Local Radiologic Technology Societies

Nearly all states and many cities and regions have local professional societies that carry out many of the functions of the larger national organizations for their states or regions. In many instances, these organizations serve as chapters or affiliates of the larger groups, although these connections may be formal or simply loose affiliations. State and local societies often make special efforts to cater to the needs of students and new members of professions with opportunities to begin a career through scholarships, student competitions, publishing, exhibits, and committee work, as well as through positions as board members.

RADIOLOGIST AND PHYSICIST ORGANIZATIONS

American Association of Physicists in Medicine

The American Association of Physicists in Medicine (AAPM) is the most prominent organization of radiation physicists. Its annual meeting is held in conjunction with the RSNA meeting each year in Chicago.

American Board of Radiology

The American Board of Radiology (ABR) was established in 1934 to conduct the certification of radiologists. The ABR has three certification divisions: radiology, diagnostic radiology, and therapeutic radiology. The basic requirement for eligibility for these examinations is a medical degree plus 4 years of residency training. A written examination must be passed before a candidate is eligible for the oral examination. The ABR also offers certification for radiologic physicists and a special competence examination in nuclear medicine.

American College of Radiology

With more than 30,000 members, the American College of Radiology (ACR) is the principal organization of physicians trained in radiology and medical radiation physics in the United States. The ACR is a professional society whose primary purposes are to advance the science of radiology, to improve service to the patient, to study the socioeconomic aspects of the practice of radiology, and to encourage continuing education for radiologists and persons practicing in allied professional fields.

American Institute of Ultrasound in Medicine

Physicians, engineers, scientists, sonographers, and other professionals involved with diagnostic medical sonography make up the American Institute of Ultrasound in Medicine (AIUM). The AIUM promotes the application of ultrasound in clinical medicine, diagnostics, and research; promotes the study of its effects on tissue; recommends standards for its applications; and promotes education in the use of ultrasonics for medical purposes.

American Medical Association

The AMA was founded in Philadelphia in 1847 and is considered the largest and most active medical organization in the world. More than 300,000 American physicians (approximately 70% of those practicing) belong to the AMA. The activities of the AMA include promotion and regulation of all aspects of medicine in the United States, including the allied health professions. The AMA publishes the most widely distributed medical journal in the world, *The Journal of the American Medical Association,* also known as *JAMA,* which is published weekly.

American Roentgen Ray Society

The ARRS is the oldest American radiologic society. Founded in 1900 in St. Louis, the society had approximately 7000 members by the early 1990s. Its primary objectives are educational, which are met through meetings and publication of the *American Journal of Roentgenology.*

American Society for Therapeutic Radiology and Oncology

The purpose of the American Society for Therapeutic Radiology and Oncology (ASTRO) is to extend the benefits of radiation therapy to patients with cancer or other disorders, to advance its scientific basis, and to provide for the education and professional fellowship of its members.

The society was formally incorporated in 1958 as an organization of physicians who believed that radiation, formerly used only as a diagnostic tool, had potential value as an interventional modality in the treatment of malignant disease. Today, ASTRO has more than 4000 members and is the leading organization for radiation oncology, biology, and physics. ASTRO publishes a newsletter and an annual membership directory. The organization also makes a major commitment to education and research through awards, fellowships, travel grants, and contributions to accredited technology programs.

International Society for Clinical Densitometry

The International Society for Clinical Densitometry (ISCD) was founded in 1993 and provides a central resource for scientific disciplines with an interest in bone mass measurement. The society has over 4000 members and offers a technical certification examination for individuals who perform bone densitometry.

Radiological Society of North America

The Western Roentgen Society was founded in Chicago in 1915 in response to a need for a national radiology organization because the ARRS had become an eastern organization. In 1920 the organization was renamed the Radiological Society of North America to reflect the nature of its membership. Since 1918 the RSNA has published the most influential journal in American radiology, known simply as *Radiology* and often referred to as *the gray journal* because of its traditional color representing the shades of gray that make up the radiologic image. In 1981 a second journal, *RadioGraphics,* was added. The RSNA had approximately 37,000 members by the year 2000, and it conducts the world's largest radiology meeting, with more than 60,000 registrants, each November.

Society for Computer Applications in Radiology

The Society for Computer Applications in Radiology (SCAR) was founded in 1980 to serve as a resource for imaging professionals interested in the current and future use of computers in medical imaging. The organization provides a focal point for picture archiving and communication system (PACS) and other radiology informatics users.

Society of Nuclear Medicine

See the section on the Society of Nuclear Medicine—Technologist Section.

SUMMARY

A major part of the fabric of a profession is its organizations, especially the accrediting agencies for educational programs, the certification bodies for individuals, and the professional societies that represent the interests of the profession to the public and government.

Radiologic technology accreditation is carried out through the various JRCs: the JRCDMS, the JRCERT, and the JRCNMT, which performs both radiography and radiation therapy accreditation.

Individuals are certified by the various registries and by state and territorial licensing agencies. The national registries are the ARDMS, the ARRT, and the NMTCB. The ARRT offers registration in radiography, nuclear medicine, radiation therapy, cardiovascular interventional technology, mammography, CT, MRI, dosimetry, and quality management.

Radiologic technologists are represented by numerous professional societies at the international, national, state, and local levels. Among the most prominent of these organizations are the AHRA, the ASRT, the AEIRS, the AVIR, the ISRRT, the SDMS, the SMRM, the SMRI, and the SNM—Technologist Section.

Radiologists and physicists are also represented by numerous organizations. Among those with the strongest ties to radiologic technology are the AAPM, the ACR, the AIUM, the AMA, the ARRS, the ASTRO, the ISCD, the RSNA, the SCAR, and the SNM. Together, these organizations constitute the full strength of the radiologic sciences profession by their activities in accreditation, certification, and representation.

BIBLIOGRAPHY

American Medical Association: *Health professions career and education directory, 2005-06,* ed 33, Chicago, 2005, The Association.

Eisenberg RL: *Radiology: an illustrated history,* St Louis, Mosby–Year Book, 1992.

3

Educational Survival Skills

Arlene M. Adler, MEd, RT(R), FAERS
Richard R. Carlton, MS, RT(R)(CV), FAERS

The real voyage of discovery consists not in seeking new landscapes but in having new eyes.

Marcel Proust

OBJECTIVES

On completion of this chapter, the student will be able to:

1. Discuss the causes and symptoms of stress.

2. Explain behaviors and thoughts that increase the fight-or-flight response.

3. Analyze interventions that can be used to reduce or buffer stressors.

4. Describe several survival techniques to reduce stress.

5. Enumerate steps to manage time through organization, setting limits, and self-evaluation.

6. Explain the benefit of uplifts in relation to hassles.

7. Identify foods that can be eaten to supply the body nutritionally with additional vitamin C, vitamin B complex, and magnesium.

8. Foster study techniques to enhance retention and to the building of information into complex concepts.

9. List the steps for successful test taking.

GLOSSARY

Buffers: activities that decrease the negative effects of stress but do not change the stressors

Fight-or-Flight Response: physiologic response resulting from anger and fear and triggered by a real or imagined threat

Hassles: unexpected negative changes or events

In-Control Language: statements that reflect an attitude of choice and evoke positive feelings

Out-of-Control Language: words or phrases that express a lack of control over a situation

Stress: demand on time, energy, and resources with an element of threat

Stressors: events, both real and imagined, that increase feelings of anxiety

Time Management: practice of self-management related to how time is used

Uplifts: planned positive activities to balance hassles

Worry: time and energy spent concerned for things over which we have little or no control

WHAT IS STRESS?

The busy world of the radiologic sciences student is filled with new ideas, concepts, demanding class and clinical schedules, and changing focus. Little thought is given to managing the stressors associated with so much change. The attention given to life in general as a student is to survive in almost any way possible. The hope is to survive midterms and finals; to survive the changing demands of clinical instructors; and to survive work, family responsibilities, and school demands. The feeling associated with this survival effort may leave the student anxious, tired, humorless, irritable, uncreative, but on rare occasions thrilled. The path through all of these emotions provides the background for finally saying, "I'm stressed out!" The focus of this chapter is on possible interventions to manage or control stressors, including time management, study habits and test-taking strategies, and other self-care interventions.

Stress is produced by events that are perceived as demands on time, energy, or resources with the threat that not enough energy, time, or resources will be available to fulfill an obligation. Studying for an important examination is difficult when a feeling exists that not enough time is available to complete the task. The pressure is on, and the result can be overwhelming anxiety. In fact, if the threat is real enough to the individual, the heart rate increases, breathing becomes shallow and rapid, and the person may have a surge of energy that seems better handled while pacing the floor. The body is ready for a big event and does not distinguish between readiness for a 100-yard dash and readiness for a paper-and-pencil test. The chemistry of the body responds to the brain's message and prepares for physical activity. When the response of the body is to stay and continue studying, the chemicals of the body have to dissipate on their own.

Usually, we deal with more than one event at a time—home and family responsibilities, school assignments, and work activities. In combination, these events produce a compounding effect. Finally, we say, "I'm stressed out!" This declaration is the plea for help when the limits of tolerance for juggling many responsibilities have been reached.

Fight-or-Flight Response

The **fight-or-flight response** is the physiologic reaction to a real or imagined threat arising from emotions of both fear and anger. It is the body's way of preparing for change that is perceived as threatening. This response served our species well many years ago when our survival was threatened. It provided a way to battle the elements. The physiologic responses include the release of hormones to increase metabolism, increases in fats and sugars for energy, and increases in heart rate and respiration. Blood flows at a greater-than-normal rate to the long muscles of the extremities, and the central nervous system is stimulated. This response is the preparation for battle or escape.

An example of triggering of the fight-or-flight response is when the telephone rings at 2 AM, waking the individual from a deep sleep. All systems are *go* as soon as the ring is heard in anticipation of bad news; the body is ready for the *battle*. The call turns out to be a wrong number. The outcome presented no emotional or physical injury, but the body readied itself automatically for a physical response. For several minutes after the event, a person is under the influence of the body's chemical response to the potential threat. Until the body readjusts to the nonthreatening environment, neither sleep nor relaxation will return. This same response occurs in the setting of threats such as missed deadlines, loss of self-esteem, poor test results, loss of friendship, overcommitment, and inability to set personal limits. Living in a state of constant alert over time can result in serious physical or emotional illness.

Attitudes about *self* and the role the environment plays in the ability to counter or cause a stress response are important to recognize. What is in the mind is in the body. If self-defeating, negative thoughts are predominant, then both consciously and subconsciously the body responds with an excessive release of chemicals; over time, these chemicals produce wear and tear on organs, resulting in serious illness. Positive thoughts and an optimistic viewpoint can actually decrease the potential for ill health and reduce the metabolism that chemically triggers the fight-or-flight response. Positive thoughts also serve as a self-fulfilling prophecy: attitudes that accurately predict gloom or happiness dictate whether we manage daily stressors positively or negatively.

Causes and Effects

The compounding effect of stress over several weeks to months can contribute to poor emotional and physical health. Examples include repeated colds, ulcers, muscle stiffness, elevated cholesterol, excessive sleeping, irritability, and headaches. Stress-related symptoms are often discounted and are not considered serious, but these problems are early warnings and can have both physical and emotional consequences.

Stress can be caused by such factors as traffic, meeting a deadline, expecting all As in school, family problems, overcommitment, a new boyfriend or girlfriend, financial problems, and car trouble. These events are **stressors.** What is stressful to one person may not affect someone else because of perspectives, life experiences, and personal circumstances. Stress is individual, and interventions used to reduce or buffer stress can be effective only when individually identified. What is helpful for one person may not be helpful to another. The important point is to recognize your stressors, to develop interventions, and to recognize the need for taking responsibility for yourself.

INTERVENTIONS

Change

For most people, major life events are stressful and, in some cases, overwhelming. Most people have observed others experiencing and coping with major changes, such as divorce, death of a family member or friend, marriage, job loss, or career change. By observing these major events, the observer makes decisions about how he or she would handle a similar situation if confronted. What has not been learned is how to handle minor changes, or **hassles.** In a busy life, these minor changes have great impact. Examples are an unexpected detour in the normal travel route to work or school, a last-minute change in examination time, a family argument, and car trouble. These unexpected events create great stress, and the body responds in the fight-or-flight mode. Once again, the body produces a chemical response, and these chemicals dissipate slowly through increased respiration, increased heart rate, muscle tension, and occasionally digestive upset. Response to these stressors may occur frequently enough that the body does not have enough time to get back to a homeostatic condition. In other words, the body can be constantly on alert as a result of the back-to-back changing conditions that are so much a part of a busy, responsible existence.

Minor changes can be countered by balancing unexpected change with planned positive activity. The minor changes often elicit negative responses in the form of anger, depression, poor self-concept, frustration, or defeat. Planned positive activities provide opportunities to experience joy, happiness, positive self-concept, optimism, and a sense of well being. These activities, or **uplifts,** are often simple and easy to carry out. Examples include complimenting someone, watching a favorite television program, taking a walk, being efficient and organized, relaxing, having fun, hugging, and laughing.

In your chosen field of study, new concepts will be introduced, the language of the art will have to be mastered, and deadlines will need to be met both for the welfare of the patient and for the efficiency of the department. As goals are accomplished, great relief and joy are experienced, but reaching these goals without some planned positive activities will take an emotional and physical toll.

SURVIVAL TECHNIQUE FOR CHANGE. Plan positive activities, called *uplifts,* to balance unexpected negative change, or *hassles.*

Language

Stress tends to be contagious. When someone is in a period of great stress, such as around the time of final examinations, his or her words often clearly express the fear and frustration felt as a result of the concern that time, energy, or resources will be insufficient to get everything accomplished. The expression of this concern may alarm others, as well as augment the individual's feeling of frustration.

Many factors influence how we feel about events occurring around us every day. Internal events (fight or flight) happen even as a result of the **out-of-control language** we use. The use of words or phrases that express a lack of control promotes this feeling of being out of control, which is apparent in such statements as "I *have* to study for a test" and "I *never* get to do what I want to do." Statements used to express a feeling of not having any control include "I have to," "I must," "I never," "it's awful," and "it's unfair."

These examples of language express not only loss of control, but also much emotion that is tied to each. Saying words such as "never," "must," "have to," "awful," and "unfair" without some strong emotion associated with each is virtually impossible. Just saying each of these words awakens feelings of anger, frustration, or despair in the speaker.

If out-of-control words can evoke negative feelings, then using **in-control language** will produce positive feelings. Substitute terminology producing feelings of more control and less fight-or-flight response includes statements such as "I decided," "I choose," "I want to," "I like," and "I can." Having strong negative feelings when uttering statements such as "I have decided to study this evening for my test" and "I choose to use this method to complete this procedure" is difficult. Each statement reflects an attitude of choice and evokes positive feelings. These statements produce the expectation of reaching an attainable goal, as well as feelings of determination, self-control, and pleasure.

In many instances, terms that maximize stress responses are used when, in fact, personal choices have been made, but they are expressed negatively: "I have to go to class." The hope is that the unsaid portion is that "I chose this field of study, and I have to go to class to reach my goal." Not only are these choices expressed negatively, but we also often lose sight of the goal. The vision of who or what we will become drives our choices; with practice, our language can reflect these decisions positively.

SURVIVAL TECHNIQUE FOR LANGUAGE. Practice language that reflects choice and expresses control over a situation. In-control language reduces the flight-or-fight response.

Worry

During high-stress times, everyone tends to be overly concerned about outcomes and to engage in a mental activity of "What will I do if . . .?" This activity is **worry.** "What will I do if I fail this examination?" "What if I do not complete all my clinical competencies in time?" "What if my family feels neglected?" "What if my car cannot last until I graduate?" "What if I lose my job? How will I pay for tuition?" Each circumstance is a real possibility for many students, but until it is a reality, it represents unnecessary energy being expended through borrowing trouble.

Worry robs energy! Less than 5% of the events about which we worry actually happen. Part of worry is time and energy spent being concerned about things over which we have no control. We often have little control over the mechanical functioning of our car, especially when preventive maintenance is practiced. We worry about situations that do not involve us directly, such as a classmate's passing an examination. We worry about possibilities that might be removed from our thoughts by taking some action. Taking no action is procrastination. If we could stop putting off an unpleasant or overly challenging activity because of laziness, poor management of time, or the fear of not being perfect, a significant part of worry would be eliminated. The big problem with procrastination is that a constant feeling of guilt goes with putting off unpleasant tasks. The best news about procrastination and the worry that accompanies it is that we have full control over it. Do something to reduce the anxiety! Doing something wrong may be better than doing nothing at all!

Consider worry this way. Most of the things about which we worry never happen or turn out better than we thought they would. A small portion of what worries us is the result of procrastination that can be eliminated by taking action. A minor part of worry is concern over matters that do not directly concern us and that may involve the worries that other people have. Less than 5% of things about which what we worry actually happen.

SURVIVAL TECHNIQUE FOR WORRY. When worrying, use this checklist to anticipate the degree of control you have over the situation:

- It probably will not happen.
- It will turn out better than expected.
- Taking action can change the outcome.
- It is not my concern.

- I have no control over the outcome.
- Am I making a mountain out of a molehill?

Managing Time

An important part of managing stress is learning to manage time. Commonly, people often believe that not enough time is available to accomplish all that needs to be done or all that we want to do. Because the amount of time available cannot be controlled, practicing **time management** is then necessary, which is self-management related to how time is used.

Many external interruptions are thieves of time. These interruptions include telephone calls, mistakes and incomplete information about assignments or jobs, and outside activities. These factors can be controlled by setting limits on the length of telephone calls if you choose to receive calls, getting a full understanding of assignments by taking a few extra minutes to clarify, and limiting outside activities temporarily.

Setting parameters on available time is also important. In many instances, too many tasks are attempted at once. This failure to set parameters on time happens to the student who has responsibilities that include not only school assignments, but also work, home, or family responsibilities. Besides attempting too much at once, other compounding issues include setting unrealistic deadlines, failing to say "no," procrastinating, and a having general lack of organization.

The biggest thief of time is indecision. The fear of making a mistake or of being imperfect prompts indecision. With much to be done in a limited time, loss of energy through worry and indecision is destructive and wasteful. If indecision is the product of fearing a mistake, consider thinking of a mistake as an opportunity to learn and improve on future activities and decisions.

Setting deadlines can provide opportunities to schedule time for study, to make and take telephone calls, to assist family members, and to socialize. Scheduling activities gives some assurance of being able to meet obligations without slighting anyone. A potential problem associated with scheduling activities is that of being trapped by the schedule. Deadlines can give rise to feelings of desperation and helplessness, especially when the number of activities that can be accomplished within the allotted time frame has been overestimated, for example, allowing 3 hours to study for a test along with some other minor activities in an evening only to discover that the 3-hour time frame was not enough. The individual is then trapped into having to meet the other obligations and yet still finding time to complete the studying.

Although scheduling activities is wise, realistic time frames must be set. Unrealistic estimates of the time needed to complete a paper, study for an examination, or travel to class can give rise to feelings of panic. This panic can trigger the fight-or-flight response, which then defeats the purpose of time management. The best way to combat the result of underestimating time needed is to build in contingency plans. "If a paper takes longer to write than expected, what alternatives do I have?" "Can I take another route to school if the street repair ties up traffic?" Providing a way out reduces feelings of panic and the negative effects of the fight-or-flight response.

The best way to manage time is to practice self-management. This goal involves four steps:

1. *Know yourself.* Evaluate your personal style, and recognize the times when you are in peaks and valleys of effectiveness. Capitalize on your peak times, and plan to do the activities that are most demanding. Ask yourself if you are a morning person or a night owl. When do you think most clearly, and how much time can you concentrate on one activity? Generally, the best results come from studying for 50 to 60 minutes in one block of time, then breaking for 10 minutes. Repeating this cycle reduces fatigue and allows more productive use of time.

2. *Prioritize responsibilities.* Identify all the roles you have that involve responsibility—that is, student, employee, or housekeeper. Prioritize all these roles from greatest to least priority. Evaluate time available after classes and after personal needs and obligations are met. Careful evaluation of activities and responsibilities should be done to determine which items can be realistically continued and which need to be delegated to someone else.

3. *Prioritize activities.* Set priorities according to goals and the length of time that will be needed to complete an activity. Setting a plan for a full week, month, or term and scheduling study, research, and social activities during these blocks of time may be helpful. By looking at a long-term plan, rushing at the last minute can be avoided, and social obligations can be met. Goals such as graduating, completing a semester, or getting a B in a course must be set so that activities will be driven by the goal.

4. *Plan for self-care.* Because we all have a need for relaxation, which includes exercise, games, rest, and socializing, this time should be anticipated and planned. For some people, planning for self-care is necessary because they learned the work-before-play ethic. Chances are, all the work will never be done;

consequently, little attention is given to social activities, leading to a negative view of life in general. For other people, the opposite may be the norm. The lack of discipline to complete work may lead to disappointing results educationally. A balance is required between work and play so that the goals can be met successfully and with enthusiasm.

SURVIVAL TECHNIQUE FOR MANAGING TIME. Plan your time, and set goals by the following:

- Knowing when you are most effective
- Prioritizing and delegating responsibility when additional resources exist
- Planning and scheduling activities as far in advance as possible to avoid last-minute rushing
- Scheduling time for relaxation and fun

BUFFERING STRESSORS

Even when all the positive steps to reduce stress are taken, stress cannot be eliminated. Because much of the stress experienced on a daily basis cannot be changed, the next best intervention is to buffer the effects of stress. Just as a mute muffles the harsh notes of a brass instrument, **buffers** are necessary to reduce the harmful effects of the fight-or-flight response.

Exercise

The fight-or-flight response readies the body for action. Circulation increases in the long muscles, and the heart rate and respiration rate increase to supply more oxygen to the muscles. Sugars and fats are dumped into the system to supply the needed energy for physical activity. If you are berated in front of your peers, then anger, rage, fear, and indignation boil in your system and can be felt immediately. A chemical, norepinephrine, is released into the body during preparation for action. This chemical heightens the emotional response that the stress causes. If irritation by someone or something is the cause, the response is anger, which is often out of proportion to the magnitude of the event. If threatened, the result may be unreasonable fear. This response accounts for the extreme reactions often elicited in the form of irritability and loss of sense of humor when someone has been under stress for prolonged periods without proper interventions.

Participation in regular aerobic activity—continuous, rhythmic activity that involves large muscles—is necessary to dissipate the undesirable chemicals in the system resulting from stress. *Aerobic* means using air to perform the activity. Examples are running, walking, biking, and other noncompetitive exercise. Because of the desire to win, exercise during a competitive event may increase tension rather than decrease it.

Exercise is not only necessary to dissipate undesirable chemicals produced by the body, but it can also be a means to prevent negative physical and emotional responses. A minimum of 30 minutes of aerobic exercise three to five times a week can have some positive health benefits. Some physical benefits are reduced risk of heart disease, decreased blood cholesterol levels, and reduced muscle tension.

Many of our efforts in society are directed at getting and keeping the competitive edge. Ego-involved activities almost never result in feelings of reduced stress. In fact, they may have the reverse effect. The noncompetitive forms of exercise are the most beneficial mentally. Exercising is done because it feels right. A sense of well being is produced as a result of the activity. This sense of well being after exercising is a result not only of reducing harmful chemicals produced under stress, but also of releasing *happy* chemicals in the brain that produce a sense of pleasure, the most notable of which are the endorphins. Endorphins released in the brain during physical activity have a relaxing effect on the body and provide a sense of well being. This feeling contributes to what is commonly called the *runner's high*. People who exercise regularly look forward to the relaxing benefits of the aerobic activity, which usually promotes improved sleep patterns, increased energy and stress tolerance, and suppressed appetite.

If possible, find a friend to participate with you. You will give encouragement to each other. Time spent walking with a friend provides some social time as well. Sharing a mutual interest is a rewarding and satisfying experience.

SURVIVAL TECHNIQUE FOR BUFFERING STRESS. Exercise aerobically three to five times per week for a minimum of 30 minutes as a buffer to the chemicals produced in the body as a result of the fight-or-flight response.

Nutrition

When we are busiest, we are least able to provide good nutrition for ourselves. Stress can be buffered by eating three well-balanced meals each day. When our body undergoes the fight-or-flight response on any regular basis, three nutritional substances that are important to us both physically and mentally—vitamin C, vitamin B complex, and magnesium—are greatly reduced.

Vitamin C has been shown to be especially important in supporting the immune system to help protect from colds, sore throats, and other infections. Frequently, when someone experiences a stressor, such as getting through final examinations, he or she may develop a cold and sore throat at that time. As vitamin C is depleted, our resistance is decreased. One way to replace the depleted vitamin C is to start a diet that includes dark-green leafy vegetables, fruits, broccoli, Brussels sprouts, potatoes, and tomatoes.

The complex of B vitamins seems to support and provide necessary energy to sustain us from day to day. When under a great deal of stress, we may oversleep or feel groggy much of the time. Lost vitamin B complex can be replaced by eating bananas, green leafy vegetables, lean meat, poultry, milk, eggs, and whole grains.

Magnesium supports the immune system also. Replacement of magnesium comes from eating bananas, fish, nuts, and whole grains. A diet rich in carbohydrates (e.g., white bread) and simple sugars tends to cause sudden rises and falls in blood sugar levels. This fluctuation can cause sleepiness, sluggishness, and mental lethargy. In addition, because of the response of insulin to the introduction of sugar into the digestive tract, blood sugar levels fall sharply. This rapid decrease in blood sugar levels provides the physiologic conditions that can lead to misinterpreting information or making mountains out of molehills. Vending machine foods and fast foods are often major sources of carbohydrates and need to be avoided or at least carefully selected.

Good nutrition includes a diet that provides proper, appropriate servings from all food groups (Fig. 3–1). The United States Department of Agriculture (USDA) has revised the historical food pyramid with *MyPyramid,* which emphasizes not only the food groups and their typical serving sizes, but also the importance of the balance between food intake and physical activity. The servings recommended on the pyramid represent an intake of approximately 2000 calories per day. For an active young adult, the appropriate daily calorie intake may need to be adjusted based on the amount of physical activity. Maintaining a good nutritional balance will not change your stressors, but it will place you at an advantage for staying both physically and mentally healthy during stressful events. For more detailed information from the USDA, visit their web site at *http://www.mypyramid.gov.*

SURVIVAL TECHNIQUE FOR BUFFERING STRESS. Eat three nutritionally balanced meals each day to replace vitamins and minerals lost through stress.

Visualization and Meditation

Other buffers to stress include visualization and meditation. Through visualization, the individual can take a minivacation by mentally revisiting a pleasant experience for 10 or 15 seconds. Maybe you recall the peace of sitting on a beach and hearing the waves lap the shore. It might be the silence and coolness of getting up early and witnessing a sunrise. Maybe it is the remembrance of a campfire, including the smell of wood burning, the sound of wood snapping, the feel of the heat from the flames, and the joy of sharing the experience with friends. Each of these mental events actually provides an opportunity to escape and relax by reliving the events momentarily; it also reduces the feeling of stress and the fight-or-flight response, thus providing a brief but real opportunity to get in touch with feelings of relaxation. This activity helps buffer day-to-day stresses.

Meditation also provides a mechanism to escape stress by emptying the mind of all thoughts and focusing on only one word or one statement. In Christian meditation, it may be the process of sharing the weight of responsibility or the blessing of support through God's love and acceptance.

Other buffers to stress include progressive relaxation, deep-muscle relaxation (usually guided by audio recordings), biofeedback, and guided imagery.

SURVIVAL TECHNIQUE FOR BUFFERING STRESS. Regularly practice visualization or some form of meditation.

STUDY SKILLS AND TEST TAKING

Study Skill Techniques

During the next few years of college and advanced-level study, you will be required to learn technical information that is tested during each term. Additionally, you will have to recall pieces of learned information much later and add them to new, more advanced concepts. Because of the building of information into complex concepts, higher-level learning, not simply a brief regurgitation of facts, must take place. An excellent way to increase the effectiveness of study time is to apply the concept of time management to develop good study skills. This process involves five techniques (Box 3-1):

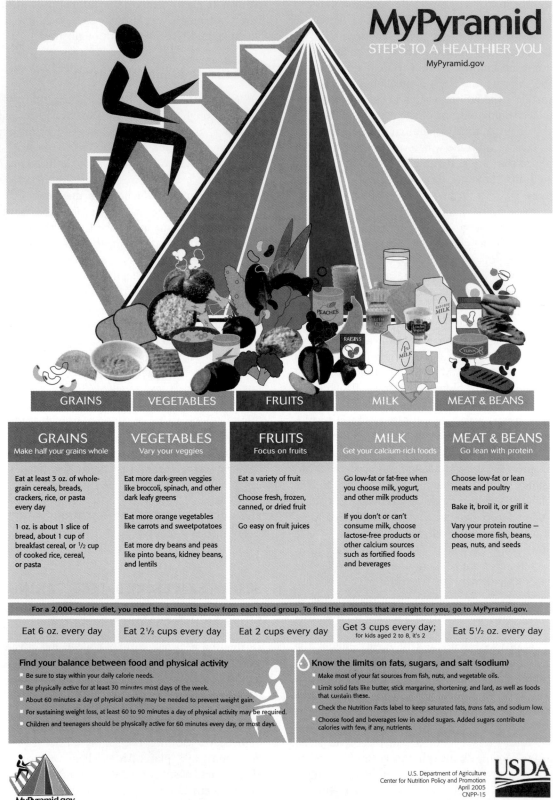

FIG. 3–1 U.S. Department of Agriculture's MyPyramid Steps to a Healthier You.

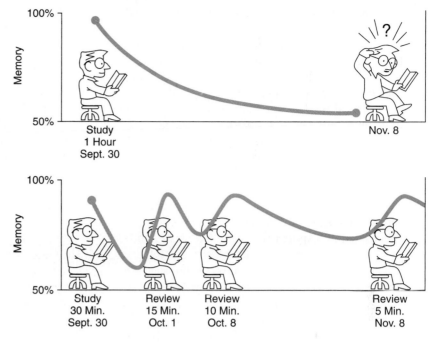

FIG. 3–2 *Top,* Massed study. *Bottom,* Spaced reviews. (From Staton TF: How to study, ed 6, Nashville, 1977, Ags Pub.)

1. *Review the material soon after it is introduced.* Most information introduced in class is forgotten within 24 hours unless steps are taken to reinforce it (Fig. 3–2). Students often do not begin to study for a test before the week of the test. Usually, a great deal of time has elapsed, and much of the material has been forgotten. A common theme expressed during last-minute study is, "The instructor didn't explain very well," or "The instructor never told us that!" If the material were reviewed immediately or within a short time after class, then the information can be reinforced and remembered longer; it would also help identify questionable areas where understanding is lacking.

2. *Use as many senses as possible.* In review of information, writing key elements or words has been shown to be beneficial. This visual stimulation through writing imprints additional and longer-lasting information in the brain, which enhances recall later. Besides writing the information, recite the material aloud. Saying the words helps formulate another dimension of the concept and allows practice at saying unfamiliar terms. The combination of seeing, saying, and hearing—using several senses—has been shown to provide opportunities for increased retention of information and recall.

3. *Plan a regular schedule of study.* Waiting until the last minute to study increases anxiety to a point that it actually may interfere with the ability to learn and recall information. Frustration sets in as the time ticks

BOX 3-1 Study Skill Techniques

Review the material soon after it is introduced.
Use as many senses as possible.
Plan a regular schedule of study.
Study in a group.
Attitude helps remembering!

away. Studying or cramming for a test at the last minute may lead to confusion about details. Cramming provides only short-term recall. Plan regular review and study of all subjects from the time the material is first introduced. This action may be as simple as planning to reread notes every other day for a short time. Studies have shown that short, regular periods of study and review result in greater recall than a long period of study followed by a long period of no exposure to the information. Studying for 1 hour per week before a test with no review in between can result in a 50% loss of recall.

4. *Study in a group.* Studying in small groups of no more than five helps test your understanding of the material. The variety of perceptions offers opportunities to conceptualize the information from more than one viewpoint. If a large amount of material has to be covered, divide it among the group, each person

preparing an area that may be within the individual's interest and expertise. Working in a group provides an opportunity to feel supported and encouraged, thus enhancing a personal expectation of success. The study group needs to focus on a goal with mutual agreement on the purpose of meeting and the task to be accomplished. This approach is necessary to avoid the temptation to use the time for socializing rather than studying. Once the business of study is completed, relaxing and enjoying the company of the group is important and appropriate.

5. *Attitude helps remembering.* Having a positive attitude about the reason for studying enhances your ability to learn and remember. You have set a goal for your professional future. Approach it with enthusiasm and a *can do* attitude. Become part of the self-fulfilling prophecy that says you are in control of your successes and failures. A feeling of control, in turn, reduces the stress response and enhances your chances for a healthy period of learning.

SURVIVAL TECHNIQUE FOR STUDY SKILLS

- Review new material soon after introduction.
- Use as many senses as possible—seeing, saying, and writing.
- Plan a regular study schedule.
- Study with a group occasionally.
- Develop a positive *can do* attitude.

Test-Taking Tips

In addition to possessing good study skills, following a few *test-taking strategies* is also helpful. Here are some useful tips for test-taking success:

1. Take the day off from study before the test to relax and prepare yourself. Last-minute cramming adds to anxiety and the possibility of *freezing* on the test.
2. Wear bright-colored clothes for the test. Color has great effect on moods and alertness; it also reflects feelings about the individual. Bright colors promote positive and optimistic feelings.
3. Avoid a diet full of carbohydrates the day before and the day of the test. *Carb loading* may be helpful to a runner preparing for a long-distance race but not for a person sitting and taking a paper-and-pencil test. The carbohydrates convert to sugar, providing the runner with extra energy as he or she runs. Carbohydrates and sugars leave the nonrunner sluggish and sleepy because of the need to metabolize all the sugar without exerting much energy. A well-balanced diet

that includes proteins and carbohydrates provides improved mental alertness necessary when taking a test.
4. Get a good night's sleep before the examination. Rest allows clear thinking and improved interpretation.
5. Get to the test early to allow yourself time to relax before beginning. Rushing at the last minute increases anxiety, which can decrease your mental effectiveness.
6. Scan the test, and answer all the questions you are sure you know. Do not waste time initially on questions that are problematic for you. Go back and repeat the procedure, allowing yourself a little more time to answer. Leave questions that are difficult to recall until the last. This way, if it is a time-limited examination, most questions will be answered even if you are caught short of time.
7. Review your test when done, and make corrections as needed. Do not be afraid to change answers. Some recall may have occurred during the test; some questions provide a key to answers for other questions. Make certain you have answered all the questions. If you are answering on an answer sheet that requires blackening circles or boxes, then be certain that the number of the question corresponds with the number on the answer sheet.
8. When the test is over, put it behind you. Use the results as an opportunity to enhance your knowledge in the future. Now, begin the study process all over again. Think positively!

SUMMARY

Stress is a demand on time, energy, and resources, with some fear of not being able to meet goals or obligations. Change is a large component of stress, and managing an ever-changing environment is the way to survive. The language we use can increase or decrease feelings of control. The issues about which we worry need to be evaluated to determine whether our worries are within our control. Are these mountains created from molehills, or can the worry energy be converted into action to diminish the problem? Much of the stress experience can be altered by practicing better time management, including prioritizing by setting limits, making decisions, establishing goals, and managing self-care.

Buffering of stress occurs when the effects of the fight-or-flight response can be offset through other activities. Most of our stressors will not go away, but we can exercise regularly, eat well-balanced meals and snacks, and use some form of meditation or visualization to reduce temporarily the physical and emotional effects of stress.

These activities will not change our stressors, but they can offer an opportunity to balance some of the negative.

For students, a great deal of stress is the result of the physical and emotional effort of preparing for classroom and clinical tests. Successful test taking depends on good time management and appropriate study skills, as well as on good nutrition and rest. Developing individualized study skills involves managing time to allow for regular review, periodic study in groups, and practicing methods to enhance learning and remembering. Letting as many senses as possible reinforce information assists in imprinting information on the brain. This approach is especially important as concepts are *built* from course to course. A systematic approach to taking the test prevents you from running out of time before all questions have been considered. Complete all the easiest questions first, and return to more difficult questions later. This method helps you relax and build confidence, and it helps trigger recall because questions are often interrelated.

Most of all, maintain a positive *can do* attitude. Attitude becomes a self-fulfilling prophecy. If you believe you can achieve your goals, you will. Associate with others who think positively. A positive attitude is contagious and needs to be fostered by you and by people around you.

BIBLIOGRAPHY

Appelbaum SH, Rohrs WF: *Time management for healthcare professionals,* Rockville, Md, 1981, Aspen Publications.

Bragstad BJ, Stumpf SM: *A guidebook for teaching study skills and motivation,* Newton, Mass, 1982, Allyn & Bacon.

Crea J: On nutrition, *Chicago Tribune,* May 28, 1992.

Ellis D: *Becoming a master student,* ed 10, Boston, 2002, Houghton Mifflin.

Fuchs NK: *The nutrition detective,* New York, 1985, St Martin's Press.

Girdano DA, Everly GS, Dusek DE: *Controlling stress and tension,* ed 6, San Francisco, 2000, Benjamin Cummings.

Hubbard R: *Stress and burnout in health care professionals,* Notre Dame, Ind, 1987, University of Notre Dame, Administrative Development Program.

Kirtbawski PA: Test-taking skills: giving yourself an edge. *Nursing '90* 20:6, 1990.

United States Department of Agriculture: *http://www. mypyramid.gov.*

4

Critical Thinking and Problem Solving Strategies

Tracy Herrmann, MEd, RT(R)
Angie Arnold, MEd, RT(R)

Education is not the filling of a pail, but the lighting of a fire.

William Butler Yeats

OBJECTIVES

On completion of this chapter, the student will be able to:

1. Define critical thinking and problem solving.

2. Discuss the importance of critical thinking and problem solving in the radiologic sciences.

3. Describe the role of critical thinking in clinical, ethical, and technical decision making.

4. Apply the steps involved in problem solving.

5. Analyze situations that require critical thinking.

6. Identify patient care situations that use critical-thinking and problem-solving skills.

7. Appreciate the need for continued development of critical-thinking and problem-solving skills for radiologic science professionals.

GLOSSARY

Analysis: determination of the cause and effect of a situation or work

Case Studies: real-life patient situations that are studied and assessed for learning purposes

Critique: a type of evaluation that provides feedback on the quality of a work or creation in the form of an opinion or review

Critical Thinking: creative action based on professional knowledge and experience involving sound judgment applied with high ethical standards and integrity

Evaluation: judgment or determination of the quality of a work or creation

Laboratory Experiments: an exercise or activity used to reinforce cognitive concepts through the performance of planned steps usually involving the analysis of data and answering of questions

Practice Standards: defining statements of the professional role and performance criteria for a practitioner

Problem Solving: answering questions in a methodical manner to resolve a challenging situation

Role Playing: acting out a situation in a realistic manner in the classroom or laboratory

Synthesis: combining multiple areas of knowledge to create a new work or understanding

WHAT ARE CRITICAL THINKING AND PROBLEM SOLVING?

In the radiologic sciences, every patient presents a new situation or challenge. No two procedures or treatments are the same. Each patient is an individual who must be cared for in a unique and often creative manner. A patient's individuality or pathologic condition can create a situation that requires a quick and inventive response from the radiologic science professional. This creative action, when performed appropriately based on professional knowledge and experience, is considered **critical thinking.** Critical thinking involves sound professional judgment applied with high ethical standards and integrity.

Critical thinking is required in most health care situations. An uncomfortable or difficult decision that must be made about a patient's care likely involves critical thinking skills. Identifying inappropriate actions or situations and correcting them also involve critical thinking. Challenges with communication, modifying procedures or treatments from the normal routine with regard to patient condition, and solving equipment malfunctions or technical problems are just a few examples of situations that involve problem solving and critical thinking.

Why Learn to Problem Solve and Think Critically in the Radiologic Sciences?

Professional standards of the radiologic sciences support and define problem-solving and critical-thinking skills expected in the workplace. Credentialing agencies such as the American Registry of Radiologic Technologists (ARRT) publish codes of ethics (see Appendix D). These codes address the expected conduct of radiologic science professionals to perform procedures while providing the highest quality of care and to act in the best interest of the patient in an ethical manner. Professional societies such as the American Society of Radiologic Technologists (ASRT) also publish **practice standards** (see Appendix A) that define specific professional expectations and responsibilities. Inherent in these professional standards are the elements of appropriate decision-making skills associated with problem solving and critical thinking. As such, future employers will expect graduates to have developed skills in these areas.

To prepare students for the workforce, educational programs reinforce the expectations of the professional standards described previously. In addition, the programmatic and institutional accrediting agencies that guide educational institutions require the preparation of students for thinking and decision making that goes well beyond memorization. For example, the Joint Review Committee on Education in Radiologic Technology *Standards for an Accredited Program in the Radiologic Sciences* requires that radiologic science programs assess the **problem-solving** and critical-thinking skills of their students. The goals and objectives of the student program may include elements of critical thinking, including **analysis, synthesis, evaluation,** and **critique.** Development and assessment of these goals may be accomplished in a variety of unique ways for each accredited program. Students are likely to encounter **role playing, case studies,** scenarios, clinical skills assessments, **laboratory experiments,** complex problems and calculations, complex multiple-choice questions, and many additional forms of learning experiences all designed to

TABLE 4-1 Steps in Problem Solving and Critical Thinking

STEPS IN ORDER	POTENTIAL QUESTIONS
Identify and/or clarify the problem.	• Does a problem exist? • What is the problem? • What is the cause of the problem? • Solving the problem is whose responsibility?
Undergo an objective examination of the problem.	• What is known about the problem? • What are all aspects of the problem, and how will these factors influence the outcome? • What are the key elements of the problem? • Who or what is or may be affected by this problem? • What are the safety, risk, and liability implications? • What are the technical considerations? • Will more than one solution or type of solution be needed?
Consider and develop all viable solutions to the problem.	• Are your decisions regarding the problem objective and based on professional knowledge, ethics, and standards? • How will these professional standards be applied and modified to fit the unique situation presented by the problem? • What additional reliable information or expertise is needed? • Do any similar problems exist that have been successfully solved that can guide you to possible solutions? • Will a creative solution be needed for this unique problem?
Select the solution with the best outcome for the patient.	• Which solution will allow for the best care of the patient and is within professional ethical standards? • Does this solution correspond with the procedures and protocol for your institution? • How quickly must the solution be enacted? • How did your solution affect the patient's outcome?

evaluate students' critical-thinking skills. Students may be asked to create products of learning or demonstrate learning through a portfolio or self-evaluation. Students must be open to unique learning experiences that require this higher order of thinking.

STEPS IN PROBLEM SOLVING AND CRITICAL THINKING

The key to mastering critical thinking is to extend learning beyond memorization of the concepts of the radiologic science profession. Students should pursue a deep long-term understanding of professional concepts and standards. Students may learn effectively by creating a scaffold of knowledge that will allow them to make additions and revisions as the students' mastery of the profession develops. Students should consider each element of their education as a building block or puzzle piece that they may need to use later to solve a complex clinical problem. After all, the knowledge base of the profession

will grow with or without the student. Table 4-1 lists the steps in problem solving and critical thinking and associated questions that are answered during the process.

Identify and/or Clarify the Problem

A key element of critical thought is problem solving. The first step in problem solving is to identify and/or clarify the problem. This step can be challenging, given that problems are often difficult to define. An unclear problem can cause frustration and discomfort. A situation or technique may not be working for you, and, as a student, you may have difficulty determining the cause.

Undergo an Objective Examination of the Problem

The next step is to undergo an objective examination of a problem. What do you already know about the problem? Review and examine all aspects of the problem and the factors that might influence the outcome. What are the key elements of the problem? Who or what is or may be affected by this problem? What are the implications of the problem that might result in safety risks and liability? What are the technical considerations? Will more than one solution or type of solution be needed? Identifying the elements of the problem is important so that you can proceed with finding the solution.

Consider and Develop All Viable Solutions to the Problem

Consider and develop all possible viable solutions to a problem. Be objective, and base decisions on professional knowledge, ethics, and standards. Look to these professional standards and modify them to fit the unique situation that the problem presents. Acquire any additional information or expertise as needed. Have you experienced similar problems that can guide you to possible solutions? Be sure to refer to your professional references or consult with an expert when necessary. Make sure your sources of information are reliable. Be creative but safe when creating solutions.

Select the Solution with the Best Outcome for the Patient

Finally, select and enact the best solution and action plan. Which solution will allow for the best care of the patient and is within professional ethical standards? Make sure that the chosen solution corresponds with the procedures and protocol for your institution. The most challenging problem solving and critical thinking occurs when an immediate decision is required, when more than one appropriate solution to the problem exists, or when no clear viable solution exists. Be sure to follow up on the problem to see how your choices affected the outcome. Reflect on this experience for use in solving future problems.

Critical Thinking in the Classroom and Laboratory

The classroom and the laboratory provide valuable experiences that allow the student to develop critical-thinking and analysis skills that involve cognitive and psychomotor learning. Cognitive and psychomotor refer to thinking and doing, respectively. In the classroom or laboratory, students are given the freedom to develop alternative ideas, test the classics, solve new problems, and increase their understanding of old problems without endangering the health of a patient. Students can also repeatedly experiment to find the answer or examine *what if* questions without irradiating a human being. The classroom and laboratory are the best places for students to begin developing the ability to apply previous knowledge to new situations (Fig. 4–1). The classroom and laboratory also allow students to begin formulating independent judgments needed for critical thinking in the rapidly changing health care environment.

Critical Thinking in the Clinical Setting

The clinical setting is where the student can transfer knowledge into action in a *real-world* environment. Students are exposed to unique real-life experiences that can be reinforced by the supervising radiologic science professional. Understanding the *why* behind a standard procedure is the key to making future decisions when a situation is not routine. Making decisions based on professional knowledge as applied to the clinical situation is important. Clinical experience provides a variety of critical-thinking situations and allows for student learning to extend well beyond *button pushing;* it permits the student to demonstrate the ability to respond when the correct decision is not clear and obvious; and it may involve recognizing when a situation is inappropriate and determining how to proceed in a professional manner.

Students who are new to the clinical setting must consider that radiologic science professionals use many variations of the standard procedures taught in the laboratory and classroom. Each radiologic science professional has developed his or her own style based on experience. These variations in practice can create a sense of frustration for the student. The student must focus on combining the best elements of each supervising radiologic science professional and then develop his or her own appropriate practice habits and professional style.

At the beginning phases of clinical experience, critical thinking may involve decisions made by the student regarding which role models to emulate or knowing when to go to program officials with concerns or problems. Early critical-thinking decisions may also involve determining whether to make independent judgments versus when to ask for help, or it may involve deciding when making a joke is appropriate and when not to do so. With experience and education, the student will be prepared to handle critical-thinking situations that may affect the life and well being of a patient under the student's care.

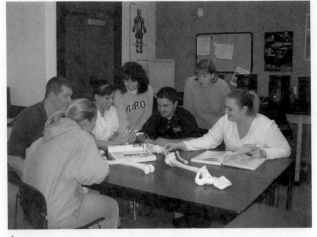

A

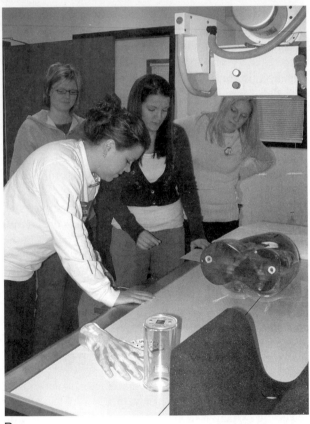

B

FIG. 4–1 The classroom and laboratory settings allow the students to develop critical thinking and analysis skills and examine *what if* questions without irradiating a human being.

Affective Critical Thinking

Analyzing personal values and feelings and managing uncomfortable ethical situations are components of affective critical thinking. Students must value the professional knowledge that serves as the foundation for their chosen profession. Students benefit by examining the ways they learn best and then taking charge of their own education. Being a creative and active learner is important in the radiologic sciences. Students often have overwhelming feelings when they first enter the health care setting. They may observe and be involved in many situations that they have not previously experienced. Feelings can be expressed through journal writing or discussions with program faculty, other students, or clinical supervisors. Students must be conscientious about maintaining patient confidentiality at all times during these types of discussions. Affective critical thinking skills are also important when dealing with the patient and his or her family, communicating in challenging situations, and working as part of the health care team. Students may also need to apply problem-solving and critical-thinking skills to manage their personal problems and issues to ensure that these do not affect their educational progress or more importantly patient care in the clinical setting.

CLINICAL APPLICATIONS OF CRITICAL THINKING AND PROBLEM SOLVING

Ethics

Many situations arise that require a radiologic science professional to make a decision based on professional ethics. These situations require the radiologic science professional to act accordingly regarding patient safety and/or radiation safety of patients and other health care personnel. At all times, the radiologic science professional is expected to act within the guidelines of the ARRT Code of Ethics (Appendix D). Chapter 22, entitled "Professional Ethics," provides specific examples and information about problem solving for ethical dilemmas, including potential situations that a radiologic science professional may face.

Technical Skills

A patient rarely arrives to the department prepared and able to cooperate as needed for a procedure or treatment. Some patients cannot stand for an upright procedure, or they cannot lay face down (prone) for an examination that requires them to be in that position. A treatment plan may need to be altered to accommodate a patient's condition or ability. In these situations, the radiologic science professional must evaluate and adjust the procedure or treatment according to the patient's ability and still produce the same outcome: adequate treatment or a diagnostic radiographic image. Advanced technical critical-thinking skills of a radiologic science professional may involve handling patients in trauma or critical care situations or recognizing an inappropriate treatment plan (Fig. 4–2). The development of technical critical-thinking skills is an ongoing process that requires extensive knowledge of the profession. Students must learn the foundation of professional knowledge to develop future technical critical-thinking skills for use in practice.

Patient Care

A radiologic science professional is responsible for interacting with and caring for each patient until his or her procedure or treatment has been completed. He or she observes the patient and looks for physical and mental changes that may occur as a result of the treatment or procedure. While communicating with the patient, the radiologic science professional will need to consider any human diversity issues that may play a part in the care of the patient. Adapting to any emergency situation that may arise during the procedure or treatment is also necessary to ensure safe and successful completion.

The following decision-making scenarios have been created as examples of situations that call for critical thinking and problem solving. Keep in mind that these are only a few examples of situations that a radiologic science professional may encounter on a day-to-day basis. The first case scenario provides an example of how the steps are used.

CASE 1: PATIENT INTERACTION AND HUMAN DIVERSITY.
"Your next patient does not understand English." You need to escort the patient from the waiting room and give them instructions for their procedure, including removing all clothing from the waist up and any metallic objects from the chest and abdomen area. You then need to bring him or her into the examination room and place him or her in the correct position for the procedure. After completing the procedure, you need to give the patient exit information.

Identify and/or clarify the problem. You only speak English and your patient does not.

Objectively examine all aspects of the problem. What instructions will need to be given to the patient? What technical considerations must be evaluated? Does the

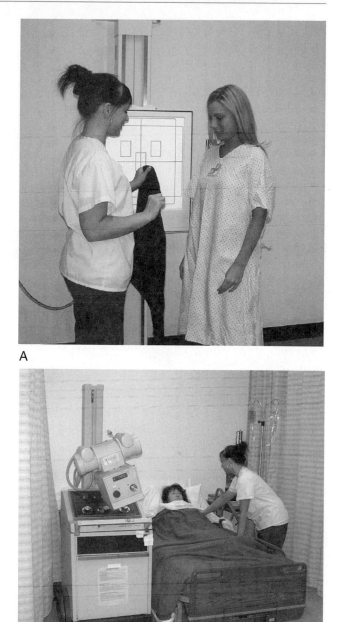

A

B

FIG. 4–2 Radiologic science professionals must use advanced critical thinking skills when handling all patient care situations.

patient speak any English? What are the cultural considerations?

Consider and develop possible solutions. You will need to develop a creative way to communicate your instructions to the patient. Can you identify someone else who can speak the language? Does anyone around the department speak the same language as the patient? Does the health care institution have an interpreter available? If the answer to all of these questions is *no,* what do you do next?

Select and enact the best solution. In this case, no interpreter is available, and the patient understands minimal English. You will need to use a variety of methods of communication such as demonstration and pantomime, as well as maintain your composure and patience while performing the procedure. All aspects of cultural diversity education and communication skills must be used in this instance. This type of situation occurs often, therefore keep in mind that it is just as frustrating for the patient as it is for the radiologic science professional.

CASE 2: RADIATION PROTECTION. *"Does any chance of pregnancy exist?"* You are taking a history from a female patient who has been sent to your department for radiation treatment, and one of the first things you ask is whether she is pregnant. The patient hesitates when asked about pregnancy, then finally states, "No, there is no chance I'm pregnant—it really doesn't have anything to do with my treatment, right?"

Identify and/or clarify the problem. Do you take the patient at her word? Does her hesitation in answering draw a red flag? Considering what you have learned about radiation protection, is knowing whether she is pregnant really necessary?

Objectively examine all aspects of the problem. What implications might arise if you continue with treatment as scheduled and you find out later that the patient actually is pregnant? What risks would you take by administering treatment without knowing for sure? Can you be held liable for any damage caused? After all, the patient denied that she was pregnant when initially asked.

Consider and develop possible solutions. Do you go ahead with treatment? Do you decide not to administer treatment? Do you have any other choices?

Select and enact the best solution. Can you find any guidance in the ARRT code of ethics regarding your responsibility to the patient, specifically in the area of radiation protection? Which principle, if any, applies to this situation, and does this principle help you in enacting your final solution? Does a solution exist that will help you accomplish your goals without compromising patient safety? What solution is in the best interest of the patient?

CASE 3: PATIENT ASSESSMENT. *"Your patient is unable to stand for x-rays."* Your patient has arrived from the emergency department for an acute abdominal series. The history provided on the requisition states that the patient is having sharp abdominal pain in his abdomen. When you ask the patient if he is able to stand for the upright abdominal radiograph, he replies, "Yes, I'll try."

Identify and/or clarify the problem. Should you permit the patient to stand? Could the patient's condition cause him to be weak or lightheaded if he stands? Could he have been given medication for his pain, and, if so, could it further affect his ability to stand? Even though he said that he would try to stand, do you allow him to do so?

Objectively examine all aspects of the problem. What might happen if the patient is forced to stand? What are the ethical and legal implications if you have the patient stand when he really should not? If the patient falls, is the patient at fault for telling you he would try to stand, or are you at fault for allowing him to try?

Consider and develop possible solutions. Do you allow the patient to stand? What are the other alternatives to the upright abdominal radiograph? Does the alternative projection demonstrate the same anatomic structures as that shown with the upright radiograph?

Select and enact the best solution. Keeping in mind that patient safety is always the first and foremost concern, if an alternative to the upright projection exists, should you use it? In the end, the decision you make must provide quality radiographs to aid in the patient's diagnosis but must also be in the best interest of the patient and his safety.

CASE 4: EMERGENCIES. *"Ma'am, are you feeling OK?"* Your patient is in the department receiving a scheduled radiation treatment to her skull for a pituitary tumor. Because of the nature of the treatment and the fact that the patient's head must remain perfectly still throughout the treatment, an immobilizing mask is being used. While the radiation is being administered, the immobilizing mask is placed over the patient's head and secured to the treatment table. While watching the patient on the monitor during the treatment, you notice that she appears pale, and her eyes are watering. By the look on her face, you recognize that she is extremely nauseous, and her head is locked in place flat on the table within the immobilizing mask.

Identify and/or clarify the problem. What is your first course of action? The patient is nauseous and needs assistance quickly, but her head is clamped to the table. What medical concerns do you have at this time?

Objectively examine all aspects of the problem. What might happen if you run immediately into the room? What will happen if the patient actually becomes ill while immobilized with her head flat on the table?

Consider and develop possible solutions. Do you run into the room and immediately remove the patient from the mask and assist her? Do you call for another radiation therapist or perhaps a physician to come and help you? Should anything else be done, or should anyone else be called before assisting the patient? What about the radiation treatment currently being administered? What about the treatment itself? Do you continue if she stabilizes?

Select and enact the best solution. Should the patient's need for immediate assistance be the first priority in this situation? Should the fact that the patient is receiving radiation treatment be considered? Should the radiation oncologist assess the patient and decide if the treatment can be continued, or should the procedure be rescheduled for another day? Do you need to contact the physician to consider whether future treatments are to be performed with some type of antinausea medication? After the decision is made about the treatment, should the physicist be consulted to compensate for the missed dose? The immediate assessment and follow-up attention to the situation by the radiologic science professional is critical in situations such as this.

After completing a radiologic science program, students will have practiced addressing scenarios such as these in the laboratory, classroom, and even clinical setting and will be prepared to handle challenging situations. Providing students with all potential challenges that may arise while working in the field of radiologic sciences is impossible for a radiologic science program. However, providing each student with the tools and information necessary will prepare him or her when faced with this type of situation.

MAINTAINING CRITICAL-THINKING SKILLS

Radiologic science professionals are an integral part of the health care team. Many critical-thinking skills revolve around working cooperatively and effectively with other members of the health care team. These skills may involve decisions related to working within your scope of practice and supporting other health care professionals. Students must learn to work cooperatively and in sync with physicians, physicists, nurses, and other allied health professionals.

The continuing professional development of radiologic science professionals is essential to maintaining and improving their critical-thinking skills. Keeping up with the changing technology and developments in medicine is a professional obligation for those working in the radiologic sciences. Continuing education is a key element to

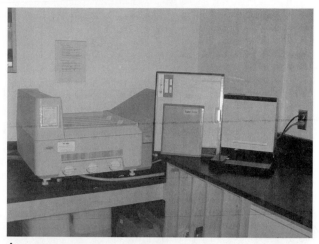

A

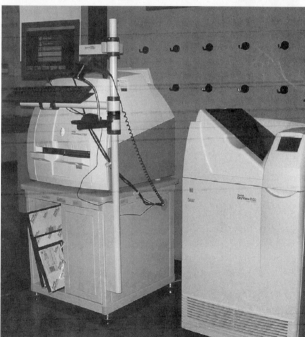

B

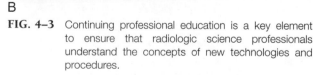

FIG. 4–3 Continuing professional education is a key element to ensure that radiologic science professionals understand the concepts of new technologies and procedures.

ensure application of up-to-date technology that allows the radiologic science professional to practice problem solving and critical thinking that will result in the best patient care (Fig. 4–3). Radiologic science professionals must also support the future of the profession by teaching and mentoring students to be competent future radiologic science professionals.

SUMMARY

Radiologic science professionals are presented with unique and challenging ethical, technical, and patient care situations every day. Critical-thinking and problem-solving skills are essential to provide quality patient care, diagnosis, and treatment in these situations. The student must learn and value the basic knowledge of the profession to develop technical critical-thinking skills for use in future practice. The steps in critical thinking involve identifying and clarifying the problem, objectively examining the problem, considering and developing all possible viable solutions, and selecting and enacting the solution with the best outcome for the patient. Professional and ethical standards, such as cultural sensitivity and communication methods, must be considered when selecting the appropriate solution. The classroom and laboratory serve as a practice field for students to develop critical-thinking skills. The clinical setting allows the student to take classroom and laboratory learning into the real world. Critical-thinking and problem-solving skills may also be used to manage personal concerns and issues. Because the technology associated with the radiologic sciences is ever changing, continued professional development is an integral part of ongoing critical-thinking and problem-solving skills development.

BIBLIOGRAPHY

Bugg N: Teaching critical thinking skills, *Radiol Tech* 68:5, 1997.

Durand KS: *Critical thinking developing skills in radiography,* Philadelphia, 1999, FA Davis.

Greathouse GF, Dowd SB: Using critical thinking to teach empathy, *Radiol Tech* 67:5, 1996.

Jackson M, Ignatavicius DD, Case B: *Conversations in critical thinking and clinical judgment,* Pensacola, Fla, 2004, Pohl Publishing.

Kowalczyk N, Leggett T: Teaching critical-thinking skills through group-based learning, *Radiol Tech* 77:1, 2005.

Pearce CE, Dowd SB: An exercise in critical thinking, *Radiol Tech* 67:6, 1996.

Ruggiero VR: *The art of thinking: a guide to critical and creative thought,* New York, 2004, Pearson Education.

Stadt R, Ruhland S: Critical-thinking abilities of radiologic science students, *Radiol Tech* 67:1, 1995.

Savin-Baden M, Major CH: *Foundations of problem-based learning,* Berkshire, Engl, 2004, Society for Research into Higher Education and Open University Press.

Stone J: The staff therapist's role in clinical education, *Radiat Ther* 11:1, 2002.

Tanenbaum BG et al: Interactive questioning: why ask why? *Radiol Tech* 68:5, 1997.

Introduction to the Clinical Environment

5

Introduction to Clinical Education

Sarah S. Baker, EdD, RT(R), FASRT

Perfect health, like perfect beauty, is a rare thing, and so, it seems, is perfect disease.

Peter Latham
General Remarks on the Practice of Medicine

OBJECTIVES

On completion of this chapter, the student will be able to:

1. Explain the purpose of the clinical education component.

2. Define terms that relate to the clinical education component of the radiography curriculum.

3. Describe the physical and human resources necessary for effective clinical education.

4. Explain the importance of adhering to major clinical education policies.

5. Discuss the methods used in effectively teaching clinical course content.

6. Describe methods of assessment that can be used to measure cognitive, psychomotor, and affective aspects of clinical education.

7. Summarize the clinical education process.

OVERVIEW OF CLINICAL EDUCATION

Planned and structured learning experiences and activities in various clinical settings are necessary for an effective educational program for radiographers. For the student to appreciate fully the actual health care setting and to allow for the observation, assistance, and performance requirements for the completion of diagnostic medical imaging procedures, learning in a clinical setting must occur. This goal is achieved in clinical education settings through clinical affiliations between medical facilities and educational institutions or in hospital-sponsored programs.

General Description of Clinical Education

PURPOSE OF CLINICAL EDUCATION. The process of developing and refining the skills required to become a competent radiographer cannot be completed without hours spent in a setting that provides a variety of medical imaging procedures. Hospitals, clinics, and surgical centers are just a few of the locations that fulfill this need.

According to the *Standards for an Accredited Educational Program in Radiologic Sciences,* developed by the Joint Review Committee on Education in Radiologic Technology (JRCERT), the curriculum is to provide competency-based educational experiences that promote synthesis of theory, use of current technology, competent clinical practice, and professional values. Furthermore, a radiologic science program should provide a well-structured, competency-based clinical curriculum. As part of an educational program, students must demonstrate competency in a variety of clinical activities. Areas of competence may include chest and thorax, musculoskeletal and trauma, cranium, spine and pelvis, abdom-

inal, fluoroscopic studies, surgical and mobile studies, pediatrics, and general patient care competencies. All policies and procedures related to clinical education should be published and provided to students, faculty, and clinical staff.

As of January 1, 2005, to be eligible for participation in the American Registry of Radiologic Technologists radiographic examination, a *minimum* number of clinical competencies must be completed, including 36 mandatory competencies, 15 of 30 elective competencies, and 6 general patient care competencies. Clinical education also may include continuing and technical competencies.

TERMINOLOGY. The **clinical** component of the radiography curriculum includes procedures and activities that occur in the clinical educational settings. Clinical experiences include one-on-one direct patient contact, rather than theoretical, simulated, or laboratory experiences. Interactions occur with inpatients, outpatients, emergency, and specialty patients of all ages.

Informational and instructional activities related to radiography make up the **didactic** portion of the curriculum. These activities occur in settings such as the classroom, laboratory, instructional media viewing area, or learning resource center. The instructional activity should be well planned, with documented goals, objectives, and learning activities provided for the students.

In the early phases of the educational program, additional time is spent in didactic instruction. Students then progress to an increasing amount of time in the clinical setting. The laboratory setting serves as a bridge to connect classroom with clinical activities (Fig. 5–1). Within the didactic and laboratory areas, the theoretical foundation of knowledge is being imparted to students.

Clinical education enables radiography students to transfer the learning from the textbooks, classroom, and laboratory environments to practical learning with real-life situations. The principle of **transfer of learning** is exemplified in the clinical education component of radiography education with the student recalling prior knowledge learned and using this knowledge in performing radiographic procedures to develop both the skills and the confidence to work with a wide variety of patients. Thus prior learning has affected the new learning within the clinical performance.

Most educational researchers agree that learning can be organized into three major categories or domains. The **cognitive** domain includes behaviors requiring various levels of thought: knowledge, understanding, reason, and judgment. The **psychomotor** domain includes behaviors involving physical actions, neuromuscular manipulations, and coordination. The **affective** domain includes behaviors guided by feelings and emotions that are influenced by an individual's interests, attitudes, values, and beliefs.

One element of the major categories or domains of learning is the performance **objective.** An objective is a description of an observable student behavior. Objectives must be concise, measurable, and achievable. They describe what behavior the student is to display, how well the student is to perform the behavior, and under what circumstances the behavior is to be achieved. Closely related to performance objectives is **competency,** the observable, successful achievement of the performance objectives.

The new student's eyes are open to anything and everything that goes on in the hospital or clinic as the clinical education segment of the program begins. This point is the *observation* phase of the educational experience and is extensive during the early portion of the program, tapering off as the new student gains confidence and can effectively integrate the appropriate cognitive, psychomotor, and affective behaviors. Throughout the length of the program, clinical situations will arise that are new to the student. After gaining knowledge of the various procedures in a didactic setting and practicing the performance of the procedures in the laboratory setting, the student is ready to watch and give critical attention to all that is occurring in the clinical setting, noting the role of the various participating health professionals. As radiographers perform various diagnostic procedures, they serve as role models for the new student. The inquisitive student makes mental notes of how the procedure is being accomplished and begins to model or imitate the actions seen, whether correct or incorrect.

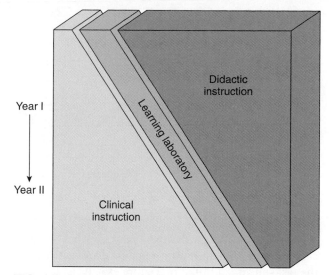

FIG. 5–1 The articulation of didactic, laboratory, and clinical instruction. (From Ford C, ed: Clinical education for the allied health professions, St Louis, 1978, Mosby.)

When the student feels confident, he or she can then proceed to *assistance,* the next phase of the educational program. In this phase, the student begins aiding and supporting the radiographer in the performance of the diagnostic procedure. The student is now gaining hands-on experience, literally placing a hand on the patient to assist in movement to the examining table or helping the patient assume a specific position for the diagnostic procedure. If numerous manipulations of the patient are required, the student should feel free to discuss with the radiographer a desire to become more actively involved in the performance of the procedure. The radiographer will then be able to determine the appropriate extent of student assistance based on an assessment of the patient's needs.

After assisting the radiographer with various aspects of the diagnostic procedure, the student eventually feels confident and is ready to proceed toward the *performance* of the entire procedure without assistance from the radiographer, clinical instructor, or clinical supervisor. During the performance of the procedure, the student should accurately demonstrate all tasks included in the entire procedure at the level of skill determined by the faculty.

In the event that the student does not have the opportunity to perform a required procedure on an actual patient, program policy may permit the procedure to be performed as a *simulation.* This provision may be made for infrequent or limited volume procedures. In this

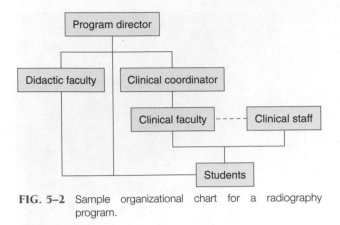

FIG. 5–2 Sample organizational chart for a radiography program.

situation, the student must accurately demonstrate all of the tasks included in the procedure exactly as described previously. The difference is that the procedure is not performed on an actual patient. A phantom patient or a live substitute patient takes the place of the actual patient. When a live substitute patient is involved in the simulation, *no radiographic exposure is to be made under any circumstances.*

The standards of quality for educational programs for radiographers are provided in the *Standards for an Accredited Educational Program in Radiologic Sciences,* often referred to as the *Standards,* adopted in 1996 and revised in 2001 by the JRCERT. The *Standards* document is used for program development and evaluation and includes criteria for program accountability.

The *Standards* document for radiography programs provides for the appropriate supervision of students. Until a student achieves and documents competency in any given procedure, all clinical assignments are carried out under the direct supervision of a qualified practitioner (radiographer). The parameters of *direct supervision* require that the qualified practitioner (1) review the request for examination in relation to the student's achievement, (2) evaluate the condition of the patient in relation to the student's knowledge, (3) be present during the examination, and (4) review and approve the procedure.

Indirect supervision means that the qualified practitioner reviews, evaluates, and approves the procedure as for direct supervision and is immediately available to assist students regardless of the level of student achievement. *Immediately available* is interpreted as the physical presence of a qualified practitioner adjacent to the room or location where a radiographic procedure is being performed. This availability applies to all areas where ionizing radiation equipment is in use.

In support of professional responsibility for the provision of quality patient care and radiation protection, unsatisfactory radiographs are repeated only in the presence of a qualified practitioner, regardless of the student's level of competency.

Resources

PHYSICAL FACILITIES. Imaging facilities must be of a sufficient number to accommodate the students enrolled in the radiography program and to provide a variety and volume of procedures for each student's clinical performance continuum and competency achievement. A variety of equipment should be available to produce diagnostic images during trauma or emergency, mobile, surgical, abdominal, gastrointestinal, genitourinary, musculoskeletal, cranium, and spine and pelvis procedures. Equipment used for computed tomography, ultrasonography, neuroradiology, cardiovascular, and interventional procedures should also be available for the educational opportunities they present.

PROGRAM OFFICIALS. A large number of individuals work together to assist the student in understanding and accomplishing the goals and objectives of the program. Included are the program director, clinical coordinator (in many programs), clinical instructor, didactic faculty, and clinical staff. Fig. 5–2 illustrates a sample organizational chart for a radiography program.

The *program director* works full time in organizing, administering, and assessing the radiography program. This person is responsible for the didactic and clinical effectiveness of the program. In a JRCERT-accredited program, program directors must hold American Registry of Radiologic Technologists certification or equivalent with registration qualifications in the pertinent discipline, have a master's degree or higher, and be proficient in such areas as curriculum design, program administration, program evaluation, instruction, and counseling.

If a program uses six or more clinical education facilities or has more than 30 students enrolled in the clinical component, a *clinical coordinator* must be among the program's officials. This person works closely with the program director in ensuring program effectiveness through a regular schedule of coordination, instruction, and evaluation. As is the case with the program director, the clinical coordinator must also possess appropriate professional credentials.

The *clinical instructor* has the unique opportunity to influence the professional development of the radiography student in a direct manner. Of all the program's officials, this person works intimately with the student in one-on-one observation, instruction, and evaluation. The clinical instructor should also possess the appropriate professional credentials.

These program officials must possess current knowledge regarding medical imaging procedures, as well as competence in instructional and evaluation techniques. Many programs are supported by a large number of individuals responsible for teaching general education, professional, and technical courses within the radiography curriculum. These *didactic faculty members* are individually qualified to teach the appropriate course work. They work closely with the program director to ensure coordination and integration of course content with the program's goals and objectives.

Members of the *clinical staff* assist the clinical instructor in one-on-one observation and instruction of radiography students. In addition to meeting patient needs, these dedicated professionals are committed to sharing their knowledge and expertise with student radiographers, their future colleagues.

MAJOR CLINICAL EDUCATION POLICIES

All participants in clinical education—faculty, clinical staff, and students—need a complete and accurate understanding of the process by which students are instructed and evaluated in the clinical setting. A clinical education handbook, student handbook, or clinical education guide is vital in providing consistent written information for all parties. The resultant benefit is improved integration of the didactic and clinical aspects of the radiography curriculum. Program faculty members develop timely policies, procedures, rules, regulations, and guidelines that are applicable to clinical education. Discussing briefly some examples of these policies is appropriate.

Supervision

An appropriately credentialed clinical staff member must monitor the activities of student radiographers. Until a student demonstrates competence in a given diagnostic procedure, all of the student's clinical assignments must be directly supervised (Fig. 5–3). The parameters for direct and indirect supervision were described earlier in this chapter. These strict requirements serve to protect the student from being used inappropriately to replace paid staff and to protect the patient from overexposure. At no time should a student radiographer be unsupervised, either directly or indirectly. Until the student completes all the program's published academic and clinical

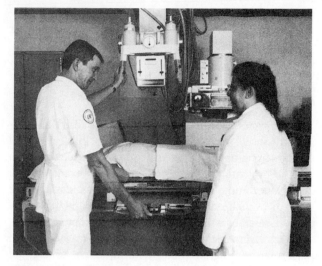

FIG. 5–3 Students need direct supervision by a qualified radiographer before demonstrating competency for a procedure.

requirements, supervision by a qualified practitioner must occur.

Performance of Actual Examinations

In a competency-based clinical education and evaluation system, the student proceeds at his or her own pace. The timing and length of the observation and assistance phases of clinical education are variable. Because most radiography programs must work within the framework of an academic grading period (semester or quarter), policies may exist that specify a suggested pace for procedure performance and proficiency.

Simulations

A simulated clinical procedure is designed to recreate an actual, real-life diagnostic examination in which no x-ray exposure is made. Simulations may involve mannequins, artificial body parts, or dramatizations (using live simulated patients). Program policy may stipulate what specific procedures may be simulated and when. Only a minor portion of the total number of clinical evaluations should be completed as simulations.

Avoidance of Using Students to Replace Staff

Students in a JRCERT-accredited program for radiographers should never substitute for, or assume the responsibilities of, regular staff. After demonstrating competency, students may perform procedures under direct or indirect supervision as determined by a qualified practitioner.

Assessments

Written examinations (paper-and-pencil tests) are frequently used to evaluate cognitive skills. Practical examinations using a checklist or rating scale are often used to evaluate psychomotor skills. Oral examinations, checklists, rating scales, or direct observations may be used to evaluate affective behaviors. A combination of these assessments is commonly used to determine the student's overall level of clinical skill, competency, and performance. Program policy determines the timing and weight of all clinical assessments, as well as the specific method by which clinical grades are achieved and documented.

Radiation Protection Practices

A radiation-monitoring device is a part of the student radiographer's uniform. Program policy may specify when and where this monitor is to be worn and the procedure to be followed if a monitor is lost or needs to be replaced. Program policy regarding the holding of patients during radiographic procedures should also be specifically documented.

Professional Ethics

The code of ethics of the American Registry of Radiologic Technologists (Appendix D) reflects the rules and standards that govern the conduct of professional technologists. Student radiographers should strive to understand, appreciate, and value these standards. To this end, program faculty members outline the standards of ethics required for all radiography students. Failure to abide by the published standards may result in disciplinary procedures.

Practice Standards

Radiography practice standards from the American Society of Radiologic Technologists (Appendix A) have been developed by the profession for judging the quality of practice, service, and education. These *Standards* define the practice of radiography for professional technologists and establish general criteria to determine compliance with the *Standards*. Similar to the code of ethics,

student radiographers should become knowledgeable of these *Standards*.

Health Insurance Portability and Accountability Act

In 1996, federal legislation was passed to improve the efficiency and effectiveness of the health care system by mandating confidentiality of health information. Among the components that affect health information are privacy, security, and the establishment of standards and requirements for the electronic transmission of certain health information. With patients being an integral part of the clinical educational setting, student radiographers must become knowledgeable of the Health Insurance Portability and Accountability Act (HIPAA) and follow confidentiality mandates. Failure to abide by HIPAA mandates may result in disciplinary procedures.

Health Professional Appearance

The program policy regarding professional appearance outlines the acceptable uniform for the student radiographer. Identifying name badges, patches, and radiation-monitoring devices are also a part of the professional uniform. Extremes are to be avoided when jewelry, hairstyles, and cosmetics are involved. Specific guidelines and program requirements are available in the published student handbook.

Attendance

The program provides clinical schedules that indicate the actual dates and times for all clinical experiences. Students are informed of schedule variations such as breaks, vacation periods, and holidays. In the event that a student is unable to participate in a scheduled clinical activity because of personal business or illness, program procedure must be followed in notifying the designated program faculty or staff. Absenteeism and tardiness are often documented and may result in disciplinary procedures.

Pregnancy

A female student is officially considered to be pregnant when she voluntarily and in writing informs program officials of her pregnancy. Informing program officials of her pregnancy is her option.

Because of the potential radiation hazard to the fetus, particularly during the first trimester, pregnancy may be reported to the program director or radiation safety officer in accordance with program policy or government recommendations. It is recommended that a pregnant student discuss her situation with her physician. The program's officials will review the program's policy with the student.

Disciplinary Procedures

Students in radiography programs are required to abide by the policies and procedures of the sponsoring institution, the program, and the clinical education centers. Students are also expected to abide by the code of ethics of the American Registry of Radiologic Technologists and HIPAA. Failure to adhere to these requirements may result in disciplinary procedures or academic sanctions. The specific steps in the disciplinary procedure are detailed in the student clinical education handbook and may include oral and written warnings. A repetition of infractions may result in suspension or dismissal from the program. Serious infractions, including, but not limited to, a threat to patient safety, gross insubordination, the disclosure of confidential information, falsification of records, cheating, theft, willful damage of property, and substance abuse, may result in immediate dismissal from the program. In all cases, students have the right of due process and the right to appeal all unfavorable evaluations, disciplinary actions, suspensions, and dismissals.

PROGRESSIVE CLINICAL DEVELOPMENT

Student clinical progress occurs when goals and objectives are clearly outlined, didactic information is integrated with the appropriate clinical experiences, and timely and objective evaluations occur. The progressive clinical development allows for the translation of theory into practice.

Process

The highlights of each clinical course are provided through a review of the course description. The description often includes the department code, course number, course title, number of credits, and the mandatory co-requisite or prerequisite courses. In two or three sentences, a brief glimpse of the course is provided. The clinical courses should be sequential, with each clinical course building on the previous ones.

The program faculty members determine the content of each clinical course. This information is then linked to the didactic material presented and to the clinical expe-

riences available to the student during a given period. The course outline or syllabus includes information such as course title and instructor, time and location of the clinical education course, a brief overview of the course, clinical competencies, specific goals and objectives, the schedule of clinical rotations and activities, grading procedures, and references. This document is distributed to all clinical instructors and students so that all parties are thoroughly familiar with the clinical course requirements and expectations.

Performance objectives are descriptions of observable student behaviors. These objectives are required for all clinical courses in the radiography curriculum. Objectives are provided for (1) the student's scheduled orientation experiences, (2) routine radiographic procedures, and (3) imaging specialties, such as pediatric, surgical, and mobile procedures. Objectives also should be provided for scheduled observations in specialty areas such as computed tomography, ultrasonography, radiation therapy, nuclear medicine, magnetic resonance imaging, and cardiovascular interventional imaging.

The first clinical education course may be structured to orient the new student to the radiology department. Students are often given assignments to observe, assist, and perform specific activities as indicated by the objectives for this course. Areas of assignment may include the film-processing area, the radiology office, patient transport areas, and the various fluoroscopic and radiographic rooms.

Subsequent clinical courses may emphasize the performance of specific radiographic procedures. Students will be required to evaluate the request for the given radiographic procedure, prepare the radiographic room before the patient's arrival, provide complete and accurate patient instructions, properly position and care for the patient, set the appropriate exposure factors, provide protection from unnecessary radiation, evaluate the processed radiographic image, and appropriately discharge the patient. The student's ability to handle the radiographic procedure completely should gradually improve as the weeks and months proceed. Eventually, the student should be able to pick up speed in doing procedures and be able to organize the activities to be completed in an assigned radiographic area.

Several instructional methods are effective in teaching clinical course content. First, the clinical instructor may use *demonstrations* to assist the students in seeing the proper way to perform the various aspects of the radiographic examination (Fig. 5–4). These demonstrations may occur in a laboratory or practice setting, as well as with actual patients. The student may be asked to

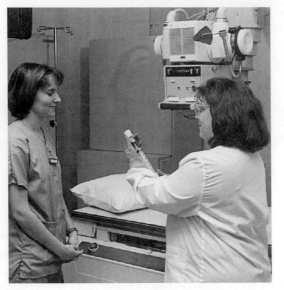

FIG. 5–4 A clinical instructor demonstrates filling a syringe.

perform a *return demonstration,* in imitation of the instructor's actions and manner. At a later time, a discussion of the performance events should occur. This review provides the instructor and the student an opportunity to critique the performance and to make mental and written notes of its strengths and weaknesses. Instructors often use additional methods to enhance the learning process and to facilitate learning.

Assessments

The clinical instructor may determine that some aspects of the radiographic procedure involve assessment of the student's knowledge or comprehension or perhaps the ability to apply, analyze, synthesize, or evaluate. These areas are the levels within the cognitive domain of learning. Measurement of the learning that has occurred within these categories usually involves an objective test of some kind: multiple choice, matching, or true-false.

Numerous cognitive, psychomotor, and affective behaviors are involved in performing a radiographic procedure, including the following:

- Assessing the requisition
- Preparing the radiography room for performance of the procedure
- Caring for the needs of the patient
- Performing the radiographic procedure
- Providing radiation protection for the patient
- Manipulating the exposure factors

- Evaluating the radiographic image
- Manipulating specialized equipment

These behaviors are assessed by the instructor's use of direct, objective observation and are documented through the use of rating scales, checklists, critical incident forms, and anecdotal notes.

Affective behaviors involving attitudes and values are also among those considered by instructors in assessing the progress of the student's clinical development. Instructors may wish to assess the student's ability to (1) communicate effectively with staff and patients, (2) perceive patient needs, (3) display maturity and confidence, (4) follow through with clinical responsibilities in a reliable and conscientious manner, and (5) display an interest in professional literature and organizations. As with the psychomotor area, these behaviors require the use of direct objective observations, documented through the use of rating scales, checklists, critical incident forms, and anecdotal notes.

SUMMARY

Clinical education is a necessary component of the radiography curriculum. It provides a structured and ordered mechanism for the student to develop and refine important skills needed in a variety of one-on-one, direct interactions with the patient. A correlation and transfer from the didactic and clinical portions of the curriculum must occur for clinical education to be successful. This correlation includes a successful weaving and integration of cognitive, psychomotor, and affective behaviors during observation, assistance, and performance of actual radiographic procedures.

The standards of quality for the educational program, described in a document called the *Standards for an Accredited Educational Program in Radiologic Sciences,* developed by the JRCERT-appropriate supervision for students in radiography programs, is essential. Direct supervision is required until a student achieves and documents competency for a given procedure. Indirect supervision is necessary once competency has been achieved and documented. At either level of supervision, unsatisfactory radiographs should be repeated only in the presence of a qualified practitioner.

In an effort to ensure a complete and accurate understanding of the clinical education process, a large number of major clinical education policies and procedures are developed and implemented by the program officials. These policies and procedures usually include those regarding appropriate supervision, procedure performance, assessments, radiation protection practices, professional ethics, HIPAA, attendance, pregnancy, and disciplinary procedures.

Progressive clinical development occurs when valid and achievable goals and objectives are clearly outlined, correlated with corresponding cognitive information, integrated with the appropriate clinical experiences, and objectively and promptly assessed. Important judgments are then made regarding a variety of cognitive, psychomotor, and affective behaviors. These areas are vital in assisting the student to ultimately assume the role of professional radiographer.

BIBLIOGRAPHY

American Registry of Radiologic Technologists: *Radiography didactic and clinical competency requirements,* St Paul, Minn, 2005, The Registry.

American Society of Radiologic Technologists: *Practice standards for medical imaging and radiation therapy,* Albuquerque, NM, 2000, The Society.

American Society of Radiologic Technologists: *Radiography curriculum,* Albuquerque, NM, 2002, The Society.

Ford CW: *Clinical education for the allied health professions,* St Louis, 1978, Mosby.

Ford CW, Morgan MK: *Teaching in the health professions,* St Louis, 1976, Mosby.

Indiana University–Purdue University Indianapolis, Radiologic Technology Program: *Radiography program clinical handbook,* Indianapolis, Ind, 2005, IUPUI.

Joint Review Committee on Education in Radiologic Technology: *Standards for an accredited educational program in radiologic sciences,* Chicago, 2001, The Committee.

Macaulay C, Cree V: Transfer of learning: concept and process, *Soc Work Educ* 18:183, 1999.

Mann KV: Thinking about learning: implications for principle-based professional education, *J Contin Educ Health Prof* 22:69, 2002.

McTernan EJ, Hawkins RO: *Educating personnel for the allied health professions and services,* St Louis, 1972, Mosby.

O'Connor AB: *Clinical instruction and evaluation: a teaching resource,* Danbury, Conn, 2001, Jones and Bartlett Publishers and National League for Nursing.

Roberts GH, Carson J: The roles instructors play in clinical education, *Radiol Tech* 63:28, 1991.

6

Radiology Administration

Larry A. Genzink, MBA, RT(R)

We can show that the number of lives that have been saved by x-rays since their discovery by Roentgen is as great as the number of lives that have been taken in all of the wars that have been fought since that time.

A. H. Compton
Nobel laureate in physics and discoverer of the Compton effect, 1927

OBJECTIVES

On completion of this chapter, the student will be able to:

1. Provide an overview of the administration of a hospital radiology department and the structure of hospital organization.

2. Describe how the radiology department fits into the hospital world.

3. Appreciate the role of the radiology administrator.

4. Define the organization of a hospital and a hospital department of radiology or medical imaging.

5. Explain the functions of management, including planning, organizing, staffing, directing, controlling, and coordinating.

Objectives—Cont'd

6. Discuss the transition from traditional functions of management to the requirements of managing radiology in the current health care environment.

7. Describe regulating agencies that affect radiology.

8. Discuss the characteristics of desirable applicants for employment in radiology imaging.

Glossary

Adverse Drug Events (ADEs): an injury, large or small, caused by the use (including nonuse) of a drug; can be as harmless as a drug rash or as serious as death from an overdose; two types of ADEs: those caused by errors and those that occur despite proper use

Board of Directors *or* Governing Board: group of people authorized by law to conduct, maintain, and operate a hospital for the benefit of the public and whose legal and moral responsibility for policies and operations of the hospital are not for personal benefit of the members

Certificate of Need (CON): certificate approved by a local (state) review board permitting hospitals to construct new or additional facilities, open new services, or make large purchases—a condition required for reimbursement by Medicare

Chief Executive Officer (CEO): person appointed by the board of directors who has full accountability for the entire hospital

Clinical Support Services: services to provide the components of patient care that collectively support the physician's plan for diagnoses and treatments

Continuous Quality Improvement (CQI): system of development in the workplace for daily improving performance at every level in every operational process by focusing on meeting or exceeding customer expectations

Department: unit of the hospital with specific functions or specialized skills such as housekeeping, surgery, radiology, or accounting

Department Chair: physician who represents a department or service to the formal organization of the medical staff and who has voting privileges on the executive committee of the medical staff

Human Resources Department (formerly Personnel): department of the hospital responsible for recruiting, selecting, supporting, and compensating employees; maintaining sklls, quality, and motivation; collective bargaining; and occupational health and safety

Joint Commission on Accreditation of Healthcare Organizations (JCAHO): national organization of hospitals and other health care providers; offers its members inspection and accreditation of the quality of operations

Medical Director: physician who has responsibility for the operation and quality of a hospital department or service; also responsible for policies and procedures and day-to-day operations of medical director's department

Medical Error: an unintended act, either of omission of commission, or one that does not achieve its intended outcome

Medical Staff: formal organization of physicians authorized to admit and attend to patients within a hospital; have authorized privileges, bylaws, elected officers, and various committees and activities (see medical director, department chair, and service chief)

Mission Statement: statement of an organization that summarizes its intent to provide service in terms of the services it offers, the intended recipients of services, and a description of the level of cost

Occupational Safety and Health Administration (OSHA): federal agency that enforces standards for safety in the workplace; conducts inspections and directs levy of fines for noncompliance with rules

Radiology Department: organization of a hospital or medical clinic that provides imaging through medical technologies such as x-ray, general diagnostics, nuclear medicine, and ultrasonography; sometimes known as medical imaging

Service Chief: physician head of a hospital service

Third-Party Payors: insurance companies, Medicare, Medicaid, and other commercial companies who are the payors of medical expenses for the patient

Total Quality Management (TQM): management of quality in the workplace from a perspective of total involvement of every employee

HOSPITAL ENVIRONMENT

Hospital Organization

Hospitals are a central part of one of the nation's largest industries, the health care industry, offering a broad range of services provided by increasingly expensive personnel, equipment, and technology. The complexity of a hospital can be compared with that of a town or city in which people work together in mutually supportive functions. For example, the building, or plan, of a hospital provides space, electricity, plumbing, and roadways that require upkeep and maintenance. A hospital employs persons in 20 or more different professions and an equal number of trades; these people require physical supports such as food service and payroll services. Supplies are needed, which are purchased from outside the hospital or produced from within the organization. Similar to a city, a hospital requires policies, procedures, administrative staff, rules, regulations, traffic laws, and plans.

The hospital-city analogy can be carried further to compare the governance and organization of a hospital with that of a city. Citizens are central to a city, and patients are central to a hospital. To ensure that its citizens are protected and to provide services necessary to living and conducting business, a city is organized through its governmental body. In a similar fashion, the hospital is organized through a board of directors and administrative staff to carry out the hospital's mission.

Hospitals have a direct relationship to the community in which they reside, comparable to the relationship a city has with the county or state where it is located. This relationship should be mutually supportive and beneficial. Single hospitals have merged into multihospital groups, similar to the way nearby cities merge activities first and later combine governance.

The medical staff and employees of a hospital find a correlate with the city's skilled and trained persons who provide services to other citizens. Volunteers in both scenarios enable many tasks to be performed at reasonable cost to the central customers. In the hospital setting, volunteers and the auxiliary organizations provide many hours of service, compassion, and assistance in an embodiment of the spirit of cooperation central to the best in human living.

The **mission statement,** or charter, is the driving and guiding force that outlines the organization's reason for existence and defines what should be done and how; but the comparison between a hospital and a city stops here. Not every citizen of a city is charged with carrying out the city's mission or charter or fully understands its meaning. Because every function of a hospital should be focused on its mission, all of its members should be familiar with the mission. The mission statement summarizes the hospital's intent to provide service in terms of the intended recipients of service, the type of care or services, and the level of quality and cost expected. If the citizens of a city can be compared with a hospital's patients, the city's elected officials, magistrates, and other civil servants might be compared with the various hospital employees who are organized to provide services.

The organizational chart of a hospital demonstrates how employees carry out the functions within the institution in an organized and logical manner. Governance of a hospital begins with the **board of directors or governing board,** which is authorized by law to operate a hospital. The board employs a **chief executive officer (CEO)** or president and defines how the operation of the hospital is maintained and conducted. The primary restriction imposed on individual board members is that their governance may not afford them personal benefit. The CEO or president then sets in place a formal reporting structure for the organization and interacts with the medical staff to ensure coordination and quality of patient care and services.

In the organizational chart in Fig. 6–1, the line of communication between the medical staff and CEO is a broken line, indicating communication but not control. The **medical staff** is the formal organization of physicians within a hospital with authorized privileges, bylaws, elected officers, committees, and organized activities. Radiologists fit into the formal organization of the medical staff; they either perform on a contractual basis to provide and supervise specific services, or they serve as paid employees of the institution.

A hospital is composed of many **departments** and services organized to provide care and **clinical support services** to its patients and clients. Most of a hospital's departments are interrelated, and some of these departments and services are directly dependent on each other. For example, all patient care services depend on the admissions department for information regarding the patients being served. Nursing, the medical staff, billing offices, and other departments rely on the medical records department for retaining records of patients and maintaining the patients' histories in charts.

The **human resources department** (formerly personnel department) is responsible for the recruitment, retention, and compensation of all employees who work in the hospital. Business offices handle the financial functions of the hospital, including billing patients and insurance companies, paying for equipment and supplies, and

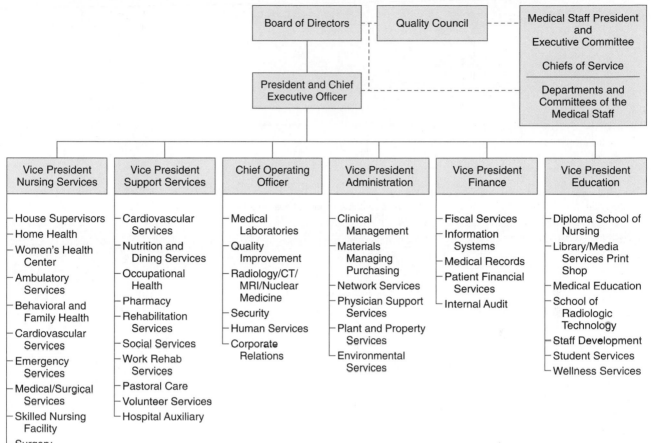

FIG. 6–1 Organizational chart.

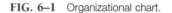

maintaining strict accounting practices. Besides nursing, medical laboratories, and radiology, other departments that support patients include pastoral care, pharmacy, cardiopulmonary services, rehabilitation services (e.g., physical therapy), nutritional services, social services, and medical clinics.

The radiology or medical imaging department plays an important role in the care of the patient. The quality of care provided to the patient by radiology (or any department) is directly related to the quality of the coordination and cooperation that exists between the department and all the other departments and services that make up the organization.

Organizational Transition in the 1990s

Social and economic conditions of the late 1980s and early 1990s have caused vast changes in health care orga-

nizations, forcing them to alter their organizational structures. Economic hardships and total quality management both have been influential in eliminating middle-management positions in many hospitals and radiology departments. These changes have continued throughout the 1990s and into the 2000s as changes in reimbursement escalated cost reductions and downsizing. Figs. 6–2 and 6-3 demonstrate the vertical and horizontal organizational structures that represent changes occurring in health care, as well as other industries, in the 1990s. The vertical structure depicted in Fig. 6–2 demonstrates a top-heavy organization, with additional layers of senior administration staff. Following reorganization, many hospital organizations resemble the flat horizontal structure in the example in Fig. 6–3. An example of continued downsizing can be seen if the positions in Fig. 6–1 are altered to eliminate the chief operating officer and vice president of administration. In Fig. 6–3, the radiology

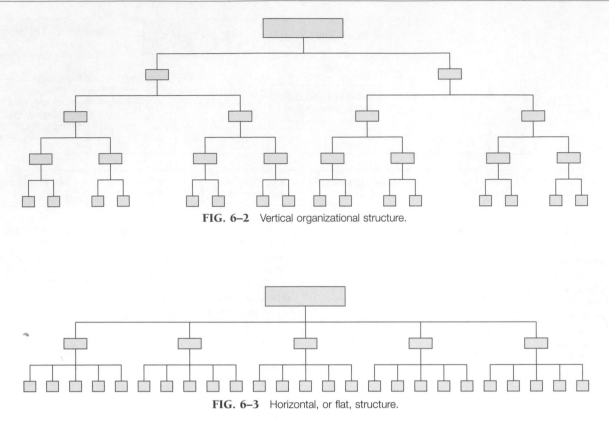

FIG. 6–2 Vertical organizational structure.

FIG. 6–3 Horizontal, or flat, structure.

administrator might be responsible for departments outside imaging, such as the laboratory or cardiopulmonary services. Similarly, for a business manager, laboratory manager, or other administrator to inherit responsibility for a radiology department is no longer uncommon.

The matrix structure pictured in Fig. 6–4 has been useful in some hospitals, as well as other industries, attempting to manage strategically the products and services that cross departmental boundaries. An example of matrix management structure that might affect radiology departments is when a manager of outpatient services or women's services interacts with many department managers in the hospital to ensure that maximum quality of care and efficiency are maintained for all patients who enter the hospital for that service.

The women's services manager would likely consult with the radiology manager about gynecologic and obstetric ultrasonography and mammography. The outpatient services manager would consult with the radiology manager on patient waiting time and the flow of patients from one department to the next (e.g., emergency department, electrocardiography, laboratory,

radiology); other managers would consult in a similar manner.

Radiology Organization

Similar to the organization of a hospital, the formal structure of a **radiology department** is a subset of the larger organization. The radiology department has the same focus on the hospital mission to serve patients and has needs similar to those of the larger organization—personnel, information, supplies, equipment, space, electricity, plumbing, upkeep, and maintenance.

SUBDEPARTMENTS OF RADIOLOGY. Larger radiology departments are often divided into subdepartments or sections such as radiography, ultrasound, nuclear medicine, positron emission tomography (PET) and computer tomography (CT), vascular ultrasound, interventional radiology, and radiation therapy and oncology (Fig. 6–5). Depending on the size of the facility, each of the subdepartments may be organized as a department within itself, with separate budgeting, reporting structure, and staffing. Examples of this structure include nuclear

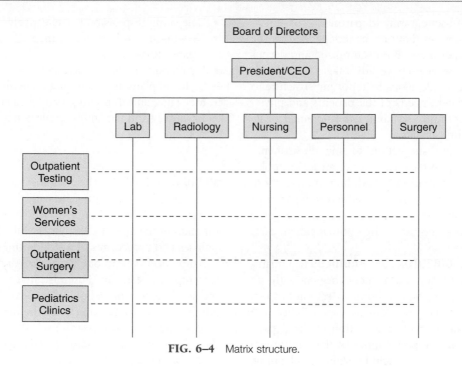

FIG. 6–4 Matrix structure.

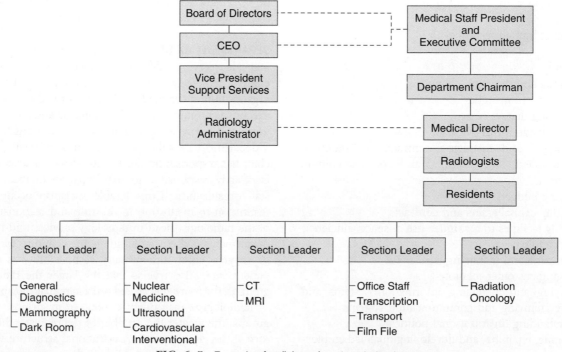

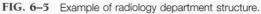

FIG. 6–5 Example of radiology department structure.

medicine and ultrasonography departments or emergency radiologic services that may be independent of the main radiology department. Both centralized and decentralized radiology services have advantages and disadvantages. Each facility develops its reporting structure to best meet the apparent needs of the patients and physicians while attempting to maximize the potential of its managers and technical staff.

Another important subsection to any department's operations is the support services area or areas. Examples of these areas are registration, scheduling, transcription, and escort services. To operate any radiology department properly, these subsections must also be carefully managed and focused on providing optimal patient care.

ADMINISTRATIVE DIRECTOR OF RADIOLOGY. Organization of the radiology department begins with an administrative director, who reports to senior hospital administration and who has direct responsibility and authority for operation and organization of the department. Key traditional responsibilities of the administrative director of radiology include staffing, planning, educating, supervising, organizing, coordinating, communicating, maintaining safety, and minimizing hazards in the workplace.

The many changes facing the health care industry of the 1990s have brought to all administrators and specifically those in radiology new challenges that require new skills and responsibilities, including the following:

- Managing limited resources
- Leading
- Coaching
- Managing and directing change
- Analyzing opportunities
- Developing market plans
- Analyzing administrative data
- Negotiating and managing contracts for purchase of equipment and supplies and for maintaining equipment
- Justifying budgets
- Managing capital assets and contracts
- Planning facilities to maximize use of space, efficiency, and technology
- Recognizing and managing legal risks
- Managing customer relations
- Specifying and managing information systems and picture archiving and communication systems
- Understanding organizational politics
- Recruiting, retaining, and developing qualified employees in the face of shortages of radiology professionals

- Delegating responsibilities effectively
- Networking other departments and professional organizations
- Maintaining technical proficiency
- Strategic planning, including technology assessment
- Managing and improving patient safety
- Effectively implementing project management methodology

MEDICAL DIRECTOR. The radiology administrator has a responsibility to communicate with the medical director, department chairman, and service chief to ensure coordination of medical staff activities with the activities and policies and procedures of the department. Considerable variation occurs from one hospital to another in the relationship between the administrative director and the medical director of radiology. In some institutions, the administrator reports directly to the medical director; in others, the medical director has little responsibility for day-to-day operations, staffing, and organization. In most cases, the **medical director** has responsibility for overseeing the quality of patient care, approving policies and procedures, and recommending improvements to quality and safety of care, equipment purchases, and technology acquisition. According to the **Joint Commission on Accreditation of Healthcare Organizations (JCAHO),** the medical director is responsible for all quality-improvement activities, although he or she may delegate responsibilities to the administrative director.

DEPARTMENT CHAIR. The medical director of radiology may also serve as department chair. The **department chair** of radiology is the department's link to the formal organization of the medical staff. He or she serves on the executive committee and other standing and ad hoc committees. Whereas a medical director has responsibility for a department or subdepartment, in some facilities, the chair has responsibility for the full range of services and is directly responsible for participation in the medical staff organization. Considerable variation occurs from institution to institution in the title and responsibilities of the radiologist head in radiology services and its subdepartments. Whether the title is medical director, chair, or **service chief,** the primary responsibility is quality patient care. Also true is that the larger the radiologist group is, the more specialized is the care that they provide.

Radiologists may practice alone or in groups. Within groups, the greater the number of radiologists, the more formal the group's own organizational structure will be. Partnerships may be established that may or may not include all the radiologists working together by agreement. When radiologists first become part of a practicing group of radiologists, they may work as employees or junior partners before becoming full partners. The function of the group's organization is to run the business of the group, which includes billing patients for services, managing and paying employees, managing group investments and benefits plans, and serving as a mechanism for decision making. Improving the quality and safety of patient care may also be functions of the group's management processes.

OTHER HEALTH CARE SETTINGS

In recent decades, the provision of radiology services has changed from primarily hospital based to include many other settings. Among the newer settings are clinics, physicians' offices, freestanding imaging centers, manufacturing plants, research centers, outpatient surgical centers, mobile imaging centers, veterinary medicine, and teleradiology services.

Clinics

Imaging in clinics includes a wide range of modalities, from radiography for orthopedic services to all modalities for major outpatient health care settings. Technologists may perform a variety of procedures and other functions or, in larger clinics, may specialize in specific procedures. Clinics may be owned or operated by physicians or by university medical centers, hospitals, health systems, or for-profit organizations.

Physician Offices

Physician offices may often be similar to clinics, but they are organized as the home base of a single physician or a group of physicians. The radiologic services offered vary from basic x-ray procedures to a full range of services, including ultrasonography, CT, nuclear medicine, magnetic resonance imaging (MRI), mammography, bone densitometry, and vascular or interventional procedures.

Imaging Centers

Imaging centers may be owned by hospitals, medical centers, radiologists, other physicians, or nonmedical investors or corporations. They may be free standing or associated with a clinic, physician office, or other medical center. The difference between a clinic and an imaging center is primarily that a clinic provides patient care by nonradiologist physicians as its primary function. The imaging center's primary function is diagnostic imaging; however, some imaging centers provide basic laboratory tests, electrocardiographic examinations, and other diagnostic testing in addition to imaging procedures.

In the early 2000s the rapid growth and variation in clinics, offices, and imaging centers have blurred these previously described definitions. The student should understand the breadth of services offered in local, nonhospital facilities.

Mobile Imaging

The 1980s saw the development of a large array of mobile imaging modalities. Mobile services provide increased access to care in remote areas and, in the case of high-priced technologies such as mammography, MRI, and PET, allow facilities to share the expense of providing access. Although the same basic skills are required of technologists and sonographers in these settings, new challenges are presented in the constant travel and interaction with medical facilities with diverse expectations and personalities. In addition, because of the remote nature of their services, patient care staff members are required to provide an increased level of independent judgment. Mobile services are also used to develop sites or regions until volume can be established to support fixed site replacement services.

Emergency Care Centers

In the 1980s a variety of freestanding emergency or urgent care centers sprang up in the United States to provide quick access in emergency situations. Shopping centers were among the many locations in which these centers were developed. Although many did not survive, some centers remain and meet important needs in their locations. Most of these centers provide primary general diagnostic radiographic procedures.

Outpatient Surgical Centers

During the 1990s, managed care and other forces influencing reduced costs in health care stimulated movement toward reduced inpatient hospital care and increased outpatient services. Surgical procedures are increasingly performed outside the traditional hospital setting. Radiology services in surgery centers represent yet another opportunity for technologists who are willing and ready to change.

Industry and Research

Less well-known settings in health care for radiology services, primarily x-ray, are those in industry and research. In recent years, health care services entered industry to protect the health of workers and lower the cost of health care. Some workplaces have their own clinics to monitor and safeguard the health of the workers. Employers are also seeking to reduce the cost of their employees' health care by negotiating lower costs with preferred hospitals, clinics, and physicians. Other industrial settings include the use of CT, x-ray, or ultrasound to examine the interiors of manufactured or used parts such as munitions or aircraft parts. Museums and archeologic facilities also use imaging to examine historical artifacts such as mummies removed from grave sites.

MANAGEMENT FUNCTIONS

The primary functions of management include *planning, organizing, staffing, directing, controlling,* and *coordinating.* In the course of performing these functions, the radiology administrator communicates with a wide range of clients, customers, employees, service providers, manufacturers, other departments, senior administration, and medical staff, as well as the community at large. As organizational transitions occur, the skills of communication take on a far greater significance. In the past, an administrator of any department or service could operate independently while focusing primarily on his or her own department. In the 2000s, new skills of communication were required to improve quality, enhance coordination, and lower the costs of doing business.

Similarly, the functions of management are evolving from the traditional roles of directing and controlling employees to leading, coaching, and supporting employees. The influence for this change comes from the movement toward **continuous quality improvement (CQI), total quality management (TQM),** or process improvement.

The concept of quality improvement moved from industry to health care in the 1980s. The impetus was derived from both the need to reduce the costs of providing health care and the rising expectations of patients, physicians, and **third-party payors.** When an institution focuses on quality or safety process improvement, it undergoes a cultural revolution, evolving over several years into a customer-focused organization. Employees are organized into work teams and trained to evaluate their work processes to reduce errors or adverse medical events and simplify work. *Doing the right things right the first time* and *meeting and exceeding the customer's expectations* become facility-wide objectives under the quality or patient safety mission. The cost savings resulting from CQI are discovered through in-depth analysis of work processes and elimination of redundant, unnecessary, and outdated work details. Improvements in productivity and efficiency may reduce the costs of doing business and may encourage employee ownership in the workplace.

Radiology departments involved in JCAHO patient safety goals or process improvement study work functions within the department, such as patient waiting time, and report turnaround time or ways to prevent medication errors. Perhaps even more significant to the overall success of the hospital are the CQI or patient safety process improvement activities conducted between multiple departments. An example of this concept would be the review of emergency services to reduce the length of stay in the emergency department. Laboratory, radiology, admissions, and nursing services all have an impact on the time required to diagnose and treat a patient in the emergency department. As these departments begin to look at each other as internal customers, they begin the cultural change of a quality or patient safety focus.

Planning

A primary management function is the process of deciding in advance what is to be accomplished. *Planning* charts a course of action for the future that enables coordinated and consistent fulfillment of goals and objectives. Without planning, activities occur at random. With planning, activities are assigned to specific employees with the skills and knowledge to achieve results.

Planning focuses attention on objectives and emphasizes efficiency and consistency. It also offsets uncertainty and change through thinking about the future and creating contingencies for what can be imagined or foreseen, as well as promoting economical operation and minimizing costs.

An example of planning in a radiology facility is the activities and forethought required to maintain sufficient supplies to accomplish the volume of radiologic procedures without expending unnecessary dollars to support a large inventory of supplies. Planning is also critical to maintaining a sufficient number of properly qualified technologists to accomplish a variety of procedures in many different subspecialties. Starting new services, efficiently performing growing or changing procedure volumes, and managing work during leaves of absence (e.g., maternity leaves, vacations) involve considerable planning skills, which vary directly with the size of the facility.

Other examples of areas in which planning is critical include developing and educating radiology employees, orienting new employees, replacing expensive radiology equipment, interpreting the hospital's goals and objectives for the accomplishment of work in the radiology department, and developing policies, procedures, guidelines, and methods for carrying out goals and objectives of the hospital and department.

Organizing

Once objectives, policies, procedures, and methods are defined through planning, administrators must define ways of carrying out those objectives. *Organizing* is the development of a structure or framework that identifies how people do their work. The division of work is essential to efficiency because it defines responsibility and authority.

Through the organizing function, the administrator defines what activities are to be performed, how they are grouped together, who has the responsibility, and who has the authority for carrying out the work. The framework created by the organizing function can be demonstrated through organizational charts such as those in Figs. 6–2 through 6–5 for a hospital and a radiology department.

Staffing

Staffing involves getting the right people to do the work and developing their abilities so they can do the work better. Because work cannot be accomplished without people, and because the quality of work is directly related to the quality of skills of the people involved, staffing is often viewed as critical.

The tools that administrators use to carry out their staffing functions are job descriptions and specifications, structured interviews, performance appraisals, the budget, wage or salary scales, orientation programs, and, most significant, the human resources department. Staffing functions include recruiting qualified employees, retaining quality employees, orienting and developing competent employees, identifying short- and long-term labor needs, and developing specifications for job qualifications.

Directing

Directing involves the stimulation of effort needed to perform the required work. Activities of directing include giving orders and promoting an understanding of what is to be done. Supervising activities relate to training, developing, and guiding employees. Through the function of leading, an administrator or supervisor inspires or influences employees to contribute toward the accomplishment of goals and objectives. Motivating encourages independent participation.

Within the function of directing, an administrator or supervisor uses communication skills to clarify and ensure understanding not only of the work to be accomplished, but also of the rationale of why and how it should be accomplished. An example of how supervisors direct through good communication is the discussion of policies and procedures. When employees understand the rationale for policies, they are more likely to enforce and support them.

While directing, an administrator or supervisor often encounters the necessity of delegating work to others. The ability to delegate well is a learnable skill that includes informing, guiding, educating, reviewing, evaluating, and giving feedback. Student radiologic technologists learn their clinical skills through a form of delegation. Work performed by others is assigned to them, and they are entrusted with the technical accuracy, patient safety, and a measure of efficiency necessary to complete radiologic procedures. The clinical instructor or registered technologist in charge of the student must understand the educational development and proficiency of the student being assigned to complete a procedure. The supervisor of a delegated task must achieve a balance that permits independence of student action to maximize the learning experience while maintaining the quality and safety of the procedure for the patient.

For students being delegated work in patient care, the issue of responsibility versus authority is often perplexing. Unless it is well defined for students in the clinical setting, the fact that a certain measure of authority is also delegated with the responsibility of caring for patients may be unclear. Examples of situations in which this concept is important include the student's authority to direct patients to follow instructions for activities such as procedure preparation, movement through the facility, and radiation safety. Students also should be instructed in their authority to solve problems, to report potential errors, and to adhere to ethical standards.

The transition in management previously described also affects the function of directing. Under the old concept of directing, some administrators or supervisors *barked* orders or issued directives. Under the new concepts of management, administrators and supervisors employ the tactics of influencing, guiding, persuading, and coaching employees.

Controlling

Just as students need instructors to observe, test, measure, and guide their educational progress, the hospital needs administrators to review daily, weekly, monthly, or annually the activities and resources used to provide care to patients. *Controlling* defines performance standards or guidelines used to measure progress toward the goals of the organization. Once the plans and goals of the hospital are formed, measures must be developed to determine whether each department or section is achieving success toward these goals. The mechanism used for reporting the defined measures creates a formal process of feedback and flow of information and are called key performance indicators. The feedback from the key performance indicators can then be used to make adjustments if needed to keep operations or expenses moving in the right direction.

The controlling process can be described in four steps: (1) establishing methods of achieving planned goals and objectives, (2) defining standards and measures to give feedback on progress, (3) measuring and reporting progress, and (4) taking action to correct variations from the expected standards. An example of controlling for radiologic technology students is the use of testing in the educational program:

1. One of the goals is the successful completion of the registry examination.
2. Defining standards is the development of curriculum, and measures are the tests used to check student progress in learning.
3. Test taking and reporting define student progress.
4. Taking action to correct deficiencies in learning helps the student move toward the successful registry examination.

In the typical radiology department, key performance indicators may include monitors such as monthly expense and revenue reports, weekly reports of employee performance, employee turnover rate, inventory of supplies, radiation safety, and quality of equipment operation.

Standards of controlling often are discussed as either managerial or technical. The standards used to control managerial functions include policies and procedures, rules, and other reports of operations or *people functions*. Standards for hiring personnel with specific job skills and

credentials fall into this category. Technical standards by comparison refer more to safety and equipment operation, such as processor sensitometry, radiation protection reports, and other measures of equipment quality control. Technical standards would then include those that govern the more technical functions such as equipment operation (quality control) and the specific routines for radiographic positioning and exposure.

Coordinating

While performing each of the other functions of management, synchronization of efforts must occur. *Coordinating* is a process by which the manager achieves orderly group activities and unity of effort by workers who are fully aware of a common purpose. In carrying out coordinating activities, an administrator communicates with other areas to facilitate work information and flow. Representing the department and being a spokesman for the department to the organization or outside the organization are critical administrative functions requiring political sensitivity to the needs of both the department and the hospital.

Optimal coordination requires superior skills in the critical areas of presentation, debate, analysis, and articulation. For example, the coordination required to bring a new service such as mobile imaging (e.g., CT, stereotactic breast biopsy, PET) to a community hospital includes at least the following departments or individuals:

- Financial management department for assistance or approval of the proposed financial plan for the project
- Hospital administration for project approval
- Board of directors for project approval
- Physicians for arranging case scheduling
- Medical staff to keep them informed of the arrival of the new service
- Human resources department if new employees are needed or if changes in job descriptions or salaries are involved
- Supervisors to inform and train employees for the new service requirements
- Plant services to plan for the location and docking of the mobile imaging truck on the hospital campus and provision of electrical, water, and telephone connections
- Service providers to coordinate the schedules of arrival and departure for the purpose of scheduling patients
- Surgery services if provision of anesthesia and monitoring equipment and nurses is required

- Nursing services for required assistance with patient care
- Postanesthesia recovery services to care for patients after treatment
- Purchasing services to ensure availability of new supplies

Project Management

The success and speed with which a new service is developed are directly related to the project management skills of the administrator and his or her team members. Coordinating the project and instilling a cooperative spirit with the interacting departments requires a special set of skills. Good project management methodology also defines outcomes, builds a plan, manages the risks of the plan, and communicates progress and results according to a schedule developed by consensus.

REGULATING AGENCIES AND COMMITTEES

The operation of a radiology department is regulated by external agencies, as well as by the governing body of the hospital. External regulating agencies include both voluntary and required regulation. Whereas government agencies usually impose required regulations on health care institutions, other regulating groups such as the JCAHO are voluntary, paid membership regulators that apply guidelines to measure quality or safety. An example of an involuntary regulating activity that is becoming tied to reimbursement is accreditation of mammography services for reimbursement by Medicare. Although participation in some external regulating agencies is voluntary, reimbursement is becoming increasingly dependent on satisfactory compliance with their guidelines.

External

External regulators and agencies that affect radiology operations today include the following entities.

JOINT COMMISSION ON ACCREDITATION OF HEALTHCARE ORGANIZATIONS. The JCAHO regulates the quality and safety of care provided to patients and the way the organization is supervised and operated. JCAHO guidelines include the assignment of responsibilities within the hospital, the development of policies and procedures for safety, and the management of continuously improving quality. Hospitals voluntarily subscribe to membership in the JCAHO, which conducts on-site visits to check hospital compliance with established guidelines and national safety goals.

STATE HEALTH DEPARTMENTS. State regulatory agencies such as the state boards of health define rules to protect the health and safety of the patients or clients that health care facilities serve. The **certificate of need (CON)** is a certificate of authority or permission granted by a state review board allowing a hospital or other health care entity to construct new facilities, develop new services, or purchase expensive equipment or technologies. The rules for cash expenditures, which vary from state to state, were developed in an attempt to control the rising costs of health care through control of duplication of services.

NUCLEAR REGULATORY COMMISSION. Radiation regulating agencies include the Nuclear Regulatory Commission (NRC) and state licensing agencies for control of equipment and technologists. A state board of health may require licensure of radiologic technologists or may leave the regulation of users of ionizing radiation to the voluntary jurisdiction of the individual health care facility. These regulating groups conduct inspections and levy fines for noncompliance with regulations, which vary from state to state. In most states, the NRC duties have been phased into state agencies such as the department of health or department of radiation safety.

OCCUPATIONAL SAFETY AND HEALTH ADMINISTRATION. The **Occupational Safety and Health Administration (OSHA)** is the federal agency that establishes standards for safety in the workplace. Some of the critical concerns of OSHA in radiology include handling and disposal of hazardous materials, universal precautions for protection of employees from infectious diseases, and eye protection from processing chemicals.

MAMMOGRAPHY ACCREDITATION. The certification of administrative, professional, and technical aspects of mammography services is provided by the American College of Radiology (ACR), the U.S. Food and Drug Administration (FDA), and various state health departments. The ACR provides voluntary accreditation; the FDA certification is required for reimbursement by Medicare. Many states also certify mammography equipment and services and in some cases have authority to inspect on behalf of the FDA.

HEALTH INSURANCE PORTABILITY AND ACCOUNTABILITY ACT. The Health Insurance Portability and

Accountability Act of 1996 (HIPAA) is intended to improve the efficiency and effectiveness of the health care system by encouraging the development of a health information system to establish standards and requirements for the electronic transmission of certain health information. The privacy standards section of HIPAA was meant to increase the public trust in the protection of health care information, prove accountability of providers and payors, facilitate the adoption of electronic management of medical data, and increase the data confidentiality integrity and availability. Many health care organizations have appointed a privacy officer to develop the policies and procedures around HIPAA and to implement these policies and procedures throughout the health care system. One of the patient benefits of HIPAA is the restricted use of protected health information (PHI). HIPAA protects the confidentiality and outlines permitted uses and disclosures of PHI in the proper health care systems. Patients must give permission to share information with a *need-to-know* basis. All external persons or entities that use or disclose PHI but are not an employee of the provider must sign a business associate agreement that further protects confidentiality of the patient.

Internal

In addition to external agencies, internal committees also regulate operations in a radiology department.

SAFETY COMMITTEE. Hospitals are required by the JCAHO to have a safety committee that directs education of employees on safety policies and procedures and ensures safe operations of the facility for patients and employees. Safety committees regulate such activities as storage and removal of hazardous or contaminated materials; physical control of chemical, radiation, and biologic hazards; special cleaning and emergency procedures; inspection of facilities to identify hazards; and correction of hazardous conditions. In the early 2000s, hospitals began to broaden the scope of the safety committee to include clinical patient safety issues such as **adverse drug events (ADEs)** and **medical errors.**

Beginning in the mid-1990s, hospital safety committees began to take on additional responsibilities for safety in the delivery of clinical services. Examples of monitoring and reducing medical errors include reduction of medication administration errors, adverse drug events, and patient falls.

INFECTION CONTROL COMMITTEE. The infection control committee regulates infection control policies and proce-

dures and conducts epidemiologic studies for patient and employee protection.

RADIATION SAFETY COMMITTEE. The radiation safety committee, required by the NRC or state radiation governing body and the JCAHO, regulates hospital activities for radiation safety and nuclear medicine activities. Radiation safety committees define safe handling of radioactive materials and policies for care of patients exposed to radiation. Policies and procedures used in the case of radiation accidents are also within the responsibilities of radiation safety committees.

PHARMACY AND THERAPEUTICS COMMITTEE. The pharmacy and therapeutics (P&T) committee is a required committee of the hospital medical staff that reviews drugs and their use in the hospital. In most hospitals, the P&T committee reviews drugs used in radiology and their protocols for use, such as ionic or nonionic contrast media. The direct control of medication hazards and safety in a radiology department is the responsibility of the radiology administrator, who writes policies and procedures, keeps records, and arranges for training in safety for all employees in the department.

RISK MANAGEMENT AND CORPORATE COMPLIANCE. Risk management was developed to control the amount of legal and financial risks to the organization and to enable a hospital to continue good financial and public standing by providing quality care to all patients. Its goal is to keep the organization, employees, and especially the patient free from any risks that may hinder their quality of care and to guarantee the safety of all its customers.

Corporate compliance was developed to prevent an organization from committing health care fraud. Most health care organizations work hard to be compliant with federal, state, and insurance regulations. Having a formal compliance program means that the health care system takes compliance seriously. It formalizes their commitment to do the right thing in all situations and interactions within the health care system.

PICTURE ARCHIVING AND COMMUNICATIONS SYSTEMS. The picture archiving and communication systems (PACS) became widely accepted as an alternative to film screen imaging devices in the late 1990s. PACS is defined as acquiring, archiving, interpreting, and distributing digital images throughout a health system enterprise. The benefits of PACS are that it allows a health care provider to access digital imaging information anytime and anywhere care is being provided. All imaging modalities are now able to be converted to PACS components, and the radiology administrator must understand the clinical and financial benefits to PACS. Briefly, the clinical benefits of PACS are the availability of digital images where care is provided, faster turnaround of imaging diagnosis, simultaneous consultation ability with the radiologist, and never losing an image, as was the case with the single original x-ray film. Financial benefits are the offset of film, storage, processor, processor maintenance, and paper supply costs. The implementation of PACS technology has dramatically changed the delivery of radiographic services in all health care settings.

CHARACTERISTICS OF GOOD EMPLOYEES

When radiology administrators and supervisors set out to hire new employees, they would like to find many characteristics in the new employee, but two specific criteria stand out in the minds of most administrators. The prospective radiology employee should have (1) a good knowledge of the required technical skills and (2) superior skills in interactive relationships.

Many administrators believe they can assist the new employee who has a solid technical knowledge base to grow and acquire an increased range of technical skills, but people skills depend on long-term training, instincts, and personality development. The employee with strong interpersonal skills cooperatively enhances patient care and workflow, thereby increasing his or her value to the workplace.

One of the most important concepts that employees in any organization or business should understand is that the customer writes the paychecks. Even in health care organizations, the hospital, clinic, or office cannot survive or succeed without a steady supply of customers who use the services provided and pay for these services. In past decades, health care facilities depended on physicians to refer patients to them. In recent years, however, patients have begun to exert influence about where they will obtain service, even to the point of changing physicians when they are dissatisfied. Therefore every employee must consider that both physicians and patients indirectly write their paychecks. If clients are dissatisfied, then they can easily carry their money down the street to a facility that provides better service. Payors are also scrutinizing satisfaction of their health plan members and holding the facility accountable through contractual arrangements. In the 1990s, health care providers began to recognize new customers in the insurance companies and other third-party payors that now contract with

health care providers for the best-quality, lowest-cost service. In the early 2000s, some third-party payors began paying reimbursement bonuses to facilities that demonstrated evidence of improved patient safety.

In 1991 the Association of Educators in Radiological Sciences (AERS), in conjunction with the American Healthcare Radiology Administrators (AHRA), conducted a survey of radiology administrators that revealed that, when hiring a recently graduated technologist, the most important skills desired were knowledge of the technical aspects of the job, customer service skills for dealing with patients, and interpersonal communication skills for dealing with co-workers, physicians, and other departments.

The same survey revealed that the most common reasons for a technologist to be disciplined, reprimanded, or terminated were poor interpersonal skills, lack of technical knowledge, and poor customer service skills. The AERS survey recommended that educators in radiologic technology programs heed the advice of radiology administrators in developing customer service–oriented technologists with interpersonal communication skills. The message for students of radiologic technology is to seek direction and personal development in sensitivities to patients and co-workers. In 1996, Akroyd and Wold surveyed AHRA members' perceptions of needed workplace skills and the ability of radiography graduates to perform them. Results indicated that the skills of students might need development. Problem-solving and critical-thinking skills, patient care skills, and customer satisfaction skills were among the top eight areas in need of development.

Quality service and communication skills are as important as technical skills in the preparation of students for future employment. Quality service can be defined as doing the right things right the first time and meeting or exceeding the customer's expectations.

Radiology administrators expect employees (including students as prospective employees) to take personal responsibility for their own motivation to seek out personal development in basic communication skills. Radiologic technologists and students should seek to achieve the following:

- Develop an ability to see their work from the patient's or the physician's point of view.
- Develop skills in handling customer complaints.
- Practice service with a smile.
- React as if the customer were always right.
- Remember that the patients and physicians write the paychecks.
- Strive to meet or exceed the expectations of all patients and physicians.

An opportunity in which the student radiologic technologist can work on developing desirable people skills is through routine clinical practice. Although technical skills can be readily learned and proficiency can be proved, the interaction with each patient offers a new opportunity for problem solving. Each difficult patient improves the student's ability to meet or exceed the next patient's expectations. When student technologists become discouraged when performing another routine chest radiograph, they should consider that the skills in interpersonal relationships are built patient by patient and that each one offers an opportunity to do it better than before.

Yet another area of opportunity for developing people skills is through interaction with employees in departments outside radiology. With each interaction, the student technologist is an ambassador of the department of radiology, an emissary of the department administrator and even the hospital president. Future cooperation and efficiency are built step by step through brief encounters in the workplace. When an investment is made in cooperation and mutual support, the dividends are paid back in many forms. When patients observe cooperative interactions between employees, their perception of the quality of the facility and the value they receive in the service provided is enhanced. Perhaps the most obvious payback to the technologist is in the satisfaction realized in working in a supportive and cooperative environment. Every encounter or interaction between two employees makes an investment—either enhancing or destroying the satisfactory environment. Each employee can make a difference.

Within the radiology department, students should be offered additional opportunities to learn the details of operations through involvement in all departmental functions. Transporting patients, filing films, processing requisitions, assisting radiologists, and assisting technologists are all important activities that develop well-rounded perspectives of the importance of all radiology employees. Students are well advised to take advantage of every opportunity to become knowledgeable, empowered employees serving and solving problems for every customer, because it will be the hallmark of both successful institutions and the sought-after employees of the future.

SUMMARY

With an understanding of how a radiology department functions within the framework of a hospital organization, the student radiologic technologist can better relate to the cooperation and interaction required to deliver quality care to patients.

The field of radiology has broadened in recent decades to include other health care settings such as clinics, imaging centers, and mobile imaging. With the new radiologic settings, the knowledge requirements for technologists continue to include solid technical skills; a higher demand, however, is placed on superior interpersonal skills.

The basic functions of management apply to all hospitals, departments, subdepartments, and work units. Each entity is required to plan and organize work, staff with workers, direct the work to be done, control the quality and outcome, and coordinate activities of workers within the unit, as well as with workers and others outside the work unit. The organization of workers within a health care facility, such as a hospital, is developed to provide service to its primary customers: the physicians and their patients.

Health care facilities, providers of diagnostic services, and users of ionizing radiation and other medical devices are regulated by mandatory and state agencies, plus voluntary agencies, to ensure the safety of patients, workers, and others in the workplace. In addition to external agencies, radiology departments must comply with internal safety committees and maintain policies and procedures for patient and employee safety.

Because radiology services provide a unique service in diagnosis and treatment, these services are usually organized within the facility under a departmental structure within which the student radiologic technologist is expected to learn and become proficient. Each activity of the student in radiology, whether directly related to developing technical skills or indirectly related to developing interpersonal skills, is an important activity that will prepare the student for future success in his or her chosen profession.

BIBLIOGRAPHY

Akroyd D, Wold B: Managers' perceptions of radiographers' skills: current and future needs, *Radiol Manage* 18(3):15, May/June, 1996.

Bouchard E: *Radiology management: an introduction,* Denver, 1983, Multi-Media Publications.

Callaway WJ: Graduate technologists and customer service: a 1991 survey, *Radiol Manage* 14(2):50, 1992.

Deming WE: *Out of crisis,* Boston, 1986, Massachusetts Institute of Technology, Center for Advanced Engineering Study.

Donabedian A: The quality of care: how can it be addressed? *JAMA* 260:1743, 1988.

Gillem TR: Deming's 14 points and hospital quality: responding to the customer's demand for the best value health care, *J Nurs Qual Assur* 3:70, 1988.

Griffith JR: *The well-managed community hospital,* Ann Arbor, Mich, 1987, Health Administration Press.

Headrick LA: *Learning to improve complex systems of care "collaborative education to ensure patient safety,"* Washington, DC, 2000, U.S. Department of Health and Human Services, Health Resources and Services Administration, Bureau of Health Professions, Division of Medicine and Dentistry.

Institute of Medicine, Committee on Quality: *To err is human: building a safer health system,* Washington, DC, 1999, National Academy Press.

Institute of Medicine, Committee on Quality: *Crossing the quality chasm: a new health system for the 21st century,* Washington, DC, 2001, National Academy Press.

Joint Commission on Accreditation of Healthcare Organizations: *Transitions: from QA to CQI: using CQI approaches to monitor, evaluate, and improve quality,* Oak Brook, Ill, 1991, JCAHO.

Juran JM: *Juran on planning for quality,* New York, 1988, Free Press.

King B: *Better designs in half the time,* Methuen, Mass, 1989, GOAL/QPC.

Leebov W: *Effective complaint handling in health care,* Chicago, 1990, American Hospital Publishing.

Leebov W: *Health care managers in transition: shifting roles and changing organizations,* San Francisco, 1990, Jossey-Bass Publishers.

Leebov W: *The quality quest: a briefing for health care professionals,* Chicago, 1991, American Hospital Publishing.

Leebov W, Vergare M, Scott G: *Patient satisfaction: a guide to practice enhancement,* Oradell, NJ, 1990, Medical Economics Books.

Peters T, Austin N: *A passion for excellence,* New York, 1986, Warner Books.

Peters TJ, Waterman RH Jr: *In search of excellence,* New York, 1984, Warner Books.

Pichert JW, Miller CS, Hollo AH, et al: What health professionals can do to identify and resolve patient dissatisfaction, *J Qual Improve* 24(6):303, 1998.

Rakich JS, Longest BB, O'Donovan TR: *Managing health services organizations,* Baltimore, 1992, Health Professions Press.

Rosenthal JS: Customer focus: The competitive edge, *Administr Radiol* 8(6):34, 1989.

Schwartz H: Managing radiology in the 1990s: part 2, *Appl Radiol* 19:20, 1990.

Stockburger W: *Radiology administration: a business guide,* Philadelphia, 1989, JB Lippincott.

Tobin E: Patient feedback, *Administr Radiol* 10(7):51, 1991.

Wesolowski CE: Let's put "care" back into health care, *Radiol Manage* 12(3):49, 1990.

7

Radiographic Imaging

Lyn Hubbard, MSE, RT(R)(M)
Tracy B. White, MS, RT(R)(T)

Four factors . . . contribute to the quality of the . . . radiograph: First, distortion; second, detail; third, contrast; fourth, radiographic density . . .

Professor Ed. C. Jerman, The Father of Radiologic Technology
An analysis of the end-result: the radiograph, Radiology 6:59, 1926.

OBJECTIVES

On completion of this chapter, the student should be able to:

1. Discuss primary, scatter, and remnant radiation.

2. Describe the fundamentals of image production.

3. Discuss radiographic quality in terms of density, contrast, recorded detail, and distortion.

4. List the major factors that influence radiographic quality.

5. Differentiate sharpness of detail from visibility of detail.

6. Perform basic calculations using milliampere seconds, inverse square law, exposure maintenance, and 15% rule formulas.

7. Describe film/screen imaging, fluoroscopic imaging, and digital imaging.

GLOSSARY

Attenuation: process by which a beam of radiation is reduced in energy when passing through tissue or other materials

Central Ray: theoretical center of a beam of radiation

Contrast: difference between adjacent densities on a radiograph

Density: degree of darkening of exposed and processed photographic or radiographic film

Distortion: misrepresentation of the true size or shape of an object

Dynamic: with motion

Fog: unwanted exposure or film densities

Grid: device consisting of thin lead strips designed to permit primary radiation to pass while reducing scatter radiation

Half-Value Layer: amount of filtration necessary to reduce the intensity of the radiation beam to one half its original value

Image Receptor: medium used to capture the image for recording, such as x-ray film or a digital imaging plate

Intensifying Screen: layer of luminescent crystals placed inside a cassette to expose x-ray film efficiently and thereby significantly reduce patient dose

Inverse Square Law: mathematical formula that describes the relationship between radiation intensity and distance from the source of the radiation

Kilovoltage Peak (kVp): measure of the potential difference, which controls the quality and quantity of x-ray photons produced in the x-ray tube

Latent Image: invisible image created after exposure but before processing

Milliampere Seconds (mAs): measurement of milliamperage times seconds, which controls the quantity of x-ray photons produced in the x-ray tube

Penetrating Ability: ability of an x-ray beam to pass through an object, controlled by the kVp of the beam

Penumbra: fuzzy border of an object as imaged radiographically

Photon: quantum or particle of radiant energy

Positive Beam Limitation (PBL): automatic collimation system used on diagnostic x-ray units

Primary Radiation: x-ray beam after it leaves the x-ray tube and before it reaches the object

Radiolucent: permitting the passage of x-rays or other forms of energy with little attenuation

Radiopaque: not easily penetrable by x-rays or other forms of radiant energy

Recorded Detail: representation of an object's true borders

Relative Speed: relative measurements of the speed of a radiographic film and intensifying screen system

Remnant Radiation: radiation resulting after the x-ray beam exits the object

Resolution: a measurement of the recorded detail on a radiograph

Scatter Radiation: radiation produced from x-ray photon interactions with matter in such a way that the resulting photons have continued in a different direction

Source-to-Image Distance (SID): the distance between the source of the x-rays (usually the focal spot of the x-ray tube) and the image receptor

Static: unmoving

Umbra: true border of an object as imaged radiographically

IMAGE PRODUCTION

When x-rays were discovered in 1895, the medical community almost immediately realized the value of this discovery. Seeing within the human body became possible. In the following years, capturing the image produced by x-rays in a format allowing for storage and repeated viewing had become the task of the radiologic technologist. Despite the almost daily advances within the field of radiology, the basic mechanism of image production has not changed a great deal. A beam of x-rays, mechanically produced by passing high voltage through a cathode ray tube, traverses a patient and is partially absorbed in the process. An interpretation device called an **image recep-**tor intercepts the x-ray photons that are able to exit the patient. Three major classifications of diagnostic radiographic imaging have been formulated based on the type of image receptor used: (1) film/screen radiography, (2) fluoroscopic imaging, and (3) digital or computerized imaging.

Basically, four requirements exist for the production of x-rays:

1. Vacuum (tube housing)
2. Source of electrons (filament)
3. Method to accelerate the electrons (voltage) rapidly
4. Method to stop the electrons (target)

The vacuum removes all of the air so gas molecules will not interfere with the production of x-rays. When the electrons strike the target, radiation photons are produced; however, only 1% of this production is actually radiation; the remaining 99% is heat.

The beam of x-ray photons is generated by the careful selection of technical exposure factors by the radiographer and exits the x-ray tube during an exposure. This beam of photons, before it interacts with the patient's body, is called **primary radiation.** When the primary beam passes through a patient, the individual x-ray **photons** interact with the various materials that make up the human body.

Depending on the characteristics of these materials, the quantities of the photons are lessened by differing degrees as they pass through matter. The resulting beam that is able to exit from the patient is called exit or **remnant radiation.** This remnant radiation produces an image on the image receptor.

Along the way, an x-ray photon may interact with the body's matter in such a way that the resulting photon continues its travel in a different direction. This type of radiation may or may not be able to reach the image receptor, but it does not carry any useful information. **Scatter radiation** is the term generally used to describe this type of nondiagnostic radiation. **Attenuation** is the process by which the nature of the primary radiation is changed (partially absorbed) as it travels through the patient. The x-ray beam is attenuated differently, depending on the type of body tissue irradiated. For example, bone tissue, being more densely packed and made of harder material, attenuates the beam to a greater degree than soft tissue of the same thickness. This difference in attenuation allows for the formation of radiographic images.

In describing the relative ease with which x-ray photons may pass through matter of different types, two terms are commonly used. **Radiolucent** materials allow x-ray photons to pass through comparatively easily, as translucent panes of glass allow the passage of light. **Radiopaque** materials are not easily traversed by x-ray photons, just as panes of frosted glass do not allow the full amount of light to pass through. Thus bone is described as a relatively radiopaque tissue, whereas air is described as relatively radiolucent.

FILM/SCREEN RADIOGRAPHY

Imaging Chain

Once the attenuated beam has exited the patient as the remnant radiation, the information it carries about the types of tissue the beam has traversed must be translated from an energy message to a visual image that can be viewed and stored. X-ray photons have the ability to produce changes in photographic film. For this reason, some people do not like to put a loaded camera through the x-ray baggage check machine at the airport. Special film, manufactured to be particularly sensitive to x-radiation and certain colors of light radiation, is used to capture the energy message carried by the remnant beam and to convert it into an image. After the energy strikes it, the film must be processed before an image can be seen. A useful analogy is that of regular photographic film, in which the camera is loaded with the film, which then receives the light reflecting off the subject. When the roll of film is finished, it is rewound into a light-tight canister, developed, and printed. The printed image can then be viewed and stored. The image is not visible before processing because it is stored in a form that is not visible.

Radiographic film is similar. The remnant x-ray photons carry an energy representation of the object of interest that strikes the film emulsion, causing a transfer of energy. This image is stored in the emulsion until it is processed. This invisible image is called the **latent image.** Once the film has been processed, a visual image appears. The correct term to describe an image produced by x-ray photons on a piece of film is *radiograph.*

Historically, the film emulsion was exposed directly by x-ray photons. Each piece of information on the radiograph was put there by an x-ray photon. This process required a great deal of radiation, particularly for large, dense body parts. Certain crystals were discovered to *luminesce,* or emit light, when struck by x-ray photons. In addition, this luminescence was at a greater than one-to-one correspondence, meaning that for every x-ray photon that hit a crystal, hundreds of light photons might be produced. By adjusting the emulsion of the radiographic film to be sensitive to the color of light emitted by a particular crystal, the photographic effect of the x-ray beam can be multiplied or intensified, resulting in the use of lower amounts of x-radiation to produce an image.

Intensifying screens are thin layers of cardboard or polyester coated with layers of luminescent phosphor crystals. The screens are mounted in a cassette, and the film is placed inside. Typically, modern radiographic film has an emulsion coating on both sides and is known as *duplitized* or double-emulsion film. Duplitized film is designed to be used with two intensifying screens for the most efficient performance. Estimates indicate that more than 99% of the photographic effect on a film/screen radiograph is due to screen light, with the remaining effect due to the direct action of x-ray photons. Most general-

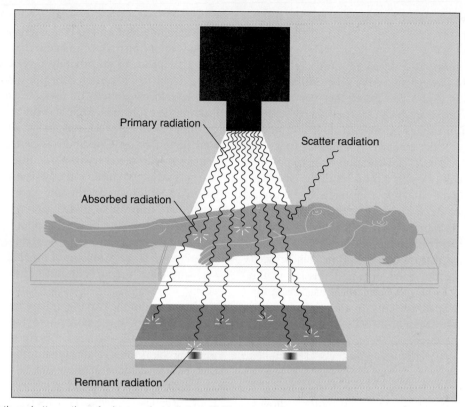

Primary radiation

Scatter radiation

Absorbed radiation

Remnant radiation

FIG. 7–1 The path and attenuation of a beam of x-radiation. (1) The primary beam exits the x-ray tube. (2) The beam enters the patient, where the individual x-ray photons' energies are altered (attenuated) by their passage through body tissues of varying characteristics. (3) The attenuated, or remnant, beam exits the patient, carrying with it an energy representation of the body tissues traversed. (4) The x-ray photons in the remnant beam strike the phosphor crystals of the intensifying screens, causing them to emit many light photons for each incident x-ray photon. (5) The light photons photographically expose the film emulsion, resulting in an invisible latent image.

purpose radiography is performed using this kind of film/screen system. Film/screen combinations may be manipulated to provide differing radiographic quality criteria when necessary. The entire path of a beam of x-radiation is shown in Fig. 7–1.

Processing

Radiographic film is similar to photographic film in that it has a silver-based emulsion. Incoming photons of light or x-ray energy is able to excite the crystals holding the silver in place, causing a rearrangement of electrons. This process results in the production of a latent image. A resultant image is produced from this latent image through a sequence of chemical reactions known collectively as *processing*. As in photographic film processing, the film must be developed, fixed, washed, and dried. Originally, each step was performed manually, which was time consuming and messy.

Moreover, if not done properly, variable results can be produced. *Automatic processing* has allowed these steps to be compressed into approximately 90 seconds, with increasingly uniform radiographs resulting. In an automatic processor, the film is carried through the chemical solutions by a series of rollers. It passes through the developer, fixer, and wash tanks, and then through the dryer compartment. The film that exits the dryer is ready to be viewed, interpreted, and then stored (archived) for later use.

Technical Exposure Factors

The radiographer directly controls radiographic quality. Selection of the proper exposure factors for each individual examination is necessary to produce a high-quality diagnostic radiograph. The exposure factors under the control of the radiographer, often referred to as *technique*, include the following, which are often called the *prime factors:*

1. *Milliamperage (mA)* is a measure of the electrical current passing through the x-ray tube. **Milliampere seconds (mAs)** is the parameter that controls the amount of radiation produced by the x-ray tube; it is the product of mA times seconds. It directly controls the *quantity* of x-ray photons produced. Time (in seconds) is a measure of the duration of the exposure.
2. **Kilovoltage peak (kVp)** is a measure of the electrical pressure (potential difference) forcing the current through the tube. It controls the penetrating ability of the beam and primarily affects the *quality but also the quantity* of the x-ray photons produced.
3. **Source-to-image distance (SID)** is the standardized distance between the point of x-ray emission in the x-ray tube (the focal spot) and the image receptor. It affects the relative intensity of the radiation as it reaches the image receptor and affects the geometric properties of the image. This measurement has also been known as *focal-film distance* or *target-to-film distance.*

Other factors that can be controlled by the radiographer include focal spot size, primary beam configuration, quantity and quality of scatter, and speed of the image receptor.

RADIOGRAPHIC QUALITY

Once processed, the finished radiograph must be evaluated for technical quality. A radiograph must exhibit proper quality to be deemed diagnostic and should demonstrate all of the desired information within the range of acceptance. Overall, the acceptance characteristics of a radiograph, termed *radiographic quality factors,* fall into two main divisions: (1) photographic qualities and (2) geometric qualities. Photographic qualities include **density,** the overall blackening of film emulsion in response to photons, and **contrast,** the visible difference between adjacent densities. Geometric qualities include **recorded detail,** the distinct representation of an object's true borders, or edges, and **distortion,** the misrepresentation of the true size or shape of an object. Each of these factors contributes to the overall radiographic quality.

A proper balance between the photographic and geometric properties of an image results in good radiographic quality. The geometric properties allow the size, shape, and edges of the object of interest to be accurately represented, whereas the photographic properties allow these carefully reproduced characteristics to be seen.

By way of illustration, imagine that you are trying to take a snapshot of an ornately carved stone. You want every detail to be captured on film, so you take extra trouble to focus carefully. To make certain of success, you make three exposures, each at a different setting. When the film has been processed and printed, you examine your three photos. One photo is perfectly exposed, and you are able to see every important detail in the carving. The second is too dark, and any detail is hard to distinguish. The third is too light, and again, the details of the carving are impossible to see. Consider the two poorly exposed photos. Just because a photograph is too dark or too light, does that mean that good detail sharpness is not present? These problems of overexposure and underexposure affect the *visibility* but not the *sharpness* of the detail.

You return to the carving, intending to use the proper exposure setting to get more photographs. This time, you forget to focus the camera properly, or you move while pressing the shutter. The resultant photograph has beautiful photographic properties but is fuzzy and blurred. This photograph can be said to possess good visibility but poor sharpness of detail. The desired image should have both characteristics (Fig. 7–2).

When evaluating radiographs, sharpness and visibility of detail must be examined to assess overall quality. The photographic factors that control visibility of detail are considered first.

Photographic Qualities

DENSITY. Commonly described as the overall darkening of a film in response to light or x-ray photons, radiographic density can be described technically as a comparison of the light incident on the film to the light transmitted through the film. With digital imaging systems, the term *density* is sometimes used to discuss the brightness of the image on a monitor. If a digital image is printed to hard copy film, then the traditional term of *density* can still be used.

When a radiograph is viewed on a viewbox, obviously, the incident light is transmitted more easily through the light gray areas than through the darker areas. The darker areas that block the transmission of light are said to have greater radiographic density. Although it can be easily measured scientifically with a densitometer, density is often a subjective measurement, judged by the human eye. A radiograph must possess the proper density to present adequate visibility of detail to the viewer in the

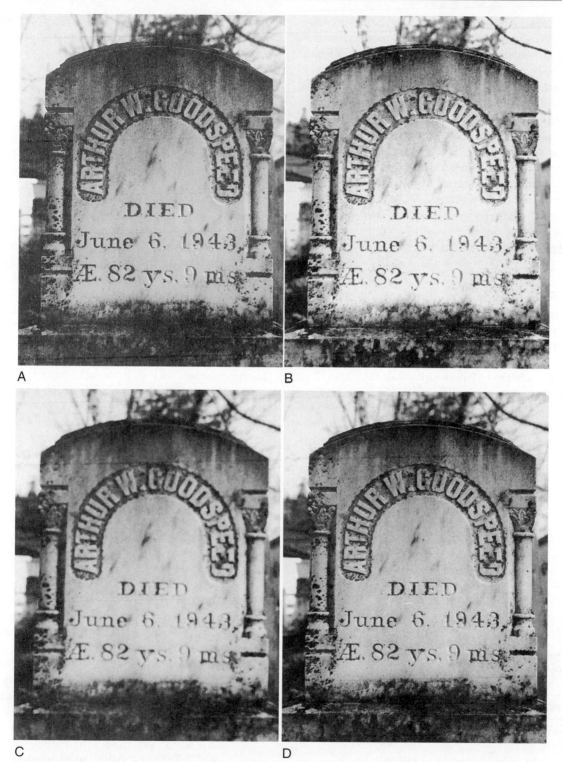

FIG. 7–2 Different-quality photographs of a gravestone: too dark *(A)*, too light *(B)*, out of focus *(C)*, perfect *(D)*.

same way that a photograph should not be overexposed or underexposed to do justice to its subject. In many instances, a radiologist's use of the term *density* refers to anatomic density and not to radiographic density. A report noting *an increased density in the right lung field* should be interpreted to mean that the lung tissue is denser than other tissues. The radiographic density in such an area would therefore be decreased because the denser tissue would absorb more of the x-ray beam than the tissue that is less dense. Many variables can affect density, including patient size and tissue composition, mAs, kVp, distance, beam modification (collimation, filtration, grids), film/screen combinations, and processing.

Milliampere Seconds. The greater the amount of x-ray photons generated, the greater the resultant image receptor exposure and film density on the radiograph will be. This ratio is a direct relation. Increasing the number of x-ray photons produced increases the exposure (in milliroentgens [mR]) and the overall radiographic density. *mAs is the chief controlling factor of exposure and density* (Table 7-1) and controls the number of electrons that flow from cathode to anode in the x-ray tube. This process, in turn, controls the number of x-ray photons produced. mAs is the product of mA and time. Any combination of mA and time producing equivalent mAs values should produce equivalent exposures and therefore densities. This process is known as mAs reciprocity.

$$mA \times time = mAs$$

Examples:

$$100 \, mA \times 1/10 \, sec = 10 \, mAs$$
$$200 \, mA \times 1/20 \, sec = 10 \, mAs$$
$$300 \, mA \times 1/30 \, sec = 10 \, mAs$$

The mAs, mA, and time factors are all directly related to image receptor exposure and film density. These effects also can be stated as follows:

TABLE 7-1 Controlling and Influencing Factors of Image Receptor Exposure/Film Density

CONTROLLING FACTOR	INFLUENCING FACTORS
Milliampere seconds	Patient factors
	Kilovoltage peak
	Distance
	Beam modification
	Grids
	Film/screen combinations
	Processing

Increasing mAs increases image receptor exposure and film density.

Decreasing mAs decreases image receptor exposure and film density.

The radiographs in Fig. 7–3 illustrate these effects. Example:

$$100 \, mA \times 1/10 \, sec = 10 \, mAs = \text{original exposure/film density A}$$
$$200 \, mA \times 1/20 \, sec = 10 \, mAs = \text{maintains exposure/film density A}$$
$$100 \, mA \times 1/5 \, sec = 20 \, mAs = \text{increases exposure/film density A}$$

Patient Factors. Diagnostic radiography makes use of the differential attenuation of a beam of radiation by various types of body tissue. In this way, information can be gained about the anatomy, physiology, and pathology of many of the body's organ systems. The degree to which the radiation is attenuated depends on tissue characteristics such as cell composition, relative atomic number, thickness, and cell density. Additionally, pathologic conditions can change the way in which the radiation is attenuated. A thick, dense tissue with a relatively high atomic number, such as bone, attenuates the beam to a greater degree than does a thin, less dense tissue with a low atomic number, such as fat. Bone prevents the easy passage of the x-ray photons; therefore, bone is represented as a lighter shade of gray, or an area of decreased radiographic density, on the radiograph.

Because radiography is actually the investigation of tissue characteristics, attempting to standardize all other factors affecting radiographic quality so that the subject is the only variable makes sense. Technique charts, automatic exposure control, accurate positioning, and standard imaging protocols are useful in this regard.

Kilovoltage Peak. In addition to the number of x-ray photons produced, the relative strength of the photons must be considered. An x-ray photon of very low energy would have difficulty passing through dense body tissue. Conversely, this same low-energy photon would pass easily through less dense tissue. This characteristic is referred to as the **penetrating ability** of an x-ray beam. Each average body part can be shown at best advantage by using an optimal kVp setting as a guideline.

The kVp setting determines the highest energy level, or the *peak,* possible for the photons within that beam. Most of the photons are, in fact, below the peak kilovoltage, covering a range from zero to peak value. The x-ray beam is described as polyenergetic or heterogeneous for this reason.

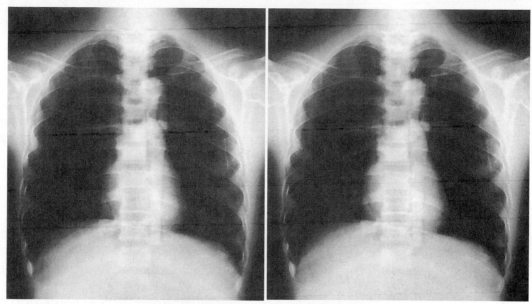

A 120 kVp at 2.5 mAs (100 mA and 0.025 s) B 120 kVp at 2.5 mAs (160 mA and 0.016 s)

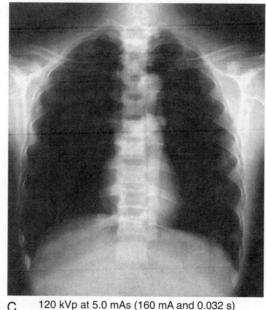

C 120 kVp at 5.0 mAs (160 mA and 0.032 s)

FIG. 7–3 Radiographs show the influence of milliamperage and time on exposure/film density. *A* and *B,* Same milliampere seconds with different milliamperage and time settings. *C,* Double the milliampere seconds.

The relationship between kVp and exposure is not as simple as that of mAs. As kVp increases, image receptor exposure increases but not in direct proportion. The general rule of thumb to account for the change in image receptor exposure relative to change in kVp is called the 15% rule: Increasing kVp 15% will double image receptor exposure. Decreasing kVp 15% will halve image receptor exposure.

For example, imagine that the original kVp is 75. Fifteen percent of the original kVp (75) equals 11.25 or approximately 11. If we want to double the image receptor exposure using the kVp, then 11 kVp should be added to the original selection (75), which would result in 86 kVp. If we want the halve the image receptor exposure using the kVp, then 11 kVp should be subtracted from the original (75), which would then equal 64 kVp.

Using this rule to change kVp while maintaining the same image receptor exposure is also possible. This process is done by changing the mAs to compensate for the exposure change caused by the change in kVp. When this adjustment occurs, the change in kVp does not change the quantity of the exposure, only the spectrum or energy of the photons. To change kVp while maintaining the same image receptor exposure:

Increase kVp 15% and halve mAs.
Decrease kVp 15% and double mAs.

Example:
To maintain the original image receptor exposure, what new value of mAs is necessary when changing from 75 kVp and 50 mAs to 86 kVp?

$$75 \times 0.15 \ (15\%) = 11.25 \ (\text{approximately } 11)$$
$$75 + 11 = 86$$

Because the kVp increased 15%, the mAs must be halved to maintain the original image receptor exposure:

$$\text{Original mAs} = 50/2 = 25 \ \text{mAs}$$

The radiographs in Fig. 7–4 illustrate these effects.

Distance. A beam of radiation obeys many of the same laws that light does. If a flashlight is projected onto a wall, then the relative intensity of the light increases as it is moved closer to the wall. *The intensity increases as the distance decreases.* As the flashlight is moved farther away from the wall, *the intensity decreases as the distance increases.* This characteristic is described as an *inverse relation.*

The same relation holds true for an x-ray beam. If all other factors are equal, the farther the distance the photons have to travel, the less chance they have of reaching the image receptor because of the divergence of the beam (Fig. 7–5). This relationship means that the same exposure factors used at a greater distance would result in reduced image receptor exposure and a radiograph of decreased density. When the effect of distance on beam intensity is measured, it is related to the distance squared. In other words, if the distance is doubled, then the intensity decreases to one fourth of the original. This relationship is described by the **inverse square law:** The intensity of a beam of radiation is inversely proportional to the square of the distance from the source. The mathematical expression of the inverse square law is:

$$I_1/I_2 = D_2{}^2/D_1{}^2$$

where:

I_1 = original intensity
I_2 = new intensity
D_1 = original distance
D_2 = new distance

Example:
If the intensity of the beam is 40 R/min (R = roentgen, a unit of radiation exposure) at the original distance of 40 cm, what will the intensity be if the new distance is 20 cm?

$$I_1/I_2 = D_2{}^2/D_1{}^2$$
$$40/x = 20^2/40^2$$
$$40/x = 1^2/2^2$$
$$40/x = 1/4$$
$$x = 160 \ \text{R/min}$$

Notice that decreasing the distance by one half causes the intensity to increase by a factor of 4.

The inverse square law describes the effect of a change in distance on beam intensity, but the radiographer would frequently like to be able to compensate for a necessary change in distance. This compensation may be accomplished by using a conversion of the inverse square law known as the *exposure maintenance formula.* This formula is actually a direct square law. The mathematical expression of the exposure maintenance formula is as follows:

$$mAs_1/mAs_2 = D_1{}^2/D_2{}^2$$

where:

mAs_1 = original mAs value
mAs_2 = new mAs value
D_1 = original distance
D_2 = new distance

Because mAs, mA, and time are all directly proportional to beam intensity, this formula may be used to derive any of these three factors.

Example:
If a radiograph produced at 72 inches SID using 20 mAs must be repeated at 36 inches SID, then what new mAs setting is necessary to maintain the same image receptor exposure?

$$mAs_1/mAs_2 = D_1{}^2/D_2{}^2$$
$$20/x = 72^2/36^2$$
$$20/x = 2^2/1^2$$
$$20/x = 4/1$$
$$4x = 20$$
$$x = 5 \ \text{mAs}$$

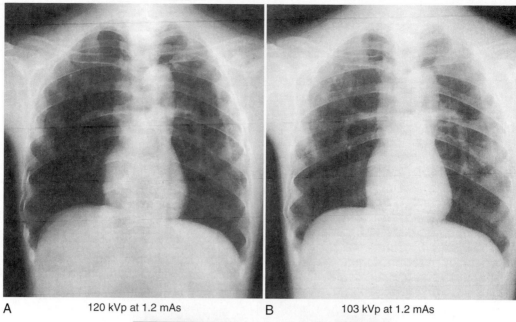

A   120 kVp at 1.2 mAs   B   103 kVp at 1.2 mAs

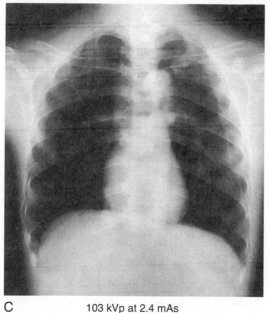

C   103 kVp at 2.4 mAs

FIG. 7–4 Radiographs show the influence of kilovoltage peak on exposure/film density. *A,* Acceptable radiograph. *B,* Fifteen percent decrease in kilovoltage peak with no change in milliampere seconds. *C,* Fifteen percent decrease in kilovoltage peak with double the milliampere seconds to maintain the same image receptor exposure/film density as in *A.*

Beam Modification. Anything that changes the nature of the radiation beam, apart from the factors already discussed, is referred to as *beam modification.* The beam may be modified before it enters the patient, in which case it is called *primary beam modification,* or after it exits the patient, in which case it is generally known as *scatter control.*

The primary beam can be adjusted by changing filtration and beam limitation. *Filtration* is the use of attenuating material, usually aluminum, between the x-ray tube and the patient. This substance mainly removes very–low-energy nondiagnostic x-ray photons in the primary beam to decrease patient exposure. As more material is placed in the path of the beam, the resultant

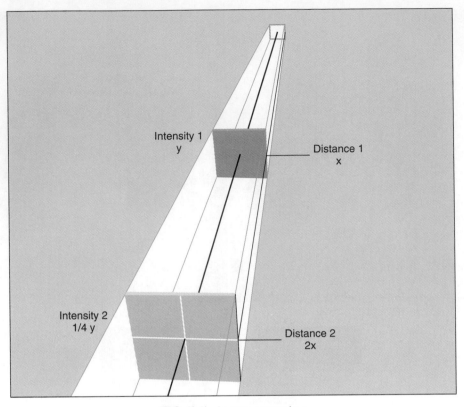

FIG. 7–5 Inverse square law.

intensity decreases. For example, a bare light bulb glows with a specific intensity. Placing a paper shade over the bulb filters out some of the light, thereby reducing its intensity. With all other factors equal, the same exposure factors used with 4 mm of filtration would produce less image receptor exposure and a radiograph with less density than if used with only 2 mm of filtration.

The amount of attenuating material required to reduce the intensity of a beam to one half the original value is referred to as the **half-value layer.** Because aluminum is the most common material used for filtration in diagnostic radiography, half-value layer is usually expressed in terms of millimeters of aluminum equivalency (mm Al/Eq).

Beam limitation is the use of devices to confine the x-ray beam to the area of interest, thereby reducing exposure to body parts other than those under examination. In addition to patient protection, beam limitation dramatically affects radiographic quality. During the transit of an x-ray photon through matter, the probability that the photon will collide with an atom is high. This collision may result in a change in direction, as well as a decrease in the energy of the photon. This scattered

photon is virtually useless from a diagnostic standpoint and contributes only to patient dose. This type of photon is usually described as *scatter radiation.* If scatter radiation reaches the film, it is not carrying information. Scattered photons that strike the film emulsion degrade the quality of the image by contributing unwanted radiographic densities known as **fog.**

By limiting the size and shape of the primary beam to the area of interest, we are decreasing the probability of the production of scatter radiation. Scatter can never be eliminated, but its effect can be lessened. In fact, scatter accounts for a large percentage of the density of any radiograph. By restricting the primary beam and decreasing scatter, we are, in effect, subtracting photons from the remnant beam. Therefore a decrease in scatter causes a decrease in image receptor exposure and film density.

Devices used to limit the size and shape of the primary beam include aperture diaphragms, cones and cylinders, and variable aperture collimators. The collimator is the device most familiar to radiographers. It consists of adjustable pairs of lead shutter leaves that allow for the use of various sized rectangular fields. **Positive beam limitation (PBL),** often referred to as *automatic collima-*

tion, is an electronic interlock system. It automatically collimates the beam to the size of the image receptor placed in the Bucky tray, the cassette holder tray within the x-ray table.

Grids. Despite the careful use of primary beam modification, once the beam enters the patient, scatter radiation is produced. As stated previously, the more scatter that reaches the image receptor as fog density, the poorer the appreciation of the details. A **grid** is a device that is designed to remove as many scattered photons exiting the patient as possible before they reach the film. A grid consists of thin lead strips interspersed with spacing material. The grid is placed between the patient and the image receptor to intercept scattered photons, which, by definition, have been diverted from their original paths. Increasing the lead in a grid increases its ability to remove scatter from the remnant beam. Decreasing the amount of scatter enhances the radiographic contrast. However, the additional lead in the grid also requires increased exposure factor settings, which increases the radiation dose to the patient.

Grids are described according to *grid ratio,* the ratio of the height of the lead strips to the distance between them. Grid ratios commonly range from 5:1 to 16:1, with the higher ratio grid able to remove more photons from the beam. Because the grid reduces the number of photons reaching the image receptor, it also causes a decrease in film density. All other factors being equal, if the same exposure factors are used with a 5:1 grid and a 10:1 grid, the 10:1 grid produces an image with less exposure or film density.

Film/Screen Combinations. The most common image receptor is a combination of intensifying screens that emit a specific color light and radiographic film that is sensitive to the same color. This matching of colors is called *spectral matching,* and it controls the efficiency of the image receptor. Using a mismatched combination results in an image receptor that does not make the greatest use of the incident x-ray photons. The careful selection of the correct film/screen combination is essential to good radiographic quality.

Image receptor efficiency is often described in terms of speed. A fast system requires less radiation to produce a certain radiographic density than does a slow system, but slower systems generally produce sharper images. System speed ratings are based on an arbitrary average **relative speed** of 100, and commonly range from 50 to 1200. The higher the relative speed number, the less radiation required to produce a given exposure or film density; however, the higher-speed film/screen combinations also produce an image with less recorded detail.

Processing. Inaccurate processing is responsible for destroying many carefully exposed radiographs. Processing errors that affect density generally fall into two major categories: (1) underdevelopment and (2) overdevelopment. Chemical changes in the film emulsion are responsible for changing the latent image into the resultant image. If the temperature of the chemical solutions is too hot, the density is increased, known as *chemical fog,* on the radiograph. If the temperature is too cool, film density is decreased as a result of insufficient chemical activity.

Automatic processing appears to be easy but in fact requires rigorous quality control to ensure consistent results. A difference of only 0.5 degree can produce a visible change in film density (see Table 7-1).

CONTRAST. The second photographic quality to be considered is *contrast.* Contrast is the visible difference between adjacent radiographic densities. An object may be accurately represented on a radiograph, but if it cannot be distinguished from the objects surrounding it, then the eye will not adequately appreciate the object. Proper contrast enhances the visibility of detail. Contrast can be understood by recalling the story of the little boy who was asked to draw a picture in art class. After laboring for some time, he presented a sheet of completely white paper to the teacher. The puzzled teacher asked what the picture was supposed to represent, to which the little boy replied, "It's a white horse eating marshmallows in a snowstorm." Of course, because no contrast existed between the different densities, the teacher failed to see the same image as the child.

Many factors affect contrast, including patient factors, kVp, mAs, beam modification, film/screen combinations, contrast media, and processing.

Kilovoltage Peak. Control of the penetrating ability of the radiographic beam allows the radiographer to manipulate radiographic contrast. More energy is required to penetrate bony tissue than soft tissue. For this reason, some technique charts are based on an optimal kVp level for a particular body part. *KVp is the chief controlling factor of contrast* (Table 7-2).

The terminology used to describe radiographic contrast can be confusing. *Contrast* is a comparison of all the various densities represented on a radiograph. These densities fall into a range from darkest to lightest gray. This range of gray tones is known as the *scale of contrast.* The

TABLE 7-2 Controlling and Influencing Factors of Contrast

CONTROLLING FACTOR	INFLUENCING FACTORS
Kilovoltage peak	Patient factors
	Milliampere seconds
	Beam modification
	Film/screen combinations
	Contrast media
	Processing

TABLE 7-3 Terms Used to Describe Contrast Relationships

FEW GRAY TONES	MANY GRAY TONES
Minimum to maximum relatively quickly	Minimum to maximum slowly
High contrast	Low contrast
Short-scale contrast	Long-scale contrast
Narrow latitude	Wide latitude
Lower kilovoltage peak value	Higher kilovoltage peak value

fewer gray tones exist, the greater the difference between individual densities will be. Consider the difference between maximum and minimum densities (D_{max} and D_{min}). In Fig. 7–6, if the 60-kVp strip goes from D_{max} to D_{min} in five steps, whereas the 120-kVp strip goes from D_{max} to D_{min} in more steps, the difference between the individual density steps in the 120-kVp strip will be less than that in the 60-kVp strip.

Radiographs with relatively few gray tones between D_{min} and D_{max} are said to possess *high contrast, short-scale contrast,* and *narrow latitude.* Radiographs with greater numbers of gray tones between D_{min} and D_{max} are said to possess *low contrast, long-scale contrast,* and *wide latitude.* Remember that contrast is a relative measure. No absolute standards of high or low contrast exist; only comparisons between radiographs can be made.

The effect of kVp on scale of contrast is that increasing kVp (the penetrating ability of the beam) lowers contrast. A higher-energy beam tends to penetrate everything in its path more easily and thus produces a wider range of gray tones. Table 7-3 outlines these relations.

Patient Factors. As described in the section on density, the tissues that make up the human body attenuate the beam of radiation to differing degrees. This differential attenuation is the basis for radiographic contrast. If two objects represented on a radiograph have similar tissue densities, then they produce similar radiographic densities, which is often the case in radiography of the abdominal organs. Distinguishing details within these similar densities would be difficult, which is an example of a body part with low subject contrast. Other body parts possess high subject contrast. In radiography of the chest, the bony tissue of the ribs has much greater tissue density than does the surrounding air-filled lung tissue. The resulting radiographic densities are therefore different and easily distinguishable.

Milliampere Seconds. Because mAs are responsible for the production of densities on the radiograph, they are considered to be a secondary influence on contrast. Changing mAs affects contrast by changing the relative density readings of minimum (underexposed) and maximum (overexposed); however, changing mAs has no effect on the penetrating ability of the beam. If an image is over- or underexposed, then contrast is affected. If exposure is maintained, then mAs will have no effect on the contrast of the image. *No increase in mAs or density can compensate for inadequate penetration.*

Beam Modification. Whether through filtration, collimation, or the use of grids, the purpose of beam modification is scatter control. Scattered radiation allowed to reach the film produces nondiagnostic densities referred to as *fog.* Removal of these fog densities results in the loss of some specific gray tones. Decreasing the number of gray tones, by definition, causes a move toward higher contrast. *Anything that decreases scatter increases contrast.*

Film/Screen Combinations. Screens and film are manufactured to produce a particular scale of contrast. Systems may be purchased to complement the inherent subject contrast of a particular area. Some common specialty systems include mammographic, chest, and extremity film/screen systems. In theory, the faster the system is, the higher the contrast will be. Film/screen system choices are made by department managers and radiologists and are often standard within a department.

Contrast Media. In areas of low subject contrast, enhancing the inherent contrast is sometimes possible through the use of contrast media. A *contrast medium* is a substance that attenuates the beam to a different degree than the surrounding tissue. Examples of contrast media used in radiography include barium and iodine compounds

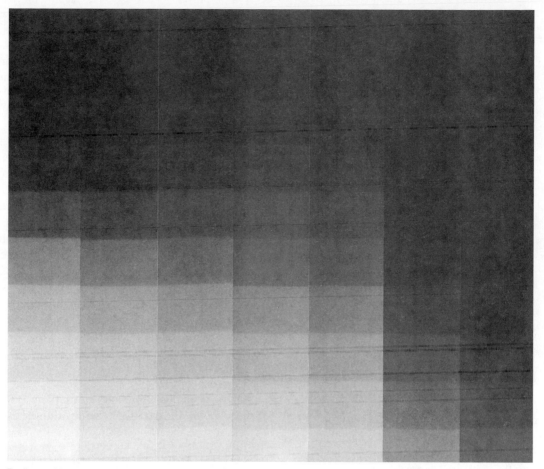

FIG. 7–6 Radiographic contrast is demonstrated with radiographs of step wedges at various kilovoltage peak settings to show variations in the number of shades of gray, also known as the *scale of contrast.*

and air. Filling the stomach and intestine with barium compound allows these structures to be visualized and examined radiographically. The kidneys filter an intravenous injection of iodine compound, allowing examination of the urinary tract as it is excreted. Because the contrast medium introduces an additional subject density to the body, technical factors, particularly kVp, must be adjusted for adequate penetration.

Processing. As previously discussed, inappropriate processing can necessitate that a carefully performed radiographic examination be repeated. Underdevelopment and overdevelopment change the range of visible densities on the finished image, which, in turn, degrades the radiographic contrast (see Table 7-2).

With digital image detector systems, the traditional relationship between the image quality properties of density and contrast to the exposure variables do not exist. Changing the exposure to the image receptor and having no effect on the density (brightness) or contrast on the monitor are possible. In digital image receptor systems, density and contrast are controlled primarily through postprocessing parameters. Despite this feature, the radiographer still must set proper exposure factors to create an acceptable image quality with a minimum of exposure to the patient.

Geometric Qualities

RECORDED DETAIL. The sharpness with which an object's borders and structural details are represented on an image is referred to as *recorded detail;* it is also described as *sharpness of detail, definition,* and **resolution.** Sharpness of detail is complemented by visibility of detail. Good radiographic quality requires a proper balance of the two.

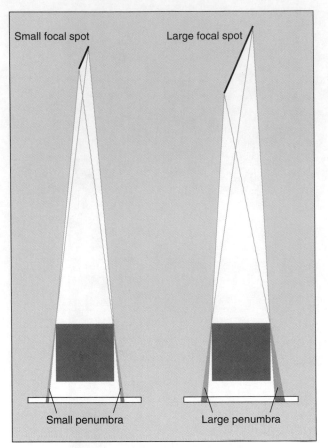

FIG. 7–7 Effective focal spot size.

The chief factors affecting recorded detail include motion, object unsharpness, focal spot size, SID, object-to-image detail (OID), and material unsharpness.

Motion. The most common cause of image unsharpness is motion. Patient motion may be voluntary or involuntary and is best controlled by short exposure times. Voluntary motion can be controlled by the use of careful instructions to the patient, suspension of patient respiration during exposure, short exposure times, and judicious use of appropriate immobilization devices. Involuntary motion, such as that caused by the heartbeat and the peristaltic movements of the intestines, is best controlled by the shortest exposure time possible. Equipment motion, such as the vibration of the tabletop during a table grid exposure, also can be decreased by the use of short exposure times.

Object Unsharpness. The fundamental problem in radiography, as in photography, is that of attempting to represent a three-dimensional object on a two-dimensional image. Objects that undergo radiography do not consist of straight edges and sharp angles. A basic unsharpness exists to the image of a three-dimensional object that cannot be eliminated. Lessening the effect of this inherent loss of detail is possible by adjusting the factors over which we have control: focal spot size, SID, and OID.

Focal Spot Size. Imagine the beam from a penlight-size flashlight. The light beam is relatively narrow and causes a sharp, well-defined shadow of an object placed in its path. Compare this shadow with that of the same object produced by a floodlight. If all the distances are the same, the image produced by the smaller source will be sharper than that produced by the larger source. In the x-ray tube, the width of the beam is controlled by the selection of the small or large focal spot. In general, the small focal spot is used when fine detail is required, as in radiography of small bones. The large focal spot is used for most general radiographic examinations. Fig. 7–7 illustrates how the focal spot size is controlled by the configuration of the x-ray tube target.

Source-to-Image Distance. In addition to its effect on the intensity of a beam of radiation, the distance from the focal spot to the image receptor is also a major influence on the size and sharpness of the image. Because a beam of radiation diverges from the source in the same fashion as light, the flashlight may again be used to illustrate the point. If an object is positioned close to a blank wall (the image receptor) and the flashlight is held at a distance from the object so that a shadow is visible, then a fuzzy border around the true shadow becomes obvious. The fuzzy border is called **penumbra,** and it obscures the true border, or **umbra.** If the flashlight is positioned closer to the object, as distance decreases, then the penumbra around the true shadow increases. If the flashlight is positioned farther from the object, then the penumbra decreases, causing the image to appear sharper (Fig. 7–8).

In radiography, the greater the SID, the better the recorded detail will be. Because radiographic rooms and equipment are not currently built to accommodate extremely long distances, SIDs are standardized so that the degree of penumbra is at least a known factor. The most common SID is 40 inches, but some procedures such as chest radiography use a 72-inch SID. Exceptions to these standards exist, but the SID of an examination should always be indicated to allow for calculation of image unsharpness.

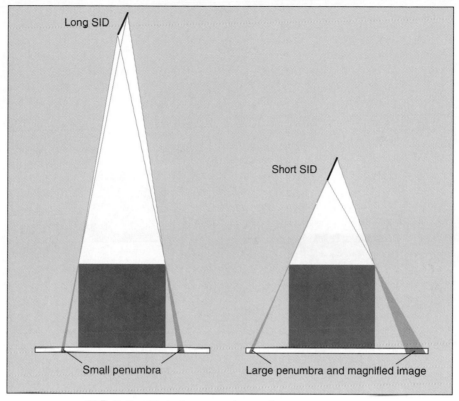

FIG. 7–8 Effect of source-to-image distance on sharpness.

Object-to-Image Distance. The flashlight experiment is used to observe what happens to penumbra when the OID is varied. When the object is moved closer to the image receptor, penumbra decreases, and image sharpness increases (Fig. 7–9). As the object is moved farther from the receptor, penumbra increases and sharpness decreases. Thus the smaller the OID is, the better the recorded detail will be. Many of the objects that must be radiographed are structures located deep within the body. Getting them close to the image receptor is often impossible. Therefore control over OID often depends on the radiographer's knowledge of anatomy and positioning.

Material Unsharpness. In addition to the inherent unsharpness of the objects that undergo radiography, the equipment that is used also contributes to the unsharpness of the image. Films and screens both have characteristics that affect their ability to represent an image accurately. Film/screen combinations must be carefully chosen to provide adequate recorded detail with consideration to patient dose. In general, faster systems produce greater unsharpness of detail but decrease patient dose.

By contrast, slower systems provide a greater degree of sharpness but at a higher patient dose.

DISTORTION. Distortion is the misrepresentation of the true size or shape of an object. Size distortion is commonly known as *magnification,* and shape distortion is sometimes referred to as *true distortion.*

Size Distortion. Magnification of the image is unavoidable but may be controlled to a certain extent by the use of proper exposure factors. The major influences on magnification are SID and OID.

The size of the image and the size of the light field covered by the flashlight vary with the distance from the source. If the distance decreases, magnification increases. Magnification decreases as SID increases (see Fig.7–8). The use of standardized SIDs allows the radiologist to assume that a specific magnification factor is present on all images. For this reason, noting any deviation from the standard SID is extremely important.

Varying the OID also influences the magnification of the resultant image. If a flashlight is kept at a standard

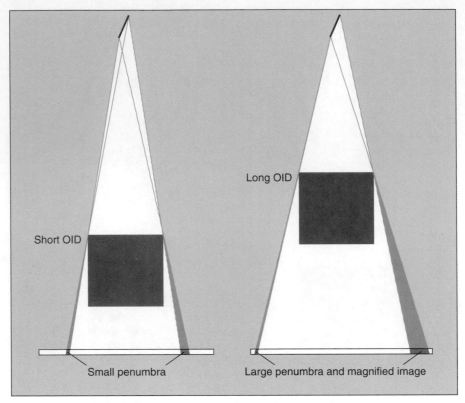

FIG. 7–9 Effect of object-to-image distance on sharpness.

distance and the object is moved closer to the receptor, the magnification of the image decreases. If the object is then moved farther from the receptor, magnification increases. Magnification decreases as OID decreases. In terms of recorded detail and magnification, the best image is produced with a small OID and a large SID (see Fig. 7–9).

Shape Distortion. The misrepresentation of the shape of radiographic image is called *shape distortion* or *true distortion*. It is controlled by the alignment of the beam, part, and image receptor. Influencing factors include *central ray angulation* and *body part rotation*.

The beam of radiation diverges from the source in an approximate pyramid shape (see Fig. 7–5). This divergence means that the photons in the center of the beam are traveling along the straightest pathway, and those at the beam's periphery are traveling at an angle. The straight, central portion of the beam is referred to as the **central ray.** The most accurate representation of an object results from the passage of photons in a straight line through the area of interest. This characteristic is the

reason for the emphasis on central ray entrance and exit points in positioning instructions.

When the central ray is angled, the relationships among the beam, part, and image receptor are altered. A sphere that is imaged by a straight perpendicular beam is represented as a circular image. An image of the same sphere, when imaged by an angled beam, appears as an oval. Objects may appear to be elongated or foreshortened (Fig. 7–10).

Because the structures of the body do not lie in exact 90-degree perpendicular relationships to one another, central ray angulation is used in many radiographic examinations to help demonstrate specific anatomic details.

Changing the orientation of the body part undergoing radiography also affects the relationship of the beam, object, and image receptor. If the object of interest is superimposed on another object, the resulting image is difficult to evaluate. By rotating or obliquing the body, the object of interest can be projected free from the interference of the overlying object. Frequently, a combination of part rotation and central ray angulation is used to best

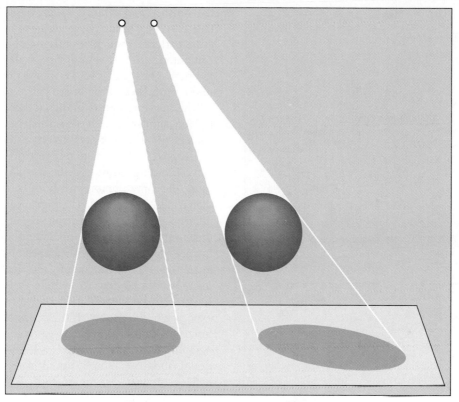

FIG. 7–10 Effect of central ray angulation.

demonstrate the anatomic details free from superimposition by overlying structures (Fig. 7–11). Ideally, the goal of a radiologic technologist is to place the anatomic part parallel to the image receptor and have the central ray aligned perpendicular to the image receptor.

FLUOROSCOPIC IMAGING

Fluoroscopic examinations often involve a combination of imaging processes. The fluoroscopic image itself is a **dynamic,** or moving, image rather than a **static** radiographic image. An analogy is that of a movie compared with a snapshot.

The fluoroscopic examination is usually divided into two portions: (1) viewing a physiologic event in real time (as it occurs) and (2) archiving images for later review. Modern fluoroscopic units are constructed so that the x-ray tube may be located either over or under the x-ray table. Opposite the tube is the image intensifier unit, a device that intercepts the attenuated beam as it exits the patient. The image intensifier is the actual image receptor in this case rather than the film image receptor previously described. When the x-ray photons reach the image intensifier, they are transformed into an electronic image. This image is then displayed on a television monitor for viewing. The radiologist is able to view a physiologic event (e.g., the passage of barium compound through the stomach) and observe abnormalities in function.

While observing the dynamic image, the radiologist frequently wishes to preserve an image as a record of the dynamic examination. A variety of image-archiving methods are available. Spot imaging is a common method of achieving this end. For spot images, the fluoroscopic unit changes instantaneously to radiographic mode for the duration of the exposure. An image receptor is placed in the image intensification device and is exposed to the remnant beam at the desired time. These spot images are then processed, viewed, and stored the same as with any other image. Roll or cut filming uses rolled or cut radiographic film of 70-, 90-, or 105-mm widths to record one image at a time in much the same fashion as with cassette spot imaging. The difference is that the roll or cut film is exposed by the light from the image intensifier tube image instead of from the fluoroscopic x-ray tube, which permits reduced total radiation dose to the

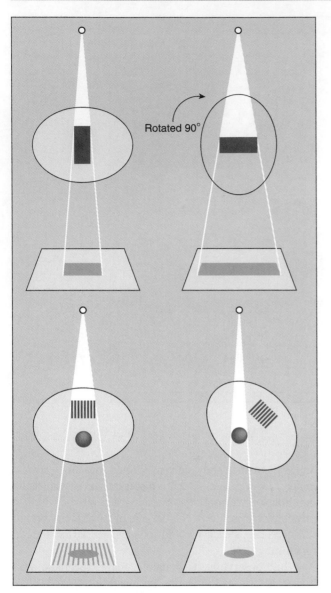

Rotated 90°

FIG. 7–11 Effect of body part rotation.

the finished radiograph. As previously indicated, mistakes in processing have ruined many radiographic examinations. In digital imaging, film is replaced by computerized sensing and storage devices as the image receptor. Thus processing errors do not affect the diagnostic properties of the image.

The image receptors in digital modalities operate in a fashion similar to that described for fluoroscopy. The attenuated beam of x-ray photons exits the patient and is intercepted by the image receptor device. These devices vary according to the specific imaging modality, but all cause the x-ray photon energy to be transformed into a digital electronic signal. This signal carries the diagnostic information and must be displayed for viewing and interpretation on cathode ray tube monitors. During viewing, the operator may change the appearance of the displayed image simply by instructing the computer as to how many shades of gray to include in the picture matrix. Images can be made darker or lighter, with no further exposure to the patient. If the operator wishes, an image from the cathode ray tube can be recorded on radiographic film to be stored as a hard copy record. Most examinations are simply stored in digital form on magnetic or optical disk or on tape. Storing the raw data allows the operator to recall the original information at a later date for further manipulation.

Digital imaging has been used in computed tomography, as well as in imaging modalities that do not use x-radiation, such as ultrasonography, nuclear medicine, and magnetic resonance imaging, for many years. Digital subtraction angiography is another application of digital x-ray technology. It uses digital computer imaging to record and manipulate radiographic images produced by a fluoroscopic unit, usually as part of an angiographic procedure. Digital radiography systems allow filmless imaging in all aspects of diagnostic radiography. These systems use photo stimuable plates that, when struck by an incident beam of x-radiation, store a latent image. Following stimulation by laser, the screens emit light that is then detected by photomultiplier tubes. The photomultipliers change the light into an electronic signal, which is the digital image. Digital imaging has become increasingly common and affordable for all aspects of radiography. The replacement of film as the primary recording medium continues to revolutionize the field of radiography.

patient. The film is then developed and mounted for viewing and storage. Today, digital fluoroscopy is replacing traditional filming and allowing for easy manipulation of the fluoroscopic images after they are converted to a digital signal.

DIGITAL IMAGING

With the advent of computerized medical technology, diagnostic imaging is advancing toward a filmless system. In the traditional image chain, a wide range of problems may occur at any point between the patient exposure and

SUMMARY

A radiograph of good quality must possess a proper balance of photographic properties (density and contrast)

and geometric properties (recorded detail and distortion). Of the many factors contributing to radiographic quality, the radiographer must be able to manipulate technical factors such as mAs, kVp, and SID; choose and operate appropriate imaging equipment and accessories; and use proper positioning and patient care skills to obtain a high-quality diagnostic radiograph. Most diagnostic radiographic examinations use some combination of film/screen imaging, fluoroscopic imaging, and digital imaging. Advances in digital imaging technology have allowed a move away from film as the primary recording medium.

BIBLIOGRAPHY

Burns EF: *Radiographic imaging: a guide for producing quality radiographs*, Philadelphia, 1992, WB Saunders.

Bushong S: *Radiologic science for technologists*, ed 8, St Louis, 2004, Mosby.

Carlton R, Adler A: *Principles of radiographic imaging: an art and a science*, ed 4, Albany, NY, 2006, Delmar Publishers.

Carroll Q: *Fuchs' principles of radiographic exposure, processing and quality control*, ed 7, Springfield, Ill, 2003, Charles C Thomas.

Cullinan AM: *Producing quality radiographs*, Philadelphia, 1994, JB Lippincott.

DeVos DC: *Basic principles of radiographic exposure*, ed 2, Philadelphia, 1995, Lea & Febiger.

Lauer OG, Mayes JB, Thurston RP: *Evaluating radiographic quality: the variables and their effects*, Mankato, Minn, 1990, Burnell Company Publishers.

8

Radiographic and Fluoroscopic Equipment

Thomas Wolfe, MSRS, RT(R)

Radiographic equipment is only a link in a system of which the end purpose is to make available a record . . . for interpretation by the physician. . . . A system is only as strong as its weakest link . . . the radiographer must understand the x-ray equipment to operate it properly.

Thomas Thompson
A Practical Approach to Modern Imaging Equipment, *1985*

OBJECTIVES

On completion of this chapter, the student will be able to:

1. Explain radiographic equipment manipulation.

2. List the generic components of a radiographic system.

3. Locate the x-ray tube in a radiographic room.

4. Describe the purpose of the collimator and its importance in radiation protection.

5. Describe the various types of radiographic tables and how they are operated.

6. Identify the major controls on the radiographic system control console.

7. Describe the various types of radiographic tube stands and how they are manipulated.

8. Describe the various planes of x-ray tube movement and how they are controlled.

9. Explain the purpose of the upright wall Bucky system and cassette holder.

10. Discuss the concept of alignment of the various radiographic system components.

11. Describe the movement of the fluoroscopic tower.

12. Describe the two major types of mobile systems.

GLOSSARY

Anode: positive electrode of the x-ray tube

Bucky Mechanism: grid that is an integral part of the x-ray table, located below the tabletop and above a cassette tray; decreases the amount of scatter radiation reaching the image receptor, which increases contrast; moves during exposure so that no grid lines appear on the image

Cassette: light-proof holder for the image receptor; for computed radiography, the cassette holds the reusable photostimulable phosphor imaging plate; for conventional film-screen radiography, the cassette contains intensifying screens and a sheet of film

Cathode: negative electrode of the x-ray tube

Collimator: diaphragm or system of diaphragms made of an absorbing material; designed to define the dimensions and direction of a beam of radiation

Fluoroscope: device used for dynamic radiographic examinations; usually consists of an x-ray tube situated underneath the x-ray table and an electronic image intensifier situated over the x-ray table

Fluoroscopy: examination by means of the fluoroscope

Longitudinal: lengthwise; along the long axis

Spot Film Device: equipment that permits the acquisition of static images during a dynamic fluoroscopic examination

Transverse: placed crosswise; situated at right angles to the long axis of a part

Tube Angulation: pivoting the tube at the point where it is attached to its support

Vertical: perpendicular to the plane of the horizon

X-ray Tube: device that produces x-rays

MANIPULATION OF RADIOGRAPHIC EQUIPMENT

A primary role of a radiographer is the manipulation of expensive, high-technology x-ray equipment. The new student must learn to master the mechanical aspects of a radiographic examination early. Becoming as comfortable as possible with the maneuvering of the x-ray equipment is important. Once this task is accomplished, the beginning radiographer can concentrate on learning to master other important skills, such as patient care, positioning, technique selection, and image quality. Generally speaking, the earlier a student masters the essential skills of equipment manipulation, the more success he or she will have in the other professional aspects of radiography. On the other hand, a student who does not learn to handle the x-ray equipment early on will have trouble moving on to advanced skills.

Generic Components

The first step in mastering equipment manipulation is being able to identify the generic components of a radiographic system. A beginning radiographer who has visited a radiology department can be overwhelmed by how different each radiography room appears. The differences are similar to those found in automobiles, which are manufactured with seemingly endless variations in outward appearance. Different models, sizes, body styles, dashboard layouts, and instruments are available; however, each one has a motor, steering column, brake

pedal, speedometer, fuel gauge, and so forth. The same is true of different types of radiographic equipment. They appear different in shape, size, and layout, but they all have common components. The new student should be able to visit different x-ray rooms at their clinical sites and identify these generic (common) components: x-ray tube, collimator, x-ray table, control console, and tube stand (Fig. 8–1).

X-Ray Tube

The **x-ray tube** is the part of the radiographic system that produces the x-rays. It is made of glass and is encased in a sturdy metal housing, which is usually a cylinder with a large electrical cable attached at each end. The x-ray tube's primary components are the **anode** and the **cathode** (see Fig. 9–1). A tube stand supports the x-ray tube and allows the radiographer to position it as needed over and around the patient.

Electrical energy is supplied to the x-ray tube through the two large electrical cables. The tube converts this electrical energy into x-rays and heat in a manner similar to energy conversion in a light bulb. Electrical energy that is supplied to a light bulb is converted into light and heat. With an x-ray tube, the radiographer controls the number and energy of the x-rays produced by adjusting the amount of electrical energy going into the tube. This adjustment is made at the radiographic system's control console.

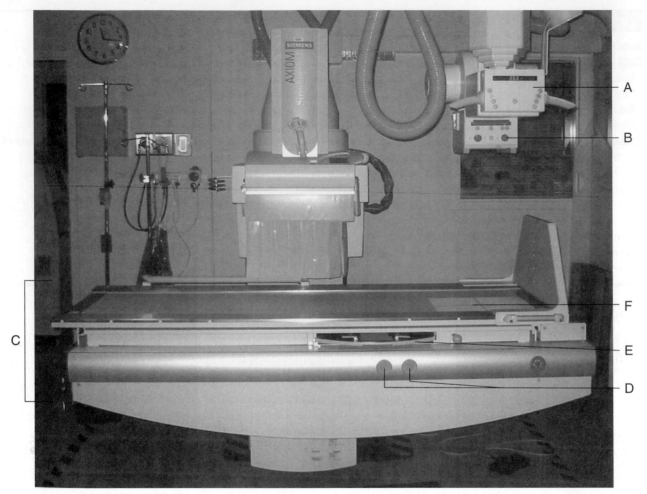

FIG. 8–1 The generic components of diagnostic radiographic equipment include the x-ray tube (A), collimator (B), radiographic table (C), top and tilt controls (D), Bucky tray for cassette (E), and moving tabletop (F). The tube is suspended from an overhead tube stand, and the control console is behind a leaded wall.

Collimator

Attached directly below the x-ray tube is an x-ray beam–limiting device called a **collimator** (Fig. 8–2). The collimator controls the size and shape of the x-ray field coming out of the x-ray tube. The radiographer determines the size of the x-ray field by adjusting two controls on the front or sides of the collimator, one for the length and one for the width of the rectangular x-ray field.

These controls move lead shutters or plates that block a portion of the x-ray beam. As an aid to adjusting the size of the x-ray beam, the operator uses a light source to project a representation of the x-ray field onto the patient. The radiographer turns on this collimator light so that the size of the x-ray field corresponds to the anatomic part to be radiographed. The collimator light automatically shuts off after a short time. Many radiographers refer to collimators as *shutters* and the act of adjusting the collimator as *coning* or *collimating*. The use of these words as verbs, for example, "I'm going to collimate [or cone] on the lateral projection," always indicates decreasing the size of the x-ray field.

Most x-ray machines are equipped with an automatic collimation system known as *positive beam limitation*. This feature allows the x-ray unit to detect the size of the image receptor the radiographer is using and automatically limit the x-ray field size to that size to minimize patient dose. Federal law no longer requires a positive beam limitation system, but permitting the x-ray beam to expose patient

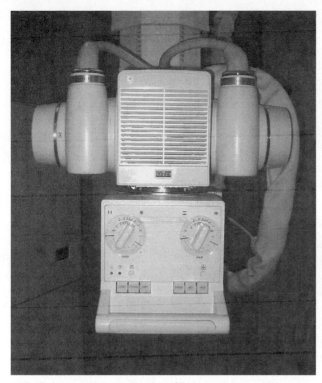

FIG. 8–2 X-ray tube collimator with control switches is used for various tube movements. The two round dials control the lead shutters of the collimator.

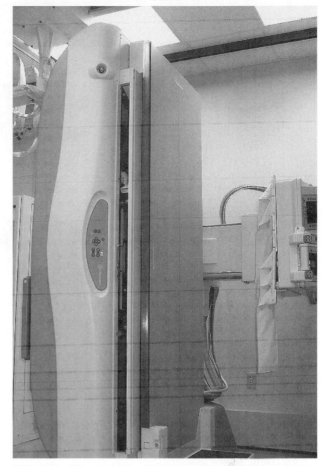

FIG. 8–3 Tilting tabletop in the upright (vertical) position is shown. Attached footboard is noted.

tissue without creating an image remains a violation of federal standards. For example, collimating to a 12 × 12-inch area when using an image receptor that is only 10 × 12 inches is against the federal standards. Most collimators are also equipped with a tape to measure the distance from the tube to the image receptor.

X-Ray Table

The x-ray table is the most obvious and recognizable component of the radiographic system. The size, shape, and location of the controls for the tables vary from manufacturer to manufacturer. X-ray tables are classified as tilting or nontilting, free-floating or stationary top, and adjustable or nonadjustable height.

Tilting tables are available in basically two types. A 90-90 table can tilt from the horizontal position to a complete vertical position in either direction. A 90-30 table can tilt to a complete vertical position in one direction and to a 30-degree tilt in the other direction. A footboard is usually attached to a tilting tabletop for patient safety. A tabletop in the upright position with a footboard

attached is shown in Fig. 8–3. Table tilt is controlled by a switch located at table or floor level on the long side of the table. The switch is usually depressed in the direction of the desired tilt. Keeping the switch depressed tilts the table to its maximal permitted degree of tilt. Releasing the switch stops the tilting action, allowing the radiographer to set the table to any desired angle. Both tilting and nontilting tables may have additional features, including a moving tabletop, a cassette tray (often called a *Bucky tray*), and a group of buttons or switches for tabletop movement and tilt control (see Fig. 8–1).

Most x-ray tables have movable tabletops that may be motorized or free-floating. Most of these tables can be moved in two directions so the radiographer can move the tabletop rather than the patient. Floating tabletops have a switch that controls a locking mechanism. If the mechanism is turned off, then the radiographer can move the top manually. Motorized tops have switches that drive

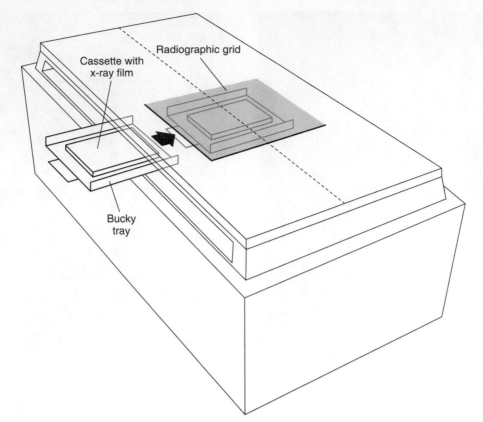

FIG. 8–4   Bucky tray holding a cassette is shown. The Bucky tray is centered to the x-ray tube underneath a radiographic grid.

the tabletop in the direction desired. The controls for the tabletop or table tilt are usually located at the end or center of the working side of the x-ray table.

The **Bucky mechanism** is located directly beneath the tabletop and is designed to hold the x-ray cassette (image receptor) stationary and to keep it centered to the x-ray tube. It also serves as the holder for the radiographic grid, which is positioned underneath the tabletop so that it forms a top to the Bucky tray when it is pushed completely into the table (Fig. 8–4). The tray is pulled out from the table, and the cassette is placed in the tray and locked into place. The Bucky mechanism can be manually moved the entire length of the table and then locked into place. A beginning radiographer should take time to practice operating the various x-ray tables and Bucky trays before attempting to position any patients.

Control Console

The control console of a radiographic system is similar to the cockpit of an airplane. It is the device that gives the operator command of the x-ray machine. Accordingly, the control console is one of the most complicated components of the radiographic imaging system. The first encounter with an unfamiliar control console can be intimidating even for an experienced technologist. Tremendous variation exists in how control consoles appear between manufacturers and even between different models from the same manufacturer. Control consoles have evolved from basic knobs, push buttons, switches, and meters to sophisticated computer screens with digital readouts. Most radiology departments have a variety of control consoles from different manufacturers (Fig. 8–5).

One of the first hands-on tasks a beginning radiographer may be asked to perform is to set the proper exposure factors on the control console. The console has five generic controls that the new student must learn: the main power, kilovoltage peak (kVp), milliamperage (mA), timer, and rotor-exposure switch. The selection of kVp, mA, and time is collectively referred to as *technique selection*. On many units, mA and time are combined into a factor known as *milliampere seconds* (mAs), which is simply mA multiplied by time in seconds.

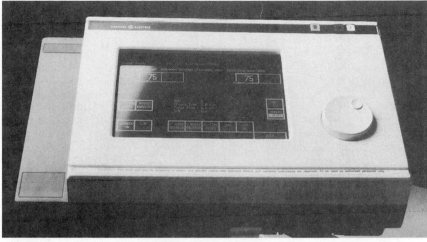

FIG. 8–5 Example of a radiographic control console is shown. (Courtesy General Electric Medical Systems.)

POWER. The first challenge when encountering an unfamiliar control console is how to turn on the x-ray machine. The main power switch supplies power to the radiographic system. Turning the power on does not activate x-ray production. The power device should be clearly marked on the control console and is usually either a switch or a push-button device. Some x-ray units require power to be activated both at the control console and at a main power box equipped with a high-voltage circuit breaker.

KILOVOLTAGE PEAK. One kilovolt is equal to 1000 volts. The kVp indicates the amount of voltage selected for supply to the x-ray tube and can range from 30 to 150 kVp. Some control consoles have major and minor kVp controls. The major kVp control allows the radiographer to change kVp settings in increments of 10 (i.e., 50, 60, 70, 80 kVp). The minor kVp control allows the radiographer to select smaller increments of 1 or 2 kVp. For example, if 85 kVp is selected, the major kVp knob is set to 80 kVp, and the minor kVp knob is set at 5 kVp. The total is then 85 kVp. Newer control consoles have digital readouts in which major and minor kVp settings are obtained with one selector, similar to changing channels on a television set with a digital remote control. The actual selection control may be a touch button or panel, a touch-screen on a computer, or a dial (Fig. 8–6). On digital readout units, these controls may simply be arrows going up and down or left and right. The exposure factor is decreased by a down or left arrow and increased by an up or right arrow (Fig. 8–7).

MILLIAMPERAGE. One mA is equal to one thousandth of an ampere. It indicates the amount of current supplied

kVp

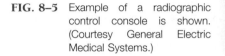

A

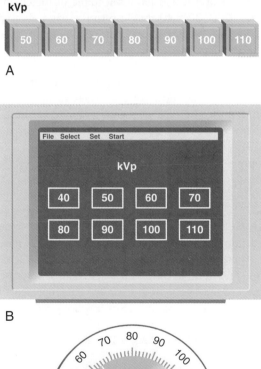

B

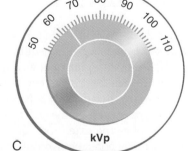

C

FIG. 8–6 Radiographic console selection controls may be touch buttons or panels (A), computer touch-screen (B), or dials (C).

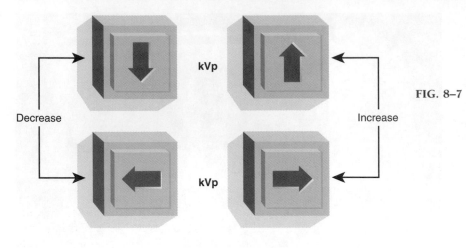

FIG. 8–7 Selection controls may be up and down arrows or left and right arrows. The factor is decreased with a down or left arrow. The factor is increased with an up or right arrow.

to the x-ray tube. Control consoles range from 10 to 1200 mA. The mA is usually selectable in increments of 100 (i.e., 200, 300, 400 mA) up to the maximum value. Most routine diagnostic radiography is done between 100 and 400 mA.

TIME. By selecting a time setting in seconds, the radiographer determines how long x-rays will be produced. Depending on the type of equipment, time settings can range from 0.001 to 6 seconds, often in increments of at least 25% (i.e., 0.1, 0.13, 0.16, 0.2, 0.25, 0.5). For example, increasing the time setting from 0.2 second to the next highest setting of 0.25 sec is a 25% increase in time.

MILLIAMPERE SECONDS. Some radiographic imaging systems do not permit independent selection of mA and time. These units use a control that combines these two factors. The number of mAs is calculated by multiplying the mA chosen by the time selected. This represents how many x-rays will be produced for how long. For example,

$$100 \text{ mA} \times 0.2 \text{ second} = 20 \text{ mAs}$$

EXPOSURE. After the x-ray exposure factors are selected and the patient, x-ray tube, and other equipment for the examination are all properly prepared, an exposure can be made. The device that begins the exposure is called the *rotor-exposure switch.* It is usually a hand-held push button or trigger-type switch connected to the control console by a telephone-type extension cord. The rotor-exposure switch actually contains two different switches that are mechanically interlocked so that one must be activated before the other. The first switch that is activated is the rotor, or *prep,* switch. The rotor switch causes

the anode to rotate and prepares the x-ray tube for the exposure factors that have been selected. The preparation process usually takes 1 to 2 seconds. After the tube is properly prepared, the second switch is activated to begin the exposure. A timer automatically ends the exposure. According to federal regulations, the termination of the exposure must be indicated both audibly and visually.

Activating the rotor-exposure switch is a skill that the beginning radiographer must master early. One common mistake that beginning students make is to start the exposure too soon before the rotor switch has done its job. The x-ray machine will not allow the exposure until the x-ray tube is ready. The beginner must develop a feeling for the rotor switch and try not to initiate the exposure switch until this tube preparation process is complete. Many manufacturers recommend complete depression of both switches simultaneously. This procedure allows the exposure to occur as soon as the tube is ready. All units include electronic interlocking circuits that prevent an exposure from occurring until the rotor has reached full speed. The rotor speed can be heard immediately before the *ready* light comes on in most units.

Another common error for the new student is releasing the exposure switch too quickly. This action ends the exposure too soon and is especially a problem with longer exposure times. To avoid ending the exposure too soon, the student must get into the habit of not releasing the exposure switch until the audible tone or light message indicates that the timer has terminated the exposure.

Tube Stands

The tube stand is the device that supports and permits the x-ray tube to be moved in different directions. Many types of tube stands are available. The floor-mounted tube stand has a steel column that runs along a track on the floor. A floor-to-ceiling or floor-to-wall system has a second track that runs along the wall or ceiling. An overhead suspension system has the x-ray tube attached to an overhead track that runs between rails on the ceiling. Another type has the tube attached and integrated with the table (Fig. 8–8).

The basic tube movements that the beginning radiographer must master are longitudinal, transverse, vertical, and tube angulation (Fig. 8–9). These basic movements can usually be accomplished with most tube stands, but they differ significantly in the degree of movement permitted. The directions of tube travel are given from the position of the technologist at the side of the x-ray table. **Longitudinal** travel is moving the x-ray tube lengthwise to the technologist's left or right or toward the patient's head or feet. **Transverse** travel is moving the tube at right angles across the table, in other words, moving the tube toward or away from the technologist or from right to left over the patient. **Vertical** travel is moving the tube up toward the ceiling or down toward the floor. **Tube angulation** is pivoting the tube at the point where it is attached to its support. For example, angulating the tube that is facing the tabletop to a position in which it is facing a wall is a 90-degree tube angulation.

Controls for Tube Movement

Most x-ray tube housings have a set of handlebars that are located between the x-ray tube and the collimator. The radiographer grips the handlebars and releases the appropriate locks to move the x-ray tube in the direction desired. For the longitudinal, transverse, vertical, and tube angulation movements, a corresponding switch is located between or on the handlebars; each switch locks or unlocks the corresponding movement. For example, if the radiographic system is energized and all the tube movement switches are in the locked position, then the tube cannot be moved. If the vertical switch is moved to the unlocked position, then the tube can be moved toward the ceiling or the floor. Locks for each of the tube movements are controlled independently, allowing the operator to make adjustments in one plane at a time. Some units also have a single switch that takes all the locks off. It is extremely important not to force the movement of the tube with the locks on. If the tube does not move easily, the proper lock must be released. A beginning radiographer should get a feel for x-ray tube movement by practicing moving, aligning and locking the tube before attempting any radiographic procedures. Patients may quickly lose confidence in a student's abilities if they observe difficulty in handling a simple task such as moving the x-ray tube.

In addition to the electrical locks, x-ray tubes can have manual locks. The tube stand that is attached to an overhead track allows rotation of the tube around the vertical tube column (Fig. 8–10). A manual lock that is released by hand often controls these movements.

Wall-Mounted Bucky System and Cassette Holders

Many radiographic rooms have a special unit that allows the technologist to obtain radiographs of standing patients. The two primary devices are a simple wall-mounted **cassette** holder and a wall-mounted Bucky system.

A simple wall-mounted cassette holder is a mechanical device that allows the radiographer to place a cassette in an adjustable holder. The cassette holder mechanism is attached to a two-rail system that permits the cassette to move up and down. A locking mechanism controlled by a knob secures the cassette at the appropriate height (Fig. 8–11).

A wall-mounted Bucky unit is similar to a miniature table that is attached to the wall. It has a surface similar to a tabletop. Beneath this surface is a Bucky mechanism. The tray is manually pulled out, and the cassette is placed in the tray and locked into place. The entire Bucky mechanism can be manually moved after releasing a locking mechanism that permits the radiographer to move it along a vertical plane. A control knob or lever operates a manual locking mechanism that permits vertical movement. Wall-mounted Bucky units typically permit only vertical movement, although some units can be tilted into a horizontal position for radiography of the head and extremities.

Alignment Concepts

The major responsibility of the radiographer is proper manipulation of the various components of the radiographic system to provide a quality image or radiograph of the anatomic area of interest. This task is accomplished by proper alignment of the various components of the radiographic system to that anatomic area of interest. The concept of proper alignment is important to the student radiographer. The x-ray tube, tabletop, and Bucky mechanism all move separately. The student must quickly learn to align the x-ray tube with the center of the cassette within the center of the Bucky tray; otherwise, a quality image will not be produced. Students often center the

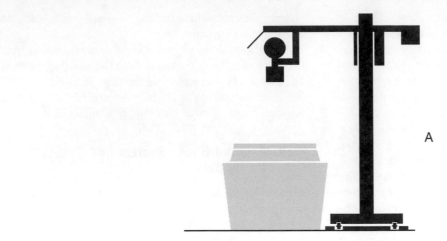
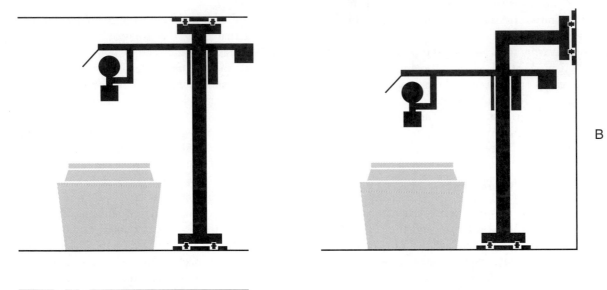
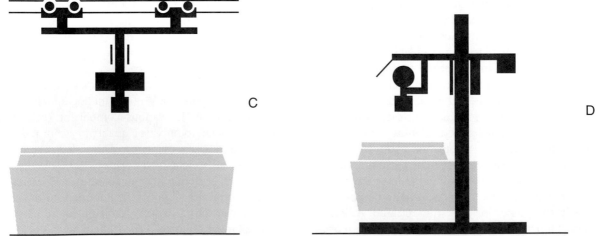

FIG. 8–8 Tube stands include those that are floor mounted *(A)*, floor to wall or ceiling *(B)*, overhead suspension *(C)*, and table supported *(D)*.

x-ray tube and then, while positioning the patient, move the tube. To avoid this error, the new student should approach the x-ray table and center the tabletop. The x-ray tube should then be centered over the table, locked transversely, and kept locked. After centering the tabletop, the student radiographer should leave it locked on center and manually move the patient. Moving tabletops are advantageous to experienced radiographers and patients in pain, but they can lead to errors for beginning radiographers.

X-ray tables used for direct digital radiography do not have a Bucky tray. The image receptor is mounted underneath the tabletop and does not need to be changed after each exposure. The image receptor moves longitudinally to stay lined up to the tube. As a result, the radiographer does not have to be concerned with tube-Bucky alignment along the longitudinal axis.

MANIPULATION OF FLUOROSCOPIC EQUIPMENT

The equipment discussed so far produces static images. Radiographs provide an image of anatomic structures at a given time. They are not designed for the study of structures that are in motion. The presentation of a continuous or dynamic radiographic image is referred to as **fluoroscopy.**

A **fluoroscope** appears similar to a radiographic system but with some additional equipment components (Fig. 8–12). Added to the table is an image-intensification unit and another x-ray tube located under the table. During fluoroscopy, the radiologist moves the image intensifier over the patient. The x-ray tube usually is located under the table and moves with the image intensifier as part of a device called the *fluoroscopy carriage.* As the radiologist moves the entire unit and activates the x-ray tube, a dynamic image is displayed on a television monitor.

When the image-intensification unit is not in use, it can be *parked* out of the way to allow the radiographer to perform routine radiography with the overhead x-ray tube. The beginning radiographer should learn how to move the image intensifier to a safe position to perform fluoroscopic procedures and to move it out of the way to perform radiographic procedures using the overhead x-ray tube. The unit usually has an interlock switch that allows the radiographer to move the image intensifier transversely from a parked position. The units are extremely fragile and expensive and must be handled carefully. Some image intensifiers are designed to shift back enough to clear the area directly over the patient for

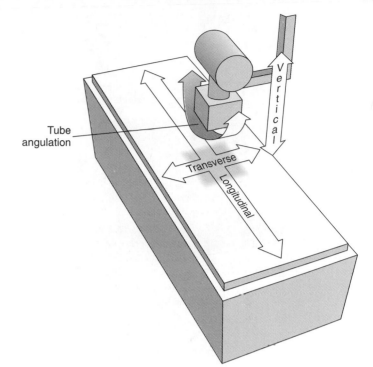

FIG. 8–9 The basic movements of a typical diagnostic radiographic tube stand are longitudinal, transverse, vertical, and tube angulation.

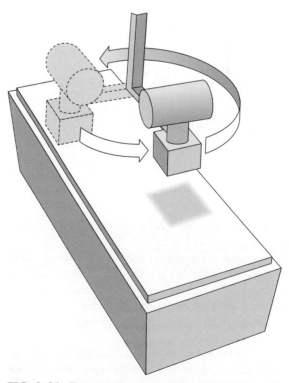

FIG. 8–10 Tube rotation around the vertical tube column is shown.

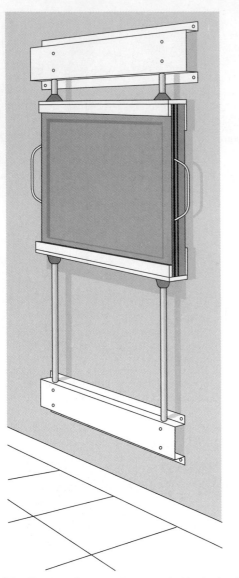

FIG. 8–11   Simple wall-mounted cassette holder is visualized.

film device contains a mechanical conveyor that accepts a variety of cassette sizes. The cassette is placed in a conveyor and automatically transfers to its parked position behind a lead shield outside the radiation field. When the radiologist makes a radiographic exposure, the conveyor moves the cassette from its protected position into the exposure field. The x-ray tube under the table exposes the cassette. The cassette then is removed for processing or returned by the conveyor to its parked position for additional exposures. Depending on the equipment, exposure formats vary. The formats range from a single exposure on the entire cassette to a series of exposures (as many as 12) on different parts of the image receptor. Most spot images are one on one (the entire image receptor as one image), two on one (the image receptor is divided horizontally or vertically to form two images), or four on one (the image receptor is divided into quarters to form four images).

Many new fluoroscopic towers are designed for digital fluoroscopy. These towers permit the electronic acquisition of spot images. Images recorded this way are stored in a computer, where they can be viewed on a monitor or printed to film. Cassettes are not needed for spot radiography with digital fluoroscopy machines.

MANIPULATION OF MOBILE EQUIPMENT

Taking radiographic equipment to the patient is often necessary. This location may be at the patient's bedside, in the surgical suite, or in the emergency department. Numerous types of mobile radiographic and mobile fluoroscopic x-ray systems are available (Fig. 8–14).

These systems are similar in components and manipulation principles to the equipment located in the radiology department. Although many units are motor driven, many must be physically pushed. A beginning radiographer should practice moving the mobile radiographic and fluoroscopic equipment until a measure of ability has been achieved. As with stationary units, practicing the various tube movements and their mechanical or electric interlocks is important.

SUMMARY

A beginning radiographer can be overwhelmed by the initial complexity of radiographic and fluoroscopic equipment. New students need to master the components of the radiographic system and how they operate. Familiarity with the x-ray tube, collimator, x-ray table, control console, and tube stand is important. The mechanical aspects of collimation, control console

the overhead x-ray tube. These units do not have to be removed from the fluoroscopic carriage for storage.

Once put into position over the table, the image intensifier can be moved in all planes with a handlebar-type switch that works similar to a joystick on a computer. Moving the handlebar switch in one direction causes the entire carriage (both image intensifier and x-ray tube) to move as one.

A major component of the fluoroscopy tower is the spot film device (Fig. 8–13). The **spot film device** permits the radiologist to obtain static radiographs during a dynamic fluoroscopic examination. The spot

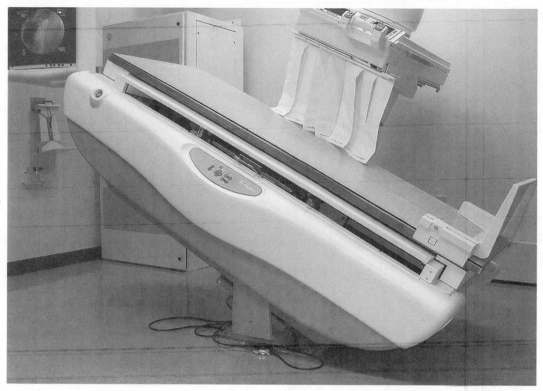

FIG. 8–12 Radiographic and fluoroscopic unit is set up for fluoroscopy. The x-ray tube is underneath the table, in alignment with the image intensifier.

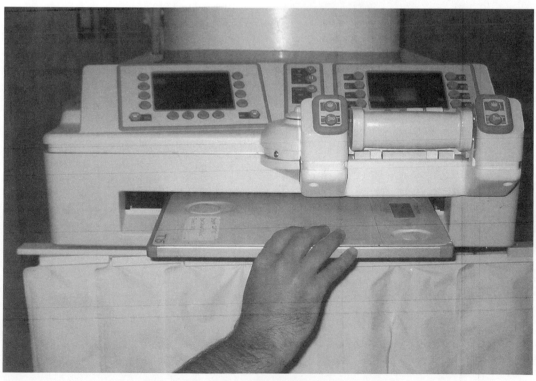

FIG. 8–13 Fluoroscopic spot film device is shown.

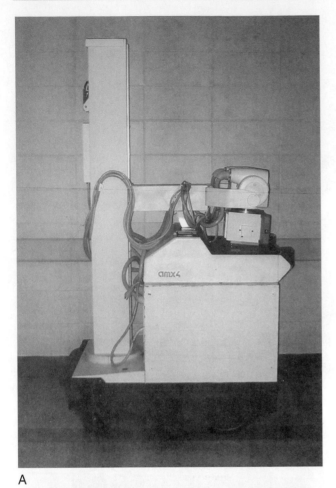

A

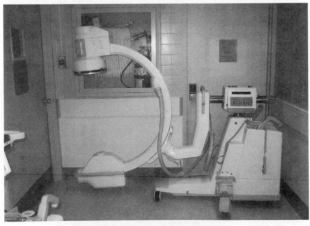

B

FIG. 8–14 Mobile units include radiographic *(A)* and fluoroscopic C-arm *(B)*.

operation, and the manipulation of the Bucky mechanism, tube stand, table, and image intensifier are essential skills that must be mastered early by a beginning radiographer. The student must become as comfortable as possible with the mechanical aspects of the x-ray examination process. Students who do well in the clinical aspects of radiography are those who master the mechanics of equipment manipulation early on.

BIBLIOGRAPHY

Bushong SC: *Radiologic science for technologists,* ed 8, St Louis, 2004, Mosby.

Carlton R, Adler AM: *Principles of radiographic imaging: an art and a science,* ed 4, Albany, NY, 2006, Thomson Delmar Learning.

Curry TS, Dowdey JF, Murray RC: *Christensen's introduction to the physics of diagnostic radiology,* ed 4, Philadelphia, 1990, Lippincott, Williams & Wilkins.

Forester E: *Equipment for diagnostic radiography,* Boston, 1985, MTP Press.

Paterson A, Thornton M, Carter PH: *Chesney's equipment for student radiographers,* ed 4, Boston, 1994, Blackwell Scientific Publications.

Seeram E: *X-ray imaging equipment,* Springfield, Ill, 1985, Charles C Thomas.

Sprawls P: *Principles of radiography for technologists,* Rockville, Md, 1990, Aspen Publications.

Stockley SM: *A manual of radiographic equipment,* New York, 1986, Churchill Livingstone.

Basic Radiation Protection and Radiobiology

Sandy L. Piehl, MPA, RT(R)(T)

Today I was reading about Marie Curie: she must have known she suffered from radiation sickness. She died a famous woman denying her wounds, denying her wounds that came from the same source as her power.

Adrienne Rich
"Power," The Dream of a Common Language: Poems 1974-1977

OBJECTIVES

On completion of this chapter, the student will be able to:

1. Identify the sources of ionizing radiation.

2. Describe the units used to measure radiation exposure.

3. Describe the nature of ionizing radiation.

4. Explain the ways in which ionizing radiation interacts with matter.

5. List the permissible limits of exposure for occupational and nonoccupational workers.

OBJECTIVES—Cont'd

6. Explain the reason for the varying sensitivity of body cells to ionizing radiation.

7. Describe the ways in which the entire body responds to varying amounts of radiation.

8. Discuss the various methods used to protect the patient from excessive radiation.

9. Discuss the various methods used to protect an occupational worker from excessive radiation.

10. Describe several devices used to detect and measure exposure to ionizing radiation.

GLOSSARY

ALARA: mnemonic meaning to keep all radiation exposure as low as reasonably achievable

Becquerel (Bq): unit of radioactivity in the International System of Units, equal to one disintegration per second

Classic Coherent Scattering: interaction with matter in which a low-energy photon (below 10 kiloelectron volts) is absorbed and released with its same energy, frequency, and wavelength but with a change of direction

Compton Effect (Scattering): interaction with matter in which a higher-energy photon strikes a loosely bound outer electron, removing it from its shell, and the remaining energy is released as a scattered photon

Curie (Ci): unit of radioactivity defined as the quantity of any radioactive nuclide in which the number of disintegrations per second is 3.7×10^{10}

Germ Cell: cell of an organism whose function it is to reproduce its kind (e.g., ovum, spermatozoon)

Gray (Gy): unit in the International System used to measure the amount of energy absorbed in any medium; 1 Gy = 100 radiation absorbed doses

International System (SI) Units: system of units based on metric measurement developed in 1948 used to measure radiation

Kiloelectron Volt (keV): unit of energy equal to 1000 electron volts

Pair Production: interaction between matter and a photon possessing a minimum of 1.02 million electron volts of energy producing two oppositely charged particles, a positron and a negatron

Photoelectric Effect: interaction with matter in which a photon strikes an inner shell electron, causing its ejection from orbit with the complete absorption of the photon's energy

Radiation: forms of energy emitted and transferred through matter

Radiation Absorbed Dose (Rad): unit used to measure the amount of energy absorbed in any medium; equal to 100 ergs of energy absorbed in 1 g of material

Radiation Equivalent Man (Rem): unit of dose equivalence; equal to the product of absorbed dose in rads and a quality factor

Roentgen (R): a unit of exposure in air; that quantity of x-radiation or gamma radiation that produces the quantity 2.08×10^9 ion pairs per cubic centimeter of air

Sievert (Sv): unit in the International System used to measure the dose equivalence, or biologic effectiveness, of differing radiations; 1 Sv = 100 rems

Somatic Cell: all of the body's cells except germ cells

X-ray: a form of electromagnetic radiation traveling at the speed of light, with the ability to penetrate matter

IONIZING RADIATION

Whenever a radiographer is applying ionizing radiation to produce a diagnostic image for the radiologist, he or she should remember the great responsibility this carries. Exposure to radiation always involves a risk of biologic changes that cannot be ignored. The benefits of improved diagnosis of disease outweigh the risk, however, as long as the radiographer is using sound judgment and always works to minimize the quantity of radiation the patient receives. The radiographer also must act to protect all persons who come in contact with radiation from any unnecessary exposure. This group includes himself or herself, the patient, and anyone else.

Sources of Ionizing Radiation

Although humans are exposed to radiation in everyday living, it is rarely given much thought. The two basic

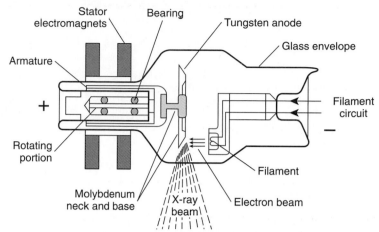

FIG. 9–1 Rotating anode tube is shown. (Modified from Carlton RC, Adler AM: *Principles of radiographic imaging, an art and a science,* ed 4, Thomson Delmar Learning, 2006, Albany, NY. Reprinted with permission of Delmar Learning, a division of Thomson Learning: *http://www.thomsonrights.com.* Fax 800-730-2215.)

sources of ionizing **radiation** are natural (or background) radiation, and human-made radiation. Background sources occur spontaneously in nature and can be affected by human activity. These forms include cosmic radiation from the sun and other planetary bodies and naturally occurring radioactive substances present on earth (such as uranium and radium), which can be inhaled or ingested through food, water, or air (radon or radiophosphorus). Sources of human-made radiation include the nuclear industry, radionuclides, and medical and dental exposures. The nuclear industry has contributed fallout from above-ground weapons testing, from accidents in nuclear power stations, and from disposal of by-products from these plants. Exposure to radionuclides results from products containing radioactive elements, such as smoke detectors, and radiopharmaceuticals used in the diagnosis and treatment of disease. Finally, medical and dental exposures constitute the greatest source of human-made radiation. Because the radiographer is primarily responsible for the application of medical ionizing radiation to patients, understanding the process by which x-rays interact with matter is important.

Human-Made Radiation

Human-made ionizing radiation, or **x-rays** as they are more commonly called, is a form of electromagnetic radiation that travels at the speed of light. Unlike particulate radiation, which is a liberated portion of the atom capable of traveling for short distances and reacting with matter, x-rays are bundles of energy moving as waves in space, depositing their energy randomly. For x-rays to be produced, three things must be present: (1) a source of elec-

trons, (2) a force to move them rapidly, and (3) something to stop this movement rapidly. These conditions are all met by the x-ray tube and its electrical supply (Fig. 9–1). The tube itself is composed of a *cathode,* or negative terminal, and an *anode,* or positive terminal, enclosed in a special glass envelope to maintain the vacuum necessary for optimal x-ray production. The filament in the cathode assembly is composed of thoriated tungsten, which provides the source of electrons. When kilovoltage (thousands of volts) is applied to the filament, it instantaneously accelerates the available stream of electrons toward the anode end of the tube. X-rays are produced when the electrons strike the anode, undergoing an energy conversion that produces both x-rays and heat. The resultant x-ray beam is heterogeneous; that is, it has many energies, measured in **kiloelectron volts (keV).** These x-rays, also known as the primary beam, are directed toward the patient through a window in the tube. Once the x-rays strike matter, three possibilities exist: (1) They can be absorbed, (2) they can transfer some energy and then scatter, or (3) they can pass through unaffected.

Interactions of X-Rays with Matter

X-rays interact with matter in five ways: (1) classic coherent scattering, (2) photoelectric interactions, (3) Compton scattering, (4) pair production, and (5) photodisintegration. Classic coherent scattering, photoelectric interactions, and Compton scattering occur within the diagnostic range of x-ray energies. Both Compton and photoelectric interactions directly influence the patient's and the occupational worker's exposure. They are the way in which x-rays transfer their energy to living tissue. They

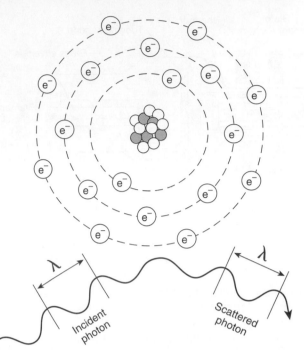

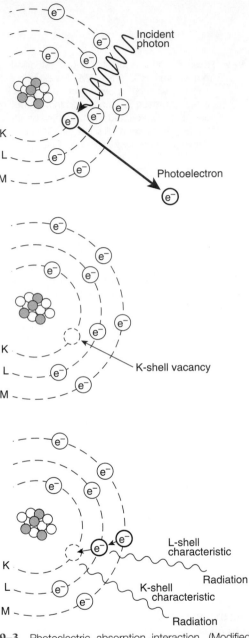

FIG. 9–2 Classic coherent scatter interaction. (Modified from Carlton RC, Adler AM: *Principles of radiographic imaging, an art and a science,* ed 4, Thomson Delmar Learning, 2006, Albany, NY. Reprinted with permission of Delmar Learning, a division of Thomson Learning: *http://www.thomsonrights.com.* Fax 800-730-2215.)

constitute the basis for all patient exposure and the reason behind the need for protective measures.

CLASSIC COHERENT SCATTERING. X-rays that possess energy levels below 10 keV can interact with matter through classic coherent scattering (Fig. 9–2). Also known as coherent or Thomson scattering, classic coherent scattering occurs when an incoming x-ray photon strikes an atom and is absorbed, causing the atom to become excited. The atom then releases the excess energy in the form of another x-ray photon, possessing the same energy as the original photon, but proceeding in a different direction. This change in direction is known as scattering. Most of these scattered photons travel in a forward direction, stopping when they strike anything in their path. More importantly, classic coherent scattering results in no energy transfer to the patient.

PHOTOELECTRIC INTERACTION. The second common interaction of x-rays with matter in the diagnostic range is the **photoelectric effect** (Fig. 9–3). Photoelectric effect occurs when an incoming x-ray photon strikes an inner shell electron and ejects it from its orbit around the

FIG. 9–3 Photoelectric absorption interaction. (Modified from Carlton RC, Adler AM: *Principles of radiographic imaging, an art and a science,* ed 4, Thomson Delmar Learning, 2006, Albany, NY. Reprinted with permission of Delmar Learning, a division of Thomson Learning: *http://www.thomsonrights.com.* Fax 800-730-2215.)

nucleus of the atom, creating an ion pair. The atom, having lost an electron, is positively charged, and the released electron, referred to as the *photoelectron,* continues to travel until it combines with other matter. All the energy from the photon is completely consumed in this interaction; it is said that the energy is absorbed by the atom. Because complete energy absorption takes place in photoelectric interactions, this constitutes the greatest hazard to patients in diagnostic radiography.

COMPTON SCATTERING. The last interaction common to the diagnostic x-ray range is the Compton effect (Fig. 9–4). The **Compton effect,** or Compton scattering, occurs when an incoming x-ray photon strikes a target atom and uses a portion of its energy to eject an outer shell electron. The remainder of the photon's energy proceeds in a direction different from the incoming photon. This process results in a Compton or recoil electron, which travels until it combines with matter, and a photon of less energy that can react with the patient through further Compton or photoelectric interactions or that can exit the patient and reach imaging equipment or the occupational worker. This interaction is extremely important because most of the occupational worker's exposure to radiation comes from Compton scatter.

PAIR PRODUCTION. The last two interactions that occur between ionizing radiation and matter require high-energy photons above 1 million electron volts (MeV). They are less relevant to diagnostic radiography because the equipment used in the production of x-rays cannot produce photons that possess this energy.

For **pair production** to occur, an incoming x-ray photon must possess a minimum of 1.02 MeV of energy (Fig. 9–5). This photon does not interact with the surrounding electron orbits; instead, it approaches the nucleus of the atom and interacts with its force field. The photon disappears, and two particles—one negatively charged and termed a *negatron* and one positively charged and called a *positron*—replace it.

Each particle possesses one half the energy (minimum, 0.51 MeV) of the original x-ray photon. The particles continue to travel, causing ionization, until the positron interacts with another electron, annihilates it, and produces two photons moving in opposite directions. Because the energy level necessary for pair production is at least 1.02 MeV, it does not normally occur in the diagnostic x-ray range.

PHOTODISINTEGRATION. X-ray photons possessing a minimum of 10 MeV of energy can interact directly with the nucleus of the atom, causing a state of excitement within the nucleus, followed by the emission of a nuclear fragment (Fig. 9–6). This process is referred to as *photodisintegration,* and it does not occur in diagnostic radiography; it occurs in the nuclear industry.

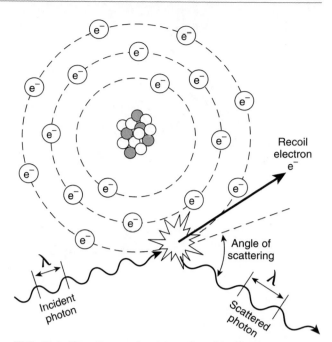

FIG. 9–4 Compton scatter interaction. (Modified from Carlton RC, Adler AM: *Principles of radiographic imaging, an art and a science,* ed 4, Thomson Delmar Learning, 2006 Albany, NY. Reprinted with permission of Delmar Learning, a division of Thomson Learning: *http://www.thomsonrights.com.* Fax 800-730-2215.)

Units of Measurement

To quantify the amount of radiation a patient or occupational worker receives, a system of units has been developed. The units most commonly used since the 1920s are listed in Table 9-1. In 1948 the International Committee for Weights and Measures developed a system of units based on metric measurement. The **SI units** (Systeme International d'Unites, or International System of Units) were officially adopted in 1985.

ROENTGEN (COULOMBS PER KILOGRAM). The **roentgen (R)** is the measure of ionization in air as a result of exposure to x-rays or gamma rays. It is defined as the quantity of x-radiation or gamma radiation that produces the quantity 2.08×10^9 ion pairs per cubic centimeter (cc) of air, for a total charge of 2.58×10^{-4} coulombs per kilogram (C/kg) (coulomb is a quantity of electric charge). The roentgen is restricted to measuring photons with energy below 3 MeV and only exposure in air. It does not indicate actual exposure to individuals when absorbed. The roentgen has no equivalent in the SI units

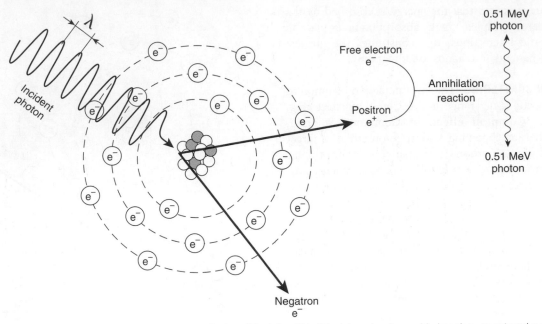

FIG. 9–5 Pair production interaction. (Modified from Carlton RC, Adler AM: *Principles of radiographic imaging, an art and a science,* ed 4, Thomson Delmar Learning, 2006 Albany, NY. Reprinted with permission of Delmar Learning, a division of Thomson Learning: *http://www.thomsonrights.com.* Fax 800-730-2215.)

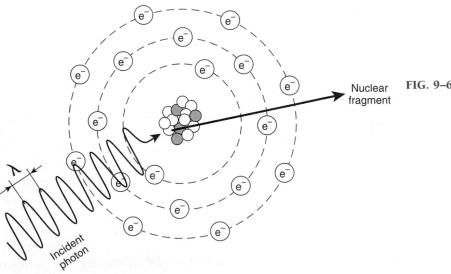

FIG. 9–6 Photodisintegration interaction. (Modified from Carlton RC, Adler AM: *Principles of radiographic imaging, an art and a science,* ed 4, Thomson Delmar Learning, 2006, Albany, NY. Reprinted with permission of Delmar Learning, a division of Thomson Learning: *http://www.thomsonrights.com.* Fax 800-730-2215.)

TABLE 9-1 Radiation Quantities and Units of Measurement

QUANTITY	TRADITIONAL UNIT	DEFINITION	SI UNIT	DEFINITION
Exposure in air	Roentgen	2.08×10^9 ion pairs/cc	Coulomb/kilogram	
Absorbed dose	Rad	100 ergs/g	Gray	1 J/kg
Dose equivalent	Rem	Rad × quality factor	Sievert	1 J/kg
Activity	Curie	3.7×10^{10} dps	Becquerel	1 dps

because exposure may be expressed directly as coulombs per kilogram, and it is being phased out as a unit of measurement.

RADIATION ABSORBED DOSE (GRAY). The need for discussing absorbed dose resulted in the development of the **radiation absorbed dose (rad)**. The rad measures the amount of energy absorbed in any medium, defined as 100 ergs of energy absorbed in 1 g of absorbing material. The rad has been replaced by the **gray (Gy)** in the SI system, which is defined as 1 joule (J) of energy absorbed in 1 kg of material. The Gy is 100 times larger than the rad; 1 Gy = 100 rads.

RADIATION EQUIVALENT MAN (SIEVERT). Not all types of radiation produce the same response in living tissue. Alpha particles, neutrons, and beta particles may produce a different degree of biologic damage compared with x-rays and gamma rays. To express accurately the biologic response of exposed individuals to the same quantity of differing radiations, the rem was developed. The **radiation equivalent man (rem)** is the unit of dose equivalence, expressed as the product of the absorbed dose in rad and a quality factor.

The quality factor varies, depending on the type of radiation being used. For example, the quality factor for x-rays is 1; therefore 1 rad of x-ray exposure equals 1 rem of dose equivalence (1 rad × 1 = 1 rem). The quality factor for fast neutrons is 10; thus 1 rad of fast neutron exposure equals 10 rem of dose equivalence (1 rad × 10 = 10 rem), meaning that neutrons are 10 times as biologically damaging as x-rays when their dose equivalents are compared. The rem has been replaced by the **sievert (Sv)** in SI units, which is defined as the product of the Gy and the quality factor. The sievert is 100 times larger than the rad; 1 Sv = 100 rem.

CURIE (BECQUEREL). Finally, the measure of the rate at which a radionuclide decays is referred to as *activity*. The **curie (Ci)** is the unit of activity, equal to 3.7×10^{10} disintegrations per second (dps). The SI unit of activity is the **becquerel (Bq)**, defined as 1 dps. Therefore 1 Ci = 3.7×10^{10} Bq. These units are commonly employed in nuclear medicine and radiotherapy.

The traditional and SI units are compared in Table 9-1.

Standards for Regulation of Exposure

Because patients and workers exposed to radiation are at risk for biologic effects, limits must be set to ensure safe

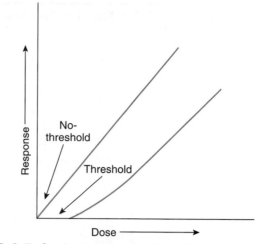

FIG. 9–7 Graph indicates no-threshold versus threshold response to radiation.

practice for both the patient and the radiation worker. Guidelines and standards set by regulatory agencies must be followed. The Center for Devices and Radiological Health (CDRH), under the direction of the U.S. Food and Drug Administration, sets and regulates the standards for radiation-producing equipment; it also continues to research possible ways of minimizing exposure to ionizing radiation. The National Council on Radiation Protection and Measurements (NCRP) is a not-for-profit organization enacted by Congress in 1964 to collect and distribute information regarding radiation awareness and safe practice to the public. It cooperates with other organizations to review on an ongoing basis the latest data on radiation units, measurements, and protection. The following information reflects the recommendations made by the NCRP, in cooperation with other organizations.

Effective dose limit recommendations have been set to minimize the biologic risk to exposed persons. The concept of a maximum permissible dose had been traditionally used to describe the maximum dose of ionizing radiation that, if received by an individual, carried a negligible risk of significant bodily or genetic damage. Maximum permissible doses were established for the occupational worker and the general population. These recommendations followed two theories: no-threshold and risk versus benefit (Fig. 9–7).

No-threshold indicates that no dose exists below which the risk of damage does not exist. *Risk versus benefit* governed the exposure to individuals when physicians ordered radiographic procedures. The benefit to the patient from performing those procedures has far

TABLE 9-2 Effective Dose Limit Recommendations

	DOSE LIMITS	
POPULATION AND AREA OF BODY IRRADIATED	SI UNIT	TRADITIONAL UNIT
Occupational Exposures		
Effective Dose Limits		
Annual	50 mSv	5 rem
Cumulative	10 mSv × age	1 rem × age
Equivalent Dose Annual Limits for Tissues and Organs		
Lens of eyes	150 mSv	15 rem
Skin, hands, and feet	500 mSv	50 rem
Public Exposures (Annual)		
Effective Dose Limit		
Continuous or frequent exposure	1 mSv	0.1 rem
Infrequent exposure	5 mSv	0.5 rem
Equivalent Dose Limits for Tissues and Organs		
Lens of eye	15 mSv	1.5 rem
Skin, hands, and feet	50 mSv	5 rem
Embryo-Fetus Exposures (Monthly)		
Equivalent dose limit	0.5 mSv	0.05 rem
Education and Training Exposures (Annual)		
Effective dose limit	1 mSv	0.1 rem
Equivalent Dose Limit for Tissues and Organs		
Lens of eye	15 mSv	1.5 rem
Skin, hands, and feet	50 mSv	5 rem

Modified from National Council on Radiation Protection and Measurements: *NCRP Report No. 116: limitation of exposure to ionizing radiation,* Bethesda, Md, 1993, NCRP.
SI units, Systeme International d'Unites (International System of Units).

outweighed the risk of possible biologic damage. Because current studies indicate that an individual's dose should be kept *as low as reasonably achievable* **(ALARA)** and that no dose is considered permissible, the term *maximum permissible dose* is no longer acceptable. Instead, the NCRP has recommended certain *effective dose* limits, summarized in Table 9-2.

The annual whole-body effective dose limit for the occupational worker is 50 mSv (5 rem). Before the NCRP issued its dose-equivalent limitations in 1987 and revised them in 1993 as effective dose limits, the lifetime accumulated whole-body dose equivalent was determined by the formula 5(N − 18) rem, where N equals the age of the worker in years. According to this formula, a 40-year-old occupational worker could have received 5(40 − 18), or 110 rem. Currently, the recommended maximum accumulated whole-body effective dose limit is 10 mSv times age in years (or 1 rem × age in years). This same occupational worker may now accumulate only 1 rem × 40, or 40 rem (400 mSv), in his or her lifetime.

Anyone exposed to ionizing radiation not as a radiation worker is a member of the general population. The whole-body dose-equivalent limit for the general population is one tenth the occupational worker's annual limit, or 5 mSv (0.5 rem).

BIOLOGIC RESPONSE TO IONIZING RADIATION

Ionizing radiation, absorbed by matter, undergoes energy conversions that result in changes in atomic structure. These changes, when considered in light of living tissue, can have major consequences on the life of any organism. To understand the necessity of protecting oneself

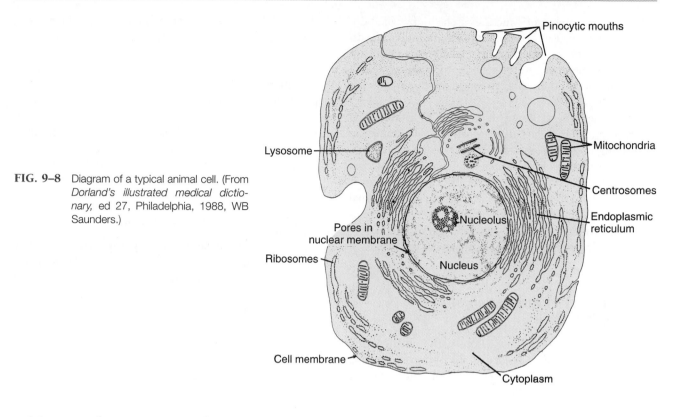

FIG. 9–8 Diagram of a typical animal cell. (From *Dorland's illustrated medical dictionary,* ed 27, Philadelphia, 1988, WB Saunders.)

and the patient from exposure to radiation, a basic review of cellular biology and how radiation interacts with cells is important.

Basic Cell Structure

The cell is the simplest unit of organic protoplasm capable of independent existence. Simple organisms are composed of one or two cells; complex organisms are *multicellular,* that is, made of many cells. Although cells may differ from each other, depending on their primary function, their structures are similar. Most cells are divided into two parts: (1) the nucleus and (2) the cytoplasm (Fig. 9–8). The nucleus is separated from the rest of the cell by a double-walled membrane called the *nuclear envelope.* This membrane has openings, or *pores,* that permit other molecules to pass back and forth between the nucleus and the cytoplasm. Most important, the nucleus contains the *chromosomes,* which are made up of genes. *Genes* are the units of hereditary information, composed of deoxyribonucleic acid (DNA). DNA, a double-stranded structure coiled around itself as a spiral staircase, is one of the molecules at risk when a cell is exposed to ionizing radiation.

The cytoplasm of the cell is separated from its environment by the cell membrane. It contains several organelles responsible for the metabolic function of the cell. The cytoplasm itself is primarily water, which can undergo changes when struck by ionizing radiation.

Cell Types

Cells are of two types: (1) somatic cells and (2) germ cells. **Somatic cells** perform all the body's functions. They possess two of every gene on two different chromosomes. Their chromosomes are paired, but each pair is different. Somatic cells possess a total of 46 chromosomes, or 23 pairs. They divide through the process of mitosis. **Germ cells** are the reproductive cells of an organism; they possess one half the number of chromosomes as the somatic cells, for a total of 23. Germ cells reproduce through the process of meiosis.

Theories for Cellular Absorption of Ionizing Radiation

When a cell absorbs ionizing radiation, two basic theories exist to explain this interaction. The first theory, known as the *direct hit theory,* occurs whenever any type of radiation transfers its energy directly to the key molecule it has struck, resulting in the formation of ion pairs or elevation to an increased, excited energy state.

Although any important structure can be hit by radiation, serious consequences arise when radiation interacts with DNA. Breaks in the bases or phosphate bonds can result in rearrangement or loss of genetic information, which can injure or kill the cell as it continues through its life cycle.

The other interaction with ionizing radiation is by indirect hit: Key molecules are affected by radiation depositing its energy elsewhere in the cell. Because cells are approximately 80% water, indirect action occurs when water molecules are ionized. This action produces chemical changes within the cell that alter the internal environment, injuring the cell, which can result in eventual cell death. With x-radiation and gamma radiation, the vast majority of cellular damage is the result of indirect hits.

Target Theory of Absorption of Ionizing Radiation

Both direct and indirect interactions with ionizing radiation apply to the target theory of absorption of ionizing radiation. Simply stated, certain molecules existing within a cell are key to the continued viability or life of that cell. Some of these molecules exist in great number, others in limited supply. If damage occurs to a molecule in abundant supply, then the effect to the cell may not be as detrimental because others exist to maintain the function of the cell. Injury to a molecule in limited supply, however, can be life threatening, because no immediate replacement is available. The term *target* is used to describe any critical molecule that has undergone some interaction with ionizing radiation, either directly or indirectly. The target whose damage has serious consequences to the life of the cell is DNA.

Radiosensitivity of Cells

To study the cell's response to radiation, a method of classification according to sensitivity was developed by Bergonie and Tribondeau in 1906. These researchers determined that mitotic activity and specific characteristics of each cell affected how the cell exhibited radiation damage. Cells are most sensitive to radiation during active division, when they are primitive in structure and function. Examples of radiosensitive cells include the basal cells of the skin, crypt cells of the small intestine, and germ cells. Cells resistant to radiation, being more specialized in structure and function, do not undergo repeated mitosis. These cells include nerve, muscle, and brain cells.

Ancel and Vitemberger, who modified this theory, stated that all cells possess the same sensitivity to radiation; the time of expression of injury is the factor that differs. This factor depends on mitosis and the external conditions in which the cell is placed. Therefore rapidly dividing cells demonstrate the injury sooner and only appear as though they are more sensitive to radiation than those whose mitotic rate is slower. Organs composed of parenchymal cells that rapidly divide, such as skin or the small intestine, exhibit injury sooner than the esophagus or spinal cord, whose cells divide more slowly.

Response of Cells to Radiation

Cells respond to radiation in many ways: They die before beginning mitosis, delay entering mitosis, or fail to divide at their normal rate. Fortunately, cells also try to repair the damage sustained through absorption of ionizing radiation. This possibility depends on how sensitive the cell is to radiation, the type of damage sustained, the kind of radiation (particulate or electromagnetic), the exposure rate, and the total dose given. Incomplete repair can result in adverse biologic effects occurring after time has elapsed.

Total Body Response to Radiation

The total body response of any organism to radiation depends on the effect to all the systems of the body. Because every system is different in its sensitivity or resistance, the total body response at a particular dose is defined by the system most affected. This response, known as *acute radiation syndrome,* occurs only when the organism is exposed fully (total body) to an external source of radiation given in a few minutes. Only then does the organism develop the full set of signs and symptoms that define each syndrome.

Three general stages of response exist for each acute radiation syndrome. The first is the *prodromal stage,* commonly referred to as the nausea, vomiting, and diarrhea (NVD) stage. The second stage is the *latent period,* in which the organism feels well; however, during this time, the body is undergoing biologic changes that will lead to the final period, the *manifest stage.* Now the organism feels the full effects of the exposure, leading to either recovery or death.

Three radiation syndromes are (1) bone marrow syndrome, (2) gastrointestinal syndrome, and (3) central nervous system syndrome. Bone marrow syndrome occurs between doses of 2 and 10 Gy (200 and 1000 rad). Total body exposure results in infection, hemorrhage, and anemia. Gastrointestinal syndrome results from doses between 10 and 50 Gy (1000 and 5000 rad). Individuals experience massive diarrhea, nausea, vomiting, and fever when subjected to these doses. Central nervous system syndrome occurs at doses above 50 Gy (5000 rad), with the individual experiencing convulsions, coma, and eventual death from increased intracranial pressure. Although these syndromes indicate serious, even lethal, consequences from exposure to radiation, an important point to remember is that these doses are far greater than those received by the occupational worker or patient.

Late Effects of Radiation Exposure

Other effects of radiation exposure are equally important, which are termed the *late effects;* these can develop over a long period after exposure. These effects result not only from high doses of radiation, but also from low doses administered over a longer time. Late effects are divided into two groups: (1) *somatic effects,* which develop in the individual exposed, and (2) *genetic effects,* which occur in future generations as a result of damage to the germ cells.

The two most frequently induced somatic effects are cataract formation and carcinogenesis. The lens of the eye is extremely sensitive to radiation, and studies have demonstrated the high incidence of cataract formation in laboratory animals exposed to radiation. Additionally, survivors of the explosion of the atom bomb developed cataracts.

The most important late somatic effect is cancer development. The first documented case was the hand of a radiographer in 1902. Early radiologists, technologists, and researchers developed skin cancer and leukemia from prolonged exposure to ionizing radiation. Watch-dial painters developed osteosarcoma from ingesting radium when they put their paintbrushes in their mouths to draw the tip to a point. Miners who inhaled radioactive dust while digging for uranium developed lung cancer. All of these cases led to today's strict limitations on radiation exposure.

Long-term genetic effects result from germ cells whose DNA has been altered by radiation exposure, meaning the effects are not seen in the exposed individual; instead, if an affected cell is fertilized and develops, the effects show up in future generations. These mutations—alterations in the DNA coding of the chromosome—are recessive. They appear only if the mutated cell is fertilized by another reproductive cell carrying the same mutation. This fact of genetics acts to minimize the appearance of possible radiation-induced changes.

PROTECTING THE PATIENT

Although the patient must be exposed to ionizing radiation for a diagnostic image to be produced, care must be exercised to minimize the quantity of radiation exposure. The radiographer has the responsibility of maximizing the quality of the radiograph while minimizing the risk to the patient. Consequently, the concept of ALARA—as low as reasonably achievable—is used to guide technical factor selection when performing examinations on the patient. In particular, the cardinal principles of protection—time, distance, and shielding—are used to minimize patient exposure.

Time

When the radiographer minimizes the length of time a patient is placed in the path of the x-ray beam, he or she is applying one of the primary rules of protection. This goal is accomplished when the radiographer accurately applies the rules of radiographic technique to produce diagnostic images and uses technique charts to help determine the correct amount of radiation to direct toward the patient. The chances of repeated exposures are minimized, reducing the patient's time in the path of the x-ray beam.

Distance

Another way to lessen patient dose is to maximize the distance between the radiation source and the patient. This increased distance lessens the entrance or skin dose to the patient. This action is not the most reasonable method to minimize patient dose because the patient must be in the path of the ionizing beam for an image to be created. Additionally, increasing distance requires an increase in technical factors to create an acceptable image.

Shielding

The last rule of protection is to shield by placing some material over the reproductive organs (gonads) of the patient whenever they are within 4 to 5 cm of the primary beam. This precaution is particularly important when performing radiography on children and adults of reproductive age. Shields are made of lead, which has an atomic number of 82. Lead absorbs x-rays through the process of photoelectric effect, thereby minimizing patient exposure. The three basic types of shields are (1) flat contact shields, (2) shaped contact shields, and (3) shadow shields.

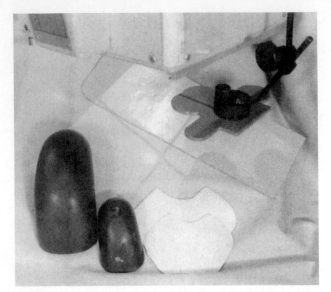

FIG. 9–9 Gonadal shields *(clockwise from top):* shadow shield, lead rubber blocker, flat contact shields, shaped shields.

Flat contact shields are made of a combination of vinyl and lead and are placed directly over the gonads of the patient (Fig. 9–9). They are made in various sizes to accommodate the age of the patient. *Shaped contact shields* are cup shaped and designed specifically to protect the gonads of male patients. Because of their shape, they can remain in place securely, even when the patient must turn to accommodate the examination. *Shadow shields* are mounted to the side of the collimator of the x-ray tube on a flexible extension arm. They can be manipulated to extend into the path of the beam and cast a shadow on the patient, indicating the area being protected. *Lead rubber blockers* also are used in some situations.

Additional Methods of Protection

Other factors specific to the production of x-rays can be manipulated with the purpose of minimizing patient exposure. These factors include beam restriction, film/screen combinations, technical factor selection, and filtration. The radiographer always must restrict the primary beam to the anatomic area of interest, never exceeding the size of the image receptor used to capture the information. This restriction limits the exposure to the area undergoing radiography and does not increase the overall patient dose. Through the use of fast film/screen combinations, a diagnostic image can be produced with reduced radiation, which minimizes patient

exposure. Additionally, selecting technical factors that use high kilovoltages increases the probability that Compton interactions will occur. This method results in a reduction of the energy being directly absorbed by the patient, creating a decrease in patient exposure. When reduced kilovoltage techniques are selected, an increase quantity of the radiation is completely absorbed within the patient, adding to the dose. Finally, using filtration in the path of the x-ray beam absorbs the low-energy x-rays that only add to the patient's entrance dose. Eliminating their presence in the primary beam does not affect the finished image because most do not exit the patient to reach the image receptor. Aluminum is the most common material used in filtration. Its atomic number and K-shell binding energies encourage photoelectric absorption of the low-energy x-rays.

PROTECTING THE RADIOGRAPHER

The same principles of time, distance, and shielding are used to reduce the occupational worker's exposure to radiation. This reduction is accomplished by minimizing the time spent in the room when ionizing radiation is being produced, using the greatest possible distance from the source of exposure, and placing a shield between the worker and the radiation source.

Time

The radiographer should always spend the least amount of time possible in a room when a source of radiation is active. This risk exists only when exposures are being made; once the exposure is terminated, no radiation remains within the room or the contents of the room. The amount of dose received is directly related to the length of time spent with the source. During fluoroscopy in which radiation is used for imaging dynamic structures, x-rays are emitted for longer periods. Therefore most units are equipped with 5-minute timers to alert the operator that a period has elapsed.

Distance

Distance is the best measure of protection for an occupational worker. The principle of the inverse square law states that the intensity of radiation varies inversely with the square of the distance. Simply stated, increasing the distance from the source of the x-ray beam greatly reduces the quantity of radiation that reaches the radiographer (Fig. 9–10). This reduction occurs because the x-rays leaving the tube spread out *(diverge)* and cover a much larger area, which, in turn, lessens their intensity. The following formula can be used to determine the exact exposure reaching the worker:

New intensity/old intensity = (old distance)^2/(new distance)^2

For example, if the intensity of radiation received by the radiographer were 20 mR at a distance of 1 m from the tube, what then would the intensity be at a distance of 2 m from the tube, all other factors remaining the same? Solving for the new intensity, we get:

New intensity/20 mR = (1)^2/(2)^2

New intensity = 1 × 20 mR/4 = 5 mR

Doubling the distance between the radiographer and the source of radiation reduces the exposure by a factor of 4.

A radiographer should not make a practice of holding a patient who cannot cooperate during a radiographic procedure. This circumstance places the radiographer closer to the beam and to the patient, who is a source of scatter radiation from Compton interactions and increases the time a radiographer is near the source of radiation.

Immobilization devices, such as sandbags or restraint bands, should be used whenever possible. If these devices are ineffective or unavailable, assistance should be obtained from a nonoccupational worker, such as a nurse, physician, or relative of the patient. The person who assists the patient must wear shielding devices to minimize his or her exposure.

Shielding

The radiographer must use shielding whenever time and distance alone cannot satisfactorily protect the worker. Lead is the material used in both fixed protective barriers and accessory devices such as aprons and gloves. Lead aprons and gloves should be worn when taking advantage of fixed barriers is impossible. They are constructed of lead-impregnated vinyl, having a content between 0.25 and 1.0 mm of lead equivalency. The greater the amount of lead used, the better the protection offered the worker will be. The greatest drawback to increased lead content is the increase in weight the device possesses. The minimum permissible amount of lead equivalency for aprons used when the peak kilovoltage is 100 is 0.25 mm. Gloves usually possess the same minimum amount.

The shielding garments must be in good condition; cracked aprons and gloves do not successfully attenuate radiation. Protective apparel must be stored properly on specially designed racks so that cracks do not develop.

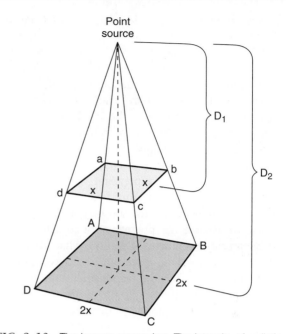

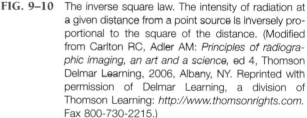

FIG. 9–10 The inverse square law. The intensity of radiation at a given distance from a point source is inversely proportional to the square of the distance. (Modified from Carlton RC, Adler AM: *Principles of radiographic imaging, an art and a science,* ed 4, Thomson Delmar Learning, 2006, Albany, NY. Reprinted with permission of Delmar Learning, a division of Thomson Learning: *http://www.thomsonrights.com.* Fax 800-730-2215.)

To determine whether aprons or gloves adequately protect the wearer, they should undergo fluoroscopy at least once a year to check for damage.

Fixed protective barriers are part of the radiographic room construction and can be divided into primary and secondary barriers. *Primary barriers* are those that can be struck by the primary beam exiting the x-ray tube. *Secondary barriers* are those that can be struck only by secondary, scatter, or leakage radiation. A diagnostic radiologic physicist, who considers the design and use of the room, determines the exact quantity of lead or the equivalent thickness of concrete.

Pregnant Student

Student pregnancy is covered under Nuclear Regulatory Commission (NRC) regulations regarding the declared pregnant worker. Radiologic sciences programs accredited by the Joint Review Committee on Education in Radiologic Technology must publish and make these regulations known to accepted and enrolled female students. Although guidelines for exposure to pregnant women has been in place for many years, in 1994 the NRC in the United States became the first regulatory agency to limit the absorbed radiation dose to the unborn child. The dose limit is 0.5 rem (5 mSv) for the declared pregnant woman. In addition, the NCRP recommends that, once pregnancy is known, a limit of 0.05 rem (0.5 mSv) per month should apply.

Study of average exposure to radiologic technologists indicates that exposure to a pregnant woman who is a student would exceed these limits is unlikely. Consequently, little reason exists for the pregnant student to decide not to declare her pregnancy or to substantially alter her clinical assignments. Deciding what the risk to her fetus may be and taking precautions to avoid excessive radiation exposure is the responsibility of the pregnant woman. Careful attention to the ALARA concepts of time, distance, and shielding is an important part of this decision.

As a result of U.S. Supreme Court litigation designed to end sex discrimination against pregnant women in the workplace, American employers may not bar women of childbearing age from jobs because of potential risk to their fetuses. Essentially, the ruling upholds the Title VII Civil Rights Act of 1964 as forbidding sex-specific fetal-protection policies. Consequently, the NRC requires that all persons frequenting any portion of a restricted radiation area be instructed in the risks of radiation exposure to the embryo and fetus. (Restricted areas include diagnostic radiologic rooms, nuclear medicine laboratories, and any other area where ionizing radiation is applied to humans.) These instructions must include the right to declare or not declare pregnancy status. A declared pregnant woman is one who has voluntarily elected to declare her pregnancy. She is not under any regulatory or licensing obligation to do so. If a declaration is made, it must be in writing, be dated, and include the estimated month of conception. Acknowledgment of a pregnancy verbally or by visual observation does not meet the requirements of these regulations. Furthermore, the woman has the right to revoke her declaration of pregnancy. Until the proper declaration has been made, the total exposure dose limit is 5 rem (50 mSv).

Current recommendations in the literature discourage moving a newly declared pregnant woman to an area of lower radiation exposure because reassignments have the potential to increase exposure to others who are not yet aware they are pregnant. If, however, students are reassigned to low exposure areas, obtaining agreement with this practice from all students at the time they begin the educational program is necessary. ALARA radiation protection philosophy supports a schedule that evenly distributes exposure risk to all students at a relatively uniform monthly exposure rate to avoid substantial variations among individuals.

The NRC regulations require that a personnel monitor be used if the declared pregnant student is likely to receive 10% of the embryo or fetus dose limit. This amount would be 0.05 rem (0.5 mSv) for the pregnancy or 0.005 rem (0.05 mSv) per month. Regulations require that the OSL badge (or other approved monitoring device) be worn at the part of the body receiving the highest exposure. No additional monitor is required if the woman has been wearing a personnel monitor at the collar or other location outside a lead apron; however, a single monitor that has been previously worn under a lead apron cannot be moved to the collar or other location. Instead, a second monitor must be worn outside lead aprons while the other monitor is worn in its usual location. This requirement is intended to avoid abnormal exposure readings from the woman's usual habits.

RADIATION MONITORING

Finally, any occupational worker who is regularly exposed to ionizing radiation must be monitored to determine estimated exposure. Any worker who is likely to receive more than one tenth of the recommended dose-equivalent limit should be monitored. Monitors measure the quantity of radiation received based on conditions in which the radiographer was placed. The most common personnel-monitoring devices are the optically stimulated luminescence (OSL) dosimeter, film badge, thermoluminescent dosimeter, and pocket dosimeter.

Optically Stimulated Luminescence Dosimeters

The Luxel OSL dosimeter is the most common method used to monitor personnel exposure (Fig. 9–11). This type of dosimeter consists of a strip of aluminum oxide, a copper filter, an open window, a tin filter, and an imaging filter. The device is heat-sealed within a laminated, light-tight paper wrapper. The entire package is then sealed in a tamper-proof plastic blister pack. The front of the dosimeter provides information identifying the person wearing it, the name of the department, and a badge placement icon. To determine the individual's exposure, the aluminum oxide is exposed to a laser light, which stimulates the aluminum oxide after use, causing it to become luminescent in proportion to the amount of

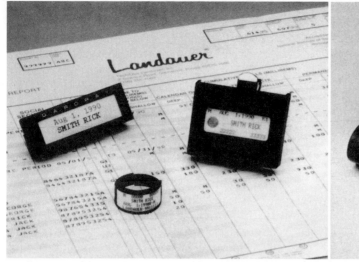

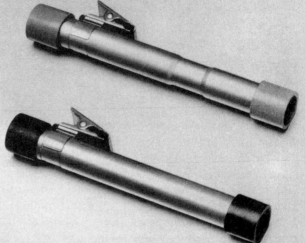

A

B

C

FIG. 9–11 *A, Left to right,* Typical film badge, thermoluminescent dosimeter ring, and collar badge. *B,* Pocket dosimeters. *C,* Luxel OSL dosimeter. (Courtesy Tech/Ops Landauer, Inc.)

radiation exposure, which determines the occupational worker's exposure.

The OSL dosimeter can detect x-rays and gamma radiation in the range of 5 keV to in excess of 40 MeV. Dose measurement range is from 1 mrem to 1000 rem. Typically, the OSL dosimeter is worn for 2 months. The holder should be worn between the collar and waist, on the front of the occupational worker. An advantage of this personal radiation monitoring device is that, because of the blister packaging, it is unaffected by heat, moisture,

and pressure. The main disadvantage of this device is the inability to get an immediate reading of the worker's exposure; the dose can be determined only when the aluminum oxide is analyzed.

Film Badges

Before the advent of OSL dosimeters, film badges were the most popular, least expensive method to monitor personnel exposure (see Fig. 9–11). The badge consists of a plastic holder containing different filters and a separate light-tight packet holding two pieces of film having different sensitivity to x-rays. Located on the front of the film packet is the identification information of the person wearing the badge. The film in the holder gets darker in response to the amount and energy of the radiation to which it is exposed. This film is analyzed to determine the occupational worker's exposure. A film badge is sensitive to doses as low as 10 mrem (0.1 mSv) and is usually worn for 1 month. Doses below 10 mrem are not detectable and are reported as *M,* or minimal. The holder should be worn between the collar and waist on the front of the occupational worker. The main disadvantage to this device is the inability to get an immediate reading of the worker's exposure; the dose can be determined only when the film is processed and analyzed.

Thermoluminescent Dosimeters

A third device to monitor personnel exposure is the thermoluminescent dosimeter (TLD). The TLD consists of a plastic holder containing crystals that absorb a portion of the energy they receive from a radiation exposure. When exposed, the absorbed energy causes the outer valence electrons to be trapped in the forbidden zone, the region immediately past their resting orbit. The number of electrons elevated to this state is directly dependent on the amount of radiation received. When the time comes to determine the dose, these crystals are heated so that the trapped electrons return to their original resting state. This process results in a release of the extra energy in the form of a light photon. The light is collected and analyzed to determine the quantity of dose received by the TLD.

The crystal most commonly used in TLDs is lithium fluoride. Once the lithium fluoride crystals have been heated *(annealed),* they can then be reused—a feature that is not possible with a film badge. The TLD provides readings as low as 5 mrem (0.05 mSv).

Pocket Dosimeters

The last device is the pocket dosimeter, which appears similar to a pen flashlight and is constructed of a central metal electrode surrounded by air and enclosed in a metal holder. The electrode is positively charged; as the dosimeter is exposed to ionizing radiation, the air in the dosimeter is ionized. Negative ions moving toward the electrode combine with some of the positive charges, neutralizing the electrode. This loss in charge is proportional to the amount of radiation, and a pointer on a scale moves upward relative to the loss in charge. The pocket dosimeter is used when an immediate reading of occupational dose is desired; however, it is subject to false readings and does not provide a permanent record.

Field Survey Instruments

Other types of instruments are used to detect the presence of radiation and give the user an indication of the intensity of the source. These devices are known as *field survey instruments.* A common instrument used to detect x-radiation, gamma radiation, and beta radiation is the Geiger-Mueller counter, which is an ionization chamber constructed of an electrode housed within a chamber. The walls of the chamber are negatively charged, and the electrode is positive. When x-rays pass through the chamber and interact with air, ionization occurs. Free electrons are attracted to the positively charged electrode, where they can be measured. The number of free electrons is directly proportional to the radiation exposure and can be displayed on a special meter that interprets this information and determines the exposure in roentgens or coulombs per kilogram.

SUMMARY

Medical ionizing radiation is a form of electromagnetic radiation capable of penetrating matter and depositing energy as it travels. Although ionizing radiation can interact with matter in five ways, of particular importance to imaging are the photoelectric interaction and Compton interaction. Both of these interactions contribute to the creation of the diagnostic radiograph, and both contribute to the exposure of the patient and the radiographer to radiation.

The quantities of radiation important in radiography are exposure, absorbed dose, and dose equivalence. The traditional units used to measure these quantities are the roentgen, rad, and rem. The SI units that correspond to the traditional units are coulombs per kilogram, gray, and sievert.

Biologic changes that occur as a result of exposure to radiation begin at the cellular level. The effects depend on what type of cell was struck, how the energy was transferred, the type of radiation, and the sensitivity of the cell. The immediate response of the cell is to repair itself; when this self-repair is not possible, other changes begin to take place. These changes have an impact not only on the cells struck, but also on all the systems that are composed of the cells. The effects resulting from exposure are either *somatic,* affecting the individual exposed, or *genetic,* affecting future generations through changes in germ cells. To minimize these changes, appropriate measures of protection must be used.

To minimize patient exposure, the radiographer must keep in mind all the principles of image production that play a role in patient exposure. Examples of these factors are kilovoltage, film/screen combinations, collimation, filtration, and repeated exposures. Shields must also be applied to protect the reproductive organs of the patient whenever possible, as long as the examination is not compromised. The radiographer must also protect himself or herself from unnecessary radiation through the use of the cardinal rules of protection: time, distance, and shielding. Finally, a record of the amount of radiation the occupational worker receives or to which he or she is exposed can be obtained by using monitoring devices such as OSL dosimeters, film badges, TLDs, and pocket dosimeters.

BIBLIOGRAPHY

Bushong C: *Radiologic science for technologists: physics, biology, and protection*, ed 8, St Louis, 2004, Mosby.

Carlton RC, Adler AM: *Principles of radiographic imaging: an art and a science*, ed 4, Albany, NY, 2006, Thomson Delmar Learning.

Curry TS, Dowdey JE, Murry RC: *Christensen's introduction to the physics of diagnostic radiology*, ed 4, Philadelphia, 1990, Lea & Febiger.

Dorland's illustrated medical dictionary, ed 3, Philadelphia, 2003, WB Saunders.

Hall J: *Radiobiology for the radiologist*, ed 5, Philadelphia, 2000, JB Lippincott.

Kane DF et al: The declared pregnant woman in nuclear medicine, *J Nucl Med Technol* 24(2):83, 1996.

National Council on Radiation Protection and Measurements: *NCRP Report No. 82: SI units in radiation protection and measurements*, Bethesda, Md, 1985, NCRP.

National Council on Radiation Protection and Measurements: *NCRP Report No. 91: recommendations on limits for exposure to ionizing radiation*, Bethesda, Md, 1987, NCRP.

National Council on Radiation Protection and Measurements: *NCRP Report No. 116: limitation of exposure to ionizing radiation*, Bethesda, Md, 1993, NCRP.

Nias AHW: *An introduction to radiobiology*, ed 2, New York, 1998, John Wiley & Sons.

Selman J: *The fundamentals of x-ray and radium physics*, ed 9, Springfield, Ill, 2000, Charles C Thomas.

Travis EL: *Primer of medical radiobiology*, ed 2, Chicago, 1989, Year Book Medical Publishers.

U.S. Nuclear Regulatory Commission: *Standards for protection against radiation.* 10 CFR Part 20, Washington, DC, September 1994, NRC.

U.S. Nuclear Regulatory Commission: *Instruction concerning prenatal radiation exposure, regulatory guide 8.13, rev 2,* Washington, DC, December 1987, NRC.

Human Diversity

Bettye G. Wilson, MAEd, RT(R) (CT), ARRT, RDMS, FASRT

"Give me your tired, your poor,
Your huddled masses yearning to breathe free,
The wretched refuse of your teeming shore.
Send these, the homeless, tempest-tost to me,
I lift my lamp beside the golden door."

Excerpted from the base of Statue of Liberty inscription, "The New Colossus,"
a poem written by Emma Lazarus

OBJECTIVES

On completion of this chapter, the student should be able to:

1. Define human diversity.

2. List some of the human diversity characteristics.

3. Describe the human diversity traits of age, ethnicity or national origin, race, gender or sexual orientation, and mental and physical ability.

4. Name the values that are prescribed to U.S. mainstream culture.

5. List the elements associated with cultural competency.

6. Discuss valuing diversity.

7. Know the empathetic practices that help foster cultural insight and produce improved outcomes.

8. Describe the six areas of human diversity that health care providers need to understand to provide quality and effective care.

9. Discuss ways in which the professional medical imaging organizations have expressed valuing human diversity.

Assimilation: process by which people of diverse backgrounds slowly give up their original cultural language and identity and melt into another, usually larger, group

Bias: prejudice; thinking negatively of others without any or significant justification; generally a combination of stereotyped beliefs and negative attitudes

Biculturalism: being able to negotiate two or more different cultures competently, individual and mainstream

Culture: all of the socially transmitted behavior patterns, arts, beliefs, institutions, and all other products of human work and thoughts by a particular class, community, or population

Cultural: of or relating to culture

Discrimination: physical actions involved in the unequal treatment of people because they belong to a certain category, group, or race.

Diverse: differing from one another; made up of distinct characteristics, qualities, or elements

Diversity: fact or quality of being diverse, different (all of the ways that human beings are both similar and different)

Ethnic: designating any of the basic groups or divisions of humankind or of a heterogeneous population, as distinguished by customs, characteristics, language, and common history; national origin

Ethnicity: ethnic affiliation or classification

Ethnocentrism: tendency toward viewing the norms and values of the individual's own culture as absolute and using them as a standard against which all other cultures are measured

Gender: chromosomal designation of female or male being

Human: people

Homophobia: irrational fear of and hostility toward homosexuality

Mental and Physical Ability: capacity to perform cognitive and psychomotor tasks with average ability

Race: population that differs from others in the relative frequency of some gene or genes; any of the different varieties of humankind, distinguished by type of hair, color of eyes and skin, stature, bodily proportions, or other characteristics

Racism: belief in racial superiority, leading to discrimination and prejudice toward races considered inferior

HUMAN DIVERSITY

The issue of human **diversity** is enjoying widespread importance throughout the United States and globally. The new millennium is perhaps the impetus for social change and acceptance, and understanding human diversity is at the heart of this issue. Human diversity, also called **cultural** diversity, addresses the entirety of the ways that people are different, yet alike, in the fact that all are human beings. Taken literally, human diversity simply means the differences inherent among people. Studies indicate that these differences are what make each person unique and valuable in their own right. Humans are divided into different **cultures**. Cultures develop behaviors, norms, and values that are suited to a specific environment and over time take on the strength of tradition. Even when conditions or environments change, cultures often do not. Lifelong habits are, in fact, a form of conditioning that is difficult to overcome.

Throughout history, the world has been composed of different nations, thus people of different cultures. Because of this composition, surprisingly, human diversity has only recently become an issue of utmost impor-

tance. Theories suggest that human diversity is more important today than ever before because of increased globalization. Globalization simply means that people now cross borders into other countries to work, go to school, receive medical care, visit, and live. This increase in globalization means that nations, societies, and businesses have become increasingly cross-cultural or multicultural.

Evidence of multiculturalism is everywhere: in cities, businesses, communities, educational institutions, and health care. With the influx of differing cultures, the need exists to understand at least broadly human diversity and to develop strategies to negotiate and mediate conflict caused by cultural differences. Colleges, universities, and businesses, as well as health care providers, institutions, and organizations, have taken the lead in fostering cultural diversity dialogue, education, understanding, and conflict resolution. Indeed, many educational institutions and businesses have developed positions and offices that deal only with diversity issues. Vice-presidents for equity and diversity, offices of equity and diversity, diversity programs for employees, and other initiatives can be found that are meant solely to foster a positive **diverse** environment. Professional health care providers, including physicians, nurses, and technologists, have addressed human diversity issues through their professional organizations. The American Society of Radiologic Technologists, American Society of Diagnostic Medical Sonographers, and the Society of Nuclear Medicine—Technologist Section have all made positive steps in addressing diversity issues within their disciplines by establishing minority scholarships, mentoring programs, and other initiatives. Most of these initiatives begin with trying to get people to understand themselves and their own cultural biases first and then to understand, accept, and value the contributions of persons from other cultures. Health care institutions and organizations are also doing the same. In these institutions and organizations, the realization exists that patients and workers alike are becoming increasingly diverse, and the key to providing quality patient care to a diverse population, by a diverse health care work force, is through organized cultural diversity initiatives. A concerted push toward cultural competency can be found throughout the United States.

Cultural competency is described as possessing a set of attitudes, behaviors, and policies that come together in a system or among individuals that enable effective interactions in a cross-cultural framework. Understanding and accepting the types of diversity is core to this process.

UNDERSTANDING HUMAN DIVERSITY

Characteristics

People have many differences, making them diverse as a whole. It has been said that no two people are exactly alike and that this uniqueness is what makes us individuals. Although the differences are intrinsic, extrinsic differences exist that further mark our diverse natures. Diversity includes many **human** characteristics that affect our perceptions of ourselves and others, individual values, opportunities, and acceptance. Some of the most prevalent characteristics are age, disability, economic status, education, **ethnicity**, family status, first language, gender, geographic location, lifestyle, organizational level, physical characteristics, political affiliation, religious preference, sexual orientation, work style or ethic, and many others.

Everyone has at least one personal **bias.** These biases, whether based on reason or simply perceptions of human characteristics, are real. Personal biases, even without conscious thought, play a major role in how individuals perceive others. Seemingly, the impact of some biases can be lessened through knowledge. The more that is known about a subject, the better the understanding of the subject will be. Examining all of the diverse human characteristics is not in the purview of this book or this chapter. The following diversity topics will be addressed because of their designation as the common and significant human diversity traits within a society:

- Age
- Ethnicity or national origin
- Race
- Gender or sexual orientation
- Mental and physical ability

AGE. Some cultures and individuals assign different values based on age. For example, some Asian cultures specifically place deference on older adults. These cultures note that without the contributions of persons now considered as old to their upbringing, education, and society, their society would not be as advanced as it is today. European and Western cultures generally do not regard older adults in this same manner. In fact, older adults are sometimes regarded as burdens on society. An upsurge in the reporting of cases of elder abuse may be considered a sign of a disregard of senior citizens.

The 2000 U.S. Census data show that individuals between the ages of 45 and 65 years comprise 23.6% of the population. In addition, 12.4% of the population is over the age of 65 years. Together, these two groups make up more than 36% of the total population, rivaling the 38% of the population between the ages of 18 and 44 years. As this so-called *baby boom generation* ages, persons considered as seniors will by most accounts overtake the current majority population. Therefore age biases must be corrected, and older individuals must be regarded for the value of the experiences and knowledge they have and continue to contribute to mainstream American business, cultural, economic, and social settings.

Americans have given names to subsets of the population. The term *baby boomer,* the most discussed subset because of sheer numbers, is applied to individuals born between 1946 and 1964. *Generation X* includes persons born between 1961 and 1981, and *generation Y* designation is applied to those born between 1981 and 1995.

The most significant subset, because of the impact they will have on the population, is the baby boomer group. Seventy-five million babies were born between 1946 and 1964. In the year 2006 the first of these individuals have begun to turn 60 years of age. This fact gives notice that, in the coming decades, a significant increase

TABLE 10-1 2003 U.S. Census Data Report on the Ethnic and Racial Make-Up of the Population

U.S. POPULATION (1000)	2000	2001	2002	2003
Caucasian alone	228,106	230,502	232,369	234,196
African American/Black alone	35,704	36,247	36,676	37,099
Native America/Alaska Native alone	2,664	2,711	2,749	2,787
Asian alone	10,589	11,105	11,515	11,925
Native Hawaiian/Other Pacific Islander alone	463	475	485	495
Combination (two or more)	3,898	4,053	4,180	4,308
Hispanic or Latino origin (may be of any race)	35,306	37,062	38,488	39,899

in the number of senior citizens and their proportion will occur to the total U.S. population. In fact, projections are that the general older adult population will increase substantially over the next three decades, with persons 85 years of age and older being the fastest-growing segment of the population.

What must not be forgotten is that the baby boom generation is considered to be overall healthy and well educated. These individuals are expected to stay in the workforce longer because they are expected to live longer than previous generations. In general, the graying of America is expected to transform many areas, including banking, health care, labor, politics, retirement systems, social services, and the stock market. This expectation forces an overview and overhaul of social mores and prejudices regarding older adults in the job market to their end-of-life care.

Time is not on the side of American society to address these issues. In 2000 Americans over the age of 85 outnumbered those at the beginning of the previous century by 26 times. At the beginning of 2000, more than 76,000 Americans were over the age of 100. Projections suggest that more than 1 million baby boomers will also live to see that age.

National policies geared toward baby boomer research and development have encountered heavy opposition because of many societal biases. Some of these biases include:

- Valuing youth over age
- Viewing of aging as something undesirable or bad
- Placing little value on contributions of senior citizens
- Favoring reactive instead of proactive approaches to policy development and implementation
- Considering all senior citizens to be mentally inferior

Continued age bias exists within the United States, especially in the realm of employment. The Age Discrimination in Employment Act, 29 U.S.C. §§ 621-634, was passed with the intent of preventing employers from exhibiting **discrimination** in hiring, promotion, job assignment, compensation, termination, based solely on age. The U.S. society, and the institutions contained within, must work to eliminate biases associated with age. This goal must be an essential element of any cultural diversity initiatives. People of all ages make positive contributions to society.

ETHNICITY, NATIONAL ORIGIN, AND RACE. Ethnicity relates to a person's distinctive racial, national, religious, linguistic, or cultural heritage. The term *race* may also be used to denote ethnicity. In the United States, the term *race* is most often used to distinguish between African Americans and Caucasians. The United States has long considered itself a melting pot of people with diverse ethnic heritages. Indeed, the Statue of Liberty beckons all people to our shores. Many people throughout the world still consider America the land of freedom and opportunity. Some of those who now call America home came to pursue the promised opportunities, others to escape persecution and oppression, while still others were brought to this country under servitude. Whatever the reason that individuals come to and remain in America, all are considered Americans. A special debt of gratitude is owed to the Native Americans who inhabited this great nation before it was *discovered*. Native Americans played an instrumental role in the successful colonization of this great nation through their assistance and friendship. The settlers and the natives were the first diverse ethnic groups in the United States. From that point on, numerous other ethnic groups have joined the ranks of American culture, although many were not born in this country. The 2000 U.S. Census data provides interesting statistics on the ethnic and racial make-up of the population, as well as growth trends among the groups from 2000 and 2003. Table 10-1 contains this information.

The census also addresses trends in growth, projecting that the U.S. Hispanic population will grow at a faster

TABLE 10-2 Some of the Core Values Exhibited by the More Prevalent Ethnic Cultures within the Population of the United States

ETHNIC GROUP	CORE VALUES
African American	Extended family
	Cooperation
	Spirituality
	Interdependence
Latino	Extended family
	Father as patriarch
	Respect
	Hierarchical relationships
Mexican American	Extended family (close knit)
	Curanderism (Mexican folk healing)
	Frequent with native country (Mexico)
	Respect
Native American	Extended family
	Spiritualism
	Collectivism
	Unified whole universe
U.S. mainstream	Individualism
	Affluence (material comfort, consumerism)
	Competition
	Personal achievement and success

rate than all other minority groups. Further projections include data suggesting that the current majority ethnic group will lose that designation within the current century because of the combined growth among the now minority groups and immigrants. This projection means that the U.S. population will become increasingly diverse, and the need to understand and accept human diversity as a fact of life is more important than ever. To understand and accept human diversity and to create and maintain a society that is mutually inclusive, ethnocentrism and racism must be eliminated. **Ethnocentrism** is regarded as the tendency of some individuals to view norms and values of their own culture as the only acceptable ones and to use them as the standard by which all other cultures are measured. **Racism** is the belief that one race or culture is superior to others and using this belief to discriminate against races they consider inferior. When ethnocentrism and racism are allowed to exist within a society, discrimination, prejudice, and oppression are often also evident and expressed. For individuals to live and work together for the mutual good of everyone,

people must learn to value the contributions of all individuals, respect all cultures, and live together as one race: human.

In the past, the interaction of culturally different individuals with mainstream (majority) culture has been that of either assimilation or biculturalism. **Assimilation** is described as the process by which persons of a diverse (different) culture, over time, give up their original cultural language and identify with, and try to merge into, another culture (usually the majority). **Biculturalism** is the ability of individuals to be able to negotiate competently two or more cultures: the mainstream culture and the individual's own culture.

Assimilation, by definition, promotes a loss of the contributions and customs of a minority culture as individuals try to become accepted by the majority or mainstream culture. Members of the U.S. mainstream culture are said to value and identify with the following:

- Activity and hard work
- Personal achievement and success
- Individualism
- Efficiency and practicality
- Affluence, consumerism, and material comfort
- Competition
- Openness, directness, and being well informed

Assimilation diminishes the accomplishments, contributions, and values of one culture in favor of those of the mainstream. People of different ethnicities have different core values, although people who reside in the United States also generally prescribe to core values of the mainstream. This tendency means that most U.S. residents are bicultural. Some of the core values of individuals within the prevalent ethnic groups within the United States are listed in Table 10-2.

As may be gleaned from the information in Table 10-2, many differences exist among cultural values. Cultural values are simply socially shared ideas about what is good, moral, and right and what is bad, immoral, and wrong. What must be understood so that generalizations and stereotyping about an ethnic group are not fostered is that not all members of a specific cultural group share the values of the group as a whole, and not all members show absolute compliance with his or her defining culture.

Ethnic and racial cultural differences are often accompanied by linguistic differences. This difference has become evident as the U.S. population grows increasingly diverse. Linguistic differences cause problems with communication. Speaking to and understanding people whose language is not the same as the majority of individuals in the mainstream culture of a society are difficult. In the United States, linguistic differences have provided fodder for controversy. Several groups in this country, who are quite vocal, have taken the position that, because the United States is an English-speaking country, policies should be adopted that require English to be spoken by every resident. What these groups may have failed to realize is that the United States has never adopted an official language. What these groups are essentially seeking is assimilation, which generally does not come easily. Many people do believe that *when in Rome, one should do as the Romans do,* meaning if you are in American, you should speak English. The answer to the linguistic cultural barrier may not be known for some time. What is known is that, to communicate with people from diverse culture, a common method of communication must be developed. This concept is particularly important in the delivery of services, especially education and health care.

The quality of health care delivery depends to a great extent on communication between providers and consumers. Individuals who are limited in English proficiency pose a real threat to quality health care. This cultural barrier subrogates patient rights and responsibilities, as well as the rights of providers. If a patient does not or cannot understand his or her health care providers, and vice versa, essential information cannot be communicated. Simple commands or questions can be difficult for a provider to convey. Table 10-3 contains some common commands and questions used in medical imaging in English with translation into Spanish, French, German, Italian, and Japanese.

One of the major concerns of linguistic differences is informed consent. A patient cannot be truly informed if he or she does not understand what is trying to be communicated to them. This failure places health care providers at great liability and serves as a barrier to medical treatment decisions. To provide improved medical care to individuals without or with limited English proficiency, many health care institutions are striving to overcome linguistic barriers to quality health care by:

- Hiring additional bilingual and bicultural staff
- Providing medical interpreters
- Providing translators
- Encouraging employees to become bilingual or multilingual
- Providing medical documents (e.g., consent forms) in different languages

TABLE 10-3 Common Commands and Questions Used in Medical Imaging

Language	Phrase
English	Hello, what is your name?
Spanish	¿Hola, cuál es su nombre?
French	Bonjour, quel est votre nom?
German	Hallo, ist was ilr name?
Italian	Ciao, che cosa è il vostro nome?
Japanese	こんにちは、あなたの名前は何であるか。
English	Take a deep breath.
Spanish	Tome una respiración profunda.
French	Prenez un soufflé profound.
German	Nehmen Sie einen tiefen Atem.
Italian	Prenda un alito profondo.
Japanese	深呼吸の取得。
English	Hold your breath.
Spanish	Lleve a cabo sue respiración.
French	Tenee votre soufflé.
German	Halten Sie ihren Atem.
Itallan	Tenga il rostro alito.
Japanese	あなたの呼吸を握りなさい。
English	Breathe.
Spanish	Respire.
French	Respirez.
German	Atmen Sie.
Italian	Respiri.
Japanese	呼吸しなさい。
English	Show me where you hurt.
Spanish	Demuéstreme donde usted lastima.
French	Montres moi où vous blessez.
German	Zeigen Sie mir Sie verletzen.
Italian	Mostrimi dove danneggiate.
Japanese	傷つくどこで私に示しなさい。
English	Radiology
Spanish	Radiologia
French	Radiologie
German	Radiologie
Italian	Radiologia
Japanese	放射線学
English	x-ray
Spanish	radiografia
French	rayon-x
German	Röntgenstrahle
Italian	raggi X
Japanese	X 線

These measures are a good start in significantly improving the quality of health care to people who do not speak or understand the majority language of the U.S. culture; however, more measures will probably need to be undertaken as additional linguistic barriers to health care are encountered. Believing that every health care provider will be able to communicate competently with every person who does not speak English is unreasonable. Complete linguistic competency may be an illusive goal but one toward which increasing progress must be made. Discrimination is often fostered in part by the inability to understand people who do not look, act, or speak the same as most of the members of the majority culture.

To lessen the impact of discrimination based on ethnicity and race, the Nineteenth Century Civil Rights Acts, amended in 1993, ensures all persons have equal rights under law. In addition, it provides an outline of the damages available to people receiving actions under the Civil Rights Act of 1964, Title VII, the Americans with Disabilities Act of 1990, and the Rehabilitation Act of 1973. Although government statutes exist to protect individuals based on ethnicity and race, such laws may not be necessary if people understand that individuals from all ethnicities and races have contributed positively to the growth and development of humankind and continue to do so. Understanding this concept is a giant step toward respecting and valuing human diversity.

"Sometimes I feel discriminated against, but it does not make me angry. It merely astonishes me. How can anyone deny themselves the pleasure of my company? It's beyond me."

Zora Neale Hurston

GENDER OR SEXUAL ORIENTATION. Human beings are genetically divided into two groups according to sex: female or male human beings. **Gender** describes the biologic or chromosomal sexual identity of an individual. Gender identity can be described as an inner sense of maleness or femaleness that may be influenced by several factors, including culture. The U.S. mainstream culture has progressed steadily in being inclusive of female contributions outside of the home and child rearing. In the early 1900s, traditional female roles outside of the home were in the areas of teaching, clerical positions, and nursing. By the end of that century, women had permeated and became accepted as executive officers of corporations, physicians, lawyers, politicians, and other professionals. However, women within these fields still often face what is known as a *glass ceiling* in which they are precluded from being promoted into high-level positions because of their gender. Just as discrimination based on age and ethnicity still exists, discrimination based on gender also exists. This tendency exists in spite of the fact that women are as capable and as educated as many men.

Women are often called the *weaker sex* and are considered as incapable of performing certain tasks at all, or

at least not as well as men. Some studies, as reported in the news media, suggest that women also do not have the intellectual capacity to solve complex analytical problems and are therefore not suited for some professions such as engineering and research.

Although the genetic make-up of men and women is different, both are equally capable. From birth, boys and girls are often treated differently. Many adults are predisposed in their thinking as to what boys should do and what little girls should do. Even the types and colors of clothes worn by an infant indicate whether the child is a boy or a girl (e.g., pink for girls, blue for boys). Little girls play with dolls and have tea parties; little boys are steered toward playing with cars, trucks, footballs, and basketballs. This steering is called gender role stereotyping. Gender role stereotyping is the expectation of how people should behave solely based on whether they are male or female beings. These stereotypes have nothing to do with the individual's capabilities, but they limit his or her alternatives. Only by recognizing, promoting, and valuing the capabilities and contributions of individuals, male or female persons can society embrace gender diversity as one of the essential elements for embracing human diversity.

Sexual orientation is another area of diversity often found under the topic of gender. This topic includes heterosexuality, homosexuality, and bisexuality. Heterosexual individuals are persons who are mentally, physically, and sexually attracted to individuals of the opposite gender. Homosexual, lesbian, or gay individuals are persons who are mentally, physically, and sexually attracted to persons of their same gender. Bisexual people are persons who are mentally, physically, and sexually attracted to members of both genders. These three groups have co-existed in society throughout history, but heterosexuality is generally the most accepted practice. However, in the latter part of the last century, homosexual and bisexual individuals have sought acceptance and recognition. They have also sought to end discrimination based on sexual preference and to seek equal treatment for themselves and their partners. This effort has been met with some societal resistance, but some successes have been reported in the area of gay rights. The fact is that individuals leading *alternative lifestyles,*—including those described as homosexual, lesbian, gay, or bisexual—live, work, and make positive contributions to society. What is problematic is that numerous individuals do not like these members of society and are in fact considered homophobic.

Homophobia is the irrational fear of homosexuality, accompanied by hostility toward individuals who are or are perceived to be homosexual, gay, lesbian, or bisexual. Although homophobia remains, the impetus for change in the way individuals in society think about homosexual and bisexual individuals began early in the 1900s.

The history of homosexuality reveals that these individuals have had a long struggle in their quest for acceptance. They have experienced and continue to experience isolation, alienation from loved ones and compatriots, ridicule, and abuse. Not until the 1930s did research on homosexuality began to be conducted in earnest and on a large scale. In 1938, Dr. Alfred Kinsey initiated what would become an unsurpassed analysis of human sexuality. Dr. Kinsey's research lasted for 20 years, with the release of his first findings occurring at midpoint in 1948. Dr. Kinsey's work is credited with providing statistical documentation and validation of homosexuality within the populus. Dr. Kinsey developed a scale that included six parameters of sexual tendencies within the population. Termed the *Kinsey Scale,* or *KSix,* the publication of the scale is considered the pinnacle of homosexuality, providing the beginning of a reversal of negative connotations associated with homosexuality. Box 10-1 describes the Kinsey rating scale of sexual orientation.

As may be noted in Box 10-1, KSix provides data on the prevalence of individuals with homosexual and bisexual tendencies, as compared with those having strictly heterosexual tendencies. For the first time, research suggested that homosexuality and bisexuality were not as rare as many people thought. People began to realize that they were working and interacting with homosexual and bisexual individuals and that these individuals were making positive contributions to society. This type of forward thinking has led to an increasingly accepting climate for persons leading alternative lifestyles within society and fosters a better understanding of human diversity.

MENTAL AND PHYSICAL ABILITY. Mental and physical abilities vary across the spectrum of the population as a whole. The intelligence quotient (IQ) is used to determine if individuals have normal, superior, or inferior intellectual capability. Physical and medical parameters are used to judge whether individuals are able to perform tasks that are considered essential to everyday life at the level of persons who are considered normal. Certainly, not everyone has the same **mental and physical ability.** However, the majority of people can just as certainly make some positive contribution to society in some form.

Throughout history, people with what are considered as less-than-normal physical or mental capacity and those having certain medical diseases have often been shunned

---

BOX 10-1 Kinsey Scale of Heterosexuality and Homosexuality (KSix)

O—Exclusively heterosexual experience(s)
1—Predominantly heterosexual experience(s), only incidentally homosexual
2—Predominantly heterosexual experience(s), but more than incidentally homosexual
3—Equally heterosexual and homosexual experience(s)
4—Predominantly homosexual experience(s), but more than incidentally heterosexual
5—Predominantly homosexual experience(s), but only incidentally heterosexual
6—Exclusively homosexual experience(s)

Note: Kinsey used this scale in the original report of his findings on heterosexual and homosexual behavior within the population. Kinsey found that American male individuals fell in the category of 1 to 2 but that the majority fell within 1 to 5, and at least appeared to be somewhat bisexual. He also reported that 10% of American males were exclusively homosexual.

---

by society. In some instances, these individuals were kept away from mainstream society for fear that they would be ridiculed, shunned, or worse. They were also seen as objects of assistance, protection, and treatment, rather than subjects of human rights. This thinking often led to these individuals being denied the equal access to the basic freedoms and rights that most people take for granted (e.g. education, employment, health care, participation in cultural and social activities).

In excess of 600 million individuals, accounting for approximately 10% of the world's population, have some type of disability. Some of these individuals have severe disabilities; others have moderate or mild disabilities. Some enjoy favorable living conditions, whereas others do not. Many are well taken care of, and others are not. Whatever their level of disability, living condition, or level of care, these individuals often share a common bond: discrimination and social exclusion.

During the last three decades, a shift in perspective has taken place regarding people with disabilities. Disabled individuals are now considered to have rights. Many nations have addressed this issue, including the United States. This profound shift in the way disabled people are treated has also been endorsed by the United Nations.

The Americans with Disabilities Act of 1990 was a profound and necessary step in preventing discrimination toward persons with disabilities. This Act provides

TABLE 10-4 **Four Core Values of Human Rights Law and How Each Relates to Individuals with a Disability**

VALUE	RELATIONSHIP TO DISABLED
Autonomy	Provides respect for the right of persons with a disability to have self-directed actions and behaviors and requires that the individual be the ultimate consideration and at the center of all decisions that affect her or him
Dignity	Provides mechanisms that recognize and support: the inestimable value of, because of her or his inherent self-worth, every individual, regardless of ability
Equality	Relates to the fair and equal treatment of everyone, regardless of perceived differences, including a disability
Solidarity	Requires society to support and maintain the freedoms of individuals with application of the appropriate social mechanisms

protection, under the law, for people with mental or physical disabilities. It also directs institutions, especially those receiving federal funds, to make *reasonable accommodations* for persons with disabilities. Facilities must also be accessible to disabled individuals.

In addition to efforts in the United States, the United Nations and other conventions have addressed the issues of persons with disabilities and have kept these issues at center stage since the U.N. General Assembly proclaimed 1981 as the International Year of the Disabled. In 1993 the U.N. General Assembly adopted a resolution: Standard Rules on the Equalization of Opportunities for People with Disabilities. The aim of the Standard Rules is to ensure that people with disabilities, as members of their societies, are allowed to exercise the same rights and obligations as all others; it also requires states to remove obstacles to equal participation.

Also in 1993 the Vienna Declaration for Human Rights reaffirmed the commitment of the world to eradicate discrimination based on disability. The declaration states that *all human rights and fundamental freedoms are universal and thus unreservedly include persons with disabilities.* This declaration placed the treatment of persons with disabilities in a human rights context.

All of these efforts are directed at enhancing, promoting, and protecting the human rights of persons with disabilities. Four essential core values of human rights law are particularly important when thinking about people with disabilities: (1) dignity, (2) autonomy, (3) equality, and (4) solidarity. Table 10-4 lists additional information on these core values.

The world and the United States are committed to promoting equality and full participation in society for persons with disabilities. Although the process may seem slow, reform in the way individuals with disabilities are viewed is underway. Nondiscrimination, equal access, and the equally effective enjoyment of all human rights by people with disabilities are long overdue. Disabilities are just one of the many diverse areas among human beings. Discrimination, inequality, and injustice applied to persons with disabilities deprive society of their active participation, as well as significant contributions. Not thinking in terms of people being called disabled, which tends to provoke a negative mind-set because of the prefix *dis,* meaning to deprive of, and thinking in terms of them being differently *abled* might promote a different mindset and alter society's perception. These differences are the core element of human diversity.

EMBRACING DIVERSITY

As mentioned in each of the preceding sections, individuals from all different cultures have contributed positively to society. A realization that everyone should learn to live and work with people who may be culturally different should also exist. In addition, goods and services are consumed and provided by people from different cultures. By recognizing, accepting, and learning about cultures that may be different from their own, people can learn ways of avoiding conflict between cultures and enjoy a more inclusive, representative, nondiscriminatory society. Only then can human diversity be fully embraced and valued.

Living and working in a diverse society is challenging. Civility and respect for others, in both areas, is expected. This respect comes from individuals and begins with first learning about other cultures. Many misconceptions exist about other groups of individuals. These misconceptions may have been developed and fostered by the beliefs and experiences of others and not as a result of personal contact. By learning ways to accommodate diversity, people can become increasingly adept at dealing with others.

"Diversity transcends race and gender, affirmative action, and equal employment opportunity. It must encompass a fundamental appreciation of one another and a respect for both our similarities and our differences. It must include a heartfelt respect in attitude and in behavior toward those of different race, gender, age, sexual orientation, and those with disabilities. All the facets that makes each individual the unique and precious resource that each of us is."

Ronald Brown, Former Secretary of Commerce

Learning is the essential element of knowledge. Understanding and accepting cannot take place if a refusal to learn exists. Interacting with different cultures personally, socially, and on a business level assists in the learning process. Knowledge itself does not automatically transcend into better outcomes; other steps also need to be taken. Policies and practices must also be put in place to allow forward thinking, acceptance, and inclusion of differing cultures. Knowledge about individuals and groups of people should be integrated and transformed into standards, policies, practices, and attitudes that are used in the appropriate cultural settings so as to increase the quality of services. This effort results in better outcomes. Multiculturalism provides an atmosphere in which everyone gains knowledge and skills that may be shared by all.

DEVELOPING CULTURAL COMPETENCY

Cultural competency is defined as possessing a set of attitudes, congruent behaviors, and policies that come together in an agency, system, or among professionals that enable effective interactions in a cross-cultural or multicultural environment. Many elements may contribute to the ability of an agency or institution to become culturally competent. Five of these elements are:

1. Valuing diversity
2. Possessing the capacity for cultural self-assessment
3. Having a consciousness of the dynamics of cross-cultural interaction
4. Institutionalizing cultural knowledge
5. Developing adaptations of service delivery that reflect an understanding of a multicultural environment

These five elements will not work in isolation within an agency or organization. They must be demonstrated at every level within the institution, including adminis-

tration, policy making, and services. Becoming culturally competent does not happen overnight; it is an ongoing process that requires reevaluation of the ways things are done within an agency or organization and how those things influence the environment and the services rendered.

To be totally culturally competent, consideration must be given to all of the areas of human diversity, including language. Linguistic competency means providing readily available, culturally appropriate, oral and written language services to individuals with limited English proficiency. This goal may be accomplished through the use of bicultural and bilingual individuals or interpreters.

In health care, including medical imaging and radiation therapy, human diversity has always been evident. To provide health care consumers (patients) with quality patient care, diagnosis, and treatment, clear and unimpeded communication must occur. Health care providers must not demonstrate bias toward any patient for any reason; rather, they must strive to understand and accept the cultural differences of patients because of their age, ethnicity, physical and mental abilities, gender and sexual orientation, and illness or disease.

Certified and registered medical imaging technologists and radiation therapists are governed by professional codes and standards that preclude discriminatory practices and provide for the delivery of quality patient care with disregard for cultural differences. The standards of ethics and the incorporated code of ethics of the American Registry of Radiologic Technologists (ARRT) (Appendix D) specifically address nondiscriminatory professional practice by persons holding ARRT credentials. The American Society of Radiologic Technologists (ASRT) has also developed initiatives to increase cultural diversity among members of the profession. One of the more notable initiatives is the establishment of the Royce Osborne Minority. This scholarship, supported by the ARRT, provides scholarships to minority imaging and therapy students in educational programs throughout the country. The ASRT has also issued several position statements in support of cultural competency and has incorporated ethical and professional attributes into documents governing those practicing in medical imaging and radiation therapy (Appendix D). The ARRT and ASRT, as well as many other professional imaging organizations, have tried to make it clear that they value human diversity and the contributions made to the profession by the diverse population of educators and clinicians alike.

Medical professionals are embracing diversity and striving toward cultural competency, but they face unique

TABLE 10-5 **Six Areas of Human Cultural Diversity Related to Health Care and the Impact They Have on the Delivery of that Care**

AREA	DEFINITION AND IMPACT ON HEALTH CARE
Communication	The ability to convey and receive information. Knowing the norm within a culture will facilitate understanding and lessen miscommunication. Miscommunication is a frequent problem among different cultures.
Space	Distance extending in all directions. Proximity to personal boundaries and comfort level—eye contact, distance and touch practices—vary between cultures. Failure to understand and respect different cultural practices, including space, may cause miscommunication and lessens regard for health care providers.
Time	A period of duration; indefinite, unlimited duration in which things are considered as happening (e.g. past, present, future). Cultures have different time orientations; for example, England and China seem to be oriented in the past, valuing tradition, and doing things as they have always been done; people from these countries may be hesitant to try new medical procedures or treatments. Present-oriented cultures (e.g. Latin American, Native American; Middle Eastern) may neglect preventive care measures because they focus on the here and now. Health care providers must work with these cultures in an attempt to get these individuals to understand that medicine is focused on both prevention and treatment and that everyone can live a healthy and long life.
Environmental control	Ability of people to control nature. Differences in health practices and definitions of health and illness are evident in the different cultures. These variation need to be understood so that the appropriate actions can be undertaken to preserve the health of individuals and provide adequate treatment while preserving cultural concepts.
Biologic variations	Ethical or racially related differences in body structure, skin color, hair texture, and other physical characteristics; it also addresses genetic variations, susceptibility to certain diseases, nutritional preferences and differences, psychologic characteristics, among others. Health care providers must understand how these biologic variations impact the health of individuals within the different ethnic cultures, and they must secure diagnosis and provide treatment based on some of these variations.
Social organizations	Patterns of behaviors related to cultures learned through the process of enculturation. Health care providers must recognize these differences and accept them. Providers need to know that, in some cultures, great value is placed on decisions made by the elders. In others, the expectations and roles of children are strictly defined.

challenges. Although they have become increasingly knowledgeable on issues of diversity in health care, medical professionals have not necessarily become effective. They know that patients, whatever their cultural background, require dignity and respect and need to feel seen and heard as individuals. Knowledge of the different cultures and empathy toward all patients are two ways that providers can become culturally competent in providing care. Empathy may be the core skill needed in health care intervention. Three critical empathetic practices help to bridge cultural insight and produce better outcomes.

- Making quick powerful connections with patient (communication)
- Gathering culturally relevant information (assessment and communication)
- Working with patients to form strategies that meet their individual needs, the needs of the provider, and the needs of the medical facility or practice (negotiating)

The application of empathy skills:

- Promotes better health care outcomes overall
- Increases patient satisfaction
- Decreases health care costs
- Decreases provider liability

Health care providers need information, and one of the best ways of obtaining cultural relevant information is by emphasizing empathy through intense listening and curiosity. The core of empathetic communication is accurately understanding patient feelings and communicating this understanding back to them effectively. Empathy is therapeutic in that it provides the patient with a feeling of being understood by their health care provider, makes them feel less isolated by their illness or disease, and gives them a sense of individuality.

To provide quality and effective care for all patients, health care providers need to understand six areas of human cultural diversity and how these areas influence the delivery of care:

1. Communication
2. Space
3. Time
4. Environmental control
5. Biologic variations
6. Social organizations

Table 10-5 provides a definition for each of these areas.

Becoming culturally competent is no easy task, but it is an essential one. Society is becoming more diverse on a daily basis. We can no longer ignore the impact of our multicultural society. Members of society must learn to value human diversity and to become culturally competent. This knowledge can only enrich society as a whole.

SUMMARY

Human diversity is a topic of importance globally. The people of the world have noticed that their societies are becoming increasingly diverse. Individuals need to learn to accept multiculturalism so that everyone can believe that they are an integral part of the society in which they live. To be accepting of human diversity, the concept of human diversity itself must first be understood. Inherent biases may hinder this understanding, but knowledge about the various cultures may help erase some of these biases. In addition, learning about the laws and statutes that help protect some cultures from discrimination is helpful as individuals in a society learn to embrace and value human diversity. That these laws and statutes were developed as a direct result of past discrimination and inequality must also be remembered. Many countries throughout the world, and the United States, are seeking ways to teach the citizens to be accepting of multiculturalism. Corporations, industry, education, and health care institutions are in the midst of a cultural diversity awareness and competency movement. Health care institutions, organization, and professionals are taking a strong lead in recognizing that patients, as well as workers, are culturally diverse. Patient care hinges on understanding, communication, and empathy, and health care is fostering the development of these skills in every practitioner because doing so will directly benefit society (the U.S. culture) as a whole. Human diversity has positively influenced society, and the recognition of this influence through cultural competency can only have greater positive impacts on society.

"Always remember that you are unique, just like everybody else."

Anonymous

BIBLIOGRAPHY

29 U.S.C. §§ 621-634—The Age Discrimination Employment Act.

42 U.S.C. Chapter 21—Civil Rights Act of 1964.

42 U.S.C. §§ 1981, 1981a, 1983, 1988—Nineteenth Century Civil Rights Acts.

42 U.S.C. §§ 102—Americans with Disabilities Act of 1990.

Bonder B, Martin L, Miracle A: Achieving cultural competence: the challenge for clients and healthcare workers in a multicultural society, *Generations* 25:35, 2001.

Gilanti GA: *Caring for patients from different cultures,* Philadelphia, 1991, University of Pennsylvania Press.

Shams-Avari P: Linguistic and cultural competency, *Radiol Technol* 76(6):437, 2005.

Townsley-Cook D, Young T: *Ethical and legal issues for medical imaging professionals,* St Louis, 1999, Mosby.

Wilson BG: *Ethics and basic law for medical imaging professionals,* Philadelphia, 1997, FA Davis.

U.S. Department of Commerce, U.S. Census Bureau: *Statistical abstract of the United States,* Washington, DC, 2001, U.S. Government Printing Office.

The American Registry of Radiologic Technologists, Ethics Division; Standards of Ethics, Available at: *http://www.arrt.org,* accessed July 19, 2005.

The American Society of Radiologic Technologists, Scholarships: Available at: *http://www.asrt.org,* accessed July 12, 2005.

Transcultural Nursing, Cultural Diversity in Nursing Assessment Measures: Available at: *http://www. culturediversity.org/assesmnt.htm,* accessed February 19, 2005.

The Freeman Institute—Diversity; The Value of Mutual Respect: Available at: *http://www.freemaninstitute.com/ diversity.htm,* accessed July 2, 2005.

The University of Alabama at Birmingham, Office of the Vice President for Equity and Diversity, Diversity; Available at: *http://www.uab.edu/equityanddiversity,* accessed May 1, 2005.

Lexico Publishing Group, Translator; Available at: *http://dictionary.reference.com/translate/text.html,* accessed March 25, 2005.

Patient Care

Patient Interactions

Bettye G. Wilson, MAEd, RT(R)(CT), ARRT, RDMS, FASRT

Once one learns to cut himself off from his feeling, it is sometimes frightening to realize how difficult it seems to get back in touch with them. This cannot always be done at 5:00 P.M. on schedule, and the student soon learns, like Dr. Jekyll, that the potion doesn't always wear off when it's time to go home.

David Reiser and Andrea Schroder
Patient Interviewing: The Human Dimension

OBJECTIVES

On completion of this chapter, the student will be able to:

1. Identify qualities needed to be a caring radiologic technologist.

2. Specify needs that cause people to enter radiologic technology as a profession.

3. Discuss general needs that patients may have according to Maslow's hierarchy of needs.

4. Relate differences between the needs of inpatients and those of outpatients.

5. Explain why patient interaction is important to patients, as well as their family and friends.

6. Analyze effective methods of communication for patients of various ages.

OBJECTIVES—Cont'd

7. Explain appropriate interaction techniques for various types of patients.

8. Discuss considerations of the physical changes of aging for radiologic examinations.

9. Discuss appropriate methods of responding to terminally ill patients.

GLOSSARY

Advanced Directive: a legal document prepared by a living, competent adult to provide guidance to the health care team if the individual should become unable to make decisions regarding his or her medical care; may also be called a living will or durable power of attorney for health care

Communication: exchange of information, thoughts, or messages; includes interpersonal rapport; also includes the accurate conveyance of information, clear self-expression, and transmitting information and ideas to others

Gerontology: pertaining to the study of the older adults

Inpatient: someone who has been admitted to the hospital for diagnostic studies or treatment

Maslow's Hierarchy of Needs: model of human needs developed by Abraham Maslow in 1954. In the original hierarchy, Maslow identifies two types of needs: deficiency and growth. These needs were further divided into seven levels, four at the deficiency needs level (physiologic, safety, belongingness and love, and esteem) and three in the upper growth needs level (need to know and

understand, aesthetic, and self-actualization). According to Maslow's concept, people fulfill their deficiency needs before seeking to fulfill their growth needs.

Nonverbal Communication: exchange of information, thoughts, or messages using methods other than the actual words of speech, for example, tone of voice, speed of speech, and position of the speaker's extremities and torso (body language)

Outpatient: patient who comes to a health care facility for diagnosis or treatment but does not occupy a bed

Palpation: application of light pressure with the fingers

Paralanguage: music of language; cadence and rhythm of speech

Patient Assessment: objective evaluation and determination of the status of a patient

Patient Autonomy: ability and right of patients to make independent decisions regarding their medical care

Verbal Communication: messages sent using spoken words; can be dramatically shaped by vocabulary, clarity, tone, pitch of voice, and even the organization of sentences

PERSONAL UNDERSTANDING

Radiologic technology is a people-oriented, hands-on profession that requires proficiency in a wide variety of **communication** techniques. Educational programs in the radiologic sciences should strive to assist students in developing effective methods of patient contact early. This approach will assist them in achieving a successful and enjoyable career.

The American population is diverse, and the importance of interacting effectively with diverse patients is critical to the radiologic technologist, as well as to the patient. These techniques greatly improve the quality of the radiologic images, as well as patient care. Obtaining the patient's cooperation is one of the most challenging parts of a radiologic technologist's role. The most seasoned radiologic technologist will sometimes have to

repeat images if the patient does not understand the procedure or does not cooperate because of poor communication.

The communication skills of the radiologic technologist often determine the patient's opinion of the radiology department. Because hospitals and clinics depend heavily on reimbursement for patient services, the use of effective interactive skills can make the patient's visit pleasant and meaningful, and it might encourage his or her return for additional medical care.

Students have needs to satisfy their career ambitions, which often include:

- Helping others
- Working with people
- Making a difference

- Thinking critically
- Demonstrating creativity
- Achieving results

Radiologic technology is capable of fulfilling all of these needs and many more. When personal needs are met, experiencing increased confidence in technical abilities as well is not unusual. The patient often perceives this concept as competence because the external appearance is that of a self-assured individual capable of smoothly carrying out procedures.

Maslow's hierarchy of needs provides insight into this type of behavior for all persons, professionals and patients alike (Fig. 11–1). Maslow suggests that people strive from a basic level of physiologic needs toward a level of self-actualization. This highest level is characterized by confidence in who the person is and what the person's goals are in life. Essentially, each level of needs must be satisfied before proceeding to the next level. Radiologic technology students often begin their education at approximately the third level, which relates to belonging or affection needs. Once instructors, classmates, and staff radiologic technologists have accepted the student, they must move toward the fourth level, which addresses self-esteem and respect needs. Many students achieve this level during the second year, once many of the required clinical skills have been mastered. As graduation and the certification examination are successfully completed, level seven, the self-actualization level, can begin in a professional context.

As jobs or roles change, moving up and down the various levels of the hierarchy and being at different levels in different roles would be normal. For example, a new husband may be at the fourth level at work but at the third level in marriage.

Patient Needs

To interact effectively with patients, understanding that patients may be in an altered state of consciousness is important. They are in an unfamiliar environment in which they are no longer in complete control. In addition, they often fear not knowing the exact state of their health. Preferring bad news to uncertainty—because, at least, plans can be made to cope with bad news—is not unusual for a patient, whereas uncertainty leaves a person without a means to attempt to control the situation. Empathizing with these feelings is difficult until they have been experienced personally.

Most patients would prefer not to be in the care of health care professionals, including radiologic technolo-

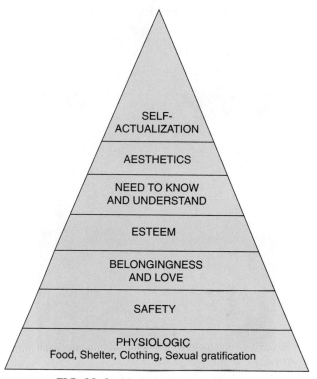

FIG. 11–1 Maslow's hierarchy of needs.

gists. Even the kindest and most cooperative patients are simply making the best of a situation they would prefer to avoid. An injury or the potential for disease or illness exists; otherwise they would not be seeking medical care. In many instances, patients' fear of what the radiologic technologist will find through the images causes them to be inconsiderate, arrogant, impatient, rude, overly talkative, or to exhibit other symptoms as they attempt to cope with their situation.

Patient Dignity

The patient may arrive for care at the first level of Maslow's hierarchy of needs, which is the physiologic or survival level. Illness or trauma may have altered many physiologic functions, which, in turn, may cause the patient to behave abnormally.

A lack of satisfaction in level-one needs can cause a patient to be unable to satisfy the other higher needs. For example, if a female patient is very sick, she might lose sleep (level one) over how she will keep her job and maintain her home or belongings (level two). When a patient arrives with a nasogastric tube (Fig. 11–2), although normally very friendly and talkative, he or she

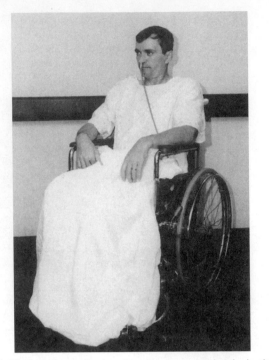

FIG. 11–2   When patients arrive with a nasogastric tube in place, although they may normally be friendly and outgoing, they may prefer to wait in a location where they do not have to face the public.

may not want to be around other patients with the nasogastric tube in place (level three).

Radiologic technologists have an awesome responsibility when interacting with patients because of the tremendous power that is held by health professionals over patients. This power is so great that it includes the most basic elements of a person's dignity and self-respect. Inconsiderate abuse of this power may seem to be difficult to avoid because of the nature of the examination procedures. Consequently, special attention is needed to ensure that the power is not abused. For example, when patients are required to wear flimsy patient gowns, when they are referred to as the *stomach* or *colon* instead of by his or her name, or when they are placed in proximity to other patients who are more critically ill, patients can feel dehumanized. Maintaining self-respect is difficult while trying to get to a toilet before evacuating barium from the bowel, when vomiting, and in other uncomfortable situations.

Professional radiologic technologists should learn about different types of patients, along with various methods of communication, that are effective with each.

Two main classifications of patients can be considered: (1) inpatients and (2) outpatients. Each type has typical characteristics that require different approaches and interaction skills on the part of the technologist. Whether the patient is an inpatient or outpatient, one of the initial patient communication skills is **patient assessment.** Initial patient assessment by the radiographer usually comes in the form of chart or procedure request review, or both. Much information can be gleaned from these two documents concerning patient history and indications for or contraindications to the requested procedure. Second, patient assessment by the radiographer usually comes in the form of verbal communication. All health care professionals should introduce themselves to their patients, explain the procedure to patients, and obtain a brief history. Many medical imaging departments have patient questionnaires requiring that the technologist ask the patients pertinent questions regarding their history and medical status before a procedure can be preformed. In other instances, if a patient is scheduled to have an invasive procedure or the use of intravascular contrast media is required, obtaining informed consent is often the responsibility of the technologist. In either instance, good communication skills are a must.

Inpatients

An **inpatient** is someone who has been admitted to the hospital for diagnostic studies or treatment. In general, these persons occupy a hospital bed for longer than 24 hours. Inpatients often move up and down Maslow's hierarchy before arriving in the care of the radiologic technologist. Gaining the patient's confidence is important, even though he or she may be in a somewhat agitated or bewildered state of mind. Previous experiences in the hospital may have shaped the manner in which the patient responds to these initial interactions with the technologist. For example, a patient with severe lower back pain who has been transferred from a bed to a cart by inexperienced nursing staff may be skeptical of a radiologic technologist's assurances of a smooth and careful transfer onto an examination table.

The inpatient may be transported to the radiology department by wheelchair or cart or by walking (ambulating). While in the waiting area of the radiology department, the patient has an opportunity to hear and see many departmental activities. Technologists should always be aware that, although they are familiar with the department and may take patients' waiting for granted, patients are listening and watching everything in anticipation of how they may be treated.

Outpatients

An **outpatient** is someone who has come to the hospital or outpatient center for diagnostic testing or treatment but does not occupy a bed. Outpatients arrive in the radiology department with prior expectations. They often expect to be seen immediately on arriving in the department because they have a scheduled appointment. Maintaining a schedule in any medical setting is difficult because of unforeseen circumstances. For example, follow-up images on a previous patient may take longer than expected; a radiologist may require extra projections to be certain of a diagnosis; or patients may become ill, refuse examinations, or be unable to cooperate fully. Apologizing for delays and trying to keep waiting patients up to date on their status is certainly appropriate and important, for example, telling a patient that it will be 20 minutes before he or she can be seen is appropriate if no emergencies exist. If something unforeseen occurs, then little extra time is required to say, "I'll be with you as soon as I finish one more patient," as you walk by 15 minutes later. Patients greatly appreciate the simple fact that you are aware they are waiting and you perceive their patience. More positive comments are received by hospitals from these types of interactions than for any other reason.

Because outpatients often have insurance or government benefits of some type, they may expect priority treatment. A professional should provide the same care and attention to all patients regardless of status. This care can be especially difficult when a patient is a famous personality, a criminal, or otherwise known.

INTERACTING WITH THE PATIENT'S FAMILY AND FRIENDS

The patient's family and friends who are visiting also must receive attention. Because they spend much time waiting, they tend to critique everything the radiologic technologist does, from appearance to tone of voice to smile (or lack of). Being courteous to visitors and relatives, as well as to the patient, is important. Relatives are justifiably concerned and may ask questions such as whether the technologist sees anything abnormal or whether a fracture is present. Thinking about how the family and friends feel or considering how concerned you would be about a member of your own family would help.

The same needs function for family and friends as for the patient and technologist. Abnormal or rude behavior may be the result of anxiety, concern, or stress. Being asked for an interpretation of images is common for the

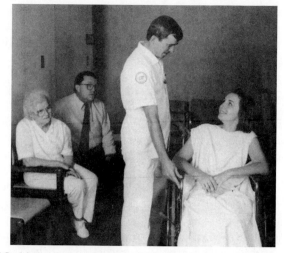

FIG. 11–3 Family members often listen closely to everything a professional says. The radiation technologist should be careful not to attempt to interpret images because this is diagnosing, which is illegal.

radiologic technologist. An important point to remember is that family and friends often listen closely to everything a professional says (Fig. 11–3). Any statements in response to this type of question may be construed as diagnosing, which is practicing medicine and is illegal without a license. The best response is usually to indicate that the findings are available to the referring physician and that only he or she can provide the information.

The radiologic technologist has a responsibility to make patients, as well as their family and friends, believe they are receiving the best possible care and that they are important and special. A smile and brief explanation of the procedure, with extra attention when delays occur, go a long way in making everyone feel more relaxed and confident.

METHODS OF EFFECTIVE COMMUNICATION

Attention to the various forms of interaction and communication techniques that have proved effective in improving relationships with patients can produce dramatic results in clinical situations. Accurate and timely communication is essential to providing quality patient care. A coordinated, team approach is required, with the patient at the center. Developing patient-provider rapport paves the way for an interchange of information that makes the patient feel at ease, leading to better cooperation. Communication comes in many forms, and health care practitioners must be aware of them all; otherwise, although they may not verbally communicate an idea or thought, other forms of communication may be conveying the message, positive or negative.

Verbal Skills

SPEECH AND GRAMMAR. The methods of **verbal communication** that are used in establishing an open relationship between the health professional and the patient are basic to the quality of the interaction. Vocabulary, clarity of voice, and even the organization of sentences must be at an appropriate level for the patient. For example, discussing units of radiation dose with a Protestant minister is probably not of interest to him or her. Conversely, telling a physics teacher that a chest x-ray dose is similar to a few minutes of sun tanning is equally inappropriate.

An important point to remember is that, whenever possible, verbal communication should occur face to face. This approach typically makes others believe as though they have your undivided attention, your concern is only for them, and they are the only person about whom you care at this specific point in time. Be polite and focus attention on the listener's perception of the manner in which you are communicating. Remember that cultural and individual differences in people may affect their perception of what you are trying to convey. Be careful not to patronize or otherwise demean an individual.

HUMOR. The value of humor in medical settings is well documented. Using humor to relax and open up conversation is acceptable, but the radiologic technologist must be extremely careful to avoid cultural slurs and references to age, sex, diseases, and the abilities of health professionals. The fact that many patients use self-deprecating humor about their disabilities or fears as an emotional release must not be construed as permission for the radiographer to joke in a similar manner. Laughter is good medicine, but when humor is used in an incorrect manner, wrong context, or is perceived as unprofessional, it becomes a tool that may prohibit good communication. For example, if a patient asks about the specifics of a medical imaging procedure, and the reply is, "I don't know, this is my first time performing this procedure," although this response may be humorous to the technologist, the patient may become apprehensive about having an unexperienced person performing his or her examination. This apprehension may lead to closure of all communication channels between the two parties.

Nonverbal Communication

PARALANGUAGE. **Paralanguage** is the music of language; it produces a form of **nonverbal communication.** Patients receive signals about your attitude toward them from the pitch, stress, tone, pauses, speech rate, volume, accent, and quality of your voice. For example, because the mind works faster than the voice, thinking of a response when someone who is talking pauses is common. This knowledge can be used to structure productive questions. For example, asking a patient "Exactly where does it hurt most?" may not produce as much information as saying "You said it hurts a lot around your stomach. Now exactly where would you say the pain is usually greatest?" The second statement gives patients time to recall what they said and to think specifically about the statement before being asked to answer.

BODY LANGUAGE. Patients quickly perceive nonverbal communication such as tone of voice, speed of speech, and the position of the speaker's extremities and torso (body language). Radiographers must be cautious to avoid giving confusing signals to patients by saying one thing and acting in a totally different manner. For example, asking a patient if he or she is comfortable but neglecting to offer a positioning sponge to hold an oblique position may call into question the sincerity, and consequently the trustworthiness, of the technologist. Positive nonverbal cues increase the quantity and quality of communication and improve the history. For example, the technologist should look at patients and show interest in their statements. Smiling, responding candidly, and using a friendly tone of voice all work toward this end. Negative nonverbal cues also can be used to improve the history. For example, looking puzzled may prompt the patient to elaborate on exactly how an injury occurred and may provide the radiologist with details on the direction of the force that caused a fracture. While speaking with patients, the radiologist should avoid standing away from them with the arms folded across the chest. This body language is generally perceived as someone who is on the defensive, has something to hide, or is repulsed by the patient.

TOUCH. The radiographer commonly uses three types of touch: (1) touching for emotional support, (2) touching for emphasis, and (3) touching for palpation. Few things are more reassuring than a gentle pat on the hand or shoulder as a form of emotional support (Fig. 11–4). Humans respond extremely well to touch, and using this technique is acceptable, as long as proper social conven-

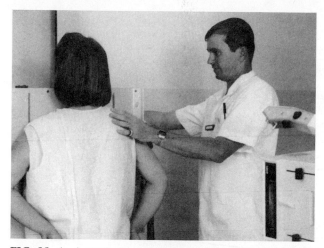

FIG. 11–4 A gentle touch at the shoulder can be reassuring without being offensive.

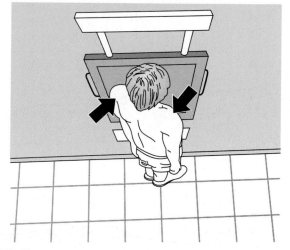

FIG. 11–5 Touching for emphasis to help a patient turn the left side toward a chest unit. A gentle touch at the posterior left shoulder accompanied by a similar touch at the anterior right shoulder accomplishes the movement quickly and efficiently.

tions are followed. The use of touch conveys to patients that the technologist is trying to understand, be empathetic, and care about them as people. Gentle support under the arm to assist patients to and from the imaging room and onto and off of the table often provides reassurance to the patient that he or she is being cared for by a professional practitioner.

Touching for emphasis involves using touch to highlight or to specify instructions or locations. For example, after a posteroanterior chest radiograph has been performed, patients can be instructed to turn their left side toward a chest unit by a gentle touch at the posterior left shoulder accompanied by a similar touch at the anterior right shoulder (Fig. 11–5). For example, after a patient states, "My stomach hurts here," and places a hand on the upper abdomen, the radiographer can elicit further information by asking, "Does it hurt more here or here?" while touching the duodenal and gastric regions.

Palpation is the application of light pressure with the fingers to the body. Palpating to locate various bony landmarks when positioning patients is often advisable. In a similar fashion, using specific palpation is often useful to determine a more exact localization during history taking. Effective and precise palpation requires the *gentle* use of fingertips (Fig. 11–6). The use of the palm or several fingers is less precise than using fingertips and may, in some instances, be painful or even offensive to patients. For example, a 14-year-old girl is usually more comfortable if a male radiographer palpates for the iliac crest with the tip of a finger than if the entire hand is used to feel the hip region. Before touching a patient, his

or her permission to do so should be obtained. Touching without consent can have legal ramifications.

PROFESSIONAL APPEARANCE. Most programs in radiologic technology have a dress code for students. Although dressing according to a code does not produce a better radiologic technologist, a professional appearance in the medical setting says as much about a person as their technical abilities say about their competence. Professional dress helps the patient feel comfortable and confident in the technologist's abilities. Gaining the patient's confidence and trust is a considerable part of being a competent radiologic technologist.

PERSONAL HYGIENE. Personal hygiene is as important as professional appearance. Personal grooming sends a powerful message. Unkempt individuals may prompt patients to suspect that the person's professional behavior is similar to his or her appearance: neglected and disheveled. Hair, nails, and teeth should be neat and clean. Nails should be kept at a manageable length, without the use of acrylics, which have been banned in many health care institutions. Body odor emanating from anyone causes others to react negatively, suggesting that the person is unclean. Daily baths or showers, good oral hygiene, and the use of personal hygiene products may be used to eliminate this problem. The use of strong perfumes, colognes, and aftershaves should be also be avoided. Patients may be allergic to certain smells or

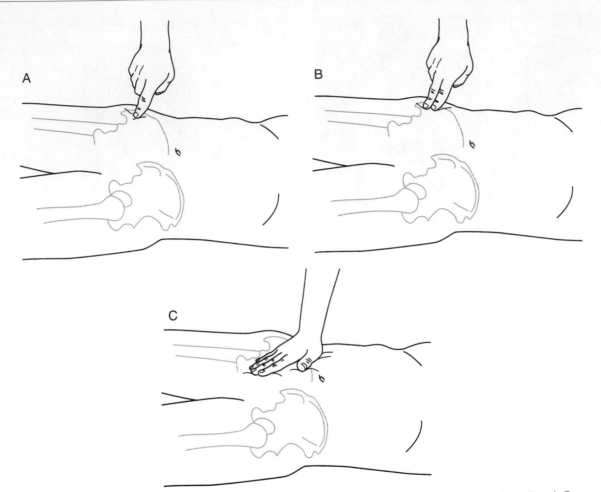

FIG. 11–6 Proper palpation is accomplished by using fingertips to provide precise and gentle localization information. *A*, Proper use of a single fingertip. *B*, Proper use of several fingers. *C*, Improper use of the palm.

nauseated, and any smell may affect them negatively. A patient will not communicate with someone with whom they do not desire to be in close contact.

PHYSICAL PRESENCE. Appearance and physical presence go together. Posture is important because it is perceived as relating to confidence and self-esteem. Facial expressions are vital nonverbal cues that give people information on the importance of instructions and questions, as well as both positive and negative reinforcement of their actions and statements. For example, confusion and frustration are easily communicated in this manner.

VISUAL CONTACT. As stated previously, eye contact may help ensure that questions, instructions, and other information have been understood. Visual inspection of a patient's condition can be critical when changes such as blood pressure and allergic reactions produce symptoms.

UNDERSTANDING THE VARIOUS TYPES OF PATIENTS

Patients in radiology often have unusual conditions in addition to the conditions for which they are undergoing examination. The medical population is as diverse as the general population and will continue to grow more diverse as time passes. An understanding of the most common special conditions can be valuable in meeting their needs.

Seriously Ill and Traumatized Patients

Not all patients with whom the technologist comes into contact want to talk or are able to cooperate during their examination. A seriously ill or traumatized patient may act differently than other patients because of pain, stress, or anxiety. In these instances, the patient must hear and understand instructions, if at all possible.

First, the technologist should try to communicate with the patient while determining his or her coherence level. This initial communication can provide cues regarding the state of consciousness and coherency of the patient. Some patients may be unable to respond, others may make incoherent statements, and still others may respond coherently but uncooperatively. Inability or unwillingness to communicate can be caused by many factors, including pain, shock, medication reaction, and disorientation. Indeed, the very nature of the illness, disease, or trauma can alter an individual's ability to cooperate or communicate, or both.

Working quickly and efficiently while continuing to communicate with the patient is important, although no response from the patient is forthcoming. Letting the patient know what is going on during an examination can be reassuring, even when no apparent sign of understanding is made.

Because seriously ill and traumatized patients may not be able to communicate effectively, watching for visual indications of changes in vital signs becomes especially important. When patients cannot tell anyone that they are having difficulty breathing, they must rely completely on the technologist to recognize potential problems promptly. Helping someone is a great feeling; however, when a seriously ill or injured patient must rely on you, the added responsibility can greatly enhance these feelings.

Radiologic technologists interact with patients who exhibit a wide variety of impairments. Combining common sense, empathy, and classroom knowledge will enable you to provide quality radiographs for patients who would otherwise receive suboptimal examinations. Remember that the patient's cooperation is one of the main factors essential to producing quality radiographs.

Visually Impaired Patients

A blind patient, a patient who has decreased vision without glasses, or an optically injured patient needs special attention. The technologist should attempt to gain the patient's confidence as soon as possible by giving clear instructions before the examination, as well as informing him or her of what is occurring at all times. Reassuring the patient through a gentle touch establishes that someone is near if needed. Continued verbal communication assists persons who are blind and visually impaired with satisfying many of the basic needs attributed to Maslow.

Speech- and Hearing-Impaired Patients

Patients who are deaf or have impaired hearing also require special attention. For persons who can read, the primary means of communication can be writing. The technologist must not insult the patient's intelligence by attempting to simplify terminology. Hearing does not control intelligence.

Pantomime and demonstration work well with hearing-impaired patients. For example, counting to three on your fingers, pinching your nose, and taking a deep breath symbolizes to the patient that you need him or her to hold the breath while you count to three. Patients should demonstrate instructions in return to make sure they understand. Many facilities offer deaf services and will provide a sign language expert as necessary.

Non–English-Speaking Patients

Imagine the frustration you would feel if you were in a foreign country where no one understood English. Effective interaction with non–English-speaking patients is greatly enhanced by using touch, facial expressions, and pantomime. Nearly all such patients understand basic words such as *yes, no,* and *stop.* Everyone appreciates any attempt to speak his or her language, even if only to say *yes* and *no.* Pronunciation and accents are quickly overlooked when good intentions are shown. Most hospitals maintain a list of bilingual employees who are available to help patients and visitors.

Mentally Impaired Patients

Working with mentally impaired patients requires a thorough knowledge of equipment and immobilization techniques, as well as interaction skills. Although degrees of mental impairment vary, using a strong yet reassuring tone of voice with these patients is important. A continuous conversation while preparing the patient for the examination usually helps keep the patient calm and aware that the technologist is working with him or her.

Substance Abusers

Radiologic technologists who work weekends, holidays, and evenings are often involved with patients who are under the influence of drugs or alcohol. These patients may not be totally aware of what they are doing and may need to be restrained from leaving the room or from playing with high-voltage cables.

The best mode of interaction with these patients often includes assessing their capabilities, attempting to establish a means of communication, using technical knowledge, and working efficiently to decrease the total examination time.

Patients who are under the influence of drugs or alcohol may be relaxed, or they may be hyperactive and irrational. The technologist must observe them closely and use immobilization techniques as necessary. If patients are hyperactive and loud, then they obviously require close supervision. Calm, quiet patients are of increased concern because they may react without warning and fall or otherwise injure themselves.

Some substance abusers respond well to firm directions about what to do, whereas others are best handled by requesting that they return for examination at a later time when the effects have diminished considerably. The technologist will always encounter some patients who simply cannot be examined properly without assistance from other medical personnel. Waiting until the patient becomes cooperative is often best. Seriously injured patients are seldom uncooperative, especially when they believe their life may be in jeopardy.

Restraints may be needed when dealing with mentally ill and other patients. Remember that using restraints can lead to legal ramifications. Using restraints must occur only as prescribed in facility procedure and policy.

MOBILE AND SURGICAL EXAMINATIONS

Many patients who require mobile examination are too sick or injured to be transported to the radiology department for examination. Patients may be unconscious and attached to an array of tubes, monitoring lines, ventilators, and other medical equipment. Except in surgery, during which the patient is normally incapable of interacting because of anesthesia, attempting to establish a line of communication with the patient is important. Begin by calling the patient's name, identifying yourself to the patient, and explaining the procedure. This approach permits assessment of the patient's condition and level of coherence.

Under no circumstances should the technologist assume that a patient does not comprehend comments that are made within the patient's range of hearing. Patients may be cognizant although they appear to be comatose. Several studies have reported instances in which patients in deep anesthesia or even long-term comatose states were able to recall jokes and derogatory comments that were made about them. Both cognizant and incoherent patients will demonstrate increased coop-

eration if they hear a kind voice of explanation before being touched. Even if the words are not understood, a caring tone of voice and a gentle touch often have a positive effect.

In interacting with the patient's family and friends, you should introduce yourself, explain the procedure briefly, and explain why they must leave the immediate area during the exposure. In most instances, no need exists to send visitors far, and explaining that the exposure is only a fraction of a second often encourages them to wait nearby while the equipment is removed. Remember that visitors sometimes arrive from distant places at considerable expense and that every moment may be precious with a dying parent or favorite aunt. Visitors appreciate courtesy and thoughtfulness.

AGE AS A FACTOR IN PATIENT INTERACTIONS

Age differences between the radiologic technologist and the patient should not be a barrier to effective communication. Nearly everyone has family members and friends of different ages, from grandparents to infants, and interactions with patients should be similar. Every patient deserves the best that all health care professionals can offer, but some require increased strategic care based on their age or condition.

Pediatric Patients

Pediatric patients always require special attention. The proper method for dealing with young children is summarized by the famous statement of Dr. Armand Brodeur, long-time chief radiologist at Cardinal Glennon Children's Hospital in St. Louis: "To stand tall in pediatrics, you have to get down on your knees." In other words, simply getting down to the child's level—physically, in language, and in spirit—establishes a positive relationship. For example, instead of picking a child up and setting him or her on an x-ray table, which is the technologist's environment, the technologist should squat at the child's eye level, which is the child's environment, to begin the relationship (Fig. 11–7). The pediatric patient can provide valuable clinical information. For example, before an examination, a 5-year-old girl may reveal that she has been battered if she is alone with a friendly and nonthreatening technologist whom she believes she can trust.

Children are special patients who are capable of presenting a challenge to the radiologic technologist's interpersonal skills. A technologist who can perform radiography effectively and competently on the pediatric patient is probably capable of handling any radiographic procedure on any type of patient. Patience, technical knowledge, understanding of the pediatric patient, and the effective use of communication skills and immobilization devices can assist in obtaining a quality image.

Many hospitals provide soft toys such as stuffed animals for children, and stocking these items in the radiology department is a good idea. Never try to separate a child from a security object such as a blanket or toy unless absolutely necessary for image quality. Even then, the object should remain within the child's sight so that he or she is assured it will be returned momentarily. If the parents accompany the child, try to sit with the parents in the waiting room while you hold the child and explain the procedure to the parents. This additional time, 2 or 3 minutes, provides the child the opportunity to become familiar with you, your uniform, and the department. Always remember that children must *never* be left alone, even if properly immobilized.

INFANTS (BIRTH TO 1 YEAR). First communications are established using facial expressions, body movements and other nonverbal behaviors, and vocalizations. Very young infants like to be held in a familiar position; observe how the parents are holding the child, or ask what the favorite position is—at the shoulder, lying on the right side, and so forth. In addition, most small infants respond well to being held closely with a tight blanket. A steady, soothing voice, male or female, also often helps. Simply repeating "It's all right; that's okay" usually works.

At approximately 8 months of age, most infants express definite anxiety when removed from a familiar person. Permitting the parents to assist with the entire examination if possible is often helpful. If separation is necessary, it should be for the minimum amount of time.

At approximately 12 months of age, children are beginning to develop memories, ideas, and feelings. A child with previous experiences with hospital personnel may rebel at the sight of a laboratory coat or surgical scrub suit. The strength a 1-year-old child is capable of mustering is amazing when a vivid memory of an injection is triggered.

TODDLERS (1 TO 3 YEARS). Although toddlers may understand simple abstractions, their thinking is basically related to tangible events. They usually cannot take the viewpoint of another (this is why statements such as "See, it doesn't hurt Mommy" is seldom effective), and they cannot understand more than one word for something.

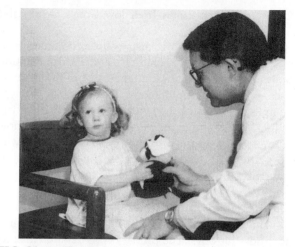

FIG. 11–7   "To stand tall in pediatrics, you have to get down on your knees." Entering the child's environment by squatting to the child's eye level can begin a rewarding relationship.

Asking a parent what word the child uses for urination is important if asking the child to urinate becomes necessary. Toddlers' concept of time is essentially now, and distance is whatever can be seen. Therefore speaking with simple words that are familiar to children is important, and expecting them to think about how they will feel in an hour should be avoided. Toddlers are often concerned only with what you are going to do to them at the moment.

PRESCHOOLERS (3 TO 5 YEARS). Preschool children are not yet able to reason logically or understand cause and effect. Telling a 4-year-old boy that he needs an examination to see if he is sick is meaningless. If his arm hurts, however, he will long remember that he broke it when he fell. Because preschoolers are very much involved with self-image, this is the age at which children may form an opinion that they are sick because they were bad. They may perceive relationships such as *big, little,* or *first* but cannot understand *next in line.* They must see or hear something to understand and must be actively involved to maintain their short attention span. They will not hold still for long, although they can be remarkably cooperative if their trust has been won.

SCHOOL-AGED CHILDREN (5 TO 10 YEARS). At approximately age 7, children begin to think logically and to analyze situations. At this point, children can reflect and develop deeper understandings. With these advancements, children often develop a special fear of bodily injury, disease, separation from loved ones, death, and punishment.

Remember that many diagnostic procedures may appear as punishment to children, and special attention is warranted to divert their attention from the negative aspects of various examinations. This task can often be accomplished by using their capacity for depth of understanding. For example, helping a child rationalize how an excretory urogram helps the physician find out why it hurts to urinate is appropriate as a method of diverting attention from the pain of the venipuncture.

ADOLESCENTS (10 TO 25 YEARS). Adolescence is not a well-defined age group, although it begins earlier for girls than it does for boys. The primary consideration in early adolescence focuses on body awareness, and modesty becomes especially important. Persons in this age group usually require special consideration to avoid embarrassment when changing clothes and during examinations. Asking unnecessary personnel to leave a room is appropriate during these examinations. Same-sex peer groups have a dominant role at this age, and conversation that focuses on friends of the same sex often eases tensions during procedures.

Middle adolescents are often bridging the gap between peer group influence and early sexual relationships. Persons in this age group are often developing their first real independence and often appreciate being treated as adults in conversation, preferences, and consultation about procedures.

Late adolescents are often focusing on mature relationships with both sexes and may be financially independent. They easily relate to adult conversation and should essentially be treated as adults, although their experiences may be limited in some areas.

Young Adults (25 to 45 Years)

Young adults are usually entering new roles of responsibility at home and in their work. They often experience problems in handling their multitude of new roles and may neglect one area while they concentrate on another. For example, focusing on childrearing at home may result in neglect of work duties. Conversation and interaction should be on the same level as that for other adults.

Middle-Aged Adults (45 to 65 Years)

In middle age, most people have found their place in life and tend to be relatively comfortable with their roles and success (or lack of it). When poor health or a threat of poor health occurs, considerable stress and special concern over how to maintain responsibilities, such as keeping a job and providing for a family, may outweigh personal health concerns.

Mature Adults (65 Years and Older)

Research shows that most persons 65 years and older do not consider themselves old. They tend to consider themselves middle aged. Because of this self-image, the radiologic technologists should not attempt to interact with them as though they are geriatric patients. Senility is not a natural part of aging, and only 10% of people in this age group demonstrate memory loss. They should be treated as middle-aged persons, with conversation centering on life activities. A much-reprinted saying, *I may be old and wrinkled on the outside but I'm young and vulnerable on the inside,* is well worth considering when phrasing statements to this age group.

Gerontology

Gerontology (geriatrics) is the study of aging and diseases of older adults. Studies show that the geriatric group will continue to increase in size and importance in American society for many years to come, primarily as a result of improvements in living standards, dietary practices, physical fitness, and medical care. At the end of the twentieth century, more than 33 million Americans were over 65 years of age, more than 12% of the total population, compared with only 4% in 1900. In addition, the elderly population itself is aging. Between 1960 and 1994 the U.S. population grew by 45%, whereas the over-65 population grew by 100%, and the over-85 population grew by almost 275%, to a total of 3 million persons. In addition, the 2000 census revealed a 49% increase in the 45-to-54-year-old category. This population surge will reach the *mature persons* category by 2010. These data have caused significant concern as young workers begin to realize that current retirement and medical care systems rely on active workers to fund care of older adults. Real concern exists that worldwide economies may not grow sufficiently to fund this increasing burden. As a result, current pressure on the medical system to find ways to decrease costs while increasing the efficiency of care for older adults is apparent.

Referring to all older patients as geriatric is inappropriate. American culture tends to be oriented toward youth, productivity, and a rapid pace. Automatically considering a person as *geriatric* results in feelings of alienation, which can be made worse by lack of respect. One author points out that, although everybody wants to live a long life, hardly anybody wants to be old because the word connotes frailty, narrow-mindedness, incompetence, and loss of attractiveness. Furthermore, the use of terms such as *senior citizens* or *golden agers* constitutes prejudice and discrimination and should be avoided. To minimize these feelings, technologists should treat geriatric patients as mature adults, with all the normal interaction that would be used with healthier or younger patients (Fig. 11–8). Talking loudly or using childish terms should be avoided with speaking with geriatric patients. At the same time, accommodating older adults by using gentle handling and extra time for movements and verbal responses is also important. This approach is identical to adjustments that must be made for other types of patients, such as a partially paralyzed patient.

Geriatric patients are now being classified as young-old, old-old, and oldest-old in an attempt to differentiate between widely varying conditions that accompany the aging process. Although these classifications can be chronologic in nature, classifying by functional age is equally appropriate. Both classifications are given in Table 11-1. The aging process itself is now divided into *primary aging* and *secondary aging*. Primary aging is the gradual and inevitable process of deterioration that begins in childhood and extends through old age. Secondary aging consists of disease, abuse, and disuse, which are often within control of the individual. Some of the changes that are especially important when patients are undergoing radiologic examinations are provided in Table 11-2. The cardinal rules when dealing with geriatric patients are patience and respect.

INTERACTING WITH THE TERMINALLY ILL PATIENT

The general agreement asserts that the primary care of the dying patient falls on the nurse; however, this concept does not release the radiologic technologist from an obligation to understand the basics of current practices toward terminally ill patients. Because few new radiologic technologists have had experiences with this type of patient, being prepared personally is important.

Unexpected death is much more complicated than anticipated death, but it is guided by a principle of trying to meet as many of the patient's needs as possible. Many radiologic technologists eventually experience patient death during radiologic examinations, often as a result of anaphylactic shock. Calling a false emergency code is always better than waiting too long to save a patient. With this guideline followed, obtaining assistance may still

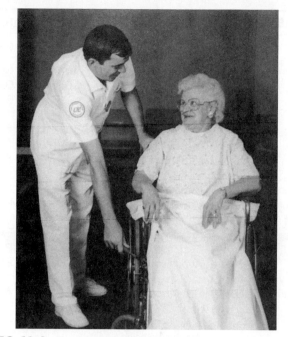

FIG. 11–8   To minimize feelings of alienation, the radiation technologist should treat geriatric patients as mature adults, with all the normal interaction that would be used with healthier or younger patients.

TABLE 11-1 Gerontologic Aging Categories

	CHRONOLOGIC	FUNCTIONAL
Young-old	65-74 yrs	Healthy and active
Old-old	75-84 yrs	Transitional
Oldest-old	85 yrs and older	Frail and infirm

become necessary when working through the personal aspects of having a patient die.

When death is expected because of age or disease, studies show that, for most people, the crisis is not death but where and how it will occur. For example, older patients who have adjusted to living at home often become anxious if they are removed from their home before death. However, by comparison, geriatric patients who have adjusted to living in an institution are much more willing to accept death in the same setting.

Patients who are kept in *closed awareness* are not told of their condition. Many of these patients deduce that they are terminally ill but lack assistance in working through the various stages of acceptance. Even heavily sedated patients may know more than the health care

TABLE 11-2 Physical Changes of Functional Aging

BODY SYSTEM	PHYSICAL CHANGE	CONSIDERATIONS FOR RADIOLOGIC EXAMINATIONS
Nervous	Slowing of psychomotor responses	Give patient time to move.
	Slowing of information processing	Give patient time to think before expecting a response.
	Decreased visual ability	Stand directly in front of patient, hold items to be seen or read at an appropriate distance without moving for a short time, and provide extra time for visual adjustments after dramatic changes in light levels.
	Decreased hearing ability	Speak directly to the patient's ear, move closer, or (as a last resort) talk louder.
Respiratory	Decreased cough reflex	Avoid aspiration by giving patient time to swallow when drinking.
Musculoskeletal	Osteoporotic loss of bone mass	Increase sensitivity to patient paranoia about potential falls with potential for permanent loss of mobility.
	Arthritis	Expect decreased joint flexibility.
	Decreased muscle strength	Prepare to provide assistance in moving if needed.
	Atrophied muscle mass	Expect decreased tolerance of positioning requirements and discomfort in placement on hard tabletops.
Cardiovascular	Decreased cardiac efficiency	Avoid orthostatic hypotension by allowing time for blood pressure adjustment when moving a patient from supine to sitting or from sitting to erect position.
	Arteriosclerosis	Avoid chilling discomfort by providing extra blankets and sheets.
Integumentary	Loss of texture and elasticity	Avoid skin lacerations (especially to the backs of hands) by not abrading skin with draw sheets during patient transfers or applying tape to sensitive areas.
Gastrointestinal	Decreased secretions	Expect difficulty when requiring a patient to drink quickly or from a recumbent position.
	Decreased gastrointestinal motility	Expect delays during completion of small bowel studies. (Prepare for long-term patient comfort via extra blankets, pillow under knees, communication of reasons for delays, and so on.)
	Decreased sphincter muscle tone	Prepare for potential loss of barium from rectum during lower gastrointestinal examinations. Expect more frequent requests for time or assistance with moving.

team suspects. Some patients develop *suspicious awareness* in that they watch for clues to their condition but attempt to keep the health care team from knowing exactly how much they understand. A state of *mutual pretense* exists when patient, staff, and family all know but are pretending not to know in hopes of avoiding interpersonal conflicts. A condition of *open awareness* is usually considered desirable because it permits everyone to work through the various stages that precede dying.

The stages delineated by Elisabeth Kübler-Ross have been generally regarded as an acceptable sequence of events. *Denial and isolation* may be the initial reactions and should be supported by silence and acceptance of the person without discussing death. *Anger* may occur as a result of the realization that life will be interrupted before everything the person planned has been accom-

plished and feelings that the person will soon be forgotten. Anger is often expressed in terms of complaints about health care, which may include radiologic services. These complaints should be addressed, and special care should be taken to avoid situations such as long waits without attention that will increase the patient's anger.

Some patients experience a *bargaining* stage that focuses on hope and may be based in religion, for example, prayers for small extensions of life to perform good deeds and heal family wounds. Supporting the patient's beliefs at this time is important because the hope itself can reduce stress. This stage may be followed by *depression,* which often occurs when remission ends and additional treatments must begin. This reaction is normal and should be encouraged by giving realistic praise while letting the patient express his or her feelings.

Preparatory depression comes with the realization of the inevitability of death and is accompanied by a desire for death as a release from suffering. The most important thing at this time is to permit the behavior. Attempting to cheer the patient may meet the needs of the health care provider but not of the patient. Touch and silence are often construed as acceptance and are appropriate at this time. *Acceptance,* which is considered the final stage, can occur only if enough time is provided and if the patient is appropriately helped through the other stages. This stage is characterized by a near-total lack of feelings.

The radiologic technologist also needs to be sure that personal feelings do not override patient concerns when caring for the terminally ill patient. Most hospitals can offer assistance in dealing with personal feelings about caring for terminally ill patients through their nursing departments. Students should consult with their program directors about assistance or appropriate courses. The technologist should not become hardened in dealing with dying and severely injured patients but learn to handle feelings appropriately during interactions with the patient, relatives, and friends.

Health care options now provide terminally ill patients with some control over their death. **Advanced directives** provide individuals a means to direct their health care should they find themselves in a situation in which they are unable to make their own decisions. These directives allow the will of the patient to be known regarding certain health care options. For instance, a person having an advanced directive stating that he or she does not wish to be placed on a ventilator should there be injury or disease requiring its use to sustain life would probably not be placed on the device if it were required. Other health care advances have supported **patient autonomy** in much the same way as advanced directives. In the past, patients with terminal illnesses were faced with few options regarding their death. The only options generally available to them were dying in pain or in a medically induced haze. Today, physicians and their terminally ill patients are making decisions together on how patient symptoms are controlled and how conscious and alert patients desire to be at life's end. Radiographers and other health care professionals should be aware that some of their patients have made these choices and should abide by their patients' wishes.

SUMMARY

The importance of interacting effectively with the patient is critical to the radiologic technologist, as well as to the patient. Maslow's hierarchy of needs provides insight into the behavior of professionals and patients alike. Maslow's hierarchy proceeds in seven levels of needs, from basic physiologic needs toward a level of self-actualization. The technologist holds significant power, including the most basic elements of a person's dignity and self-respect. Special attention is needed to ensure that the power is not abused.

The inpatient is someone who has been admitted to the hospital for diagnostic studies or treatment. Previous experiences in the hospital may have shaped the manner in which such a patient responds. Outpatients arrive in the radiology department or center with prior expectations. They often expect to be seen immediately on arriving in the department because they have a scheduled appointment. Apologizing for delays and keeping waiting patients up to date on their status is appropriate and important. Family and friends of patients who are visiting must also receive attention.

Attention to the various forms of interaction and communication techniques that have proved effective in improving relationships with patients can produce dramatic results in clinical situations. These skills include verbal skills, including humor, and nonverbal communications, such as paralanguage, body language, and touch. Touching can be used for emotional support, emphasis, and palpation. Professional appearance, personal hygiene, physical presence, and visual contact are also important.

Special consideration and techniques are necessary when dealing with seriously ill and traumatized patients, as well as impaired patients. Patients with vision, speech, hearing, and mental impairments, patients with the inability to speak English, and substance abuse patients require extra care. Mobile and surgical examinations also have special techniques for effective communication.

Age is also a special factor in patient interactions. Knowledge of growth and development differences for infants, toddlers, preschoolers, school-aged children, adolescents, young adults, middle-aged persons, mature persons, and geriatric persons can be useful in clinical practice. The cardinal rules when dealing with geriatric patients are patience and respect.

When death is expected because of age or disease, studies show that, for most people, the crisis is not death but where and how it will occur. Understanding the various stages that many terminally ill patients undergo once they have reached a condition of open awareness about their disease is helpful for the technologist. The Kübler-Ross sequence includes denial and isolation, anger, bargaining, depression, preparatory depression, and acceptance. Preparing personally for dealing with the death of a patient is important for the radiologic technologist.

BIBLIOGRAPHY

Ehrlich RA, McCloskey ED, Daly JA: *Patient care in radiography; with an introduction to medical imaging,* ed 6, St Louis, 2004, Mosby.

Freiberg K: *Human development: a life-span approach,* ed 4, Boston, 1992, Jones & Bartlett.

Gurley LT, Callaway WJ: *Introduction to radiologic technology,* ed 5, St Louis, 2002, Mosby.

Kübler-Ross E, ed: *Death, the final stage of growth,* Englewood Cliffs, NJ, 1975, Prentice-Hall.

Papalia D, Olds SW: *Human development,* ed 6, New York, 1995, McGraw-Hill.

Purtilo R: *Health professionals and patient interaction,* ed 6, Philadelphia, 2002, WB Saunders.

Torres LS: *Basic medical techniques and patient care for radiologic technologists,* ed 6, Philadelphia, 2004, JB Lippincott.

U.S. Department of Commerce, U.S. Bureau of the Census: *Growth of America's oldest-old population (profiles of America's elderly no. 2),* Washington, DC, 1992, U.S. Government Printing Office.

U.S. Department of Commerce, U.S. Census Bureau: *Profile of general demographic characteristics for the United States: 2000,* Washington, DC, 2002, U.S. Government Printing Office.

U.S. Department of Commerce, U.S. Census Bureau: *Sixty-five plus in America (current population reports, Special Studies, Series P23-178),* Washington, DC, 1992, U.S. Government Printing Office.

12

History Taking

Richard R. Carlton, MS, RT(R)(CV), FAERS
Arlene M. Adler, MEd, RT(R), FAERS

When you talk with the patient, you should listen, first for what he wants to tell, secondly for what he does not want to tell, thirdly for what he cannot tell.

L. J. Henderson
Physician and Patient as Social Systems

OBJECTIVES

On completion of this chapter, the student will be able to:

1. Describe the role of the radiologic technologist in taking patient clinical histories.

2. Describe the desirable qualities of a good patient interviewer.

3. Differentiate objective from subjective data.

4. Explain the value of each of the six categories of questions useful in obtaining patient histories.

5. Describe the importance of clarifying the chief complaint.

6. Detail the important elements of each of the *sacred seven* elements of the clinical history.

PATIENT INTERVIEW

The clinical history describes the information available regarding a patient's condition. To extract as much information as possible during a clinical history, the event must be viewed as an interview with the patient. Because the radiologic technologist's job often involves obtaining the **clinical history,** learning methods of accomplishing valid patient interviews is important.

Role of the Radiologic Technologist

Radiologists often do not have the opportunity to obtain a clinical history from the patient. Although more complex procedures such as angiography and radiation therapy permit extensive history taking by the radiologist or radiation oncologist, most patients for diagnostic radiography are never examined or interviewed by the radiologist. Because history taking is one of the most critical and valuable diagnostic tools, possessing good history-taking skills is an essential responsibility of the radiologic technologist.

Many radiologic technologists fail to appreciate the importance of this role as a clinical historian. Unquestionably, history taking is one of the most valuable opportunities to acquire clinical information that can contribute to the diagnostic process. A radiologist can be instructed to give special attention to the exact anatomic area where pain is focused. For example, stating that a patient has pain in the right hand is less focused than stating the pain is over the anterior aspect of the distal portion of the second metacarpal.

In addition, the interaction with the patient plays an important role. A unique opportunity to become part of the healing process presents itself with each new patient. Eric Cassell, a physician noted for his teaching of the art of practicing medicine, relates feeling powerless to help a patient with severe pulmonary edema late one night. While waiting for equipment to arrive, he began to talk calmly, explaining how the water would begin to ease bit by bit until, much to his amazement, that is precisely what happened. By reducing the patient's fear, he had reduced the hypertension and actually eased the pathologic process. Cassell refers to this action as the *art of healing,* and it is directly related to the role of the radiologic technologist when taking a history. Genuine interest in what the patient has to say, attentiveness, and an aura of professional competence can provide patients with a real sense of caring.

Desirable Qualities of the Interviewer

Taking a history must be a cooperative event between the patient and the radiologic technologist. Because patients wish to have a medical problem resolved, most want to help with the history; however, sick people may be combative as a symptom of their frustration. In these instances, acknowledging the patient's anger as a method of overcoming it often helps. For example, a patient who complains about already having given a history to someone and who then rants about incompetent health professionals will often become an ally if the technologist agrees with the inconvenience and suggests that, because the radiologist needs specialized information, the interview will be as short as possible and can be taken while getting ready for the x-ray examination.

Carl Rogers identified several qualities that appear to be important in establishing an open dialogue. These qualities include respect, genuineness, and empathy. When patients perceive any of these qualities to be missing, the interview may become increasingly difficult as the good faith between the two persons decreases. Patients need to believe that the information they are providing is important. When they lack these thoughts because of intimidation or lack of respect, they may withhold information as unimportant or unworthy of being mentioned. Because many patients often perceive physicians as being busy authority figures, radiologic technologists can serve a useful role in that they are usually seen as less threatening and easier to talk with than physicians.

The radiologic technologist should maintain a polite and professional demeanor during the interview, especially when introducing himself or herself to the patient, verifying the patient's name (by using Mr. or Ms. instead of first names), and explaining that a history is needed.

Notes should be added to the paperwork, usually the examination request or requisition. Most patients perceive note taking as positive because the technologist is making it clear that the information being given is important enough to be recorded. Additionally, little point exists in acquiring the clinical history if it is not written on the paperwork that will be in front of the radiologist when the images are read.

Data Collection Process

Good history taking involves the collection of accurate objective and subjective data. **Objective** data are perceptible to the senses, such as signs that can be seen, heard, or felt and such things as laboratory reports. **Subjective** data pertain to or are perceived by the affected individual only. They include factors that involve the patient's emotions and experiences, such as pain and its severity, and are not perceptible to the senses. *Objective data are not necessarily more important than subjective data.* In fact, much has been written on the therapeutic value of the interview itself. Many patients come to see the physician with a personal agenda of finding a professional to listen to and empathize with a problem, which may or may not have physical manifestations. The technologist must realize that conversation with the patient has great value by itself in addition to the diagnostic information that may be obtained. The art of radiologic technology includes this aspect of patient interaction.

An important point to realize is that an objective approach to the collection of subjective data is also necessary. For example, never disregard anything the patient says, *especially* if it does not fit with the opinion you are forming about the patient's symptoms. Disregarding some comments constitutes subjective collection of the data. Asking patients to define and clarify the words they use can considerably accelerate the diagnostic process. For example, the word *pain* can often provide significant additional information if it can be localized and a chronology established.

Questioning Skills

Adult patients usually are experienced in providing medical histories, especially if they have been hospitalized previously. The student can use this experience to advantage by simply letting the patients tell their stories. Listening instead of asking more questions often provides the necessary information. Effective histories result when the following questioning techniques are used:

- Open-ended questions (nondirected, nonleading) let the patient tell the story.
- Facilitation (nod or say *yes, okay, go on* . . .) encourages elaboration.
- Silence (to give the patient time to remember) facilitates accuracy and elaboration.
- Probing questions (to focus the interview) provide more detail.
- Repetition (rewording) clarifies information.
- Summarization (condensing) verifies accuracy.

All histories should begin with open-ended questions to encourage the patient's spontaneous associations about the clinical problem. For example, "What type of chest problem are you having?" These questions should be followed with increasingly focused and directed probing questions based on what the patient has already said. For example, "When you breathe deeply, exactly where does it hurt on the left side of your chest?" This technique permits the radiologic technologist to pick up where the patient stops telling the story and provides medically specific information that might not occur to the patient otherwise.

The use of *precise and clear wording* cannot be overemphasized. Words do not always mean the same thing to patients as they do to radiologic technologists. For example, many patients refer to the entire abdomen as the *stomach*. Therefore recording *gastric pain* when a patient says the left side of the stomach hurts may be inaccurate. If this information is verified by asking the patient to point to the area, the technologist may discover that the complaint the patient is actually experiencing is left lower-quadrant abdominal distress. The medical terms that are learned in radiologic technology are professional ones and will not be understood by all patients. On the other hand, some patients will understand medical terms, and they should not have their intelligence offended by the use of overly simplified words. For example, no need exists to tell a high school biology teacher that the esophagus is a tube leading to the stomach.

The ability to assess the patient's background can be a difficult skill to develop. Probably the most helpful technique is to begin with a question that provides an opportunity for the patient to respond in a manner that reflects his or her life experience and educational background. For example, a patient who responds to a question about the location of pain with a specific anatomic term such as *epigastric* clearly signals that medical terminology may be used. Conversely, a response using the word *belly* may indicate lack of knowledge about abdominal organs and should signal the use of simpler terms.

The use of **leading questions** should be avoided whenever possible because they introduce biases into the history. For example, "Does the pain travel down your leg?" may lead the patient to a description of sciatica. Asking the question "Does the pain stay deep within your hip, or does it move?" provides a more reliable indication.

A useful tool is to *repeat information* obtained as a part of the history for two reasons: (1) to verify that the radiologic technologist perceived the information correctly and (2) to ensure that the patient has not changed his or her mind.

ELEMENTS OF THE CLINICAL HISTORY

Determining the Chief Complaint

Physicians attempt to determine the patient's **chief complaint.** This effort is valuable because it focuses the history toward the single most important issue (Box 12-1). In many instances, the chief complaint is directly related to the first symptom that is discussed; however, a danger exists in becoming too focused on determining a single chief complaint. Permitting the patient to add more than a single complaint when multiple complaints are apparently valid is important. Ignoring all symptoms except the most predominant can obscure other important clinical information.

BOX 12-1   Sample Patient History Guide

Review the Chief Complaint
Indications for This Examination
Localization
Chronology
Quality
Severity
Onset
Aggravating or alleviating factors
Associated manifestations

Has There Been Any Trauma?

Has There Been Any Previous Surgery?

Depending on the Chief Complaint
Skeletal System
Pain location
Injury location
Injury chronology

Central Nervous System
Pain
Unconsciousness or lethargy
Bleeding location
Vision
Vertigo
Convulsions

Respiratory System
Cough
Dyspnea
Hemoptysis
Infection
Pain location
Pain duration

Gastrointestinal and Genitourinary Systems
Pain location
Gastric
Nausea
  Vomiting
Bowel
  Constipation
  Diarrhea
  Stool description
Date of last bowel movement
Urinary
  Known allergies and contrast media reactions
  Blood pressure
  Hematuria
  Blood urea nitrates
  Creatinine
  Burning
  Frequency

Sacred Seven

The radiologic technologist typically does not need to compile a complete medical history on patients. The physician or the nursing staff who first saw the patient will have completed this job. The technologist's role is to collect a focused history specific to the procedure that is to be performed. Seven elements are recognized for a complete history. These elements are often referred to as the *sacred seven:*

- Localization
- Chronology
- Quality
- Severity
- Onset
- Aggravating or alleviating factors
- Associated manifestations

LOCALIZATION. Localization is defining as exact and precise an area as possible for the patient's complaint. It requires the use of carefully worded questions accompanied by proper touching of the patient. By consenting to the procedure, patients give implied consent for the technologist to touch their bodies for both information and positioning. Remember that the patient can use verbal or nonverbal communication to withdraw this permission at any time. Two types of touch that the technologist commonly uses in gathering a clinical history are (1) touching for emphasis and (2) touching for palpation.

Touching for emphasis involves using touch to highlight or to specify instructions or specify locations. A history can be clarified by a light touch to specify the region. For example, after a patient states "My stomach hurts here" and places a hand on the upper abdomen, the radiologic technologist can add information by asking, "Does it hurt more here or here?" while touching the upper left side and then the upper middle region. *Palpation,* or applying the fingers with light pressure, can also be useful in history taking. For example, palpating the olecranon process of the elbow can assist the patient in the localization of pain within that region.

Sometimes localization is not possible because of the nature of the problem. For example, a radiating pain may also be a deep pain that the patient cannot localize. When this confusion occurs, the radiologist should be informed that the pain is not localized. This description tells the radiologist that attempts were made to confine the complaint to a specific region. The term *nonlocalized* then becomes valuable clinical information.

CHRONOLOGY. The **chronology** is the time element of the history. The *duration since onset, frequency,* and *course* of the symptoms should be established. This information should be described in seconds, minutes, hours, days, weeks, or months. For example, the onset of a chest problem may have been several weeks before the examination, the duration of coughing may average 10 to 15 seconds, the frequency may be several times per hour, and the course may reveal that it is worse during the night and in the morning. Radiologists may derive important diagnostic clues from a good chronology. For example, a stress fracture may first be visualized 10 to 20 days after the onset of symptoms.

Students should avoid giving dates or days as a chronology. For example, reporting that an injury occurred last Thursday or on July 14th requires that the radiologist find a calendar to determine how much time elapsed between the trauma and the examination.

QUALITY. The **quality** describes the character of the symptoms. Examples include the color and consistency of body fluids, the presence of clots or sores, the size of lumps or lesions, the type of cough, and the character of pain.

When pain is involved, it must be described carefully. This description should include either the word *acute,* meaning having a sudden onset, or the word *chronic,* meaning having a prolonged course. It should also include specific descriptors such as *burning, throbbing, dull, sharp, cutting, aching, prickling, radiating, pressure,* and *crushing.* Again, the patient's understanding of medical terms is important. For example, a patient may describe acute pain as *sharp* or *recent.* Gaining this additional information often requires the use of focused, probing questions, such as, "When did the pain begin?"

SEVERITY. The severity of a condition describes the intensity, the quantity, or the extensiveness of the problem. Examples are the intensity of pain, the number of lesions or lumps, and the extent of a burn. A patient may say that a light burning sensation versus a very intense burning sensation exists.

ONSET. Describing the onset of the complaint involves the patient's explaining what he or she was doing when the illness or condition began. A review of the onset can help determine whether predictable events occurred that preceded the recurrence of a symptom. For example, a patient might have had a series of mild headaches before a convulsion.

AGGRAVATING OR ALLEVIATING FACTORS. The circumstances that produce the problem or intensify it should be well defined, including anything that aggravates, alleviates, or otherwise modifies it. For example, heartburn may occur only after a full meal or a stressful day on the job and may be aggravated by certain foods and alleviated by assuming a right anterior oblique position with the head elevated slightly.

ASSOCIATED MANIFESTATIONS. Determining whether other symptoms accompany the chief complaint may be necessary to determine whether all the symptoms relate to the chief complaint or are related to a separate condition. For example, the patient may describe gastrointestinal symptoms as a part of, or separate from, a cardiac condition.

SUMMARY

The radiologic technologist who sees himself or herself as a clinical historian realizes the value of this service. Understanding the fine art of accomplishing patient interviews can often assist in gaining increased insight and information that can add significantly to the radiologist's ability to diagnose.

Good history taking involves the collection of accurate objective and subjective data. Objective data are perceptible to the senses. Subjective data pertain to or are perceived by the affected individual only.

Thorough histories result from using such techniques as open-ended questions, facilitation, silence, probing questions, repetition, and summarization. Physicians need to determine the patient's chief complaint. This effort is valuable because it focuses the history toward the single most important issue. Seven elements are recognized as producing complete history. These elements are often referred to as the *sacred seven* and are localization, chronology, quality, severity, onset, aggravating or alleviating factors, and associated manifestations.

BIBLIOGRAPHY

Aldich C: *The medical interview: gateway to the doctor-patient relationship,* ed 2, New York, 1999, Parthenon Publishing Group.

Bates RC: *The fine art of understanding patients,* Oradell, NJ, 1972, Medical Economics Book Division.

Billings JA, Stoeckle J: *The clinical encounter: a guide to the medical interview and case presentation,* Chicago, 1989, Year Book Medical Publishers.

Cassell E: *Talking with patients, vol. 1: theory of doctor-patient communication,* Cambridge, Mass, 1985, MIT Press.

Cassell E: *Talking with patients, vol. 2: clinical technique,* Cambridge, Mass, 1985, MIT Press.

Cassell E: *The healer's art: a new approach to the doctor-patient relationship,* Philadelphia, 1976, JB Lippincott.

Carlton R: Radiographers as clinical historians, *RT Image* 4(29):16-17, 1991.

Carlton R, Adler AM: *Repeating radiographs: setting imaging standards. Postgraduate advances in radiologic technology,* Berryville, Vir, 1989, Forum Medicum.

Carnevali DL, Mitchell PH, Woods NF, et al: *Diagnostic reasoning in nursing,* Philadelphia, 1984, JB Lippincott.

Cole S, Bird, J: *The medical interview: the three-function approach,* ed 2, St Louis, 2000, Mosby.

Coulehan JL, Block MR: *The medical interview,* ed 4, Philadelphia, 2001, FA Davis.

Enelow A, Forde, D, Brummel-Smith, K: *Interviewing and patient care,* ed 4, New York, 1996, Oxford University Press.

Engel G, Morgan W Jr: *Interviewing the patient,* Philadelphia, 1973, WB Saunders.

Feinstein A: *Clinical judgment,* Baltimore, 1967, Williams & Wilkins.

Hillman R, Goodell BW, Grundy SM, et al: *Clinical skills: interviewing, history taking, and physical diagnosis,* New York, 1981, McGraw-Hill.

Levinson D: *A guide to the clinical interview,* Philadelphia, 1987, WB Saunders.

Park C, Morrell RW, Shifren K, eds: *Processing of medical information in aging patients: cognitive and human factors perspectives,* Mahwah, NJ, 1999, Lawrence Erlbaum.

Prior JA, Silberstein JS, Stang JM: *Physical diagnosis: the history and examination of the patient,* St Louis, 1981, Mosby.

Purtilo R: *Health professionals and patient interaction,* ed 6, Philadelphia, 2002, WB Saunders.

Reiser D: *Patient interviewing: the human dimension,* Philadelphia, 1980, Williams and Wilkins.

Transfer Techniques

Jan Bruckner, PhD, PT

At no time in the day is the patient in more peril than when being transferred from bed to wheelchair. More injuries of consequence occur to patients, and health care personnel serving them, during transfer than at any other time.

Marilyn Rantz and Donald Courtail
Lifting, Moving, and Transferring Patients, 1981

OBJECTIVES

On completion of this chapter, the student will be able to:

1. Define the terms associated with body mechanics.

2. Describe the cause, signs, symptoms, and treatment of orthostatic hypotension.

3. Describe the basic principles of proper lifting and transfer techniques.

4. Explain four types of wheelchair-to-bed transfers.

5. Explain a standard cart transfer procedure.

6. Identify five standard patient positions.

BODY MECHANICS

The application of proper lifting and transfer techniques increases job safety. Radiologic technologists who use these techniques can reduce their injuries and minimize low back pain. Low back pain causes major disability in adults ages 45 years and younger and results in major activity limitations in people ages 45 to 64 years. The annual cost of this disability to Americans was recently estimated at $14 billion. Much of this pain, suffering, and expense might be avoided if health professionals would learn and use basic principles of body mechanics.

Biomechanics is a branch of science that applies the laws of physics to living creatures. Biomechanics examines the action of forces on bodies at rest or in motion and can be used to optimize exercise programs, promote greater athletic skills, and design relatively safe work environments. Biomechanical studies also yield insights into the mechanisms of injury and help researchers discover how people get injured and what can be done to prevent injuries.

For radiologic technologists, an understanding of the basic aspects of biomechanics can help prevent back injury while promoting safe and effective patient transfers. Fundamental to good patient transfer techniques are the concepts of the base of support, center of gravity, and mobility and stability muscles.

Base of Support

The **base of support** is the foundation on which a body rests. When a person is standing, the feet and the space between the feet constitute that person's base of support (Fig. 13–1, *A*). Standing with the feet wide apart enlarges the base of support (Fig. 13–1, *B*). Standing on one foot provides the person with a narrow base of support (Fig. 13–1, *C*). Narrow bases of support characterize unstable and mobile systems. Wide bases of support characterize stable systems. When transferring a patient, the health professional needs to establish as stable a base of support as possible. Standing with feet apart to increase the base of support improves stability.

Center of Gravity

Center of gravity is a hypothetical point at which all the mass appears to be concentrated (Fig. 13–2), and gravitational forces appear to act on the entire body from this specific point. In humans aligned in the anatomic position, the center of gravity is at approximately sacral level two (S-2), with slight variations between men and women. Moving heavy objects is relatively easy and safe if the object is held close to the mover's center of gravity. Stability can be achieved when a body's center of gravity is over its base of support (Fig. 13–3, *A*). Instability results when the center of gravity moves beyond the boundaries of the base (Fig. 13–3, *B*). For safe, stable lifting, the center of gravity always must be over the base of support.

Mobility and Stability Muscles

The body contains muscles that are designed for mobility and other muscles that are designed for stability. **Mobility muscles** are found in the limbs. Typically, these muscles have long white tendons and cross two or more joints. Examples include the biceps muscles, which flex the elbow, and the hamstring muscle, which flexes the knee (Fig. 13–4). **Stability muscles** are found in the torso. Typically, stability muscles are large expanses of red muscle that provide postural support. Two examples are the latissimus dorsi girthing the back and the rectus abdominis supporting the abdomen. For effective transfers, technologists should use white mobility muscles for lifting and red postural muscles for support. Lifting

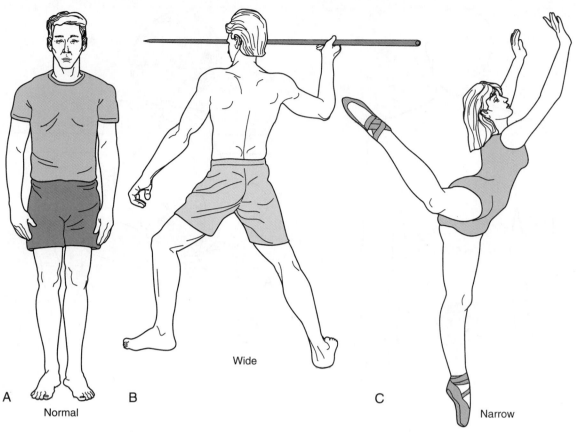

FIG. 13–1 Variations in base of support: *A,* normal; *B,* wide; *C,* narrow.

should be done by bending and straightening the knees. The back should be kept straight or in a position of slightly increased lumbar lordosis.

PRINCIPLES OF LIFTING

When performing a transfer, let patients do as much of the work as possible (Box 13-1). Before attempting a transfer, always ask patients whether they can do the transfer independently. Patients can often transfer on their own or with minimal assistance. If assistance is required, then let the patient help. This approach minimizes the trauma to the patient and avoids stress on the technologist. In addition, this approach enhances rapport and mutual respect between the patient and the technologist.

Patients may be unsure whether they need assistance. Patients sometimes believe that they are capable of transferring themselves when they are incapable. Before executing the transfer, check the patient's chart and verify

---

BOX 13-1 Principles for Safe Transfers

Let the patient do as much of the transfer as possible.

Check the chart for precautions, such as weight-bearing status and joint disease, before executing the transfer to minimize patient discomfort and harm.

Establish a wide base of support for your stability.

Hold the patient's center of gravity close to your own center of gravity for a better mechanical advantage.

Hold the patient with a transfer belt around the patient's waist to minimize stress on the patient's shoulder girdle.

Lift the patient with your legs. Avoid back bending.

Avoid trunk twisting during transfer.

Never lift more than you can. Ask for assistance when needed.

Watch the patient for signs of orthostatic hypotension and take precautions to minimize its effects.

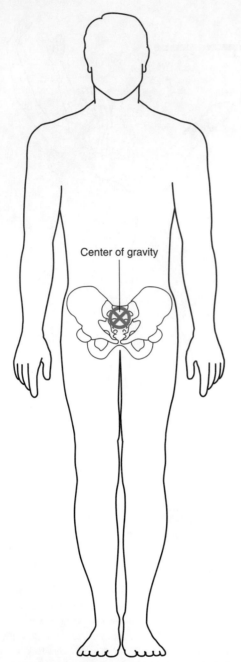

FIG. 13–2 The center of gravity for most people is located at approximately S-2.

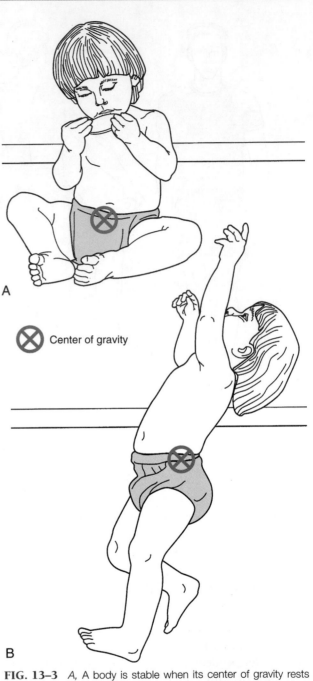

FIG. 13–3 *A,* A body is stable when its center of gravity rests over its base of support. *B,* A body is unstable when its center of gravity is not over its base of support.

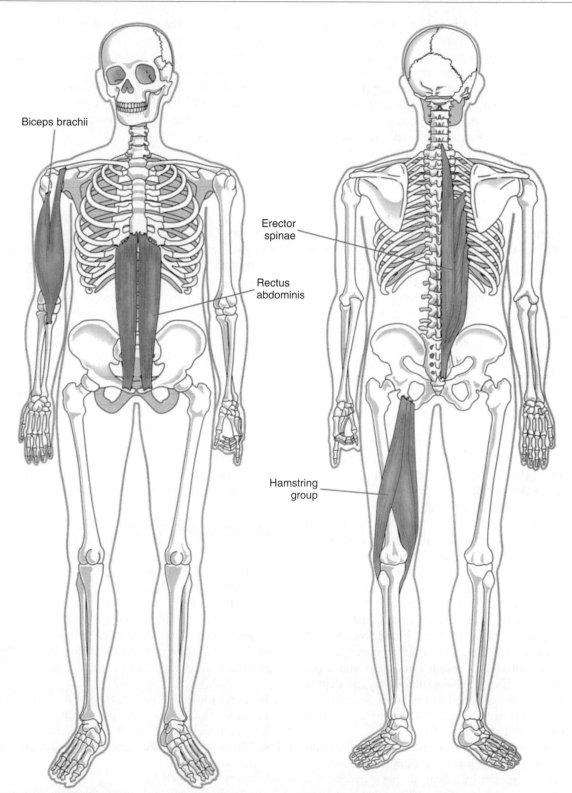

Biceps brachii

Erector spinae

Rectus abdominis

Hamstring group

FIG. 13–4   Mobility muscles include the biceps brachii and the hamstring group. Postural muscles include the rectus abdominis and the erector spinae muscles.

whether he or she has a restricted weight-bearing status. Be especially protective of patients with diagnoses such as lower-extremity or pelvic girdle fracture; painful, inflamed, or unstable joints; or any weakened or debilitated condition. If any of these conditions appear, handle the patient gently, and offer assistance as required. Always inform the patient of what you are going to do and how you intend to proceed. For example, tell the patient you are going to assist him or her move from the table to the wheelchair then list the specific steps: stand up from the table, turn your back toward the seat of the wheelchair, and sit down gently. Let patients perform as much of the transfer as they can. Execute the transfer slowly enough for the patient to feel secure.

Safe, effective transfers rely on proper body mechanics. When lifting a patient, the person performing the transfer should stand with feet apart to increase the base of support. The patient's center of gravity (S-2) should be held close to the transferrer's center of gravity (S-2). This positioning provides the best mechanical advantage for lifting. Some patients may be wearing bathrobes or hospital gowns. Loose clothing inhibits the mover's ability to hold a patient securely. One solution is to place a transfer belt around the patient's waist. Transfer belts are usually made of webbing or muslin and can provide a good grip with minimal trauma to the patient. Taking a transfer belt is a good practice when planning to perform transfers. When lifting patients, *keep the back stationary and let the legs do all of the lifting.* Twisting should be avoided. After the patient is standing, help him or her to pivot around to a bed or x-ray table and to sit down.

Technologists should be aware of **orthostatic hypotension,** the drop in blood pressure that occurs when a person stands. A slight drop in blood pressure occurs normally when any person rises quickly from a recumbent to an upright position. This condition becomes increasingly serious when patients have been in bed for long periods and have a debilitated status. These weakened patients tend to have blood vessels with decreased vasomotor tone and other problems in their circulatory systems. As a result, circulation and blood pressure may be affected. Rising too quickly can deprive patients of oxygen-rich blood to the brain. Symptoms of orthostatic hypotension include dizziness, fainting, blurred vision, and slurred speech.

To minimize the severity of orthostatic hypotension, have the patient stand slowly. Encourage the patient to talk during the transfer by asking simple questions. For example, "How are you feeling?" or "Can you turn toward the bed now?" Slowing or slurring of speech may be indicative of decreased blood flow to the brain. If symp-toms do occur, then slowing down the speed of the transfer is important; ask the patient to take slow, deep breaths, and provide additional assistance in the execution of the transfer. If patients report symptoms when returning to a wheelchair, then let them pause for a few moments until they feel better. *Do not send symptomatic patients on their way* and risk having them faint on the way to their rooms.

WHEELCHAIR TRANSFERS

Radiologic technologists use four types of wheelchair transfers: (1) standby assist, (2) assisted standing pivot, (3) two-person lift, and (4) hydraulic lift. Begin by determining whether the patient has a strong side and a weak side or whether both sides are equal. Look at the patient. A long leg cast, a severe foot deformity, or a lower-extremity amputation clearly indicate a unilateral problem. For less easily observed transfer precautions, check the patient's chart, ask the patient, or inquire of staff about restricted weight-bearing status, generalized weakness, or arthritic conditions. If the patient has a strong side and a weak side, then *always position the patient so that he or she transfers toward the strong side.* If patients have equal strength on both sides, then the transfer direction may be determined by convenience or space limitations. In all wheelchair transfers, be sure that the wheelchair wheels are locked and that the footrests are elevated and not obstructing the patient.

Standby Assist Transfer

Some patients have the ability to transfer from a wheelchair to a table on their own. Position the wheelchair at a 45-degree angle to the table (Fig. 13–5). Talk to the patient before he or she moves to determine how much, if any, assistance is required. Divide the transfer into single-step components and talk the patient through each step. Give the following commands to the patient to provide verbal assistance for a wheelchair-to-table transfer:

1. "Move the wheelchair footrests out of the way."
2. "Be sure that the wheelchair is locked."
3. "Sit on the edge of the wheelchair seat."
4. "Push down on the arms of the chair to assist in rising."
5. "Stand up slowly."
6. "Reach out and hold onto the table with the hand closest to the table."
7. "Turn slowly until you feel the table behind you."

8. "Hold onto the table with both hands."
9. "Sit down."

If the table is too high for the patient to sit comfortably, then after step 6, give the patient a footstool. Provide assistance as needed for the patient to step up on the stool and sit on the table.

Assisted Standing Pivot Transfer

For patients who cannot transfer independently, a standing pivot technique is used. Position the wheelchair at a 45-degree angle to the table with the patient's stronger side closest to the table. If the patient is wearing loose-fitting clothes, place a transfer belt around the patient's waist (Fig. 13–6, *A*). Having a secure grip on the patient without traumatizing any of the patient's joints is important. Execute the following steps one at a time:

1. Move the wheelchair footrests out of the way.
2. Be sure that the wheelchair is locked.
3. Have the patient sit on the edge of the wheelchair seat (Fig. 13–6, *B*). Provide assistance as needed.
4. Have the patient push down on the arms of the wheelchair to assist in rising (Fig. 13–6, *C*).
5. Bend at the knees, keeping your back straight, and grasp the transfer belt with both hands. The patient's feet and knees must be blocked to provide stability, especially for paraplegic and hemiplegic patients who are partially paralyzed and may not be able to move or feel sensation in a lower extremity. This task is accomplished by placing one foot outside the patient's foot while the knee is placed at the medial (inside) surface of the patient's knee (Fig. 13–6, *D*).
6. As the patient rises to a standing position, rise also by straightening your knees (Fig. 13–6, *E*).
7. When the patient is standing, ask, "Are you feeling all right?" If the patient reports any feelings of dizziness or exhibits any of the other signs of orthostatic hypotension, let him or her stand for a moment until recovered.
8. When the patient is ready, both of you pivot toward the table until the patient can feel the table against the back of the thighs (Fig. 13–6, *F*).
9. Ask the patient to support himself or herself on the table with both hands and to sit down (Fig. 13–6, *G*).
10. Help the patient to sit by gradually lowering him or her to the table. Be sure that your back remains straight and that the lowering occurs from the knees.

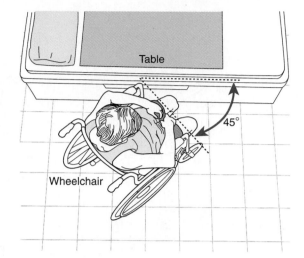

FIG. 13–5 Angle the wheelchair to be 45 degrees from the table.

Two-Person Lift

Some patients cannot bear weight on their lower extremities and must be lifted onto the table. If the patient is lightweight, then a two-person lift can be executed. The stronger person should lift the patient's torso while the other person lifts the patient's feet. The person lifting the patient's torso is usually in charge of the transfer and directs the other person's actions.

Prepare for the transfer by verbally planning out the procedure. This verbal planning enables a coordinated effort among the people doing the transfer and the patient. Verbal planning also allows for troubleshooting before the execution of the transfer.

Before the patient is moved, lock the wheelchair, remove the armrests, and swing away or remove the leg rests. The patient is asked to cross his or her arms over the chest. The stronger person stands behind the patient, reaches under the patient's axillae, and grasps the patient's crossed forearms. The second person should squat in front of the patient and cradle the patient's thighs in one hand and calves in the other hand (Fig. 13–7, *A*). On command, the patient is lifted to clear the wheelchair and is moved as a unit to the desired place (Fig. 13–7, *B*).

Hydraulic Lift Techniques

Some patients are too heavy to lift manually and require a hydraulic lift. Lift transfers have multiple steps and

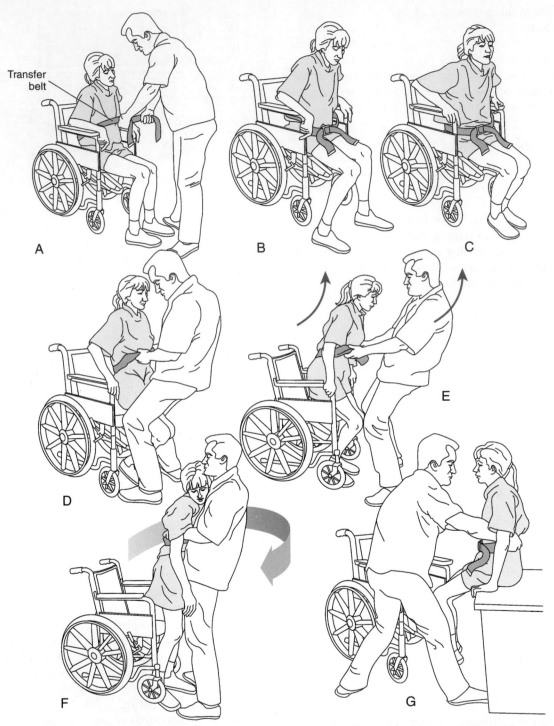

FIG. 13–6 An assisted standing pivot transfer is used when transferring a patient from a wheelchair to a table. *A,* Use a transfer belt to hold the patient securely. *B,* Have the patient sit on the edge of the wheelchair seat. Provide assistance as needed. *C,* Have the patient push down on the arms of the wheelchair to assist in rising. *D,* Bend at the knees, keeping your back straight, and grasp the transfer belt with both hands. *E,* As the patient rises to standing, rise also by straightening your knees. *F,* When the patient is ready, pivot toward the table until the patient can feel the table against the back of the thighs. *G,* Ask the patient to hold onto the table with both hands and to slowly sit down.

require some skill. Health professionals should familiarize themselves with the equipment and practice using it before attempting to lift a patient.

Most hydraulic lifts have several basic features. To facilitate moving, they often have four caster wheels but no wheel locks. The lift's base of support can be widened or narrowed by means of a lever. Most lifts have two handles for steering, a manual pump for raising the support arm, a release valve for lowering the support arm, and a spreader bar for the sling attachment (Fig. 13–8). Identify these features and learn their operation before attempting to use the lift.

For patients who need to be transferred using a hydraulic lift, prior arrangements should be made with the nursing staff to have these patients arrive in the radiology department sitting in a wheelchair on a transfer sling. If the patient arrives without a sling, then assistance should be requested. Sending a patient back to the ward to return sitting on a sling is better than risking injury to the patient, the transferrer, or both by attempting transfer without using one.

The sling attaches to the spreader bar by hooks and chains. The chains have a short segment for attachment to the sling back and a longer segment for attachment to the sling seat. Adjust the chain length according to the size of the patient. Hook the chains to the sling from the inside out (Fig. 13–9, A). This precaution minimizes the risk of a patient being injured by the hooks.

Check that the release valve is closed and that the patient is positioned comfortably in the sling. Gently begin to raise the patient (Fig. 13–9, B). When the patient has cleared the wheelchair seat, the wheelchair can be removed and the patient can be positioned on the table. Manual assistance may be required to position the patient's legs appropriately.

To lower the patient, open the release valve and gently lower the patient. Guard the patient's head from contact with the spreader bar. Remove the chains with care; they have a tendency to swing and must be steadied to avoid patient injury. After the patient has achieved a safe, stable position, the lift can be removed. If possible, leave the sling under the patient in anticipation of the return transfer.

CART TRANSFERS

Many patients are transported by cart (also called a stretcher or gurney). To move a patient from a cart onto a radiographic table, position the cart alongside the table on the patient's strong or less affected side. The cart must be as close to the table as possible and then secured.

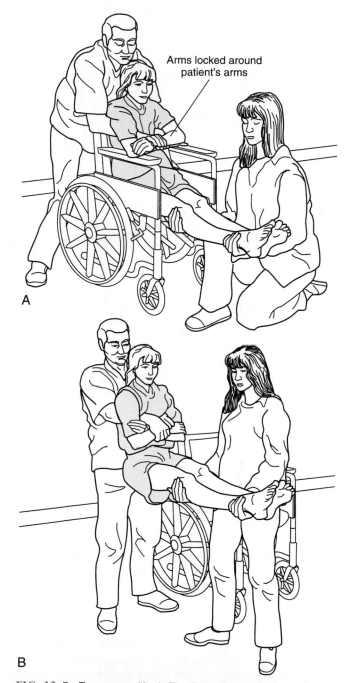

FIG. 13–7 Two-person lift. *A,* The first person asks the patient to cross his or her arms over the chest. The person making the transfer stands behind the patient, reaches under the patient's axillae, and grasps the patient's crossed forearms. The assistant squats in front of the patient and cradles the patient's thighs in one hand and the patient's calves in the other. *B,* At the command of the person supporting the patient's upper body, the patient is lifted to clear the wheelchair and moved as a unit to the desired place.

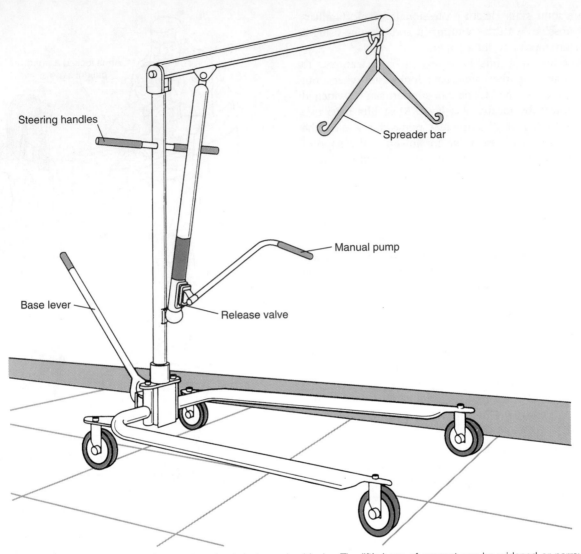

Steering handles

Spreader bar

Manual pump

Base lever

Release valve

FIG. 13–8 Hydraulic lifts often have four caster wheels but no wheel locks. The lift's base of support can be widened or narrowed by means of a lever. The lift has two handles for steering, a manual pump for raising the support arm, a release valve for lowering the support arm, and a spreader bar for the sling attachment.

Simply depressing wheel locks may not be sufficient to keep a cart from moving. Placing sandbags or other devices on the floor is often necessary to block the wheels satisfactorily.

If the patient can assist with the transfer, then all that may be required is stabilization of the cart and support for the involved body part. For example, a patient may move his or her body if a leg in a cast is supported during the transfer. If the patient cannot assist, then a moving device should be used. If no moving devices are available, then three people can be used for a cart-to-table transfer.

Numerous commercially manufactured moving devices are available. Some devices are smooth, thin sheets of plastic, and others are composed of canvas or plastic over small rollers, but all are designed to be used as aids during cart-to-table transfers. To do the transfer, begin by rolling the patient onto his or her side away from the direction of the transfer. Place the moving device in the midpoint of the patient's back. Roll the patient supine so that he or she is positioned on the moving device. The draw sheet is used to move the patient slowly onto the table (Fig. 13–10). If necessary, the patient can be rolled to remove the moving device.

A second type of moving device is a low-friction polyester sheet that enables health practitioners to slide rather than lift their patients during transfers. The Arjo Company manufactures such products under the names of MaxiSlide, MaxiTube, and MaxiTransfer. A patient must be placed on a double thickness of this fabric and then glided from one place to another. The top layer moves with the patient so that the patient's skin is protected from abrasions. Because the patient is pushed or pulled into position rather than lifted, each transfer requires less effort and fewer personnel.

To perform a lateral transfer from, for example, a gurney to a radiographic table, two sheets are needed. One sheet must be directly under the patient and the second sheet must be under the first sheet to serve as a track on which the patient will slide. If the patient arrives without a transfer sheet, one can be placed under the patient easily. Roll the patient to one side, place a double thickness of the sheeting under the patient, and then roll the patient on top of the transfer sheets.

For the actual lateral transfer, both transfer surfaces must be side to side, as close to each other as possible, and at the same height. The wheels of the gurney must be locked so the two surfaces cannot separate during the transfer. The transfer sheets have handles. Two technologists, one at the patient's head and chest and a second at the patient's pelvis and legs, can grasp the top sheet and slide the patient laterally into the desired position.

To perform a cart-to-table transfer without a moving device, a draw sheet is needed. Begin by checking that the sheet is properly positioned for the transfer. Then, roll up the draw sheet on both sides of the patient (Fig. 13–11, *A*). The person directing the transfer should support the patient's head and upper body from the far side of the radiographic table. Another person should support the patient's pelvic girdle from the cart side. A third person should support the patient's legs from the tableside. The patient's arms should be crossed over the chest to avoid injury or interference with a smooth transfer (Fig. 13–11, *B*).

The person supporting the pelvic girdle stands on the opposite side of the cart and makes sure that the cart does not move away from the table during the transfer. The person in charge, at the patient's head, gives the commands and directs the transfer. On command, everyone grasps the rolled-up draw sheet and slowly pulls the patient to the edge of the cart. Depending on the length of their reach, the assistants may need to reposition themselves in anticipation of moving the patient from the cart onto the table. When everyone is ready, the person in

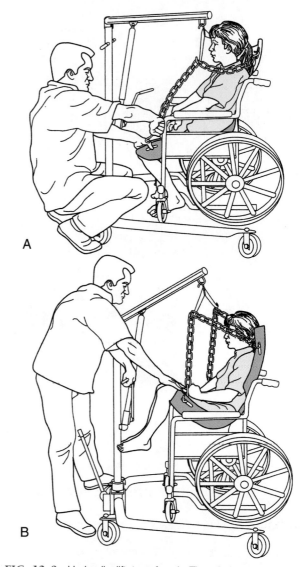

FIG. 13–9 Hydraulic lift transfer. *A,* The chains have a short segment for attachment to the sling back and a longer segment for attachment to the sling seat. Adjust the chain length according to the patient's size. Hook the chains to the sling from the inside out. This precaution minimizes the risk of a patient's being injured by the hooks. *B,* Check that the release valve is closed and that the patient is positioned comfortably in the sling. Gently begin to raise the patient.

charge again issues the command and the patient is slowly lifted and pulled onto the table.

The transfer without a moving device is difficult. Because of the potential of strain and injury to the persons performing the maneuver, it is generally not recommended for most patients, especially those who are heavy or who have serious injuries. The transfer personnel are

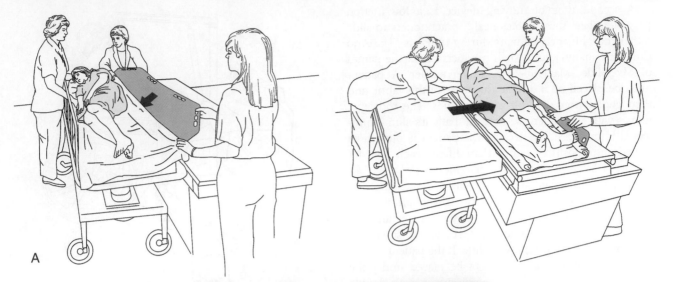

A

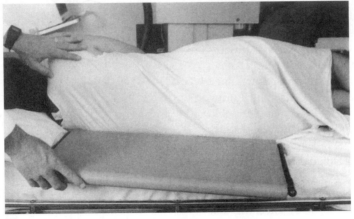

B

FIG. 13–10 Cart-to-table transfer with a moving device. The preferred method of moving a patient from a cart to a table is with a moving device. The patient should be rolled away from the table while the device is placed halfway underneath both the patient and the draw sheet. The patient is then returned to a supine position, and the draw sheet is gently pulled to move the patient onto the table. If necessary, the patient may be rolled again to remove the moving device. *A,* A plastic moving device in use. *B,* A roller moving device in use.

never recommended to attempt to kneel or stand on the radiographic table to perform this type of transfer.

POSITIONING

To examine the desired body part, patients need to be moved into a variety of different positions. In general, the patient needs to be transferred as a single unit, placed on the table in a safe and secure position, and then moved segmentally into the desired body position. Before executing the move, talk through the steps to prepare the patient and any assistants. Let the patient assist as much as possible. To minimize trauma and discomfort for the patient, take an extra moment to make sure that the patient is ready to make the move. When moving a patient, always roll the patient *toward* you. Provide positioning sponges to support the patient comfortably in the desired position. The proper terms for the most common positions are given in Fig. 13–12. All radiologic technologists should become familiar with both the positions and the appropriate methods to assist patients in achieving them.

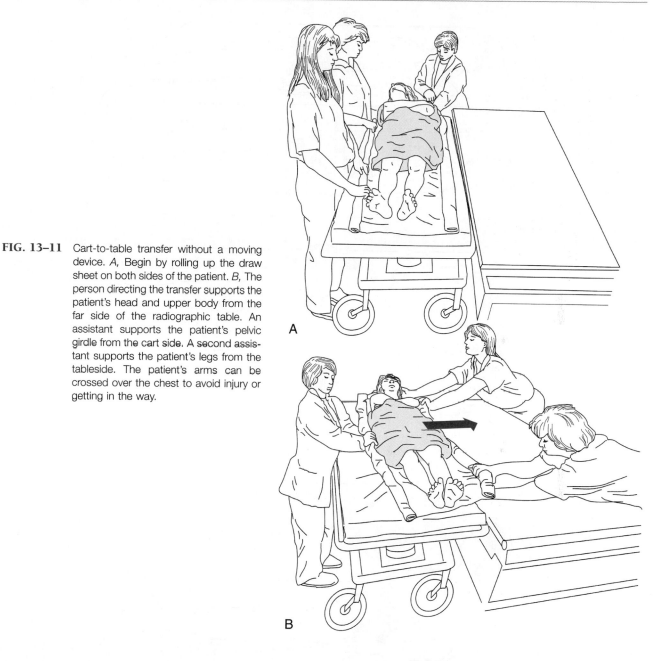

FIG. 13–11 Cart-to-table transfer without a moving device. *A,* Begin by rolling up the draw sheet on both sides of the patient. *B,* The person directing the transfer supports the patient's head and upper body from the far side of the radiographic table. An assistant supports the patient's pelvic girdle from the cart side. A second assistant supports the patient's legs from the tableside. The patient's arms can be crossed over the chest to avoid injury or getting in the way.

A

B

SUMMARY

To execute safe, efficient patient transfers with minimal stress and discomfort for health professionals and patients, the radiologic technologist must maintain a wide base of support, hold patients close to the center of gravity, avoid trunk twisting, keep the back stable, lift from the knees, and let the patients assist as much as possible. Prepare both patients and assistants for transfers by verbally planning out and rehearsing the procedures. Take the time to be gentle and safe and to move slowly. These extra moments might prevent a serious injury.

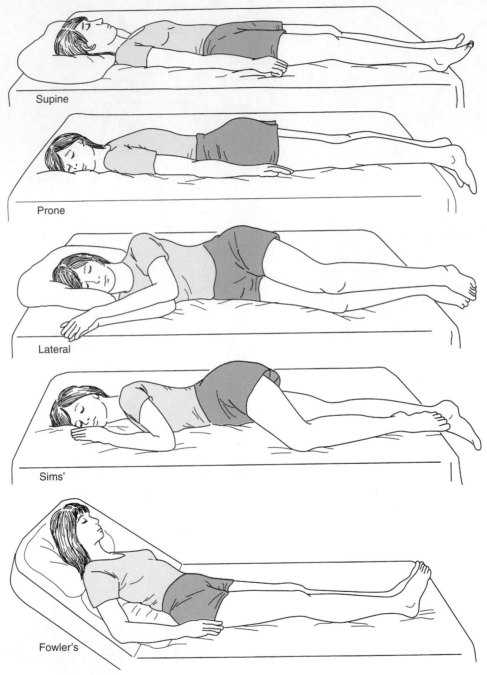

Supine

Prone

Lateral

Sims'

Fowler's

FIG. 13–12   Patient positioning.

BIBLIOGRAPHY

Delitto RS, Rose SJ, Apts DW: Electromyographic analysis of two techniques for squat lifting. *Phys Ther* 67:1329, 1987.

Ehrlich RA, McCloskey E: *Patient care in radiography,* ed 6, St Louis, 2004, Mosby.

Hollis M, Davis PR: *Safer lifting for patient care,* ed 3, Oxford, UK, 1991, Blackwell Scientific Publications.

Kelsey JL, White AA, Pastides H, et al: The impact of musculoskeletal disorders on the population of the United States, *J Bone Joint Surg [Am]* 61:959, 1979.

Minor MA, Minor SD: *Patient care skills,* ed 4, Upper Saddle River, NJ, 1999, Prentice Hall.

Norkin CC, Levangie PK: Biomechanics. In Norkin CC, Levangie PK, eds: *Joint structure and function: a comprehensive analysis,* ed 4, Philadelphia, 2005, FA Davis.

Rantz MF, Corntial D: *Lifting, moving and transferring patients: a manual,* ed 2, St Louis, 1981, Mosby.

Smidt GL: Biomechanics and physical therapy: a perspective, *Phys Ther* 64:1807, 1984.

Sullivan MS: Back support mechanisms during manual lifting, *Phys Ther* 69:38, 1989.

Torres L: *Basic medical techniques and patient care in imaging technology,* ed 6, Philadelphia, 2004, Lippincott, Williams & Wilkins.

White AA, Gordon SL: Synopsis: Workshop on idiopathic low back pain, *Spine* 7:141, 1982.

14

Immobilization Techniques

Robin Jones, MS, RT(R)

Uncooperative behavior can be viewed as active resistance, a defensive action which serves to preserve self-esteem and ward off the invasiveness of intervention. . . . Resistance is therefore a sign of strength; . . . the therapeutic solution is not to confront resistance, but to honor it.

Helen Burr, 1987

OBJECTIVES

On completion of this chapter, the student will be able to:

1. Demonstrate a range of immobilization techniques.

2. Explain the importance of quality communication with the patient.

3. Describe reduction of patient radiation exposure by using proper immobilization methods.

4. Apply immobilization techniques in routine situations.

5. Use immobilization devices effectively.

6. Describe trauma immobilization techniques as they pertain to specific anatomic involvement.

7. Explain the importance of establishing rapport with pediatric patients.

8. Use various methods of pediatric immobilization.

9. Describe appropriate application of immobilization techniques pertinent to geriatric patients.

SCOPE OF IMMOBILIZATION TECHNIQUES

When discussing **immobilization** techniques, the effect of motion and positioning inaccuracy on the diagnostic quality of the procedure is important to understand. One of the many factors that affect diagnostic quality is motion. When attempting to photograph a fast-moving object (a sprinter or a race car, for example), a good possibility exists that the image on the developed film will appear streaked or blurry because of the motion of the object photographed.

The same phenomenon occurs when radiographing a wiggly 3-year-old patient's chest or the shaking hand of a badly injured accident victim. The movement of the toddler or the shaking hand results in a blurred image and necessitates a repeat exposure, which increases patient dose. The important fact is that the motion of the subject does not have to be considerable or exaggerated to affect the procedure. Even the slightest movement can seriously compromise the radiograph.

Another important factor affecting diagnostic information is inaccuracy when positioning the patient during an examination. Many positions for procedures require exact degrees of rotation of the patient or body part. Use of positioning aids such as sponges or supports enables the radiologic technologist to position the patient accurately. At the same time, this support of the patient significantly lessens the possibility of motion.

A thorough knowledge of the various methods that can be used to reduce the possibility of motion problems and positioning inaccuracies is therefore extremely important when studying the art and practice of radiologic technology.

Simple versus Involved Immobilization Techniques

Although some forms of immobilization techniques can be intricate, understanding that immobilization techniques cover a wide range of applications, from minimal to highly sophisticated, is important. The simplest techniques involve the use of a positioning sponge to support the anatomic area of interest or gently laying a sandbag across a patient's forearm to minimize shaking caused by patient anxiety. More complex techniques might involve completely wrapping an infant or small child in a sheet (often referred to as a *mummy wrap*) or securing an accident victim to a backboard to facilitate transport of the patient to the emergency department and to minimize the possibility of more severe complications, such as spinal cord damage, during the transport process. In the latter case, the radiologic technologist has not applied the immobilization device but must recognize the importance of the device and be able to use it to the best advantage.

Protection from Radiation

A conscientious, professional radiologic technologist strives to produce the most diagnostic film possible with the least amount of radiation to the patient and others. If the patient moves, either voluntarily or involuntarily, then the radiographs may be of less than optimal quality and therefore need to be repeated. By repeating the projection, the patient is receiving an additional dose of radiation. Voluntary movement can be controlled by the patient and most often occurs as a result of inadequate communication by the technologist. Involuntary movement is the result of many contributing factors (e.g., examination room temperature, medication, posttraumatic shock) and cannot be controlled by the patient. To minimize the radiation dose to the patient, performing the procedure correctly the first time is important.

Communication

Various physical **restraints** can be used to reduce the possibility of motion, but perhaps one of the most effective means of reducing motion on the part of the patient is also one of the most simple and, unfortunately, one of the most overlooked. The method is *communication.*

The art of communication is a skill that is often used ineffectively. Ineffective or unskillful communication can occur at all levels: between radiologist and radiologic technologist, from one technologist to another, from clinical instructor to student, from department manager to secretary, from technologist to patient, and so forth. Keeping in mind the objective of reducing repeated procedures and exposure to radiation, the most important communication that occurs in a radiology department may take place between the technologist and patient.

The patient is often capable of cooperation and would be more than willing to facilitate the examination if he or she were simply informed of what was going to happen and apprised of the importance of cooperation in producing an accurate diagnosis. A key component to effective communication with the patient is the establishment of rapport.

Rapport is a relation of harmony and accord between two persons, as between patient and physician. This harmony and relationship building should begin as soon as the technologist comes into contact with the patient. It begins as the radiologic technologist introduces himself or herself to the patient and continues throughout the history-taking process. While obtaining the history, the technologist has the opportunity to display empathy, respect, and concern for the patient as a person, as well as to ascertain the clinical facts behind the examination. Once the radiologic technologist has established rapport with the patient, the patient becomes increasingly comfortable, a sense of trust and confidence is established, and the patient is able to focus on the explanation of what will occur during the examination.

Whereas a good explanation of the examination is important and will better enable the patient to cooperate, the explanation generally need not be highly technical or filled with professional jargon. A simple explanation, in lay terms, stressing the importance of cooperation on the part of the patient, is usually all that is needed. Care must be taken, however, that in simplifying the explanation the patient is not insulted by underestimation of his or her intelligence. A proper assessment of the patient's replies and questions allows the technologist to explain the examination at a level appropriate to each patient. The explanation should emphasize that cooperation on the part of the patient will make the examination proceed quickly and result in the highest possible diagnostic information. Keeping the explanation simple is important, but make sure the patient understands that his or her cooperation is essential.

The radiologic technologist will not always be able to communicate effectively in a verbal sense, as in the case of a very young child or someone who is highly stressed because of the nature of his or her injury or condition. If the technologist is truly genuine in his or her **empathy** for the patient, then communication of a subtle nature will occur. For example, a newborn infant often senses and responds positively to warmth, gentle holding, a soft calm voice, and a sense of security.

ROUTINE APPLICATIONS

Although some immobilization methods may seem mundane to the experienced technologist, their dedicated use results in fewer repeated procedures as a result of patient motion.

Positioning Sponges

One of the most common methods of reducing patient motion involves the use of positioning sponges. These sponges come in a variety of shapes and sizes and are designed to support the patient or the anatomic area of interest by reducing physical strain on the patient from having to hold a position that might otherwise be difficult to achieve (Fig. 14–1). Positioning sponges also allow for increased accuracy in positioning by supporting the patient or anatomic area of interest in the correct position and in relation to the film. The use of positioning sponges is limited only by the creativity of the technologist.

Velcro Straps

Although often not considered a form of restraint, Velcro straps can be effective as restraining or positioning devices. A good example of the use of straps is provided by an upright lateral chest position (Fig. 14–2). The patient should be standing for a chest examination if at all possible. Although capable of standing, a patient who

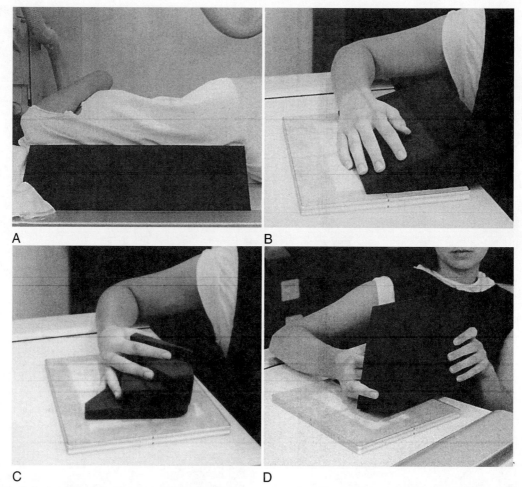

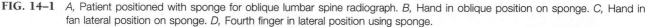

FIG. 14–1 *A,* Patient positioned with sponge for oblique lumbar spine radiograph. *B,* Hand in oblique position on sponge. *C,* Hand in fan lateral position on sponge. *D,* Fourth finger in lateral position using sponge.

has not been regularly **ambulatory** for a time may be unsteady when standing at the upright cassette holder. Placing Velcro straps across the patient's upper chest can help the patient hold still and also provides a sense of security. Holding the arms up out of the way on a lateral chest position raises the center of balance and can cause slight swaying even in the steadiest subject.

Velcro straps also can be used in immobilizing only the area of interest during the procedure. For example, an **axial projection** of the calcaneus requires extreme dorsiflexion of the ankle to produce an optimally diagnostic radiograph (Fig. 14–3). The use of the strap beneath the **plantar surface** of the foot allows the patient to maintain the extreme **flexion** required and at the same time reduces the possibility of motion that may result from maintaining an uncomfortable position.

Velcro straps can serve as a safety precaution when performing a procedure on a patient who is not completely cognizant, such as those who are heavily medicated or intoxicated or who have diminished mental capacities. This type of patient should never be left unattended; the straps serve only to facilitate protection of the patient from injury. With straps in place, sudden or unexpected movement by the patient would not result in injury to the patient and would allow the attendant to respond to the situation.

Velcro Strap Restraints

Velcro strap restraints are designed to be attached easily to the radiography table. These types of restraints include two brackets that mount to each side of the table with a

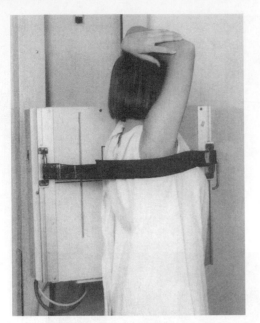

FIG. 14–2 Patient positioned for lateral upright chest radiograph with straps in place.

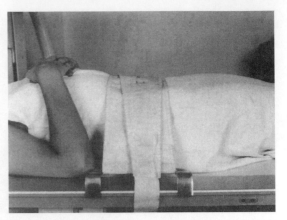

FIG. 14–4 Patient supine on table with Velcro straps in place.

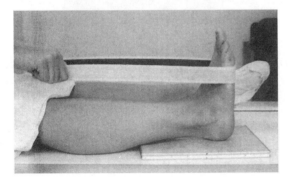

FIG. 14–3 Patient positioned for axial calcaneus radiograph using strap.

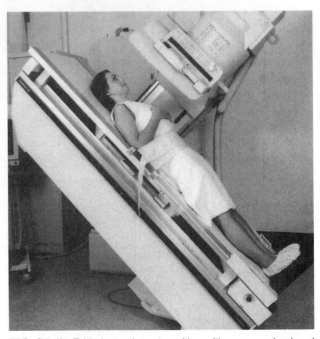

FIG. 14–5 Table in semi-erect position with compression band over patient. If more support is needed, then additional bands may be applied to the chest, hips, and knees.

strap that is adjustable to any size patient. It can be adjusted to cover any part of the body, such as the chest, abdomen, and legs (Fig. 14–4). These restraints can also be used for compression. By tightening the strap a little further, gentle pressure can be applied to the abdomen to enhance diagnostic information in certain procedures.

When performing gastrointestinal procedures, for example, placing the patient in the semi-erect position may be desirable. In these circumstances, when a patient is too weak to stand unassisted, Velcro strap restraints can be applied across the patient's upper and lower abdomen to support the patient firmly during the procedure (Fig. 14–5). This precaution helps reassure the patient that he or she will not fall.

Sandbags

Sandbags are useful positioning and immobilization devices and can be used in a variety of ways. By themselves or in combination with positioning sponges, sandbags are extremely helpful in reducing voluntary motion (Figs. 14–6 and 14–7). Sandbags, unlike radiolucent positioning sponges, are radiopaque (i.e., radiation does not pass through easily). As a result, they cannot be

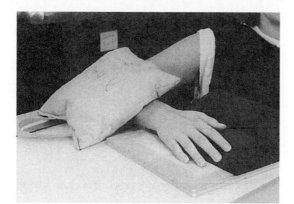

FIG. 14–6 Hand in oblique position on sponge with sandbag across forearm.

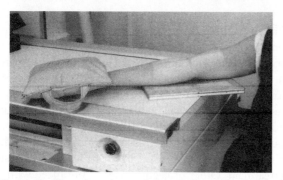

FIG. 14–7 Elbow in anteroposterior position with sandbag on palm.

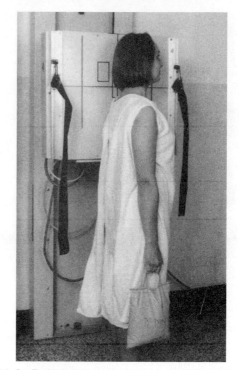

FIG. 14–8 Patient in erect lateral cervical position with sandbags.

placed in such a way that diagnostic information is obscured within the anatomic area of interest. They must be placed gently on or against the areas adjacent to the anatomic area of interest so as not to injure or cause further damage.

A common use of sandbags as positioning aids is in performing examination of a lateral cervical spine or of the acromioclavicular joints. Both examinations require that the shoulders lie in the same transverse plane and have the patient hold sandbags of equal weight. For the lateral cervical spine, the patient must depress the shoulders as much as possible to demonstrate the lower cervical vertebrae (Fig. 14–8).

Here again, as in the case of positioning sponges, the variety of uses for sandbags is limited only by the technologist's imagination.

Head Clamps

Head clamps can be attached to radiographic imaging devices (e.g., radiographic table, upright cassette holder) and are designed strictly for use in positioning various projections of the skull. When applied safely and appropriately, head clamps serve more as positioning aids than as immobilization devices. A patient so desiring can easily pull away from the head clamps. Head clamps serve as a reminder to the patient of the importance of remaining as still as possible, and they ensure the reduction of voluntary movement on the part of the patient (Fig. 14–9).

SPECIAL APPLICATIONS

Immobilization techniques are often required for use with trauma, pediatric, and geriatric patients. Each type of patient provides unique opportunities to apply immobilization techniques.

Trauma Applications

Methods for safely and expeditiously performing examinations on badly traumatized patients involve entirely different concepts. Immobilization is one of the most critical considerations when working with seriously injured patients. In these instances, the technologist is faced with immobilization devices that already have been applied to the **trauma** victim by the emergency medical team to

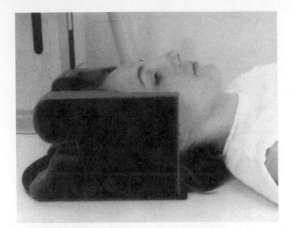

FIG. 14–9 Patient positioned for anteroposterior skull radiograph with head clamps in place.

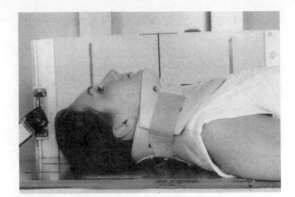

FIG. 14–10 Patient positioned for recumbent lateral cervical spine radiograph with a cervical collar in place.

stabilize the area of injury and to facilitate safe transport to the trauma center. The technologist must be familiar with the various types of traction and immobilization techniques and devices used by emergency medical personnel. This familiarity must include knowledge of which devices are radiolucent, which must be left in place for initial examinations, and when these devices can safely be removed for more detailed procedures.

In many situations, the technologist must consider performing the initial examination with immobilization devices left in place. In fact, more often than not, the technologist has no choice but to perform the procedure in this manner. Fortunately, manufacturers of emergency traction devices are designing equipment to use radiolucent materials whenever possible. This equipment permits initial studies to result in increased diagnostic information without endangering the accident victim by necessitating the removal of immobilization devices.

In most instances, initial images can and should be produced without removing immobilization devices. Only after a radiologist or an attending physician reads the initial radiographs and approval has been given should the technologist remove the immobilization device for a more complete examination.

Immobilization devices should be removed gently while maintaining patient comfort and safety by immobilizing the injured area above and below the device. Positioning sponges should be placed to support the anatomic area of interest. Depending on his or her condition, the patient may be moved or rolled slightly to facilitate removal of the device. If help is available, safety and comfort for the patient is enhanced if two people, working together, remove immobilization devices.

SPINAL TRAUMA. The most common spinal trauma traction device encountered by a technologist is probably the cervical collar. This device is designed to place traction on the cervical spine to prevent further life-threatening movement in this vital area. The lateral position is the most important when performing a cervical trauma examination and is essential in evaluating cervical trauma. After evaluating this radiograph, the attending physician or neurosurgeon can determine the next step in treatment. Other projections can be produced with the cervical collar in place, but the most critical diagnostic information is obtained from the lateral position (Fig. 14–10). In all instances, the cervical collar must be left in place until a physician has seen the initial radiographs and has approved removal of the collar.

The backboard or spineboard is another spinal immobilization device often seen in trauma situations. Although the backboard is mentioned here under spinal trauma considerations, its uses are by no means limited to spinal injury. It is used to immobilize and support the victim's entire body. A backboard can be used if the thoracic or lumbar spine is involved. Additional trauma situations in which the backboard is used include injuries to the pelvis, hips, and lower extremities or when multiple injuries in addition to spinal trauma are present.

Most backboards are made from radiolucent materials (e.g., wood, plastic), making radiography of patients relatively easy. With assistance, one end of the backboard can be lifted and a cassette placed under the area of interest beneath the board (Fig. 14–11). All **anteroposterior** projections from head to toe can be accomplished in this manner.

Another advantageous way of using the backboard is to transport a stable trauma patient to the radiology

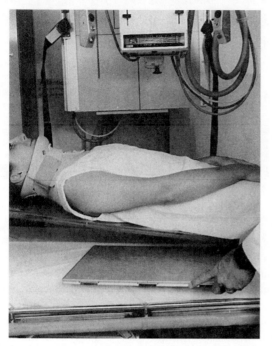

FIG. 14–11 Patient on backboard with grid cassette placed under backboard for anteroposterior lumbar spine radiograph.

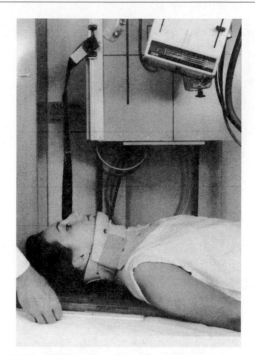

FIG. 14–12 Patient on backboard positioned for acanthoparietal projection with cervical collar in place.

department for the initial examination. Moving the patient onto the table by sliding the entire backboard onto the examination table is relatively easy for the movers and comfortable for the patient. Once the radiologist has evaluated the initial radiographs, the backboard can be moved from under the patient for further projections. Conversely, if the findings indicate the presence of fracture or other traumatic involvement, then the patient can be safely moved back onto a stretcher for transport to surgery, the emergency department, or the appropriate treatment area.

HEAD TRAUMA. The technologist will encounter trauma immobilization devices applied to other areas of interest besides the spine. In many instances, examining the skull of a patient wearing a cervical collar or similar immobilization device is necessary. Because of the presence of the cervical collar, a radiographer must become versatile in the production of skull radiographs. Instead of being able to rotate and tilt the head or flex and extend the neck so as to position the patient correctly, the radiographer must be able to manipulate the radiographic equipment to compensate for the patient's lack of mobility (Fig. 14–12). The cervical collar cannot often be removed for more difficult skull projections until after approval by a physician.

EXTREMITY TRAUMA. Other anatomic areas of interest that may involve the use of traction devices are the extremities, particularly the lower extremities. In these cases, the traction devices are in the form of splints, most often inflation or traction splints.

An inflation or air splint is simply an inflatable plastic cuff that is slipped over the affected limb and inflated to provide stability for transport by the emergency team (Fig. 14–13). These splints are readily radiolucent, and routine radiography usually can be achieved with little discomfort or danger to the patient. An exception would be when a patient has multiple injuries that complicate the procedures.

Traction splints are designed for use on the lower extremities. They exert a steady force on the affected limb by applying pressure against the pelvis and groin area (Fig. 14–14). Although traction splints often contain radiopaque materials, satisfactory initial radiographs can be obtained with the splint in place. Most splints designed for use on the upper extremities are made from radiolucent materials and do not present any great obstacles for the procurement of diagnostic radiographs.

An antishock garment might also be occasionally encountered. The antishock garment is a pair of inflatable trousers applied to the victim. This garment is used

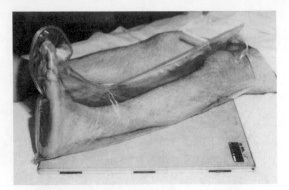

FIG. 14-13   Inflation (air) splint on lower leg.

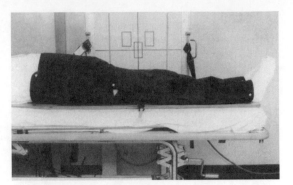

FIG. 14-15   Patient wearing antishock garment.

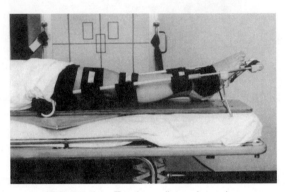

FIG. 14-14   Traction splint on lower leg.

in instances in which the patient has sustained trauma to the abdomen, pelvis, or lower extremities and internal hemorrhage is suggested. Once the antishock garment is in place around the patient, the garment is inflated to slow the rate of hemorrhage. Performing radiography is sometimes necessary on these patients for pelvic or other fractures with the garment in place. Because the trousers are radiolucent, they can be left in place while the examination is being performed (Fig. 14-15).

Pediatric Applications

Special problems are encountered when performing radiographic examinations on **pediatric** patients. Although many methods and devices are available to facilitate pediatric radiography, perhaps the most overlooked aspects of positioning and immobilizing children are communication and the establishment of rapport. In many instances, children as young as 3 or 4 years of age can be convinced to hold still without immobilization when communication is well done. This rapport is established with kindness, patience, honesty, and understanding. Although this communication may not be difficult to convey under normal circumstances, an entirely different situation arises within the context of a busy radiographic department with a child who is injured or sick. Kindness, patience, honesty, and understanding are best conveyed to children literally on their level by dropping to one knee to talk with the children face to face. To quote Armand Brodeur, former chief radiologist at Cardinal Glennon Children's Hospital in St. Louis, "To stand tall in pediatric radiology, you have to get down on your knees." A diagnostic examination will be obtained relatively quickly if a little time is spent in establishing rapport with the child. Speak in a calm, soothing voice, perhaps while offering a toy to the child. Young children often respond well to making a game of having their *picture taken* or seeing how long they can hold still. Allow the child time to explore the new surroundings and ask questions. Threats and force must be avoided at all times, with restraints being applied gently.

Another preliminary consideration for pediatric radiography is how to manage parents while the examination is being performed. Some possibilities include having the parent accompany the child into the radiography room to assist the radiographer, having the parents wait outside the radiography room during the procedure, or having a parent accompany the child but observing only. With the use of department protocol and experience, the radiographer must decide what option will yield the best results.

As is often the case, when departmental policy or the situation calls for parents to be present during the examination, the radiographer absolutely must share the importance of cooperation and understanding with the parents. Being objective is difficult for parents when they observe their child being placed in a pediatric immobilization device. Although a child who is confined in an upright chest immobilization device or strapped to a restraint board may appear uncomfortable, the parent must be made to understand that the technique or device used for immobilization is the safest, surest way to produce optimal diagnostic radiographs with a minimal amount of discomfort and radiation exposure to the child.

Pediatric positioning and immobilization are increasingly appropriate for **neonates** and small children. If well done and genuine, rapport and communication should be all that is necessary for older children. The radiographer must determine what methods are required according to the situation.

SHEET RESTRAINTS. One of the most effective, simple, inexpensive, and reliable methods of restraining or immobilizing a child is mummification. Although this method can be used on children 4 or 5 years of age, it is beneficial for children who are still too young to understand cooperation. Basically, the child is wrapped in a sheet, which effectively limits the movement of the extremities and also gives the technique its name (Fig. 14–16). Sheets or blankets can be used in many ways for immobilizing infants and small children, and other mummification variations exist. Again, the technologist is limited only by imagination.

COMMERCIAL RESTRAINTS. Commercial restraints usually take one of two forms: (1) upright restraint devices or (2) restraint boards. One of the most common and useful upright restraint devices is the Pigg-O-Stat (Fig. 14–17). This device is made of radiolucent materials and can be useful for upright chest and abdominal radiographic examinations. It is large enough to accommodate children up to approximately 3 years of age. Once secured, the patient can be rotated 360 degrees to demonstrate various oblique and lateral positions. A built-in, adjustable lead shield facilitates examinations for gonadal protection, respiration phase indicators, and left and right markers. Because the Pigg-O-Stat is made of clear plastic, patient movement can be easily observed during exposures. It holds the child securely and safely and greatly reduces the need for repeated exposures or the necessity of having someone hold the patient. One disadvantage of the device is possible **artifacts** caused by the plastic sides, which can overlap the anatomic area of interest.

Another type of commercial restraint device occasionally used in radiology departments is the restraint board (infant immobilizer). Even though several variations of restraint boards exist, all of them consist basically of a contour-fitting pad, mold, or sponge with attached Velcro straps for securing the patient (Fig. 14–18). The restraint board is a good way to immobilize an infant or small child when radiographic studies of the abdomen are desirable. Similar to the upright restraint device, these restraint boards allow the child to be safely and securely immobilized while eliminating the need for someone to hold the child.

A modification of the Velcro strap restraint board is the Octastop board (Fig. 14–19). Octagonal metal frames are attached to the end of the board, and the child is restrained on the board with Velcro straps around the limbs and across the torso and head. The patient can be rotated 360 degrees into eight different positions (Fig. 14–20). The disadvantage of the regular restraint board and the octagonal framed version is size. Only infants and small children up to 1 year of age should be immobilized with these devices.

NONCOMMERCIAL RESTRAINTS. A clever means of immobilizing the hands, fingers, feet, and toes of young patients is the use of a radiolucent Plexiglas paddle (Fig. 14–21). Pediatric patients have a tendency to wiggle fingers and toes. Applying gentle pressure to the affected area of interest aids the child in holding still while at the same time allowing the production of a diagnostic radiograph of the entire subject with one exposure.

One other immobilization technique worthy of consideration is the use of Velcro straps and tape. Velcro straps can be used in pediatric situations in much the same way as for adult applications. Because children are curious, they tend to be easily distracted by the new surroundings of a radiographic room with all its new information. With their attention wandering from one new wonder to another, even the best rapport and communication may not be able to overcome entirely a slight bit of motion as the child continues to investigate the surroundings during the examination. Using Velcro straps for a 5- or 6-year-old child during an upright chest examination not only keeps the patient more still, but it also serves as a reminder to the child that he or she should hold still.

Tape is also sometimes used when immobilizing pediatric patients. Tape should be used more as a reminder to the patient to hold still than as an absolute restraining device. The radiographer should keep in mind that the skin of infants and young children is much more tender

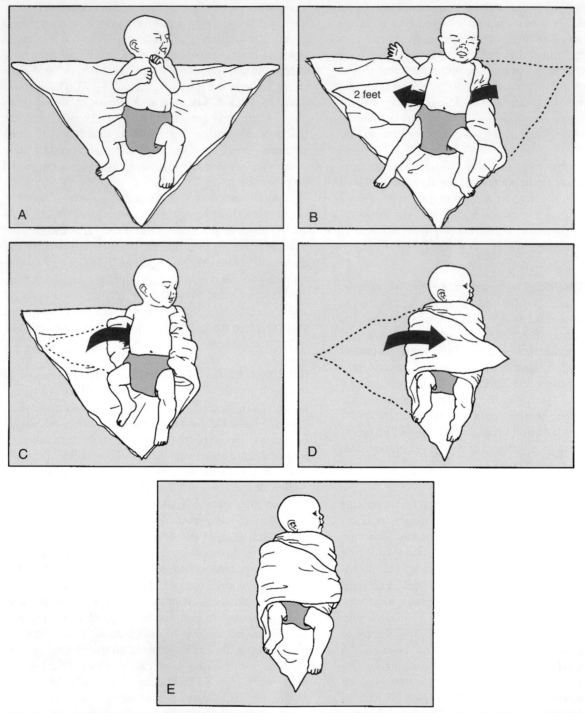

FIG. 14–16 Sheet restraint (mummification technique) sequence. *A,* The child is placed in the center of a triangular folded sheet as shown so that the shoulders are just above the top fold. *B,* The left corner of the sheet is brought over the left arm and under the body so that approximately 2 feet of the sheet extends beyond the right side of the body. Make sure the child is not lying on the left arm. *C,* Tuck the 2 feet of sheet over the right arm and under the body. Again, make sure the child is not lying on the arm. *D,* Bring the remaining sheet over the body. *E,* Tuck the sheet securely under the left side of the body. Remember that this technique restrains most movement but is not satisfactory as a complete immobilization procedure. Restraint bands are still required, and the child should not be left alone, even for the amount of time needed to make a radiographic exposure.

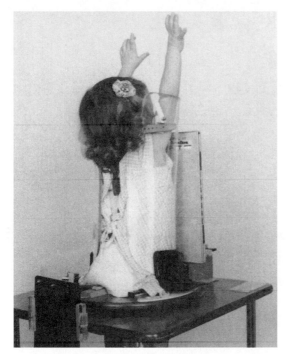

FIG. 14–17 Patient positioned in Pigg-O-Stat for posteroanterior chest radiograph.

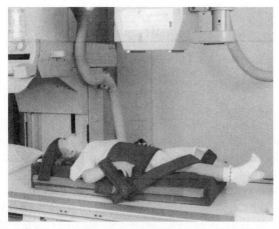

FIG. 14–18 Pediatric patient in a Velcro strap restraint board.

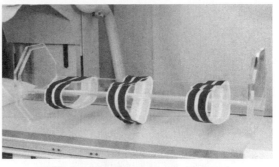

FIG. 14–19 Octastop restraint board.

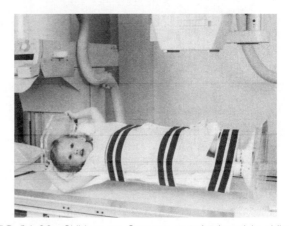

FIG. 14–20 Child on an Octastop restraint board in oblique position.

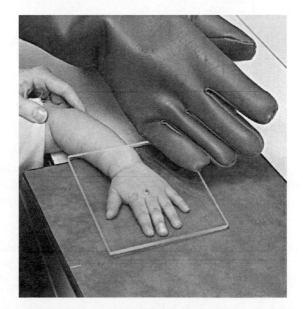

FIG. 14–21 Positioning for pediatric posteroanterior hand radiograph using Plexiglas paddle.

and sensitive than that of an adult. Caution should be taken when using tape to restrain so as not to abrade the skin of the child. When tape is used, it should be twisted where it comes in contact with the skin so that the nonadhesive side is in contact with the skin (Fig. 14–22, A). Another technique to protect the skin is to place a gauze pad between the skin and the tape (Fig. 14–22, B).

A stockinette is also an invaluable pediatric immobilization device. A stockinette is stretchable cotton fabric

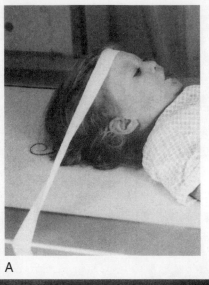

A

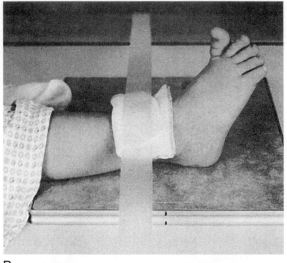

B

FIG. 14–22 *A,* Patient positioned for anteroposterior (AP) skull radiograph with tape twisted across the forehead. *B,* Gauze pad between the skin and tape for an AP ankle radiograph.

in the shape of a sleeve that is pulled over a fractured extremity before a plaster cast is applied. Its purpose is to prevent chafing and irritation of the skin while the limb is in the cast. It comes in a roll and can be cut to any length. A stockinette is effective as a restraint when pulled over the upper or lower extremities of a child and secured with tape. This technique is good for immobilizing the upper limbs above and behind the child's head (Fig. 14–23).

Pediatric radiography is an art in itself, and it is a special radiographer who is its master. Conversely, radi-

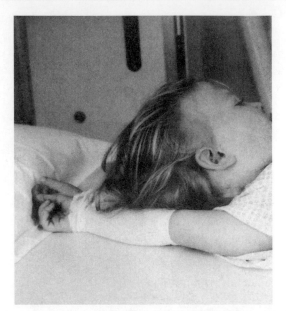

FIG. 14–23 Pediatric patient with stockinette applied to the upper extremities.

ography of a patient who is at the other extreme of age also requires a skillful and professional radiographer.

Geriatric Applications

Radiographic studies on **geriatric** patients can be difficult, but the radiographer can make the examination go smoothly if a few considerations are kept in mind. The first of these considerations is security.

In many instances, one of the greatest concerns of an older person is fear of falling. A natural part of the aging process is loss of mobility, agility, and sense of balance. What would be considered a minor fall for a younger person often has catastrophic results for an older adult. Therefore in addition to communication and rapport, the radiographer must take extra care to make a geriatric patient feel secure. This measure always includes patience in allowing for extra time during the examination so that the geriatric patient does not feel rushed or hurried. Using an extra assistant or two to help move the older patient onto the radiographic table can increase the patient's feeling of security. Always take extra care not to make the geriatric patient feel disoriented by rushing through the examination or by quickly moving from one radiographic position to another. This precaution will allow the geriatric patient to feel more relaxed and better able to concentrate on holding still, thus reducing the need for repeated exposures.

An often overlooked consideration of geriatric radiography that goes along with security is keeping the patient warm. Older persons tend to become chilled easily. This fact, along with the necessity of wearing thin hospital gowns and robes, can add to the difficulty of a geriatric radiographic examination. If the patient is cold and concentrating on trying to keep warm, then he or she will be less likely to be able to cooperate by maintaining a radiographic position. If the older patient is going to be in the department for a long time or is undergoing a lengthy examination such as an excretory urogram, which requires an extended time on the radiographic table, the radiographer should cover the patient or offer extra blankets between radiographic exposures.

A third factor that can interfere with an older patient's ability to cooperate and maintain position is comfort, and this factor too must be considered during the radiographic examination. Just as security and warmth are part of patient comfort, consideration must be given to how long the geriatric patient must lie on the radiographic table. Radiographic tables are hard and cold. Many older patients are thin and are therefore conscious of the hardness of the table. To enable the geriatric patient to cooperate easily and fully, a radiolucent pad should be placed on the table before the examination (Fig. 14–24). A radiographic examination that might take 20 to 30 minutes can seem as an eternity on an unpadded radiographic table. Additionally, a sponge or radiolucent pad beneath the patient's knees can greatly reduce strain on the patient's back and increase the patient's ability to cooperate during the examination. A disadvantage of using a pad is the possibility for slight artifact production or loss of radiographic detail because of increased object-to-image receptor distance. In some instances, a pad might be objectionable to a radiologist.

Although the previously mentioned aspects of security, warmth, and comfort should be considered for all patients, these elements are of extra importance for geriatric patients and can greatly reduce the amount of stress to the patient and radiographer during a radiographic examination if extra emphasis is placed on them.

SUMMARY

Although patient immobilization is only one of many factors in the production of a successful radiographic study, awareness of the various elements to be considered in immobilization techniques must be a part of the radiographer's professional repertoire.

Before learning the various methods of immobilization and restraint that are pertinent to radiographic studies,

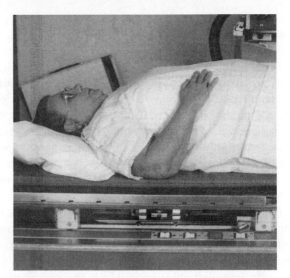

FIG. 14–24 Geriatric patient on a radiolucent pad.

the radiographer must first understand that immobilization techniques are used to eliminate or minimize movement by the patient and to enhance the proper positioning of the anatomic area of interest. Appropriate use of immobilization or restraint techniques can greatly reduce the negative effects of movement or improper positioning on the diagnostic quality of the finished radiograph.

The skill that may be the single most important technique in patient immobilization and the one that must be developed by all radiographers is high-quality communication. Quality communication allows the patient to become an active participant and assistant in the radiographic examination, thus accelerating the examination and reducing the need for repeated exposures. Two key essentials for effective communication are explanation of the procedure and establishment of rapport with the patient.

The range of immobilization techniques runs from simple involvement, such as the use of a positioning sponge or sandbag to reduce patient motion, to rather involved techniques, such as sheet restraints in pediatric radiographic studies or making decisions about removal of traction splints in trauma situations. Within this range are a significant number of different immobilization techniques and considerations for their use. The radiographer should be familiar with all these applications and be able to adapt them to fit each radiographic situation and each patient's condition.

Some of the commonly used routine immobilization methods are positioning sponges, Velcro straps, Velcro strap restraints, sandbags, and head clamps. Many ways exist to use these methods of immobilization, and their use is limited only by the creativity of the radiographer.

Because immobilization is one of the most critical aspects of trauma radiography, the radiographer should be familiar with numerous trauma immobilization devices, methods for producing diagnostic radiographs with these devices in place, and when removing these devices for further radiographic studies is appropriate. Some of these trauma immobilization devices are cervical collars, backboards, air splints, traction splints, and antishock garments.

One area of radiography that often requires the use of immobilization methods is pediatric radiography. Perhaps the most effective method of immobilization is establishing rapport with the young patient. Methods for pediatric immobilization with which the radiographer should be acquainted are sheet restraints, upright and board restraint devices, radiolucent paddles, stockinettes, and the correct use of tape.

Although radiographic examination of geriatric patients can be difficult, certain considerations can greatly facilitate these studies. In addition to communication, rapport, and respect, key considerations for successful geriatric radiography are security, warmth, and comfort.

Familiarity with various immobilization techniques is one aspect of the art of radiography that enables the radiographer to attain the highest levels of professional standards—that is, the production of optimal diagnostic quality images with the least amount of radiation exposure to patient, radiographer, and ancillary personnel.

BIBLIOGRAPHY

Ballinger P, Frank E: *Merrill's atlas of radiographic positions and radiologic procedures,* ed 10, St Louis, 2003, Mosby–Year Book.

Bontrager K: *Textbook of radiographic positioning and related anatomy,* ed 6, St Louis, 2005, Mosby.

Campbell J: *Basic trauma life support,* ed 2, Englewood Cliffs, NJ, 1988, Prentice-Hall.

Darling D: *Radiography of infants and children,* ed 3, Springfield, Ill, 1979, Charles C Thomas.

Ehrlich R, Givens E: *Patient care in radiography,* ed 6, St Louis, 2004, Mosby.

Gurley L, Callaway W: *Introduction to radiologic technology,* ed 6, St Louis, 2002, Mosby.

Torres L: *Basic medical techniques and patient care in imaging technology,* ed 6, Philadelphia, 2004, Lippincott, Williams & Wilkins.

Wilmot DM, Sharko GA: *Pediatric imaging for the technologist,* New York, 1987, Springer-Verlag.

Vital Signs, Oxygen, Chest Tubes, and Lines

Denise E. Moore, MS, RT(R)

Life is only known as the complex of many functions, and health as the integrity of these functions, each in itself and in harmony.

Peter Latham
General Remarks on the Practice of Medicine

OBJECTIVES

On completion of this chapter, the student will be able to:

1. Discuss the significance of homeostasis.

2. Explain the mechanisms that adapt and maintain homeostasis.

3. Discuss the significance of each of the four vital signs: temperature, respiration, pulse, and blood pressure.

4. Identify the normal range for each of the vital signs.

5. Explain the implication of abnormal vital signs.

6. Describe how vital signs are assessed.

7. Explain the indications for administering oxygen therapy.

8. Differentiate high-flow and low-flow oxygen-delivery devices.

OBJECTIVES—Cont'd

9. Explain why caution must be used when performing radiographic procedures on patients receiving oxygen therapy.

10. Describe the uses of, or indications for, the following thoracic tubes and lines to manage compromised patients: endotracheal tubes, thoracostomy tubes, and central venous lines.

11. Describe the radiographic appearance and proper placement of endotracheal tubes, thoracostomy tubes, and central venous lines.

12. Differentiate various types of central venous lines.

13. Recognize the clinical complications associated with use and placement of tubes and lines used in the thorax.

GLOSSARY

Apnea: cessation of spontaneous ventilation

Auscultation: listening to sounds of the body, typically through the use of a stethoscope

Atelectasis: absence of gas from part or the whole of the lungs as a result of failure of expansion or reabsorption of gas from the alveoli

Body Temperature: measurement of the degree of heat of the deep tissues of the human body

Bradycardia: slowness of the heartbeat as evidenced by slowing of the pulse rate to less than 60 beats per minute

Bradypnea: abnormal slowness of breathing

Diaphoresis: profuse sweating

Diastolic: pertaining to dilation, or a period of dilatation, of the heart, especially of the ventricles

Dyspnea: difficult or labored breathing

Febrile: pertaining to or characterized by fever

Homeostasis: constancy in the internal environment of the body, naturally maintained by adaptive responses that promote healthy survival

Hypertension: persistently high arterial blood pressure

Hyperthermia: abnormally high body temperature, especially that induced for therapeutic purposes

Hypotension: abnormally low blood pressure; seen in shock but not necessarily indicative of shock

Hypothermia: low body temperature

Hypoxemia: decreased oxygen tension (concentration) in the blood

Hypoxia: the reduction of oxygen supply to the tissue

Intubation: insertion of a tubular device into a canal, hollow organ, or cavity

Pleural Effusion: increased amounts of fluid within the pleural cavity, usually the result of inflammation

Pneumothorax: presence of air or gas in the pleural cavity

Pulse Oximeter: photoelectric device used for determining the oxygen saturation of the blood

Sphygmomanometer: instrument for measuring blood pressure

Systolic: pertaining to contraction, or a period of contraction, of the heart (myocardium), especially that of the ventricles

Tachycardia: rapidity of the heart action, usually defined as a heart rate greater than 100 beats per minute

Tachypnea: abnormal rapidity of breathing

Ventilation: mechanical movement of air into and out of the lungs

VITAL SIGNS AS AN INDICATION OF THE PATIENT'S HOMEOSTASIS STATUS

Homeostasis is a relative constancy in the internal environment of the body that is naturally maintained by adaptive responses that promote healthy survival. The primary mechanisms that maintain homeostasis are the heartbeat, blood pressure, body temperature, respiratory rate, and electrolyte balance. These adaptive response mechanisms identified as homeostasis are continuously interacting with and adjusting to changes originating inside or outside the body to maintain the constant internal environment. Every health care professional should have a fundamental comprehension of the mechanisms that maintain homeostasis. For example, *vital signs* are primary mechanisms that adapt to responses, inside or outside the body, to maintain homeostasis. Collectively, the vital signs are body temperature, pulse rate, blood pressure, and respiratory rate. In addition, assessment of the patient's mental alertness (*sensorium*) is often reported along with the vital signs.

Vital signs can be assessed quickly in the clinical setting and serve as objective, noninvasive evidence of the patient's immediate condition; similarly, vital sign measures are physiologic indicators of a patient's response to therapy. Most notably, vital signs provide important information because they often reveal the first clue of adverse reactions to treatment. Improvement in a patient's vital signs is strong evidence that a treatment is having a positive effect. For example, a decrease in the patient's heart rate and respiratory rate, toward normal, after oxygen therapy suggests a beneficial effect.

BODY TEMPERATURE

Description

Body temperature is a measurement of the degree of heat of the deep tissues of the human body. The normal mean body temperature is approximately 98.6°F (37°C), with a daily variation of 1° to 2°F (0.5° to 1.0°C). Because humans are warm-blooded animals, the cells of the human body function best within a narrow range of temperature variations. Body temperature must maintain a relatively constant level despite extremes in environmental temperatures. *Thermoregulation* is the term used to describe the body's maintenance of heat production and heat loss. The hypothalamus plays an important role in regulating heat loss and can initiate peripheral vasodilation and sweating **(diaphoresis)** to dissipate body heat. Similarly, the respiratory system plays an important role by removing excess heat through ventilation. The hypothalamus also plays an important role in the preservation of heat by initiating shivering (to generate heat) and vasoconstriction (to conserve heat).

Measurement

Five routes are commonly used to measure body temperature: (1) oral, (2) axillary, (3) tympanic, (4) temporal, and (5) rectal. Oral measurements are obtained by placing a thermometer under the patient's tongue. Depending on the type of thermometer used, electronic or glass bulb, the thermometer stays in place for 20 seconds to 3 minutes until a stable reading is obtained. Oral temperature readings are the most common method of determining the body temperature of an adult or a cooperative child (Fig. 15–1).

Axillary temperatures are obtained by placing the thermometer high between the upper arm and the torso. This method, used for children and infants, is notoriously inaccurate and time consuming. The thermometer must

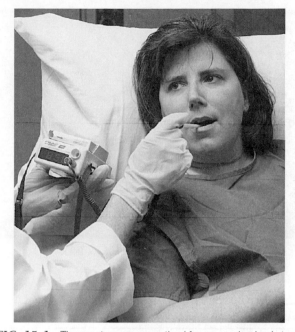

FIG. 15–1 The most common method for measuring body temperature is the oral route; the thermometer is placed under the tongue.

remain in place 5 to 10 minutes to obtain a stable reading. Its shortcomings make this technique almost useless. Tympanic temperatures are obtained by placing an electronic thermometer in the ear (Fig 15–2). A stable reading is displayed within 3 seconds. To obtain rectal temperatures, the bulb of a rectal thermometer is lubricated and placed in the rectum of the patient for 2½ to 5 minutes.

Until recently, tympanic and rectal temperatures were the preferred assessments for all infants, as well as for adults, when oral measures were not feasible. Even today, rectal thermometry is believed to be the most accurate reflection of core body temperature, and tympanic measures closely correlate to rectal measures; however, newer *temporal artery (TA) thermometers* have recently been introduced. TA thermometers are believed to be more closely equivalent to rectal measures, and, as a noninvasive assessment, the convenience of sweeping the device along the forehead with instantaneous display of body temperature makes these thermometers attractive devices. The TA lies superficial in the temporal region of the skull. A swipe of the thermometer along the forehead and across the temporal region provides immediate, accurate measures closely correlating to core body temperature. TA thermometry is gaining popularity.

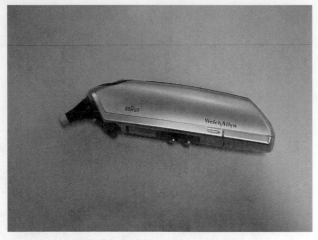

FIG. 15–2 Tympanic thermometer.

TABLE 15-1 Normal Vital Signs

SIGN	RANGE
Temperature	97.7°-99.5° F (36.5°-37.5° C)
Respirations	
Adult	12-20 breaths per minute
Child	20-30 breaths per minute
Pulse	
Adult	60-100 beats per minute
Child	70-120 beats per minute
Blood pressure	
Systolic	<120 mm Hg
Diastolic	<80 mm Hg

Body temperature readings may be measured in either degrees Fahrenheit (°F) or degrees Celsius (°C). Oral temperature readings in healthy adults and children are within the narrow range of 97.7° to 99.5°F (36.5° to 37.5°C) (Table 15-1). Axillary temperatures register slightly lower, and rectal and TA temperatures register approximately 1°F higher than oral readings.

Significance of Abnormalities

When the oral temperature is higher than 99.5°F, a fever exists **(hyperthermia).** A patient with a fever is said to be **febrile.** When the body temperature falls outside the normal range, for example, with an illness or a head injury, the metabolic rate changes accordingly, and the demands on the cardiopulmonary system also change. For example, when the body temperature increases, the metabolic rate also increases, resulting in increased oxygen consumption and carbon dioxide production at the cellular level. As the metabolic rate increases, the cardiopulmonary system must work harder to meet the additional cellular demands by providing more oxygen and eliminating carbon dioxide. As a result of increased body temperature, an increase in cellular metabolism occurs; therefore, any event that increases cellular metabolism also increases body temperature.

Conversely, when the patient's temperature falls below the normal range, **hypothermia** is said to be present. Although not common, hypothermia may be present in patients exposed to cold environmental temperatures and in those with trauma to the hypothalamus. In addition, medically induced hypothermia is used during heart surgery to decrease the metabolic demands, thereby decreasing the demand on the cardiopulmonary system.

Fevers are common with viral and bacterial infections as a natural response of the human body to increase cellular activity to combat the invading organism. Similarly, a patient may become febrile for a day or two after a surgical procedure as the body responds to initiate healing. Prolonged fever in these patients is evidence of postoperative infection. The culprit is often an infection in the wound, lungs, or urinary tract. Patients suffering from a myocardial infarction might be febrile because of increased cellular activity. Hyperthermia also may result from injury to the temperature-regulating center of the hypothalamus, causing it to set the thermostat at a higher level. This injury may occur as a result of a cerebrovascular accident, cerebral edema (swelling), or tumor.

Despite the increased body temperature in some disease states, cellular function is optimal within only a narrow temperature range. Prolonged hyperthermia can lead to serious complications and resultant cellular damage. Patients suffering from hyperthermia may become confused, dizzy, and even comatose. Conversely, hypothermia may be medically induced or the consequence of accidental exposure. Medically induced hypothermia is performed to therapeutically decrease the body's need for oxygen. Because temperature is an easily obtained indicator of the presence of disease, it is routinely followed as a yardstick of response to therapy for many conditions.

RESPIRATORY RATE

Description

While assessing a patient's respiratory rate, the health care professional obtains a general impression of the func-

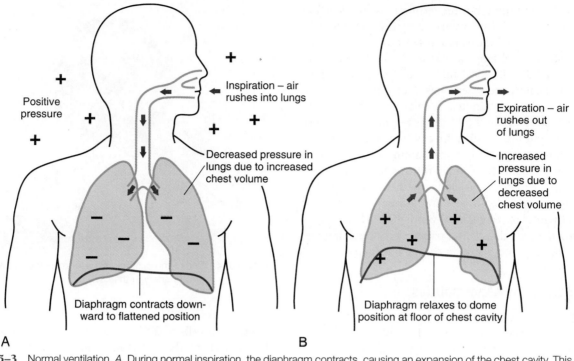

FIG. 15–3 Normal ventilation. *A,* During normal inspiration, the diaphragm contracts, causing an expansion of the chest cavity. This expansion decreases the pressure in the lungs to below the atmospheric pressure; consequently, air rushes into the lungs. *B,* During normal expiration, the diaphragm relaxes, returning to its original position at the floor of the chest cavity and causing a decrease in the volume of the chest cavity. The decrease in chest cavity volume increases the pressure of air in the lungs to above atmospheric pressure so that air flows out of the lungs.

tional status of the respiratory system. The respiratory system is responsible for delivering oxygen (O_2) from the environment to the tissues and eliminating carbon dioxide (CO_2) from the tissues to the environment. The cells of the body require a constant supply of oxygen for cellular metabolism. As a result of cellular metabolism, the waste product carbon dioxide is produced. Unless oxygen is continually supplied and carbon dioxide is continually eliminated, death will occur. Consequently, failure of the respiratory system is a life-threatening event.

Measurement

The major muscle of **ventilation** is the diaphragm. During inspiration, the diaphragm contracts, moving downward in the abdominal cavity and pushing the abdominal contents outward. The downward movement of the diaphragm causes an expansion of the chest cavity, along with a decrease in chest cavity pressure. With decreased internal pressure, air rushes into the lungs. Expiration is achieved by simple relaxation of the diaphragm. As the diaphragm relaxes, it returns to its

original position at the floor of the chest cavity. This action causes an increase of pressure and, subsequently, air flows out of the lungs to the environment (Fig. 15–3).

In a healthy adult, a single respiration consists of an inspiratory phase and an expiratory phase. Because the diaphragm is responsible for the movement of air in and out of the lungs, respirations often are counted by observing the movement of the abdomen. A respiratory rate is also assessed by observing the rise (*inspiration*) and fall (*expiration*) of the chest; however, abdominal and chest wall movement may be difficult to detect by observation alone, particularly with patients who are breathing shallowly. In these cases, the hand of the health care professional may be placed on the patient's abdomen or chest to assist in assessing each ventilation. However, obtaining a patient's respiratory rate without the patient's knowledge is best because, when aware, patients often alter their breathing rate and pattern. Therefore, after obtaining a pulse rate, many health care professionals leave their hand on the patient's wrist and count the respiratory rate; the patient assumes that a pulse rate is still being assessed.

In the healthy adult, normal respirations are silent and effortless, automatically occurring at regular intervals. Respiratory rates are measured as the number of breaths per minute; normal range at rest is 12 to 20 breaths per minute (see Table 15-1). Children under the age of 10 years have slightly increased rates, averaging between 20 and 30 breaths per minute. Newborn respiratory rates average between 30 and 60 breaths per minute. Because respiratory rates are higher in children than in adults, counting respirations for a minimum of 1 minute is important to obtain an accurate measurement. Additionally, while counting respirations, the health care professional assesses the depth (shallow, normal, or deep) and pattern (regular or irregular) of ventilation. Therefore, by assessing the rate, depth, and pattern, an overall impression of the respiratory system can be obtained.

Significance of Abnormalities

Any deviation from normal indicates a change in the status of the respiratory system. If cellular metabolism increases, then the demand for oxygen increases, as does the production of carbon dioxide. The respiratory system responds by increasing the respiratory rate to deliver additional oxygen to the blood. Similarly, with increasing respiratory rates, more carbon dioxide will be exhaled by the lungs. **Tachypnea** is the term used to describe respiratory rates greater than 20 breaths per minute in the case of an adult patient. Common causes of tachypnea include exercise, fever, anxiety, pain, infection, heart failure, chest trauma, decreased oxygen in the blood, and central nervous system disease.

Bradypnea is the term used to describe a decrease in the respiratory rate. Bradypnea occurs much less frequently than tachypnea. Bradypnea results from depression of the respiratory center of the brain common with drug overdoses, head trauma, and hypothermia. **Dyspnea** is a common term used to describe difficult breathing. **Apnea** is the term used to identify the absence of spontaneous ventilation; it is an ominous sign.

PULSE

Description

The cardiovascular system is a closed fluid system composed of a pump (the heart) and many blood vessels. When the left ventricle of the heart contracts, blood is pumped out of the heart into the aorta and throughout the arteries of the body. The function of the cardiovascular system is to transport oxygenated blood from the

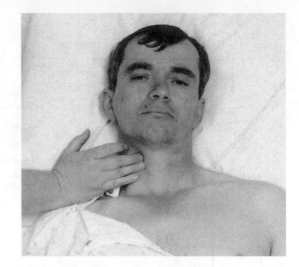

FIG. 15-4 One of the common sites for measuring pulse is the carotid artery in the neck.

lungs to the cells of the body and to return deoxygenated blood back to the heart and lungs to become reoxygenated. Additionally, the cardiovascular system transports carbon dioxide from the cells to the lungs for removal.

As previously stated, the cells of the human body require a constant supply of oxygen to effectively function, and any impairment to the cardiovascular system will result in decreased oxygen to the cells and injury; furthermore, if the heart stops beating, death is imminent.

Measurement

Under normal conditions, the pulse can be palpated at superficially located arteries. Three common sites are used for measuring pulse rate: (1) the radial artery on the thumb side of the wrist, (2) the brachial artery in the antecubital fossa of adults and the upper arm of infants, and (3) the carotid artery in the neck (Fig. 15-4). In addition, listening to the chest with a stethoscope (**auscultation**) and counting each heartbeat can also measure pulse rates. Pulses obtained in this manner are called *apical* pulses (Fig. 15-5).

During cardiopulmonary resuscitation, the pulse is routinely assessed at the carotid artery; however, peripheral pulse points—the femoral, pedal, and radial arteries—are also assessed to verify the effectiveness of chest compressions. Presence of a peripheral pulse indicates a systolic blood pressure of at least 80 mm Hg and verifies effective chest compressions.

Pulse rates reflect the rapidity of each heart contraction and are recorded as the number of beats per minute. Counting the pulse rate for 1 minute is important for an accurate measurement. Resting pulse rates in the normal adult vary from 60 to 100 beats per minute (see Table 15-1). A normal pulse range for children under the age of 10 years is between 70 and 120 beats per minute.

In critical-care settings, patients' arterial oxygen saturation (SAO_2), respiratory rate, and pulse rate are continuously monitored. Examples of devices that can provide continuous monitoring are electrocardiograms, arterial lines, and pulse oximeters. Electrocardiograms continually monitor the patient's heart rate and rhythm. Electrodes placed on the patient's chest monitor the electrical activity of the heart and transform this electrical activity to rate values and waveforms visible on a monitor (Fig. 15–6).

An arterial line is a catheter that is inserted into an artery. The catheter is connected to a pressure transducer that is attached to a monitor. A continual measurement of the patient's heart rate and blood pressure is visible on the monitor.

A **pulse oximeter** is a noninvasive device used to provide ongoing assessment of the hemoglobin oxygen saturation of arterial blood and the patient's pulse rate. A light-emitting probe is placed on the finger, foot, toe, earlobe, temple, nose, or forehead of the patient. Arterial oxygen saturation and pulse rate are determined by measuring absorption of selected wavelengths of light by the circulating blood. The oximeter converts the light intensity information into oxygen saturation and pulse rate values (Fig. 15–7). Normal pulse oximeter values for a healthy person would be between 95% and 100%.

Several factors can affect the accuracy of electronic devices used to monitor pulse rates. For example, patient movement can give rise to inaccurate readings. In addition, misplaced or loose electrodes, lines, or probes also yield inaccurate values. Poor peripheral perfusion caused by low blood pressure, nail polish, and acrylic nails are common causes of pulse oximetry inaccuracies. When the factors or situations that limit the device's precision are corrected, however, these monitoring instruments

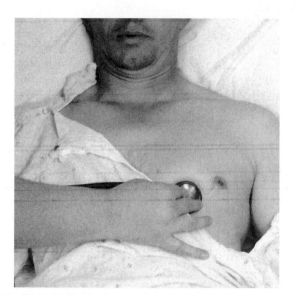

FIG. 15–5 Apical pulses can be obtained by listening to the chest with a stethoscope.

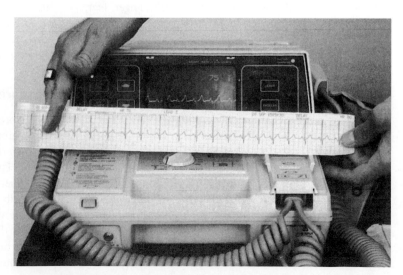

FIG. 15–6 Electrodes placed on the patient's chest transform the electrical activity into pulse-rate values and waveforms visible on a monitor.

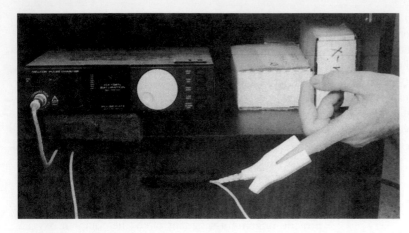

FIG. 15–7 A pulse oximeter can be used to display a patient's pulse and oxygen saturation.

provide reliable, continual, and rapid assessment of patients.

Significance of Abnormalities

Because the cardiovascular system is responsible for delivering oxygenated blood to the cells, when cellular demand for oxygen increases, the heart responds by sending more blood to the tissues. The heart accomplishes this task by increasing the number or force of each myocardial contraction. When heart contractions, and therefore pulse rates, increase by more than 20 beats per minute in the resting adult or reach a rate greater than 100 beats per minute, the patient is said to be experiencing **tachycardia.** Exercise, fever, anemia, respiratory disorders, congestive heart failure, hypoxemia, and shock can cause a patient to become tachycardic because of the increased cellular demands for oxygen. Pain, anger, fear, anxiety, and medications may also induce tachycardia, but the stimulus is through the nervous system, not through an increased demand for oxygen.

Bradycardia refers to a decrease in heart rate. Although initially pain can cause tachycardia, unrelieved, severe pain in fact can lead to bradycardia and subsequent heart problems and even heart failure. Bradycardia may also be seen in hypothermia and in physically fit athletes.

If no pulse can be felt at the wrist, or if cardiac arrest is thought to occur, the pulse should be assessed at the carotid artery for a full 5 seconds while emergency help is summoned. If pulse irregularities are accompanied by patient complaints of palpitations, dizziness, or feeling faint, then a physician should be notified because these irregularities can be life threatening.

BLOOD PRESSURE

Description

Blood pressure is a measure of the force exerted by blood on the arterial walls during contraction and relaxation of the heart. An analogy can be made to water being pumped through a hose. A constant pressure is exerted on the inner surface of the hose by the water. When pumping occurs, the pressure increases as more water is added to the system, causing the water to flow. A similar situation exists in the human body. The pump is the heart, arterial blood vessels are analogous to the hose, and the fluid component is blood instead of water. A constant pressure is exerted on the arterial vessels by the blood when the heart is relaxed. This pressure is called the **diastolic** pressure. During a contraction of the heart, blood is ejected from the ventricles into the arterial blood vessels, creating an increase in pressure. The peak pressure present during contraction of the heart is known as the **systolic** pressure.

Measurement

Blood pressure readings are obtained with the use of a **sphygmomanometer** and stethoscope. The sphygmomanometer consists of a cuff, tubing, valve, and bulb (Fig 15–8). The cuff of the sphygmomanometer is placed on the upper arm midway between the elbow and shoulder. The bulb is used to inflate the cuff with air. Inflation of the cuff above the patient's systolic pressure stops blood flow to the arm by collapsing the brachial artery. With the stethoscope placed over the brachial artery in the antecubital fossa of the elbow, opening the valve slowly

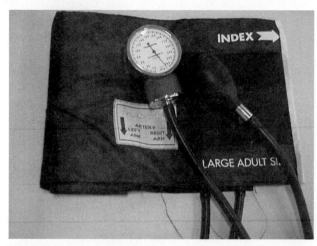

FIG. 15–8 Aneroid-style sphygmomanometer consisting of an air bladder (cuff), bulb and valve to control airflow in and out of the cuff, and a calibrated pressure gauge or dial.

deflates the cuff of the sphygmomanometer. When cuff pressure no longer exceeds the internal pressure of blood in the brachial artery, blood flow returns and can be heard through the stethoscope. The first sound of blood flow (heartbeat) indicates the systolic pressure. When the sound of blood flowing through the arm can no longer be heard, the diastolic pressure is reached (Fig. 15–9). Blood pressures are recorded in millimeters of mercury (mm Hg), with systolic measurements recorded over diastolic measurements (systolic/diastolic).

Normal blood pressure in the healthy adult includes a systolic pressure of less than 120 mm Hg and diastolic pressure of less than 80 mm Hg (see Table 15-1). Pressures are most often recorded with the patient in a sitting position and the arm at approximately the level of the heart. Variations of these conditions can cause some difference in blood pressure readings.

Significance of Abnormalities

The persistent elevation of blood pressure above 140/90 mm Hg is known as **hypertension**. Hypertension is common, but patients are usually unaware of its existence because no symptoms exist. Hypertension causes a significant increase on the workload of the heart. Extreme elevations in the blood pressure can damage the brain within minutes. Moderate degrees of hypertension can cause damage to the heart, brain, kidneys, lungs, and other organ systems. In addition to various disease states, stress, medications, obesity, and smoking can contribute

to hypertension. The incidence of hypertension is higher in men than in women, and it is more common in African-Americans compared with Caucasians.

Hypotension is defined as low blood pressure and may be identified by a blood pressure of less than 95/60 mm Hg. Low blood pressure is generally desirable and is usually not problematic unless it produces symptoms (e.g., syncope). In other words, in a healthy adult without any accompanying symptoms, hypotension presents no cause for alarm. A hypotensive patient complaining of dizziness, confusion, or blurred vision may have an inadequate circulating blood volume, and further evaluation needs to be initiated immediately. A patient in shock from severe bleeding, burns, vomiting, diarrhea, trauma, or heat exhaustion is hypotensive as a result of a decrease in total blood volume. These persons require immediate care.

OXYGEN THERAPY

The moment-to-moment sustenance of human life depends on a single external substance. This substance is so important that its absence in the environment causes irreversible damage to the brain in approximately 6 minutes. In its absence, production of cellular metabolism is grossly inadequate, and death ultimately occurs. This substance is, of course, oxygen, which is essential to each of the billions of cells making up the human body. Oxygen is a colorless, tasteless, and odorless gas that plays a critical role in efficient cellular metabolism. Although oxygen is not flammable, it does support combustion and constitutes 21% of atmospheric gases.

The need for oxygen becomes critical to patients when the internal environment of the body is not consistent. Normally, the 21% of oxygen supplied in room air maintains homeostasis; however, when oxygenation levels become low, the metabolic rate is compromised, and the patient's homeostasis is altered. Accordingly, the patient's cardiopulmonary system has to adapt to maintain homeostasis caused by **hypoxemia.** Approximately one-third of all patients in acute-care settings receive oxygen therapy of some type. The overall goal of oxygen therapy is to maintain adequate tissue oxygenation while minimizing cardiopulmonary work.

Indications for Oxygen Therapy

The primary clinical indications for oxygen administration are to correct hypoxemia or possible tissue hypoxia and to prevent or minimize the increased cardiopulmonary workload (increased heart rate, blood pressure,

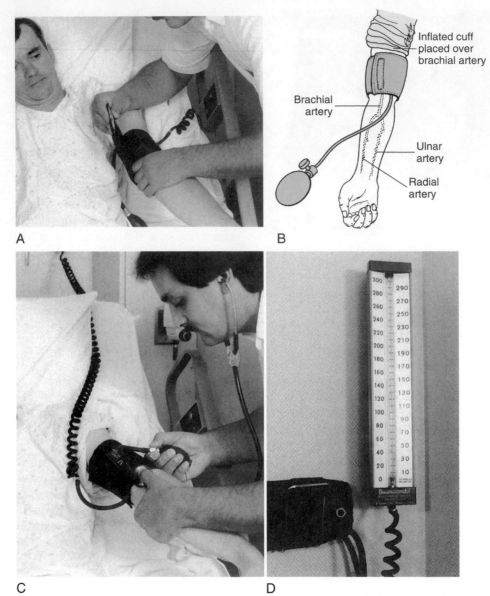

FIG. 15–9 Blood pressure is measured by using a sphygmomanometer and a stethoscope. *A,* The cuff of the sphygmomanometer is placed on the upper arm midway between the elbow and shoulder and then is inflated. *B,* Proper placement of the cuff. *C,* The stethoscope is placed over the brachial artery, the cuff pressure is gradually released, and pulse changes are listened for through the stethoscope. *D,* A Mercury-style sphygmomanometer gauge. (Part *B* from Craig M: *Introduction to ultrasonography and patient care,* Philadelphia, 1992, WB Saunders.)

and respiratory rate). Tissue **hypoxia** is a term used to describe an inadequate amount of oxygen at the cellular (tissue) level. The tissues most sensitive to hypoxia are the brain, heart, lungs, and liver. When hypoxia is present, the metabolic rate of the body is compromised, resulting in altered homeostasis.

To compensate for hypoxia, respiratory rates, depth of breathing, blood pressure, and heart rates increase. A patient with hypoxia feels short of breath and has to work harder to breathe, thereby allowing the body's adaptive response mechanisms to maintain homeostasis. During this event, oxygen therapy is administered to alleviate the cardiopulmonary work. As a result, blood pressure, heart rate, and respiratory rate and depth may return toward normal.

Oxygen as a Drug

Oxygen is listed in the *U.S. Pharmacopeia* and is defined as being a drug in the Federal Food, Drug, and Cosmetic Act of 1962. Similar to any drug, oxygen has both good and bad biologic effects. As such, the minimum dose should always be given to obtain the desired result, and no more. Therefore a physician must prescribe oxygen. In terms of dosage and depending on equipment, oxygen is usually ordered either in liters per minute (LPM) or as a concentration. When a concentration is prescribed, it may be either a percentage, such as 24%, or a fractional concentration of oxygen (FiO_2), such as 0.24. Once the desired result is achieved, the dosage is maintained, and the patient's response is continually monitored.

OXYGEN DEVICES

The radiologic technologist will encounter a variety of devices used to deliver oxygen. Most of these devices in no way hamper the technologist's ability to perform radiologic procedures, although sometimes repositioning the devices is necessary to avoid artifacts on the film. If the oxygen device must be repositioned, the responsibility of the technologist is to ascertain that any tubing leading to the device is not kinked or disconnected and that the device is properly repositioned on the patient at the conclusion of the radiologic procedure. *Under no circumstances should an oxygen device be completely removed from the patient for the purpose of taking a radiograph without the consent or supervision of a physician, respiratory care practitioner, or attending nurse.*

Supplemental oxygen administration for patients requires an oxygen-delivery device, a gas source, and a means by which the two can be connected. Oxygen-delivery devices are designed to operate at a certain LPM. An oxygen flowmeter is a reducing valve that permits flows (LPM) safe for patient use and serves as the connection between the oxygen-delivery device and the gas source. The oxygen flow meter is green in color (or has green labeling) and has the word OXYGEN on it (Fig. 15-10).

In portable oxygen tank operation, including liquid oxygen systems, a regulator attached to the tank consists primarily of a flowmeter and pressure manometer. Although various configurations of flowmeters may be

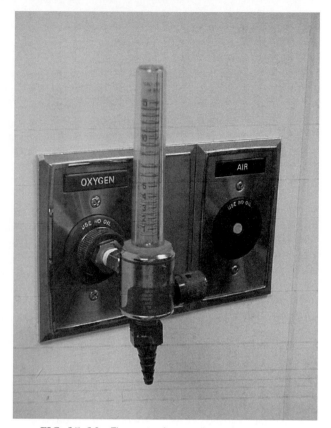

FIG. 15–10 Flowmeter for a wall supply of oxygen.

seen on the regulator, all serve as a means of setting the LPM flow of oxygen required (Fig. 15–11).

Oxygen devices are divided into low-flow and high-flow delivery systems. A low-flow, or *variable-oxygen concentration*, device does not meet the entire inspiratory needs of the patient. An unknown amount of room air is entrained through the nose or mouth of the patient and mixes with the constant amount of 100% oxygen delivered. The precise oxygen concentration or FiO_2 the patient receives is unknown and can vary as the patient's breathing pattern changes. As the patient takes in more air (either by deeper breaths and normal respiratory rate or by normal volume breaths and faster respiratory rates) the oxygen concentration decreases as more room air dilutes the 100% oxygen source. Oxygen concentration increases if the patient takes in less air (either by smaller volume breaths and normal respiratory rate or by normal volume breaths and decreased, slower respiratory rates) because less room air is entrained to dilute the 100% oxygen coming from the flowmeter. Consequently, in the low-flow delivery systems, the percentage of oxygen that

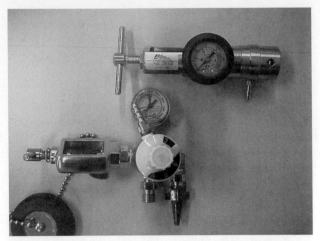

FIG. 15–11   Oxygen tank regulators for small portable (E-size) tanks. Each regulator has a flowmeter (dial and knob styles). Also note the small bore connectors for hooking up oxygen tubing.

piratory rate and has irregularly increasing and decreasing inspiratory volumes, then the high-flow device is designed to mix a known amount of entrained room air with the 100% oxygen supply to produce a consistent concentration of oxygen. The constant ratios used in the mixing of the gases (oxygen and room air) will provide the patient a precise oxygen percentage or FiO_2 regardless of the breathing pattern.

Table 15-2 provides a summation of low-flow and high-flow oxygen therapy systems. The flow rates and FiO_2 ranges described in the table are the generally accepted values; however, patient-specific physician prescription is to be followed.

a patient receives may fluctuate with a change in depth of respiration, respiratory rate, or breathing pattern.

A *high-flow* device, sometimes referred to as a *fixed* or *precise oxygen concentration* device, does meet or exceed the inspiratory needs of the patient. The inspired concentration of oxygen does not change with altered breathing patterns because high-flow systems function on an air-entrainment principle; that is, room air gases are precisely mixed with 100% oxygen before reaching the patient. For example, if a patient exhibits a variable res-

Nasal Cannula

The most common device used to deliver low concentrations of oxygen is the nasal cannula (Fig. 15–12). The nasal cannula delivers oxygen through short prongs inserted into the nares. Because the patient inhales oxygen from the cannula as well as room air, this device is classified as a low-flow device. Usually, oxygen flow rates of 1 to 4 LPM are used, delivering approximately 24% to 36%. Flow rates greater than 6 LPM generally should not be used because high-flow rates can dry out the nasal mucosa and cause severe sinus pain. The nasal cannula is well tolerated by the patient because talking, eating, and sleeping are not hindered. In addition, because oxygen is extremely drying to the respiratory mucosa, humidifiers can be used in combination with the nasal cannula apparatus (Fig. 15–13).

TABLE 15-2 Summary of Oxygen Devices

CATEGORY	DEVICE	LITERS PER MINUTE (LPM)	FiO_2 (%)
Low-flow	Nasal cannula—adult	0.25 to 8	22-45
	Nasal cannula—infant	<2	22-45
	Nasal catheter	0.25 to 8	22-45
	Transtracheal catheter	0.25 to 4	22-35
	Simple mask	5-12	35-50
	Partial rebreathing mask	6-10	35-60
	Nonrebreathing mask	6-10	55-70
High flow	Air-entrainment mask	Varies; should provide >60 LPM	24-50
	Air-entrainment nebulizer	10-15; should provide >60 LPM	24-50
Enclosure	Oxyhood	>7	21-100
	Isolette	8-15	40-50
	Tent	12-15	40-50

Adapted from Scanlan CL, Wilkins RL, Stoller JK: *Egan's fundamentals of respiratory care,* ed 7, St Louis, 1999, Mosby.
FiO_2, Fractional concentration of oxygen.

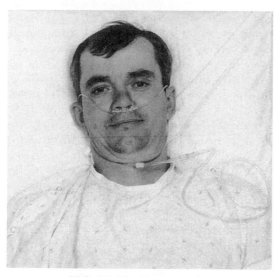

FIG. 15–12 Nasal cannula.

Masks

Various kinds of masks, including simple, nonbreath-ing, partial rebreathing, aerosol, and air-entrainment masks, are used for oxygen therapy. A mask is generally not tolerated as well as a nasal cannula. Masks can be hot, and because they are made of plastic, they tend to stick to the patient's face. Masks need to be removed for eating. They muffle speech, and frequently the head strap does not fit well around the patient's head. Therefore masks often become dislodged during sleep. Masks also increase the risk of aspiration in the patient who vomits. Despite these disadvantages, masks provide an effective way to deliver accurate, as well as high, concentrations of oxygen.

Simple oxygen masks, low-flow devices, cover the patient's nose and mouth (Fig. 15–14). They require oxygen flow rates greater than 6 LPM to prevent an accu-mulation of carbon dioxide. Simple oxygen masks are capable of delivering 35% to 60% oxygen, depending on the oxygen flow rate and the respiratory pattern of the patient. Although not commonly used, simple masks are convenient for short-term oxygen therapy.

A nonrebreathing mask can deliver a higher percent-age of oxygen (Fig. 15–15). These masks have bags attached to them known as *reservoirs* and are filled with oxygen. As disposable units, these nonrebreathing masks are constructed with one-way valves at the opening of the reservoir bag, preventing exhaled air from being rebreathed and ensuring that only oxygen from the device is inhaled. A partial rebreathing mask is similar to a

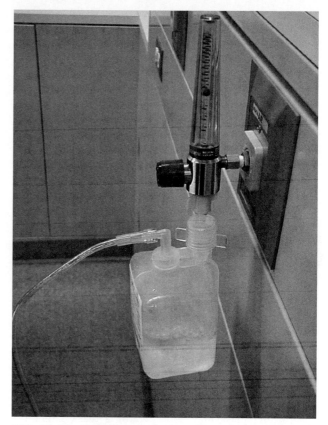

FIG. 15–13 Humidifier attached to a flowmeter in a wall supply of oxygen.

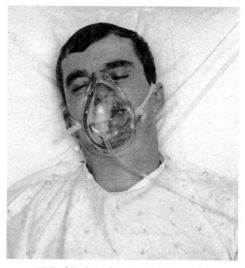

FIG. 15–14 Simple oxygen mask.

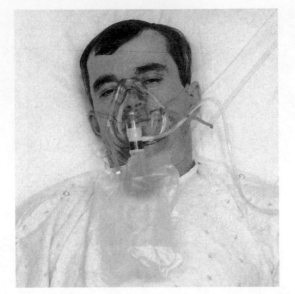

FIG. 15–15 Nonrebreathing mask. (A partial rebreathing mask looks similar to this.)

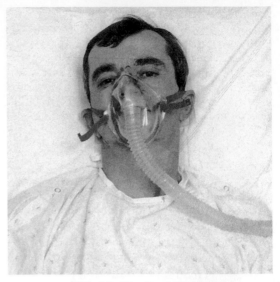

FIG. 15–16 Aerosol mask.

nonrebreathing mask, but it does not contain the valve. Because of the small volume of the reservoir, the partial rebreathing mask and nonrebreathing mask might not necessarily meet the total inspiratory demands of a patient exhibiting variable respiratory rates or variable inspiratory volumes. The masks should always be maintained with a liter flow high enough to keep the reservoir bag inflated. Theoretically, a high liter flow and a tight seal against the face should provide 100% oxygen; however, clinically, these devices may deliver as little as 60% or as much as 90% oxygen, depending on how tightly the mask is affixed to the face.

Aerosol masks are commonly used when both high oxygen concentrations and humidity are needed (Fig. 15–16). Because therapeutic gases are extremely drying to the respiratory mucosa, to provide humidification, the mask is attached, through corrugated tubing, to a *nebulizer* containing normal saline solution (Fig. 15–17). To prevent carbon dioxide accumulation under the mask, the oxygen flow should be adjusted to a minimum of 6 LPM. Aerosol masks can deliver oxygen concentration values of 21% to 100%. The aerosol device can be adapted to fit face masks, tracheostomy collars, or patients with endotracheal tubes.

The air-entrainment mask, a high-flow device, is constructed to provide an accurate concentration of oxygen to the patient by propelling a high velocity of source oxygen through a narrowed opening near the mask

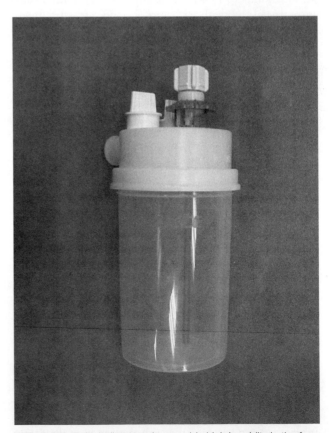

FIG. 15–17 Nebulizer used to provide high humidity in the form of a mist.

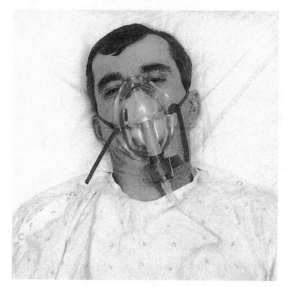

FIG. 15–18 Air-entrainment mask.

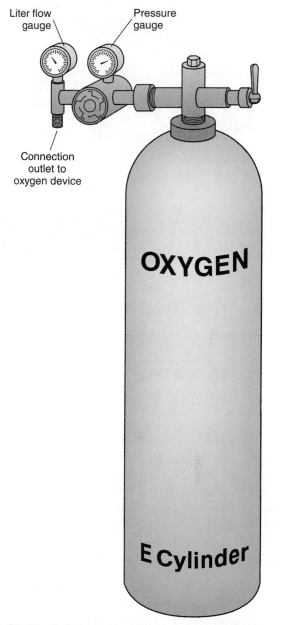

FIG. 15–19 Typical portable oxygen cylinder-small size (E-tank).

(Fig. 15–18). This method results in room air being drawn into the mask. The source oxygen, along with the entrained room air, provides a flow of gas that is capable of meeting the total need of the inspiratory capacity of the patient. Therefore, the set liter flow must not be altered for the purpose of maintaining accurate oxygen concentrations. Air-entrainment masks provide consistent concentrations of oxygen, even though the patient's respiratory pattern may change. Depending on the manufacturer, air-entrainment masks generally can provide consistent oxygen concentration values at 24%, 28%, 35%, 40%, and 50%.

In the patient's hospital room, these oxygen devices are usually attached to a wall outlet through which oxygen is piped; however, a patient who requires oxygen must often be transported to the radiographic examination room. This task is accomplished by attaching the tubing from the oxygen device to a portable oxygen cylinder that has two regulator valves (Fig. 15–19). One of the valves reads the pressure and indicates how full the cylinder is, and the other valve indicates the rate of oxygen flow, in liters, to the patient. Although oxygen cylinders and regulators are extremely durable, they should be secured during transport and used to prevent them from falling and possibly developing cracks or leaks.

Tent and Oxyhood

Pediatric patients requiring oxygen therapy and additional humidity can be placed either in oxygen tents or in oxyhoods. An oxygen tent covers the child's bed. Con-

trolling the oxygen concentration is difficult in a tent because the frequent openings necessary for childcare allow oxygen to escape. Because oxygen supports combustion, care should be exercised, and machines that are likely to produce sparks should not be used in the vicinity of oxygen tents or free-flowing oxygen. Therefore the technologist is responsible for ascertaining that the mobile x-ray unit is safe for use in combustible situations.

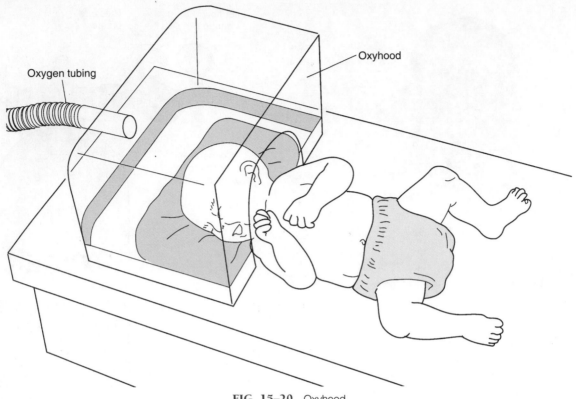

Oxygen tubing

Oxyhood

FIG. 15–20 Oxyhood.

Oxyhoods are generally used on infants. The oxyhood consists of a disposable or permanent plastic box that fits over the infant's head (Fig. 15–20). Oxygen concentrations between 21% and 100% can be delivered in an oxyhood.

Ventilators

When the cardiopulmonary system of a patient is unable to supply adequate oxygen to the tissues, a patient may have an artificial airway inserted into the trachea, which is then connected to a mechanical ventilator (Fig. 15–21). The ventilator delivers a minimum set respiratory rate, preset inspiratory volume, and consistent FiO_2. A radiograph of the patient's chest is frequently required to determine whether the artificial airway is in the proper place (Fig. 15–22). The attending nurse or respiratory care practitioner must be informed before the initiation of any radiologic procedure because care must be taken not to dislodge the artificial airway when positioning the patient or when adjusting the ventilator tubing. The radiographer must also be aware that proper head position is critical because flexing or extending the head can adversely influence artificial airway placement, particularly in neonatal patients.

If a mobile procedure is to be performed on a mechanically ventilated patient, the radiographer must carefully observe the rise and fall of the patient's chest to determine full inspiration or full expiration.

Audio and visual alarms on the ventilator monitor the patient's response. Occasionally, the alarms sound when the patient is repositioned. *These alarms should not be silenced or altered on the ventilator.* The nursing staff or respiratory care practitioners should assist the technologist in positioning the patient, thereby preventing accidental disconnection and patient endangerment.

CHEST TUBES AND LINES*

Provided they are well informed, radiographers can play an important role in the early detection of problems associated with malpositioned lines. As experts in radiographic quality, radiographers have a clear responsibility

---

*This section is extracted from Moore DE: ET, CV, VAD, PA, Swan: What's it all about? *Semin Radiol Technol* 5(2):49, 1997.

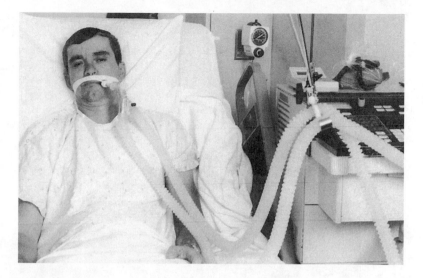

FIG. 15–21 Mechanical ventilator.

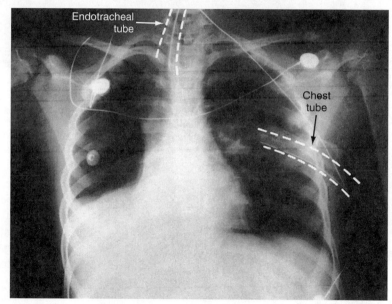

FIG. 15–22 Chest radiograph of an 8-year-old girl demonstrating a properly placed endotracheal tube and a chest (thoracostomy) tube.

in this area that is separate from the issue of interpretation of images. Without any expectation of the radiographer to interpret the image from a pathologic diagnostic standpoint, when malpositioning is thought to occur, alerting the appropriate authority (e.g., radiologist, attending physician) is both appropriate and beneficial to the patient.

Endotracheal Tubes

Endotracheal tubes are used to manage a variety of respiratory complications (Fig. 15–23). Indications for use include (1) a need for mechanical ventilation or oxygen delivery because of inadequate ventilation (breathing), inadequate arterial oxygenation, severe airway obstruction, shock, and parenchymal diseases that impair gas exchange; (2) upper-airway obstruction; (3) impending gastric acid reflux or aspiration; and (4) provisions for tracheobronchial toilet (lavage).

Tracheal **intubation** is accomplished most often using a translaryngeal approach via the mouth or nose, but in certain cases, the use of a tracheostomy is necessary (Fig. 15–24). The nasal tracheal approach is preferred except during emergency situations or when anesthesia is

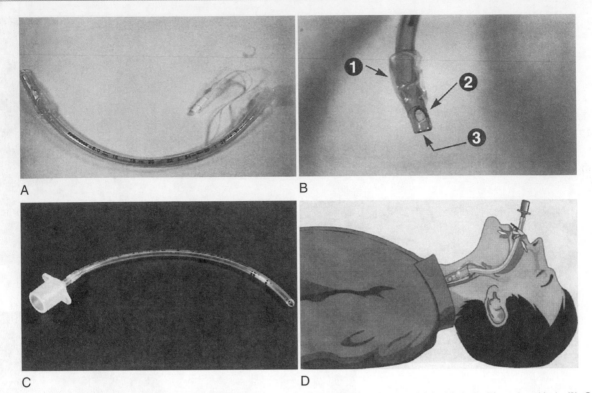

FIG. 15–23 *A,* Adult endotracheal tube. *B,* Distal end of endotracheal tube with cuff deflated *(1);* side hole *(2);* and end hole *(3). C,* Pediatric endotracheal tube; note the absence of cuff. *D,* Patient intubated with an endotracheal tube. (From Moore DE: ET, CV, VAD, PA, Swan: What's it all about? *Semin Radiol Technol* 5[2]:49, 1997. Part *D* originally from LifeART Collection Images, copyright ©1989-1997 by TechPool Studios, Inc., Cleveland, Ohio.)

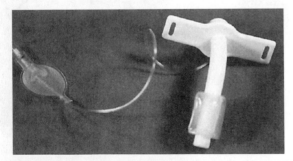

FIG. 15–24 Tracheostomy tube. (From Moore DE: ET, CV, VAD, PA, Swan: What's it all about? *Semin Radiol Technol* 5[2]:49, 1997.)

administered. Historically, cuff structure and its pressure often damaged the tracheal mucosa, especially during long-term care; thus, in extended-care settings, tracheostomies were often substituted. Today, endotracheal cuffs are softer and exert lower pressure on tracheal tissues and as such are more compatible with long-term use.

Once an endotracheal tube is inserted, placement of the tube is confirmed by chest radiography and is assessed periodically thereafter. Properly positioned tubes will show the distal tip 1 to 2 inches (3 to 5 cm) superior to the tracheal bifurcation (Fig. 15–25). The cuff is inflated with air and is positioned at midtrachea; however, the cuff is not radiographically apparent. The most common example of malpositioning involves intubation of the right main-stem bronchus because it originates at the trachea at a lesser angle compared with the left main bronchus. Complications may include overventilation of the right lung and potential airway obstruction of the left. When the tip of the tube slides into the right main bronchus, its shaft may occlude the left main bronchus, causing severe **atelectasis** of the left lung (Fig. 15–26).

Occasionally, endobronchial tubes are used to provide ventilation to one lung, as in the case of pneumonectomy, or to use two mechanical ventilators, one for each lung. Endobronchial tubes are designed so that the tip is inserted in one of the main-stem bronchi. In such cases, the tip will be located in either the right or the left system.

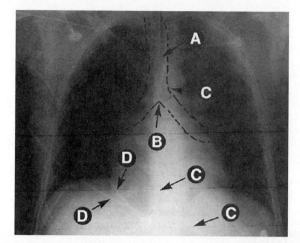

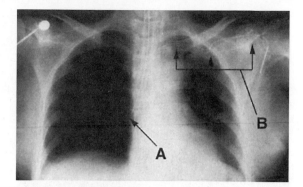

FIG. 15–25 Anteroposterior mobile chest projection showing trachea *(dotted line)* with endotracheal tube *(A)* positioned approximately 2 inches superior to the carina *(B)*; nasogastric tube *(C)*; cardiac monitor leads/electrodes *(D)*. (From Moore DE: ET, CV, VAD, PA, Swan: What's it all about? *Semin Radiol Technol* 5[2]:49, 1997.)

FIG. 15–27 Distal tip of endotracheal tube in right main bronchus *(A)*; central venous catheter in the left subclavian vein *(B)*. (From Moore DE: ET, CV, VAD, PA, Swan: What's it all about? *Semin Radiol Technol* 5[2]:49, 1997.)

1. Bronchial intubation, most often involving the right main-stem bronchus (Fig. 15–27)
2. Intubation not far enough so that cuff inflation damages vocal folds and inadequately provides ventilation
3. Erosion of the tracheal mucosa as a result of cuff trauma causing subcutaneous or mediastinal emphysema
4. Pneumothorax

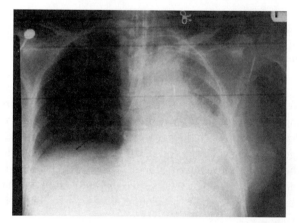

FIG. 15–26 Intubation of right main-stem bronchus with complete occlusion of the left bronchus causing left lung atelectasis. (From Moore DE: ET, CV, VAD, PA, Swan: What's it all about? *Semin Radiol Technol* 5[2]:49, 1997.)

Thoracostomy Tubes

Thoracostomy (intrapleural) tubes, more commonly called *chest tubes* (Fig. 15–28), are used to drain the intrapleural space and the mediastinum (Fig. 15–29). Fluid or air accumulation, or both, in either space will have deleterious effects and may be life threatening, depending on volume.

The pleural cavity is a potential space where parietal and visceral pleurae meet. A minimal amount of serous fluid exists to provide a lubricant for ease of movement between the two pleural layers during breathing. Negative pressure in the intrapleural space provides a suction-type mechanism between the lung and thorax that facilitates lung expansion. When fluids or air accumulate in the space, negative pressure is lowered or lost, and the lung fails to fully expand. If pressure falls too low, then the lung will collapse.

Thoracostomy tubes are inserted through the chest wall to reestablish negative intrapleural pressure in cases of **pneumothorax**, hemothorax, **pleural effusion**, and empyema. In addition to chest tubes, mediastinal drains (usually small chest tubes) are used after cardiac surgery

Once inserted properly, two cuffs are inflated to anchor the endobronchial tube in position, one at the bronchial end and one in the trachea. When dual ventilation is used, a side hole in the endobronchial tube is positioned adjacent to the nonintubated bronchus to facilitate ventilation to the contralateral lung.

Radiographic demonstration of complications associated with tracheal intubation and mechanical ventilation includes the following:

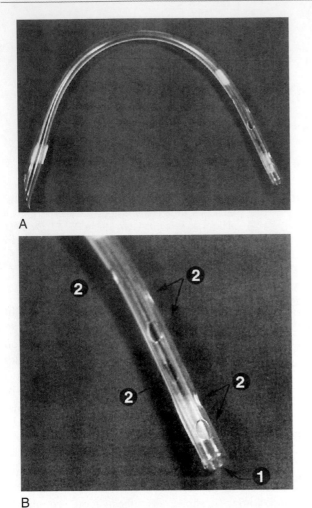

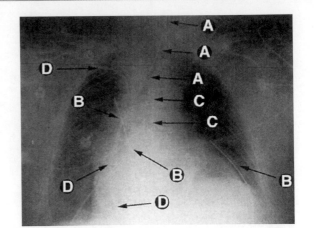

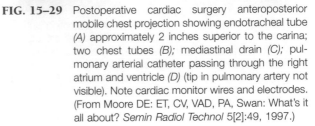

FIG. 15–29 Postoperative cardiac surgery anteroposterior mobile chest projection showing endotracheal tube *(A)* approximately 2 inches superior to the carina; two chest tubes *(B)*; mediastinal drain *(C)*; pulmonary arterial catheter passing through the right atrium and ventricle *(D)* (tip in pulmonary artery not visible). Note cardiac monitor wires and electrodes. (From Moore DE: ET, CV, VAD, PA, Swan: What's it all about? *Semin Radiol Technol* 5[2]:49, 1997.)

FIG. 15–28 *A,* Thoracostomy tube. *B,* Thoracostomy tube: end hole *(1)* and side holes *(2)*. (From Moore DE: ET, CV, VAD, PA, Swan: What's it all about? *Semin Radiol Technol* 5[2]:49, 1997.)

to drain residual blood from the mediastinum. Postoperative blood accumulation around the pericardium can cause cardiac tamponade, which is a life-threatening event.

Insertion sites for thoracostomy vary with the intrapleural substances to be removed. In the case of hemothorax and pleural effusions, fluids flow with gravity and tend to accumulate near the lung base. Typical insertion sites in these instances are the fifth to sixth intercostal spaces and laterally at the midaxillary line. Tubes also can be inserted as high as the fourth and as low as the eighth rib. In cases of pneumothoraces, air will rise to the upper pleural spaces, requiring higher insertion sites in the apical region. Generally, the second

to third intercostal space at the midclavicular line is preferred.

Pleural fluid accumulation becomes apparent radiographically when enough fluid is present to show costophrenic blunting. Once radiographically apparent, the angles typically show medial displacement. Costophrenic fluids may approach 300 ml or more before becoming radiographically evident on posteroanterior or anteroposterior chest projections, but as little as 150 ml of fluid may be visible on lateral decubitus views. Supine filming may obscure visualization of pleural fluids and should be avoided when possible.

Causes of pneumothorax include a break in the continuity of the visceral pleura (rupture of an emphysematous bleb, fractured rib, central venous line insertion error), penetration of the external chest wall seen in trauma, or in rare instances a gas-producing microorganism *(empyema)*. When air accumulates in the intrapleural space, creating a loss of negative pressure, the lungs cannot fully expand, creating a space between the lung edge and the costal border.

Radiographically, pneumothoraces are shown when the increased density of the collapsed lung is contrasted with a lateral radiolucency that is absent of lung markings (Fig. 15–30). During inspiration, the lung expands laterally and meets the lateral rib edge, rendering small pneumothoraces that are difficult to detect. Therefore pneumothoraces are best shown by expiratory posteroanterior or anteroposterior projections of the chest. Lateral decubitus filming with the ipsilateral side up may also be useful.

After thoracostomy, sutures are applied to anchor the tube so that patients can move with caution. Radiographic studies require erect or semi-erect filming whenever possible, and care must be exercised to avoid dislodging the tube. Partially dislodged tubes, leaks at the insertion site, and extracostal insertions may lead to subcutaneous emphysema (see Fig. 15–30).

Various degrees of pneumothoraces exist. Small pneumothoraces are typically classified as *simple* and *spontaneous,* usually caused by a ruptured bleb, and may resorb naturally. *Secondary* pneumothoraces are complications of parenchymal disease, or they may be caused iatrogenically during central venous catheter insertion. Because of coexisting conditions and the fact that these patients are already in a compromised state, secondary pneumothoraces require chest tube evacuation of the pleural cavity.

Tension pneumothorax is a dramatic event that requires aggressive care. In these cases, air continues to enter the pleural cavity through either a valvelike opening in the external chest wall (trauma) or a similar opening in the visceral pleura whereby air continues to enter the pleural space but cannot escape. Pressure increases on the ipsilateral side, causing a shift of the mediastinum toward the opposite side and producing a life-threatening event.

Tension pneumothorax may occur during mechanical ventilation. Rupture of the visceral pleura allows air to enter the pleural space without escape. Immediate aspiration of the intrapleural air relieves pressures and is standard treatment for tension pneumothorax.

Central Venous Lines

Central venous (CV) lines are catheters that are inserted into a large vein. They have a multitude of uses and descriptive terms. Initially, CV lines were developed to administer chemotherapeutic drugs and parenteral nutrition. Today, they may also be used to administer a variety of drugs, manage fluid volume, serve as a conduit for blood analysis and transfusions, and monitor cardiac pressures.

Known commonly as *central venous catheters* and *venous access devices,* the developer also names venous lines. One of the first modern CV lines was developed by Broviac and later enlarged by Hickman. Leonard and Groshong catheters are also widely used. Groshong catheters have a unique rounded, closed-end tip with a

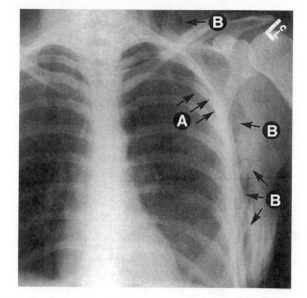

FIG. 15–30 An expiratory, anteroposterior projection showing an approximate 10% pneumothorax on the left *(A);* also note moderate subcutaneous emphysema in the left chest wall extending up to the neck *(B).* (From Moore DE: ET, CV, VAD, PA, Swan: What's it all about? *Semin Radiol Technol* 5[2]:49, 1997.)

three-way valve mechanism that reduces the risk of blood loss and air embolism during withdrawals and infusions.

Catheters generally vary by size and composition and are available in single, double, and multiple lumens for short- and long-term care use. They are available as percutaneous catheters (subclavian insertion catheter), totally implanted access ports (Infusa Port, Port-a-Cath, Mediport), peripherally inserted central catheters (PICCs) (Fig. 15–31), and externally tunneled catheters (Broviac, Hickman, Groshong) (Fig. 15–32). In cases of chronic illness, implantable ports are desired when access is required intermittently over a long period; however, PICC insertion into the basilic or cephalic veins near the antecubital area also allows for long-term intravenous treatments especially for patients receiving intravenous therapy home care.

Regardless of the style used, the goal is to position the catheter tip in a central vein. The preferred location is the superior vena cava, approximately 2 to 3 cm above the right atrial junction (Fig. 15–33). Superior vena caval placement is preferred because of its size. Infusions of intravenous fluids are much less caustic in central veins than in smaller, peripheral veins.

The most common insertion site for central venous catheters is the subclavian vein (see Fig. 15–33, *A*). Other

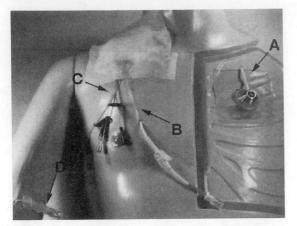

FIG. 15–31 Various central venous catheters inserted in a model. Subcutaneously implanted port *(A)*; tunneled catheter into subclavian vein *(B)*; triple-lumen subclavian line *(C)*; peripheral catheter in the antecubital area *(D)*. (From Moore DE: ET, CV, VAD, PA, Swan: What's it all about? *Semin Radiol Technol* 5[2]:49, 1997.)

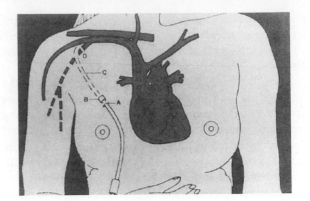

FIG. 15–32 Tunneled catheter. Subcutaneous insertion site *(A)*; catheter cuff *(B)*; subcutaneous tunnel *(C)*; subclavian insertion site *(D)*. (From Infuse-a-Cath: *Central venous catheter nursing manual*, Beverly, Mass, 1992, Strato Medical Corp.)

common sites include the internal jugular (see Fig. 15–33, *D*) and femoral veins. Recent technologic advancements in catheters and safer insertion techniques now provide the opportunity to access the subclavian vein from a peripheral approach. When percutaneous subclavian and internal jugular approaches are contraindicated, the antecubital area may be accessed for line insertion, as is the case with PICC line insertions. Ports used in conjunction with peripherally inserted central catheters are smaller than those used in a subcutaneous pocket in the thorax but functionally are identical.

Pulmonary arterial (PA) lines are commonly called Swan-Ganz catheters, so named for the developers of the catheter. PA lines are specialized, single, or multilumen CV lines that incorporate a small electrode at the distal end used to monitor pulmonary arterial pressures (Fig. 15–34).

Pulmonary arterial lines are used to estimate left ventricular end-diastolic pressure. Access to the left ventricle requires an arterial approach. Because catheter placement in the left ventricle has major physiologic consequences, the safest way to assess left heart pressure is to extrapolate its value by monitoring right-sided heart and pulmonary pressures. Cardiopulmonary circulation is a continuous network of vascular structures interconnected by valves. Some valves are open, whereas others are simultaneously closed. When atrioventricular valves (tricuspid and bicuspid) are open, semilunar valves (pul-

monary and aortic) are closed; when the semilunar valves open, the atrioventricular valves close.

Pulmonary arterial catheters have a balloon located at the distal end. During pressure monitoring, this balloon is inflated, allowing the catheter tip to float and wedge in a small pulmonary artery. During this interval, the electrode, at the most distal end of the catheter, measures pulmonary arterial (wedged capillary) pressures. PA-wedged pressure is indicative of left atrial pressure, which, in turn, is indicative of left ventricular pressure. PA lines are routinely used to monitor discretely or continuously venous oxygenation.

Other than PA lines, no central catheter should appear beyond the superior vena cava. In the case of PA lines, the distal tip will locate in one of the two pulmonary arteries (Fig. 15–35). During pressure recordings, the balloon floats and wedges in a small arterial branch. Balloon wedging is synchronized with the cardiac monitor and lasts momentarily to avoid potential ischemia and infarction of the lung. The cardiac monitor generates pressure tracings during the wedge procedure. Once the measurement is complete, the balloon is deflated, and blood flow beyond the catheter tip is resumed (Fig. 15–36).

Central venous access devices can improve and extend quality of life for many patients, but the potential for complications demands the attention of all members of the health care team. Reported incidence of CV complications varies, but that related to the management of CV lines by health care workers is significant. Examples of complications include catheter dislodgment and occlusions resulting from the accumulation of blood clots or

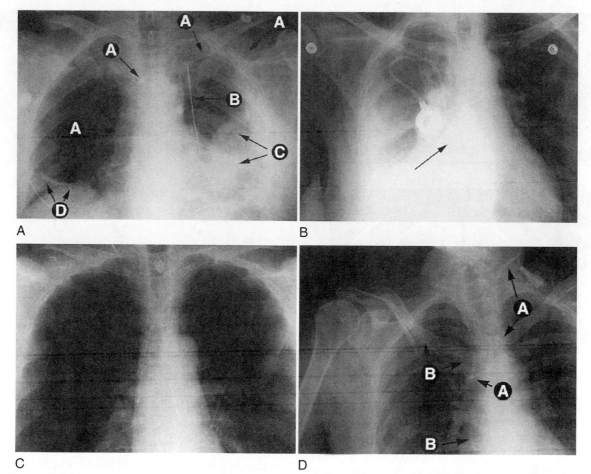

FIG. 15–33 *A,* Anteroposterior projection of the chest shows a subclavian catheter inserted from the left side and advanced to the superior vena cava *(A);* a thoracostomy tube *(B)* with moderate pleural infiltration in the left lung *(C)* and some atelectasis noted in the right lung base *(D). B,* Implanted central venous port with its tip in the superior vena cava. The catheter does not cross midline when advanced from the right side. *C,* Groshong catheter subcutaneously tunneled into the left subclavian vein and advanced to the superior vena cava. *D,* Two central venous catheters are seen. A catheter is inserted into the internal jugular vein with its tip positioned in the proximal portion of the superior vena cava *(A).* A tunneled catheter is inserted from the right subclavian vein with its tip positioned lower in the superior vena cava *(B).* (From Moore DE: ET, CV, VAD, PA, Swan: What's it all about? *Semin Radiol Technol* 5[2]:49, 1997.)

drug precipitates. Catheter flushing procedures conducted by nursing staff help prevent occlusive problems. One of the most critical concerns of radiographers is catheter dislodgment, which can be prevented only with increased awareness of the catheter's presence. Care must be exercised when handling patients with CV lines. Assessing the patient before performing radiographic procedures is essential to avert the possibility of line displacement (Fig. 15–37).

Regarding insertion problems, Eisenburg estimates that up to one third of CV catheters are placed incorrectly at insertion time. Malpositioning, pinching, or kinking also occur with significant frequency. Pneumothorax and hemothorax are potential complications associated with catheter insertions (Fig. 15–38).

Radiographic confirmation of line placement is essential at the time of insertion and thereafter as needed. Aberrant tip location is one of the most common complications associated with CV catheters. Additional medical imaging modalities also may prove useful when catheter placement is difficult or complications occur. For example, complications involving catheter fracture and subsequent migration can be resolved using angiography and fluoroscopy.

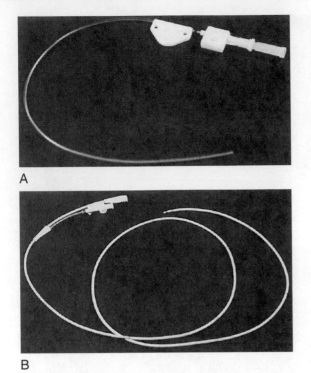

A

B

FIG. 15–34 *A,* Single-lumen central venous catheter. *B,* Single-lumen pulmonary arterial catheter. Note the distal tip with a deflated balloon and electrode. During pressure measurement, the balloon is inflated, drifting the catheter into a small pulmonary artery, where it wedges. The electrode at the tip of the catheter measures pulmonary pressure. (From Moore DE: ET, CV, VAD, PA, Swan: What's it all about? *Semin Radiol Technol* 5[2]:49, 1997.)

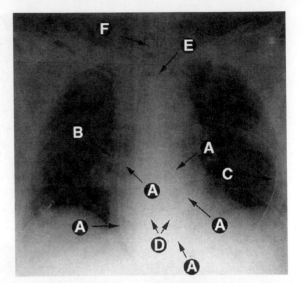

FIG. 15–35 Postoperative anteroposterior chest projection showing several lines: pulmonary arterial catheter with the tip in the right pulmonary artery *(A);* a second central venous line seen in the superior vena cava *(B);* thoracostomy tube in the right lung *(C);* mediastinal drains *(D);* nasogastric tube in the esophagus *(E);* and endotracheal tube *(F).* (From Moore DE: ET, CV, VAD, PA, Swan: What's it all about? *Semin Radiol Technol* 5[2]:49, 1997.)

Recognition of catheter malposition requires thorough knowledge of CV structures and their branches. Typically, CV lines inserted from a right-sided approach will follow the course of the subclavian vein in a lateromedial direction and then descend through the right brachiocephalic vein. From the right brachiocephalic vein, the catheter passes into the superior vena cava, where it should terminate above the right atrium. Because of the right-sided position of the superior vena cava, as the catheter advances, its image should remain to the right of the vertebral column and should not cross midline (see Fig. 15–33, *B*).

A left-sided approach involves a slightly longer catheter that is advanced lateromedially through the left subclavian vein to the left brachiocephalic vein. Because the left brachiocephalic vein courses in a relatively horizontal fashion as it crosses to the right of midline (see Fig. 15–33, *C*), the catheter will traverse from left to right,

where it terminates in the superior vena cava with a short descending pattern. One problem associated with a left-sided approach is placement of the catheter tip in the thoracic duct. In this instance, the catheter does not cross midline. Checking for catheter position in orientation to the midline can be a simple way to assess catheter position; right-sided approaches never cross midline, whereas a left-sided approach should always cross midline.

Although recognition of problems related to tubes and line use is not specifically identified in the radiographer's scope of practice, an implied responsibility certainly exists. As techniques for patient care become more sophisticated, and as the team concept of health care management takes greater hold, practicing radiographers must direct attention to expanded learning opportunities to maintain clinical competency. In this regard, radiography remains a vital component of the health care team, and improved patient care will result.

SUMMARY

Vital signs represent the primary mechanisms that maintain homeostasis. These mechanisms can adapt to changes inside or outside of the body to maintain home-

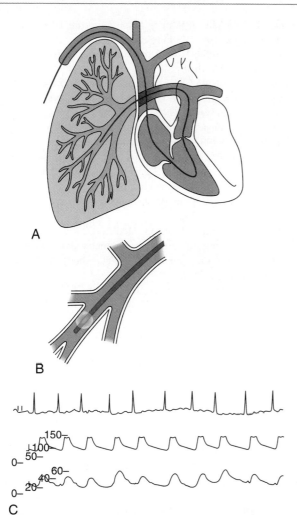

A

B

C

FIG. 15–36 *A,* Pulmonary artery catheter passes through right atrium, right ventricle, and main pulmonary artery into right pulmonary artery. *B,* Balloon of a pulmonary artery catheter inflated and wedged in a small pulmonary branch for wedge pressure measurement. *C,* Pulmonary artery pressure tracing. (From Moore DE: ET, CV, VAD, PA, Swan: What's it all about? *Semin Radiol Technol* 5[2]:49, 1997. *A* and *B* originally from LifeART Collection Images, copyright ©1989-1997 by TechPool Studios, Inc., Cleveland, Ohio.)

FIG. 15–37 Right hydrothorax caused by displacement of a central venous line during dressing change; 1300 ml of intravenous fluids were evacuated via thoracentesis. (From Moore DE: ET, CV, VAD, PA, Swan: What's it all about? *Semin Radiol Technol* 5[2]:49, 1997.)

ostasis. Therefore the vital functions provide a relative constancy in the internal environment of the body to promote healthy survival. Assessment of vital signs is an objective. noninvasive evaluation of the patient's immediate condition or response to therapy. Every health care professional should be competent in obtaining vital signs and understanding the significance of any abnormalities. Because the primary mechanisms that maintain home-

ostasis are represented by vital signs, accuracy in obtaining and recording the data is crucial.

The need for oxygen becomes critical to patients when the internal environment of the body is not consistent. Normally, room air gases containing 21% of oxygen is sufficient to maintain homeostasis; however, when vital signs are abnormal, supplemental oxygen therapy is necessary. Supplemental oxygen therapy relieves the increased stress on the cardiopulmonary system.

Oxygen therapy can be administered by high-flow devices, such as air-entrainment masks, which deliver consistent concentrations of oxygen and supply entire inspiratory volumes as required by the patient. Low-flow devices, such as nasal cannulas, simple masks, aerosol masks, and partial rebreathing and nonrebreathing masks, can also deliver oxygen therapy. Because of the variance of the patient's respiratory rate or change in breathing pattern, these devices provide neither consistent concentrations of oxygen nor the entire inspiratory volumes required by the patient.

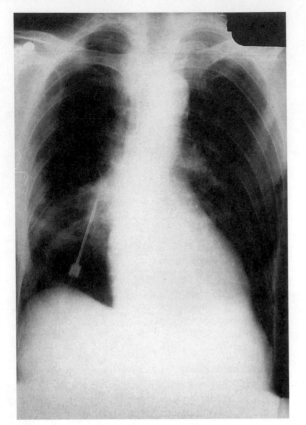

FIG. 15–38 Pneumothorax on the right resulting from complications associated with central venous line insertion. Note a small angiographic catheter inserted to evacuate the pleural cavity and the oxygen tube across the lower field creating an artifactual distraction. (From Moore DE: ET, CV, VAD, PA, Swan: What's it all about? *Semin Radiol Technol* 5[2]:49, 1997.)

Oxygen tents and oxyhoods are used to deliver oxygen to children requiring supplemental oxygen or humidity.

Patients on ventilators require special care in handling, and the radiographic technologist must never alter ventilator alarms and settings.

Radiographers must understand the use and radiographic appearance of common chest tubes and lines, including endotracheal tubes, thoracostomy tubes, and central venous lines.

BIBLIOGRAPHY

Bard Access Systems: *Groshong catheters,* Salt Lake City, Utah, 1993, Bard Access Systems.

Burton GC, Hodgkin J, Ward J: *Respiratory care,* ed 4, Philadelphia, 1997, JB Lippincott.

Cairo JM, Pilbeam SP: *Mosby's respiratory care equipment,* ed 7, St Louis, 2003, Mosby.

Carrasco C, Richli W, Charnsangave C, et al: Technical note: repositioning misplaced central venous catheters, *Cardiovasc Intervent Radiol* 10:234, 1987.

Des Jardins: *Cardiopulmonary anatomy and physiology,* ed 3, Albany, NY, 1998, Thomson Delmar Learning.

Eisenburg R: Fluid, electrolyte, and nutritional management of the surgical patient. In *Diagnostic imaging in surgery,* New York, 1987, McGraw Hill, p 1.

Erickson R: Mastering the ins and outs of chest drainage, *Nursing* 89:37, 1989.

Exergen Corp. Medical Division, Medical Education Center: Technology, temporal artery thermometry. Available at: *http://www.exergen.com/medical/eductr/technology.htm.* Accessed August 3, 2005.

Ferguson D: Cardiogenic shock. In Bennett C, Plum F, eds: *Cecil textbook of medicine,* Philadelphia, 1996, WB Saunders.

Freedman S, Bosserman G: Tunneled catheters: technological advancements and nursing care issues, *Nurs Clin North Am* 28:851, 1993.

Heckman JD, Crosby L, Lewallen D: *Emergency care and transportation of the sick and injured,* ed 6, Chicago, 1995, American Academy of Orthopaedic Surgeons.

Infuse-a-Cath: *Central venous catheter nursing manual,* Beverly, Mass, 1992, Strato Medical Corp.

Kacmarek RM, Mack C, Dimas S: *The essentials of respiratory care,* ed 3, St Louis, 1990, Mosby–Year Book.

Kozier B, Erb G, Berman A, et al: *Fundamentals of nursing,* ed 7, Upper Saddle River, NJ, 2004, Pearson Education.

Levitzky MG, Cairo J, Hall S: *Introduction to respiratory care,* Philadelphia, 1990, WB Saunders.

LifeART: *CD-ROM Collections,* Cleveland, Ohio, 1994, TechPool Studios Corp.

Potter PA, Perry AG: *Basic nursing theory and practice,* ed 2, St Louis, 1991, Mosby–Year Book.

Recht M, Burke D, Meranze S, et al: Simple technique for redirecting malpositioned central venous catheters, *AJR Am J Roentgenol* 154:183, 1990.

Scanlan CL, Wilkins RL, Stoller JK: *Egan's fundamentals of respiratory care,* ed 7, St Louis, 1999, Mosby.

Scott W: Complications associated with central venous catheters, *Chest* 94:1221, 1988.

Shapiro BA, Kacmarek R, Cane R, et al: *Clinical application of respiratory care,* ed 4, St Louis, 1991, Mosby–Year Book.

Sheldon R: Clinical application of the chest radiograph. In Wilkins R, Krider S, Sheldon R, eds: *Clinical assessment in respiratory care,* St Louis, 1995, Mosby.

Summerell N: Chest traumas: Causes of impaired gas exchange. In *Nurse review: a clinical update system, vol 2,* Springhouse, Pa, 1989, Springhouse Group.

16

Infection Control

Jody L. Ellis, MMS, PA-C, RT(R)

What man does not avoid contact with the sick, fearing lest he contract a disease so near?

Ovid, 43 BC to AD 17

OBJECTIVES

On completion of this chapter, the student will be able to:

1. Define the terminology related to infection control.

2. Categorize the four basic infectious agents along with their unique characteristics.

3. Explain the steps involved in the establishment of an infectious disease.

4. Discuss the four factors involved in the spread of disease and the chain of infection.

5. Describe the various sources of nosocomial infection.

6. Explain the constituents of microbial control within the host.

OBJECTIVES—Cont'd

7. Contrast medical and surgical asepsis.

8. List the chemical and physical methods of asepsis.

9. Demonstrate the medically aseptic handwashing technique.

10. Describe the basic premises of standard precautions.

11. Relate types of transmission-based precautions with appropriate clinical situations.

12. Demonstrate the contact precautions technique.

GLOSSARY

Asepsis: freedom from infection

Bacteria: in former systems of classification, a division of the kingdom Procaryotae, including all procaryotic organisms, except the blue-green

Blood-borne Pathogens: disease-causing microorganisms that may be present in human blood

Chemotherapy: treatment of disease by chemical agents

Cyst: stage in the life cycle of certain parasites during which they are enclosed in a protective wall

Dimorphic: occurring in two distinct forms

Disease: any deviation from or interruption of the normal structure or function of any part, organ, or system (or combination thereof) of the body that is exhibited by a characteristic set of symptoms and signs and whose cause, pathologic mechanism, and prognosis may be known or unknown

Disinfectant: chemicals used to free an environment from pathogenic organisms or to render such organisms inert, especially as applied to the treatment of inanimate materials to reduce or eliminate infectious organisms

Eucaryotes: organisms whose cells have a true nucleus

Flora: microbial community found on or in a healthy person

Fomite: object, such as a book, wooden object, or article of clothing, that is not in itself harmful but is able to harbor pathogenic microorganisms and thus may serve as an agent of transmission of an infection

Fungi: general term used to denote a group of eucaryotic protists—including mushrooms, yeasts, rusts, molds, and smuts—that are characterized by the absence of chlorophyll and by the presence of a rigid cell wall

Host: animal or plant that harbors or nourishes another organism

Iatrogenic: resulting from the activities of physicians

Immunity: security against a particular disease

Infection: invasion and multiplication of microorganisms in body tissues that may be clinically inapparent or result in local cellular injury as a result of competitive metabolism, toxins, intracellular replication, or antigen-antibody response

Medical Asepsis: reduction in numbers of infectious agents, which, in turn, decreases the probability of infection but does not necessarily reduce it to zero

Microorganism: microscopic organism; those of medical interest include bacteria, viruses, fungi, and protozoa

Nosocomial: pertaining to or originating in the hospital; said of an infection not present or incubating before admittance to the hospital but generally occurring 72 hours after admittance

Pathogen: any disease-producing microorganism

Procaryotes: cellular organisms that lack a true nucleus

Protozoa: a subkingdom comprising the simplest organisms of the animal kingdom, consisting of unicellular organisms that range in size from submicroscopic to macroscopic; most are free living, but some lead commensalistic, mutualistic, or parasitic existences

Reservoir: alternate or passive host or carrier that harbors pathogenic organisms, without injury to itself, and serves as a source from which other individuals can be infected

Standard Precautions: precautions to prevent the transmission of disease by body fluids and substances

Sterilization: complete destruction or elimination of all living microorganisms, accomplished by physical methods (dry or moist heat), chemical agents (ethylene oxide, formaldehyde, alcohol), radiation (ultraviolet, cathode), or mechanical methods (filtration)

Surgical Asepsis: procedure used to prevent contamination by microbes and endospores before, during, or after surgery using sterile technique

Vaccine: suspension of attenuated or killed microorganisms (bacteria, viruses, or rickettsiae) administered for the prevention, improvement, or treatment of infectious disease

Vector: carrier, especially an animal (usually an arthropod), that transfers an infective agent from one host to another

Virion: complete viral particle found extracellularly and capable of surviving in crystalline form and infecting a living cell; comprises the nucleoid (genetic material) and the capsid; also called viral particle

Virus: any of a group of minute infectious agents not resolved in the light microscope, with certain exceptions (e.g., poxvirus), and characterized by a lack of independent metabolism and by the ability to replicate only within living host cells

MICROBIAL WORLD

Well over 300 years have passed since Anton van Leeuwenhoek first observed what he called *wee animalcules* under his crude microscope. At the time, he reported his findings to the Royal Society of London; the fact that these tiny creatures, known as *microbes,* could be anything more than a mere curiosity was beyond anyone's imagination.

At the beginning of the twentieth century, the major causes of death in the United States were microbial infectious diseases. These **diseases** included pneumonia, tuberculosis, gastroenteritis, and diphtheria. Although today most microbial infections are under control, microbes still present a major threat to survival for the immunosuppressed person. Furthermore, the threat of microbial disease in less developed countries still constitutes the major causes of death. Millions of people still die annually of illnesses such as malaria, cholera, and dysentery.

The last century saw an explosion in knowledge of the sciences. The tiny amusing creatures of Leeuwenhoek's time have proved to be literally a matter of life or death. Microbes are essential to life through their ability to recycle organic and inorganic matter and are devastating through their ability to produce disease. Most important, by studying these microbes at the molecular level, scientists have learned to identify them and determine their capabilities. Using this knowledge, many microbial functions can be controlled, making them beneficial or preventing potential harm.

The health care practitioner must have an understanding of what infectious diseases are, how they are spread, and how they are controlled. Health care providers have been granted the responsibility not only to the patients entrusted to their care, but also to the entire public sector.

Many **microorganisms** can grow in or on a host organism and cause disease. These diseases are known as *infections.* **Infection** refers to the establishment and growth of a microorganism on or in a host. Only when the infection results in injury to the host is the host said to have a disease. Pathogenic microorganisms cause *infectious diseases.* Most often, **pathogens** have the ability to do one of three functions extremely well: (1) They can multiply in large numbers and cause an obstruction, (2) they can cause tissue damage, and (3) they can secrete organic substances called *exotoxins.* These exotoxins can produce certain side effects such as an extremely high body temperature, nausea, vomiting, or shock. Pathogens are divided into four basic infectious

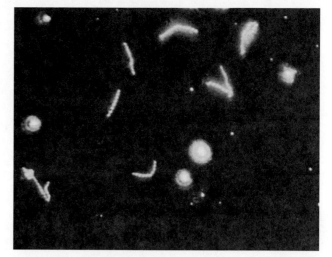

FIG. 16–1 Dark-field photomicrograph shows the tightly coiled characteristics of the spirochete *Treponema pallidum.* (From Atlas RM: *Principles of microbiology,* St Louis, 1995, Mosby. Forbes BA, Sahm DF, Weissfeld AS: *Bailey & Scott's diagnostic microbiology,* ed 11, St Louis, 2002, Mosby, p 131.)

agents: (1) bacteria, (2) viruses, (3) fungi, and (4) protozoan parasites.

Bacteria

Bacteria are microscopic, single-celled organisms with a simple internal organization (Fig. 16–1). Bacteria are procaryotic rather than eucaryotic organisms. **Procaryotes** lack nuclei and membrane-bound organelles, whereas **eucaryotes** have a true nucleus. Most of the cellular metabolic activities take place on the cytoplasmic membrane. Procaryotes do not have the capacity to ingest particulates or liquid droplets. Although bacteria are single celled, they may reside in the host in a group or cluster called a *colony.*

Bacteria are identified and classified according to their morphology, biochemistry, and genetic constitution. Morphology is considered a major criterion for classification. *Morphology* is the size or shape of the bacterium and is routinely determined by a simple staining technique called *Gram staining.* The medically important bacteria are classified into three general morphologies: cocci or spheres, bacilli or rods, and spirals.

Some bacteria have the ability to produce a highly resistant resting form known as an *endospore.* This structure is internal, as reflected in its name. Endospores are metabolically dormant structures that are highly resistant to the external environment. Spores possess extreme

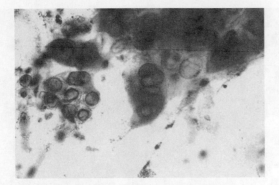

FIG. 16–2 Papanicolaou (Pap)-stained smear showing multinu-cleated giant cells typical of herpes simplex or vari-cella-zoster viruses. (From Forbes BA, Sahm DF, Weissfeld AS: *Bailey & Scott's diagnostic microbiology,* ed 11, St Louis, 2002, Mosby, p 835.)

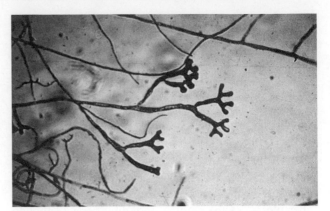

FIG. 16–3 Antler hyphae showing swollen hyphal tips resem-bling antlers, with lateral and terminal branching (favic chandeliers) (500×). (From Forbes BA, Sahm DF, Weissfeld AS: *Bailey & Scott's diagnostic micro-biology,* ed 11, St Louis, 2002, Mosby, p 743.)

resistance to chemical and physical agents. They can remain viable for many years and then germinate in response to specific requirements. The endospore is a survival form of the bacterium that is produced, most often in response to nutritional deprivation. Of all the bacteria able to produce endospores, only two genera, *Bacillus* and *Clostridium,* are of medical importance. Some common bacterial infections encountered today are strep-tococcal pharyngitis (strep throat), *Klebsiella pneumoniae* infection (bacterial pneumonia), and *Clostridium botu-linum* infection (food poisoning).

Viruses

Viruses are much simpler in form compared with bacte-ria or animal cells (Fig. 16–2). Viruses are neither pro-caryotic nor eucaryotic. They are considered obligate intracellular parasites. Viruses cannot live outside a living cell. They lack the components necessary for their own survival because of their inability to synthesize specific required proteins. Viruses depend on the host cell to provide these missing factors. A virus carries its own genetic information in the form of deoxyribonucleic acid (DNA) or ribonucleic acid (RNA), but never both. A protein coat called a *capsid* surrounds the viral DNA or RNA.

Viruses are characterized generally by the chemical nature of their nucleic acid, their size, and their symme-try. Nucleic acids within a virus are, as stated earlier, either DNA or RNA, but these nucleic acids may be double or single, positive or negative stranded. Nucleic acids of differing viruses also possess varying weights. The size of a virus may vary from 20 to 250 nm. A *nanometer* is equal to 10^{-9} m; therefore direct observation

of a virus is possible only through an electron microscope.

Viral infection is the result of a viral particle, also called a **virion,** which attaches to a host cell and inserts its genome or genetic information into the host. The viral genome then redirects the host cell. The virus uses the organelles and metabolic functions of the host cell to produce new viruses. Once this process is completed, the new viral particles are released from the host cell, some-times resulting in the destruction of the cell. Some viruses have the ability to travel within the nervous system. They reappear sporadically and emerge at the nerve ending, causing various symptoms. They then leave the site and travel up the nerve again. This pattern can be repeated several times and is known as a *latent* or *dormant* infec-tion. A cold sore caused by herpes simplex virus is an example of a latent viral infection. Common viral diseases in humans include the common cold caused by the rhi-novirus, infectious mononucleosis caused by the Epstein-Barr virus, and warts caused by the papillomavirus.

Fungi

Fungi (singular, *fungus*) can be macroscopic, as in the case of mushrooms and puffballs, or microscopic, such as yeasts and molds (Fig. 16–3). They are eucaryotic organisms with a nucleus and membrane-bound organelles. Fungi can be distinguished from bacteria by the fact that intracellular organelles can be visualized within the fungal cell. Fungal cells differ from animal cells in the type of sterol present in the cell membrane. The sterol present in animal cells is cholesterol. Fungi are also much larger than bacteria. Medically important pathogenic fungi are **dimorphic**; that is, they have the ability to grow in two distinct forms, either as a single-celled yeast or as filamentous hyphae. A filamentous hypha is better known as *mold*. Whether the organism is present in either form depends on the growth conditions. Fungi are classified according to the type and method of sexual reproduction.

A photomicrograph of a typical mold would reveal a structure similar to that of a plant or small tree. The molds produce tiny branches that extend into the air. These branches are where spores are formed. These spores are called *conidia*. They are lightweight and resistant to drying, and they are easily dispersed to new habitats. Diseases caused by fungi can be of four different classifications. The first is a *superficial* infection, which usually causes discoloration of the skin. *Tinea nigra* is a fungal infection that results in a painless black or brown discoloration of the palmar surface of the hand and the plantar surface of the foot. Second are the cutaneous infections, which involve the keratinized tissues of the hair, nails, and skin. The most common clinical infection in this group is *tinea pedis,* or *athlete's foot*. The growth pattern of this fungus forms a ring and is also known as *ringworm*. The third type is a subcutaneous fungal infection that enters the human host as a result of trauma to the skin. The fourth type is characterized by a systemic infection, which enters the circulatory and lymphatic systems and may be fatal.

Protozoan Parasites

Protozoa are unicellular organisms that are neither plants nor animals (Fig. 16–4). They are distinguished from bacteria by their greater size and by the fact that they do not possess a cell wall. Protozoa are generally motile organisms and are eucaryotic. They are able to ingest food particles, and some species are equipped with rudimentary digestive systems.

Protozoa are classified according to their motility. The first group is classified by its slow cellular flowing called *amoeboid locomotion*. Few amoebas are pathogenic. The motility of the second group is facilitated by long *flagella*, a protein tail. The third group moves by the action of numerous short protein tails called *cilia*. Sporozoans constitute the fourth group. This group is unique in that they are nonmotile and, despite their name, do not form spores as bacteria and fungi do.

Some protozoa are able to form **cysts**, which permit them to survive while the parasite is out of a host. Cysts are resistant to chemical and physical changes.

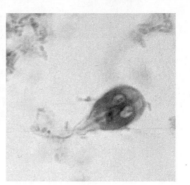

FIG. 16–4 *Giardia lamblia* trophozoite. (From Forbes BA, Sahm DF, Weissfeld AS: *Bailey & Scott's diagnostic microbiology,* ed 11, St Louis, 2002, Mosby, p 664.)

Typical protozoan infections include *Trichomonas vaginalis* infection, a sexually transmitted disease that infects both male and female hosts, and *Plasmodium vivax* infection (malaria).

ESTABLISHMENT OF INFECTIOUS DISEASE

From the time the infectious agent comes in contact with the host until the devastation of a disease is apparent, several complicated processes must be completed. These processes can be categorized into six steps. These six steps are the (1) encounter, (2) entry, (3) spread, (4) multiplication, (5) damage, and (6) outcome (Fig. 16–5). Remember, all six steps require breaching of the host.

Encounter

The encounter involves the infectious organism coming in contact with the host. Each encounter varies according to the host and microorganism. Every individual and every microbe will respond differently. Some organisms can infect an unborn child, although this is difficult because the mother's womb is, microbially speaking, a sterile environment because of the selective passage allowed by the placenta. Still, some microorganisms are able to pass through the placenta to create what are called *congenital* infections. Examples of these infections are rubella and syphilis.

The initial encounter with infectious microorganisms takes place during the normal birthing process. The child comes in contact with the microbial world that is present in the mother's vaginal canal. Fortunately, the newborn is born with antibodies obtained from the mother. These antibodies, plus those acquired through the mother's

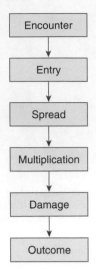

FIG. 16–5 The establishment of an infectious disease is a six-step process.

breast milk, provide the newborn with a sufficient immunologic base to cope with infection until its own immune system has matured.

During the entire human life span, the body comes in contact with new organisms; some are quickly eliminated, and others are efficient colonizers. The colonizers either become part of the microbes normally found in the body or cause disease.

Entry

Much of the body is in contact with the external environment. The digestive, biliary, urinary, and respiratory systems are in direct connection with the exterior. In women, the peritoneal cavity is also exposed via the fallopian tubes. An infectious microbe can gain entrance into the human body by either ingression or penetration.

Ingression does not involve deep-tissue penetration. Instead, these microorganisms adhere to the surface of the cell and excrete toxins that cause a distressed state within the system. Through the digestive system, infectious agents are ingested, most commonly through contaminated food or water. If the organism has the ability to survive the lower pH of the stomach and the small intestine, then it may become anchored on the colon and cause a diseased state. The most common example of a symptom caused by an ingressive organism is diarrhea. Ingression can also take place in the respiratory system. Inhalation of contaminated aerosols or dust particles that are able to evade the powerful retrograde movement of

the ciliary epithelium can lead to colonization within the lower respiratory tract. Pneumonia is contracted in this manner.

Penetration involves the microorganism invading past the epithelial barrier. This action can take place in various forms. Some microbes are equipped with a special apparatus, such as flagella. The bacteria that cause syphilis are able to penetrate using this mechanical device. Other microbes use vectors, such as mosquitoes or fleas, to penetrate into the tissue. Still others gain entry through tissue cuts and wounds. A *phagocyte,* which engulfs a foreign microbe, can transport it deeper into the tissue. In this instance, the human body itself is used to aid in penetration.

Spread

Spread, the propagation of the infectious organism, can take place before or after multiplication. In either case, the most important barrier for the microbe to overcome in this step is the host's immune defenses. Dissemination is dictated by the logistics of both the host and the microbe. In other words, the site of microbial entry or the site where the microbe has taken up residence and the human anatomy at that site determine the spread of the microbe. For example, the viruses that cause the common cold are easily spread as aerosols through coughing and sneezing.

Multiplication

The number of microbes that gain entrance into the host is usually much too small to cause the symptoms of a disease. Most infectious agents must first multiply for their impact to be recognized. The time frame applied to this phenomenon is termed the *incubation period,* and its parameters are defined from the time the host's defenses have been overcome until the time a substantial population has been achieved.

Damage

Virtually uncountable ways exist in which an infectious agent can cause damage to a host. Damage can be either direct or indirect. Cell death caused by destruction of the host cells or by toxins or poisons secreted by the infectious agent are examples of direct damage. The growth phase of a microbe is characterized by exponential growth, and in a matter of hours enough organisms may be present to cause a complete obstruction in a major organ system.

Infectious microbes can also damage a host indirectly by altering the metabolism of the host. These infections are represented by some of the most life-threatening diseases. Once a person has ingested the toxins secreted by the organism that causes botulism, death can result in only a matter of hours.

A microbe can also induce host responses. Indirectly, the host's inflammatory and immune responses can cause further cell destruction than that already achieved by the microbe. This destruction is usually minimal compared with the overall devastation that an infectious agent can induce. The sacrificing of a few cells is justified when the integrity of the entire human body is at stake.

Outcome

An encounter with an infectious agent can result in one of three outcomes: (1) the host gains control of the infectious agent and eliminates it, (2) the infectious agent overcomes the host's immunities to cause disease, or (3) the host and the infectious agent compromise and live in a somewhat anxious state of symbiosis.

CHAIN OF INFECTION

In 1876, Robert Koch, a physician, introduced the germ theory of disease. Before this point, the assumption was that something was transmitted from an ill person to a well person. Up until the sixteenth century, evil spirits were a popular explanation for illness. In the sixteenth century, however, diseases were assumed to be spread by an unknown entity called a *contagion,* and the disease was said to be *contagious,* a term still in use today. Through scientific experimentation, Koch was able to prove that specific organisms caused specific diseases. He was able to prove that a precise series of events must occur for microorganisms from an infected person to be transmitted to an uninfected person. His postulates forever changed the relationship between microorganisms and humans.

According to the postulates of Koch, four factors are involved in the spread of diseases. Each factor is considered a link in the chain, and each link is connected to the next to form a ring. If at any point in the infection the chain is broken, the cycle cannot continue, and infection will cease. For infections to be transmitted, the following must exist: (1) a host, (2) an infectious microorganism, (3) a mode of transportation, and (4) a reservoir (Fig. 16–6).

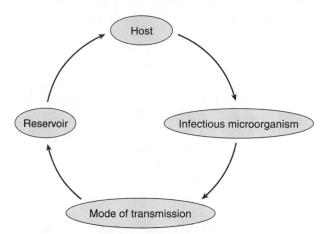

FIG. 16–6 The chain of infection. For infections to be transmitted there must be (1) a host, (2) an infectious microorganism, (3) a mode of transmission, and (4) a reservoir.

Human Host

Humans provide a favorable **host** environment for the growth of many microbes because of the abundance of organic nutrients and metabolites found within the human body. Each region or organ of the body offers a different temperature, pH, or body fluid for microbial growth to occur. This diversity is optimal for the microbe with limited metabolic or aerobic requirements.

Infectious Microorganisms

Microorganisms include bacteria, viruses, fungi, and protozoa. These organisms have already been discussed.

Mode of Transmission

Microorganisms can be transmitted either *exogenously,* from outside the body, or *endogenously,* from inside the body. Exogenously acquired diseases are those that result from an encounter with a microbe in the environment. This transmission can occur by either direct or indirect host-to-host contact. Indirect transmission may also occur through a vector or a fomite.

Direct host-to-host transmission occurs when an infected individual transmits an infection by any number of methods, such as handholding, coughing, or sexual contact, to name just a few. Most important, direct contact involves touching of some sort. Sexually transmitted diseases use this route. Skin pathogens also are spread by the direct route. Staphylococcal infections can be spread by direct contact with the infected area, as demonstrated in impetigo infections.

Infective microbes are usually transported in a liquid medium. Secretions and excretions pick up organisms from infected areas and remove them during normal body functions. Body secretions such as phlegm and aerosols from sneezes and coughs are common transportation media.

Respiratory pathogens transmitted in the aerosols do not remain airborne and viable for long. Transmission is therefore considered to be of the direct route. Excretions, including urine and feces, are also pertinent carriers of microorganisms.

Some microorganisms require a **vector** to enter and exit the human host. A vector is usually an arthropod (mosquito, flea, tick, and so forth). When it consumes its blood meal from its human host, it can ingest an infectious microbe from the blood. When the vector goes on to obtain its next meal from a different individual, it can transmit the infection to that individual. A vector, the deer tick, transmits Lyme disease.

A **fomite** is an inanimate object that has been in contact with an infectious organism. Food and water, radiographic equipment, and latex gloves can all serve as fomites.

Endogenous transmission is the result of encounters with organisms already present in or on the body, the normal flora. This transmission usually happens when the normal flora of a specific area is transported to a different area. Staphylococci on the surface of the skin can invade deeper tissue through a laceration. In this case, the initial encounter with staphylococci may have been years earlier, but the infection was initiated as a result of the trauma. The primary encounter is termed the *colonization* and denotes the presence of a microbe. Do not assume that because colonization exists that disease is present. Disease implies tissue damage and related symptoms.

Reservoir

A **reservoir** is the site where an infectious organism can remain alive and from which transmission can occur. People, animals, and inanimate objects can all serve as reservoirs.

A person who serves as a reservoir is called a *carrier.* A carrier is an infected person who does not display the disease symptoms. Typhoid Mary is a classic example. Mary Mallon was a chronic carrier of *Salmonella typhi,* the organism that causes typhoid fever. She was employed in numerous households and institutions as a cook. She

daily exposed other people to the pathogen, which led to an epidemic. After extensive investigations of numerous outbreaks, she was revealed as the source of each one. When tested, her bacteria count for this specific species was incredibly high. She continued to shed the organism for many years. The assumption is that her infected gallbladder supplied a continuous wave of organisms to her colon. Public health officials offered to remove her gallbladder, an operation she refused. Their only recourse was to imprison Mary to prevent further epidemics. After 3 years in prison, Mary was released on the promise that she would cease to handle food and that she would continue to be monitored on a regular basis. Mary never appeared for her checkups. She changed her name and continued to cook. For 5 more years, she caused another epidemic of typhoid fever. After another epidemiologic investigation, the source of infection was, once again, traced to her. She was imprisoned and remained there for 23 years until her death in 1938.

Animals can also serve as reservoirs. A common animal reservoir is the cow. Some diseases can be passed from the cow to a human host through the ingestion of milk. Pasteurization has helped obliterate most of these pathogens.

Insects are another common reservoir. After an insect ingests a blood meal infected with pathogens, protozoa may complete their life cycles within the insect and are introduced into the host in a different stage of life. Such is the case for malaria, which is spread primarily by a mosquito vector. A dusty corner, contaminated linen, and food can serve as inanimate reservoirs.

NOSOCOMIAL INFECTIONS

The statement that the hospital is a place where sick people can go to get better is a general concept, and, for the most part, this statement is true. Approximately 5% of all hospital patients acquire an additional condition while in the hospital, however. These hospital-acquired conditions are known as **nosocomial** infections (*nosocomium* is the Latin word for hospital). These hospital pathogens follow the chain of infection, but the links are limited to persons who are in contact with the microenvironment we know as the hospital. In the United States, billions of dollars are spent annually on nosocomial management, and such infections represent the eighth leading cause of death.

Within the health care field, yet another microenvironment can be found: between patient and physician. An infection that is the result of intervention with a physician is an **iatrogenic** infection. This type of infection is strictly limited to the physician, whether he or she is in the hospital or not. For example, a patient may develop pneumonia following the performance of a lung biopsy by a physician.

The same organisms that cause nosocomial and iatrogenic infections may be found elsewhere in the community, but the healthy population can usually combat these pathogens. Nosocomial pathogens are opportunistic. Given the right conditions—a patient with an impaired immune system; the ability to bypass anatomic barriers through burns, wounds, or surgery; and introduction through a catheter, syringe, or respirator—these pathogens thrive and exert their maximum biologic effects. Hospitals and their patients provide this optimal environment.

Compromised Patient

Hospital patients have a greater sensitivity to infection. Many patients have weakened resistance to infectious organisms because of their admitting illness. These patients are said to be *compromised* or *immunosuppressed.* For example, organ transplant patients are intentionally given drugs to suppress their immune system. This action is taken to prevent rejection of the transplanted organ, but it provides the opportunistic pathogen with a suitable host at the same time. The severity of the admitting condition corresponds to the risk of acquiring a nosocomial infection and vice versa. An outpatient having a mole removed has an extremely small chance of acquiring an infection compared with a patient having emergency open-heart surgery.

Sources

Cross-infection within the hospital can come from a multitude of sources. The complexity of the hospital environment provides innumerable opportunities for the encounter of patients with infectious microbes.

MEDICAL PERSONNEL. Transmission between the hospital staff and the patient may be by direct skin-to-skin contact or through indirect contact, by ingestion or inhalation. Unusual epidemics have been traced to hospital personnel. Food handlers can contaminate food eaten by the patient, and a nurse can sneeze onto his or her hands and then touch a patient. Surgeons have been known to carry organisms in their facial hair. In one epidemic, the organisms were harbored in the carrier's vagina and were presumed to be aerosolized through normal body movement. The possibilities of transfer are endless. Medical personnel can continually serve as active colonizers or transient carriers, or they can become infected themselves.

PATIENT FLORA. Microorganisms are almost always found in regions of the body that are exposed to the external environment, such as the skin, gastrointestinal system, genitourinary system, and respiratory system. Potentially harmful bacteria such as staphylococci and streptococci are harbored in the nasopharynx of almost every healthy person. When a person is healthy, the relationship between the host and the microbe is either beneficial or neutral; but when this person is compromised, the microbe seizes the opportunity to flourish and is harmful.

CONTAMINATED HOSPITAL ENVIRONMENT. Many microorganisms are endemic to the hospital environment. An example would be fungal infections acquired from the mildew that grows on moist walls. Infection can also be acquired through improperly sterilized surgical equipment or contaminated intravenous solutions. Contamination through the hospital environment is often through fomites, such as instruments, fluids, food, air, and medications.

BLOOD-BORNE PATHOGENS. Blood-borne pathogens are disease-causing microorganisms that may be present in human blood. They may be transmitted with any exposure to blood or other potentially infectious material. For this reason, these pathogens will be considered nosocomial infections.

Two blood-borne pathogens are of concern within the hospital setting: hepatitis B virus (HBV) and human immunodeficiency virus (HIV). Numerous other blood-borne pathogens exist, such as those that cause hepatitis C, hepatitis D, and syphilis, but they are not as prevalent as HBV and HIV.

HBV causes illness that primarily affects the liver. This infection results in swelling, soreness, and loss of normal function in the liver. HBV is a major cause of viral hepatitis.

The symptoms of hepatitis B include weakness, fatigue, anorexia, nausea, abdominal pain, fever, and headache. As the illness progresses, a yellow discoloration of the skin, called *jaundice,* may develop. In some patients, the disease may be asymptomatic and therefore may not be diagnosed.

A person's blood will test positive for the HBV surface antigen 2 to 6 weeks after symptoms of the illness develop. Approximately 85% of persons infected will recover in 6 to 8 weeks, and yet a blood test will always reveal that they have been exposed to the virus because of the presence of the HBV surface antigen.

A major source of HBV is the chronic active carrier of the virus. The carrier has the surface antigen present at all times. This presence may be the consequence of a problem with the immune system that prevents complete destruction of virus-infected liver cells. Estimates suggest that 1.25 million persons in the United States have chronic HBV and are potentially infectious to others. The carrier can unknowingly transmit the disease to a susceptible host through a contaminated needle or other penetrating injury and through intimate contact. Each year, 5000 people die as a result of liver disease caused by HBV.

HIV is a virus that specifically infects the immune system CD4+ T cells in the human host. The presence of the virus renders the cells decreasingly effective in preventing disease. HIV is responsible for acquired immunodeficiency syndrome (AIDS).

Symptoms of HIV infection may include weight loss, fatigue, glandular pain and swelling, muscle and joint pain, and night sweats. People with HIV infection may feel fine and not be aware of their previous exposure to HIV for as long as 10 years. As long as 1 year may be required for the results of a blood test to become positive for HIV antibodies. Therefore more than one test over a specified period may be required to determine infection after exposure to HIV.

INVASIVE PROCEDURES. Invasive diagnostic or therapeutic interventions allow a microbe to gain entrance into an area of the body where it may not normally be able to overcome that person's defenses. These procedures give the microbe a free ride. The most common nosocomial infection, a urinary tract infection, is introduced by a Foley urinary catheter.

Other invasive procedures include any surgery and the insertion of such devices as needles, vascular catheters, endotracheal tubes, and endoscopes.

MICROBIAL CONTROL WITHIN THE HOST

Microbes can be controlled within the host by different mechanisms. Some of these defenses are part of the normal anatomic and physiologic mechanisms of the host. Others are introduced into the host, and microbes themselves control others.

Constitutive Defenses of the Body

The human body has defense mechanisms with which a host can protect itself from microbial invasion. These defenses are categorized as mechanical, chemical, or cellular. The intact skin and the mucous membranes provide a mechanical and chemical barrier through which a microorganism must first pass. The sebaceous and sweat glands secrete moisture and fatty acids onto the skin that kill many bacteria and fungi. In addition, the mechanical process of the shedding of cells caused by friction from rubbing the hands together during washing also provides a strong defensive system. Trauma such as a burn, abrasion, or another type of wound provides the obvious breaches to this barrier.

The mucous membranes of the respiratory, gastrointestinal, and genitourinary tracts and conjunctiva of the eye secrete a gel-like substance called *mucus* that traps foreign particles and prevents them from invading the adjacent tissue. Some epithelial cells are ciliated. The beating action of the cilia on the mucous membranes provides for the continuous movement of the fluid mucus to the exterior.

Tears continually bathe the eyes, and urine cleanses the urinary tract. Both tears and urine are rich in *lysosome*, an enzyme that destroys the bacterial cell wall. The acidity of the stomach and the vagina also provides a competent barrier to invasion.

Despite these efficient chemical and mechanical barriers, microbes penetrate the bloodstream and connective tissue daily. They gain entrance through everyday activity such as eating, brushing teeth, scratching, and bowel movements. These daily attacks are survived through the cellular mechanism of defense, the *phagocytic cell*. The phagocyte is responsible for removing foreign particles, engulfing and destroying them through a process called *phagocytosis*. Phagocytosis is part of the inflammatory response.

Normal Microbial Flora

The human body contains thousands of species of microorganisms. Each of us is unique in that the types and amounts of each organism vary. Normal **flora** is defined as the microbial community found on or in a healthy person. The normal flora for one person may be completely different from that of the next. Because of this microbial uniqueness, pathogenicity is not a *black and white* issue. What constitutes the normal flora of one person may be life threatening to another. Although the normal flora may serve as the source of many opportunistic infections, in many areas of the body, the normal flora inhibits the attachment and colonization of many pathogens. The old saying that *possession is nine tenths of the law* also applies to microbes. Invaders who have found their niche are reluctant to concede their occupancy to another organism, maintaining their physical advantage. Others secrete toxins that are inhibitory to other microbes.

Chemotherapy

Killing a microorganism outside the human body is a fairly simple task. To kill a microbe within the host requires the selective toxicity of a drug, also called selective **chemotherapy.** Most antimicrobial drugs have a single primary target, which most often are specific proteins, nucleic acids, and, in bacteria, the cell wall. Clinically useful antimicrobials must have the ability to inhibit reactions within the microbe but not interfere with the human cell with which the microbe is associated. Some chemotherapeutic drugs are termed *static* because they inhibit growth but do not cause killing. Tetracyclines are examples of bacteriostatic drugs. Others are termed *-cidal* because of their ability to kill susceptible microbes. Penicillins are examples of bacteriocidal drugs.

Immunization

The awareness that persons who survived an epidemic did not contract that disease again has been evident in history for many centuries. As early as the tenth century, the Turks were inoculating their infant daughters with extracts from the pustules of smallpox patients. If they survived, their value on the market as concubines for harems was increased because their bodies were not pocked or scarred from the disease.

Modern immunology began with the experiments of Louis Pasteur, who developed vaccines for diseases, including anthrax and rabies. A **vaccine** is a mixture used to induce active **immunity** (the production of antibody). The importance of immunization is reflected in the marked drop in incidence of that specific disease after vaccination. The degree of immunity varies according to the patient and the quality and quantity of the vaccine. An important point to remember is that immunization rarely lasts throughout life. In many cases, booster vaccines must be administered.

ENVIRONMENTAL CONTROL

Up to this point, the primary concern has been with the intimate relationship between the infectious microbe and the host. The constituents of the body, other microbes, medicines, and immunizations all contribute their defenses in the constant battle against infection. Each of these factors is important in ensuring the integrity of the host, but another important step not yet considered exists. In a world populated with millions and millions of people, each with their own millions of microbes, focusing attention on the larger picture of environmental control is important. When the number of microbes is considered, the problem of environmental control seems overwhelming, and yet it is one of the easiest methods of control.

Within the United States, recommendations and guidelines for environmental control of infectious diseases are issued by the U.S. Department of Health and Human Services (HHS) and by the Centers for Disease Control and Prevention (CDC). The U.S. Department of Labor's Occupational Safety and Health Administration (OSHA) enforces the established policies. All rules and regulations are strictly enforced at both the state and the federal levels. At the international level, the World Health Organization (WHO) issues recommendations for infection control.

Asepsis

As radiologic technologists, we have the ability and the responsibility to prevent the spread of infectious organisms. Knowledge of the principles of sterilization and disinfection is fundamental. **Asepsis** means freedom from infection and can be divided into two categories: *surgical* asepsis and *medical* asepsis. **Surgical asepsis** is the procedure used to prevent contamination of microbes and endospores before, during, and after surgery using sterile technique. The absolute killing of all life forms is termed **sterilization.** If proper sterilization techniques are used, the probability of infection is theoretically zero. **Medical asepsis** involves a reduction in numbers of infectious agents, which, in turn, decreases the probability of infection but does not necessarily reduce it to zero. The microbes are not eliminated, however. Instead, their environment is altered so that it is not conducive to growth and reproduction.

Each microbial species has an optimal temperature range for growth. Any variation above or below this range results in a blockage of growth. Most organisms that infect humans survive best at 37° C (98.6° F). An increase in metabolic activity, within the range, results in an increase in growth. Once above this range, the proteins or enzymes cannot perform their normal functions. A decrease within the range results in a slowing down of growth; once below the range, the protein loses its flexibility. This factor is one of the reasons the operating room is kept so cold.

Another important environmental effect on microbial growth is pH. Most human infectious microbes grow best at a neutral or slightly alkaline pH (7.0 to 7.4). Some microbes prefer acidic or alkaline conditions and seek parts of the body that provide these conditions. Microbes are also sensitive to the presence or subsequent absence of oxygen. Consequently, environmental microbial control can be achieved through both chemical and physical means.

CHEMICAL METHODS. Chemicals that alter the environment available to the microbe are called **disinfectants.** This term is an ambiguous term referring to either the inactivation or the inhibition of microbial growth. Disinfection may or may not entail the removal of bacterial endospores. If the disinfectant is applied topically, it is termed an *antiseptic*. Not only can disinfectants be classified according to whether they can be used on a living body, they also can be classified as to whether they kill or do not kill microbes. A *bacteriostatic* agent stops bacterial growth, and a *bacteriocidal* agent causes cell killing.

Chemical disinfectants common to the radiology department include the halogens chlorine and iodine, which are bacteriocidal. Chlorine is found in bleach. Because it is such a strong oxidizing agent, bleach is ordinarily used on inanimate objects. Iodine is used as the antiseptic in Betadine and Surgidine and is used in conjunction with alcohol swabbing. This antiseptic method is commonly used with invasive procedures. Alcohol cannot be used independently; although it is lethal to all vegetative cells, it cannot destroy endospores. Also common to the radiology department is hydrogen peroxide. This substance is used in a 3% solution as an antiseptic and is most effective in deep wounds. Ammonium-containing detergents are used as surface-active disinfectants throughout the hospital, and ethylene oxide is used for sterilization in the gas phase. Gas sterilization is used for electronic and plastic equipment that may be damaged by heat.

The effectiveness of chemical disinfectants is subject to concentration, temperature, time of exposure, types and numbers of microbes, and the nature of the object or person being treated. Reading all manufacturers' labels carefully is important to ensure maximal effectiveness.

PHYSICAL METHODS. Heat is the most frequently used method of sterilization. Moist heat is much more effective and rapid at killing than dry heat. Moist heat involves using steam under pressure. This task is accomplished in a device known as an *autoclave*. Effective killing of vegetative cells and endospores is accomplished at 121°C (250°F) at a pressure of 15 lb/in^2 for 15 minutes. Sterilization by dry heat is achieved in an oven. Compared with wet heat, dry heat requires a higher temperature for a longer time (160°C [320°F] for 120 minutes). *Pasteurization* involves moderate heating followed by rapid cooling. This process is used to kill heat-sensitive organisms in milk, beer, and wine. Pasteurization does not sterilize the liquid involved. Freezing can also kill certain organisms but is not a reliable form of sterilization. Ultraviolet (UV) light at 260 nm can produce maximal killing of microbes. UV light is used in germicidal lamps for control of airborne contaminants. UV light is restricted in its usage by its inability to penetrate glass, paper, body fluids, and thin layers of cells.

A host need not be a patient. The health care provider can also serve as a host. One of the simplest physical methods of microbial control, for the health care provider or the patient, is the use of barriers. Gloves, gowns, masks, protective eyewear, or face shields all serve as barriers and defend against invasion by an infectious microbe.

Hand Washing

The importance of hand washing in preventing the spread of infection is credited to Dr. Semmelweis of Vienna in 1846. He noted that when the medical students of the hospital went directly from class, in this case autopsies, to rounds in the hospital, the incidence of infection was high. What drew his attention to this practice was that, when the students were on vacation, the incidence of infection dropped significantly. He noted that the nurses attending the patients were not permitted in the autopsy room. He established a policy that no medical students would be allowed to examine patients until they had cleansed their hands with a solution of chloride of lime.

Hand washing is a routine practice in all patient care settings. It is the single most important means of preventing the spread of infection. Washing or scrubbing the hands involves removal of contaminants (transients), as well as resident microorganisms. Hand washing is both a chemical and a physical process. Many soaps and detergents are bacteriocidal, but their application during hand washing is usually too brief to kill microbes. Depending on the condition of the skin and the numbers of microbes present, as long as 7 to 8 minutes of washing may be required to remove the transients; and resident microbes

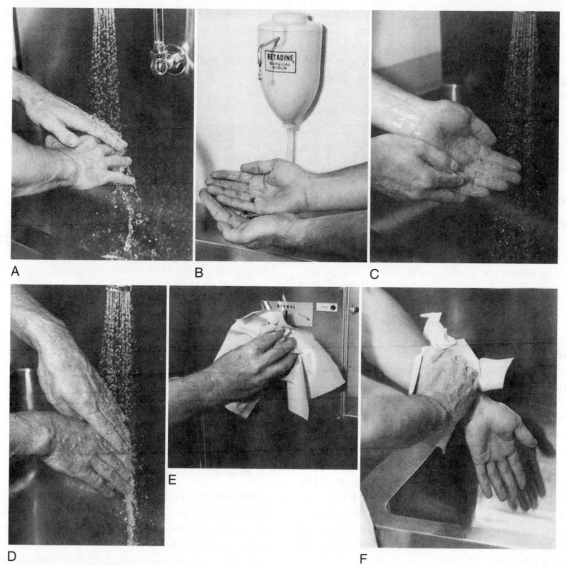

FIG. 16–7 Proper hand washing. *A,* Wet hands thoroughly with water. *B,* Apply soap. *C,* Rub hands using a firm, vigorous rotary motion. *D,* Rinse, allowing the water to run down over hands. *E,* Turn off the water, using toweling on handles. *F,* Dry hands from elbow to fingertips.

are even harder to remove because they are so firmly embedded. Soaps are effective at removing some fragile bacteria, such as pneumococci and meningococci. An important and effective portion of hand washing appears to be the mechanical action of rubbing the hands together.

Because a radiologic technologist comes in contact with a myriad of patients on a daily basis, hand washing absolutely must be performed *before and after attending to each patient.* This practice provides the simplest method of environmental control. A specific protocol should be followed that is accepted as medically aseptic (Fig. 16–7):

1. Approach the sink. Consider it to be contaminated. Avoid contact with your clothing. Use foot or knee levers when available. If not, use toweling to handle all controls. Adjust water flow to avoid splashing. Adjust water temperature to comfort.
2. Wet hands thoroughly with water. During the entire procedure, keep the hands lower than the elbow. This advantageous use of gravity allows organisms to flow down the arm and off the fingertips.
3. Apply soap. Soap should be available in liquid form and can be applied by using foot or knee levers. Soap can also be dispensed from a pump.

4. Use a firm, vigorous, rotary motion. Begin at the wrist and work toward the fingertips. Rub palms, back of hands, between fingers, and under the nails.
5. Rinse and allow water to run down over hands.
6. Repeat the entire process to cleanse from the elbow to the fingertips.
7. Turn off the water. Use toweling on handles if foot or knee levers are not available.
8. Dry from the elbow to the fingertips, never returning to an area.

Standard Precautions

The CDC and the Hospital Infection Control Practices Advisory Committee (HICPAC) recently revised the isolation precautions for hospitals and other health care facilities. To clarify the confusion of such terms as *universal precautions, body substance isolation precautions,* and the old disease-specific *isolation precautions,* the CDC and HICPAC reclassified infections, standardized terminology, and simplified precautions.

Standard precautions incorporate the features of both body fluid precautions and body substance isolation. Standard precautions should be used when performing procedures that may require contact with blood, body fluids, secretions, excretions, mucous membranes, and nonintact skin. Also included in this category are items soiled or contaminated with any of these substances. Because most patients in the radiology department have an unknown serostatus, all patients should be regarded as potentially infectious. Apply standard precautions to all patients, regardless of diagnosis and infection status. Biosafety in the radiology department using standard precautions includes, but is not limited to, the following guidelines.

HAND WASHING. Hands must be washed before and after performing invasive procedures and after touching body fluids, blood, secretions, excretions, and contaminated items, regardless of whether gloves are worn. Gloves may have undetectable defects and may also be torn or damaged during use.

GLOVING. Gloves must be worn during procedures that may involve contact with any patient's body fluids, blood, secretions, excretions, mucous membranes, nonintact skin, and contaminated items. Gloves must be worn during all vascular access procedures. Gloves must be promptly removed after use, before touching noncontaminated surfaces, and, of course, between patients.

PERSONAL PROTECTIVE EQUIPMENT. Personal protective equipment is provided by the hospital at no cost to the health care worker. This equipment provides a barrier between the patient and the health care provider to prevent exposure to the skin and mucous membranes. This equipment includes gloves, fluid-repellent gowns, facemasks, protective eyewear, and resuscitation masks and bags. Personal protective equipment must be used when contact with body fluids, blood, secretions, and excretions is possible.

NEEDLE RECAPPING. An estimated 800,000 needlestick injuries and other injuries from sharp objects occur to health care workers annually in the United States. Recapping used needles should be avoided. If recapping is necessary, the one-handed *scoop* technique or a needle-recapping device that holds the needle sheath can be used. All used sharps must be placed in the designated puncture-resistant container, commonly called a *sharps container.*

BIOSPILLS. To clean biospills, gloves and the appropriate personal protective equipment must be worn. Paper towels can be used to blot the spill and are then discarded into a designated medical waste container. The contaminated area can be cleaned with a bleach solution or a hospital-grade disinfectant.

Transmission-Based Precautions

Transmission-based precautions are applied whenever a patient is infected with a pathogenic organism or a communicable disease. Transmission-based precautions must also be applied when the patient is at risk of becoming infected, such as those who are immunosuppressed.

Transmission-based precautions are used along with standard precautions, serving as a double protection, protecting both the patient and the health care practitioner. The transmission-based precautions have replaced the old category of specific isolation precautions, such as contact and respiratory isolation. Isolation techniques have been revised and combined into three sets of guidelines. An important point to keep in mind is that, under these guidelines, some infections and conditions fall into two categories.

AIRBORNE PRECAUTIONS. Pathogenic organisms that remain suspended in air for long periods on aerosol droplets or dust include tuberculosis, varicella (chickenpox), and rubeola (measles). Patients infected with pathogens that disseminate through the air are to be placed in a negative-pressure isolation room with the door closed. Health care practitioners should wear respiratory protection when entering the room. This type of respiratory protection should filter inspired air. An infected patient leaving his or her room should wear a surgical mask, which filters expired air.

DROPLET PRECAUTIONS. When caring for patients who are infected with such pathogenic organisms as rubella, mumps, influenza, and adenovirus, droplet precautions should be used. These pathogens disseminate through large particulate droplets expelled from the patient during coughing, sneezing, or even talking. The pathogens infect another person through contact with the mouth, nasal mucosa, or conjunctiva.

Patients infected with these pathogens are placed in private rooms or with another patient who is infected with the same disease. The door can remain open because large droplets typically travel 3 feet before dropping to the ground. Health care practitioners should protect themselves by wearing a surgical mask when within 3 feet of the patient. Special ventilation precautions are not necessary. The patient should wear a surgical mask when leaving the room.

CONTACT PRECAUTIONS. These precautions must be used when caring for a patient infected with a virulent pathogen that spreads by direct contact with the patient or by indirect contact with a contaminated object, such as patient's dressings or bed rails. Conditions that require using contact precautions include methicillin-resistant *Staphylococcus aureus,* hepatitis A, impetigo, varicella, and varicella zoster.

This patient will be housed in a private room or with another patient who is infected with the same disease. The health care practitioner should properly don gloves before entering the room. The gloves are removed and hands washed before leaving the room. A gown should be worn if the practitioner anticipates contact with the patient or his or her environment; the gown is removed before leaving the room. All radiographic equipment placed in the contaminated environment should be cleaned with an antiseptic solution.

When a patient requiring contact precautions is sent to the radiology department, the patient must wear appropriate barriers. In many cases, the patient will wear a mask and an impervious gown. Staff in the department should be notified before receiving the patient. All radiographic equipment should be decontaminated with an antiseptic after the radiographic procedure is completed.

Contact Precautions Technique. In many instances, a radiologic technologist is required to perform examinations on patients who are on contact precautions. Maintaining contact precautions usually requires teamwork. Acquiring the assistance of another health care provider is important. Contact precautions are maintained by the following steps (Fig. 16–8):

1. Determine the correct number of cassettes needed for the examination. Place each cassette into a protective bag, which may be either a plastic or a cloth isolation bag. These bags should be available in the radiology department.
2. Move the portable machine to the isolated room.
3. Locate the isolation supplies for the room.
4. Remove all ornamentation (including watch, rings, earrings) and place them in a pocket.
5. Put on a lead apron.
6. Wash your hands as described previously.
7. Put on a clean gown, making sure it is sufficiently long to cover most of the uniform. Pick up the gown from the inside near the armhole openings and gently shake it open. Put one arm in and then the other. First tie the neck strings and then tie the waist strings.
8. Put on a mask, tying it securely, and then a cap. Goggles may also be worn, if available.
9. Put on the gloves, which should be clean but need not be sterile. (See Chapter 17 if sterile gloving is required.)
10. Have the assistant put on a gown, gloves, and a cap.
11. Enter the isolated area and explain to the patient who you are and what you are doing. You will appear intimidating. A gentle word will go a long way at this point.
12. Position the patient and the cassette.
13. Have your assistant manipulate the machine and make the exposure.
14. Remove the cassette from behind the patient. Fold the edge of the protective bag back, never touching the inside. Have your assistant remove the cassette, never touching the outside. Place the covering into an appropriate container. Have your assistant remove the portable equipment from the room.
15. Untie the waist ties of the gown.
16. Remove your gloves. Remove the first glove with the other gloved hand, never touching the inside of the glove. Grasp the top of the glove and pull it inside out. Remove the other glove with the exposed hand, touching the inside only. Discard into an appropriate container.

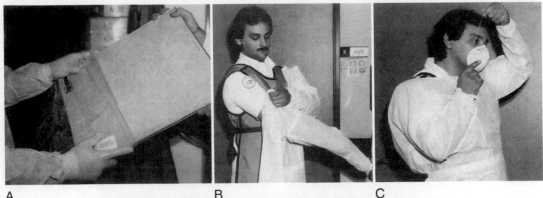

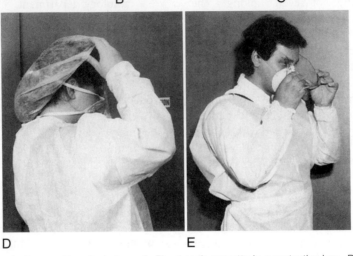

FIG. 16–8 An appropriate contact precautions technique. *A,* Place each cassette in a protective bag. *B,* Put on a lead apron and then gown, never touching the outside of the gown with your hands. *C,* Put on a mask. *D,* Put on a cap. *E,* Put on protective glasses, if recommended.

17. Remove the cap and then untie the mask, touching the ties only, and remove the mask.
18. Untie the neckties of the gown, and pull the gown forward and down from the shoulders. Pull the gown off so that the sleeves are inside out and the front of the gown is folded inward. Avoid touching the front of the gown. Discard into an appropriate container.
19. Wash your hands.
20. Have your assistant follow the same protocol. Clean the portable equipment with an antiseptic.
21. Wash your hands one last time.

SUMMARY

Infection involves the establishment and dissemination of a microorganism on or in a host. Disease results when an infection causes physiologic damage to the host. Infectious diseases are caused by pathogenic microorganisms, which are divided into four basic infectious agents: bacteria, viruses, fungi, and protozoan parasites.

For an infectious agent to become established in a host, a breach of the host's defenses must occur. The establishment of infectious disease involves six steps: encounter, entry, spread, multiplication, damage, and outcome.

Four factors are involved in the spread of infectious diseases: the microorganism, the host, the mode of transmission, and the reservoir. Each factor is considered a link in the chain of infection. A break at any point in the chain results in the infectious disease's losing its ability to spread.

Nosocomial infections are those acquired in the hospital setting. Hospitals and compromised patients provide the optimal environment for nosocomial infections. Sources of this specific type of infection include the hospital proper and the medical personnel within,

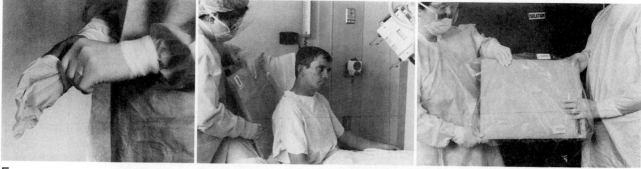

F   G   H

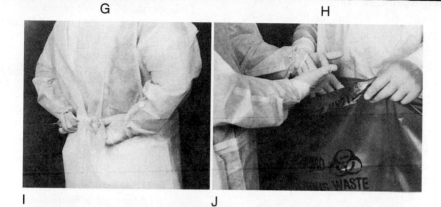

I   J

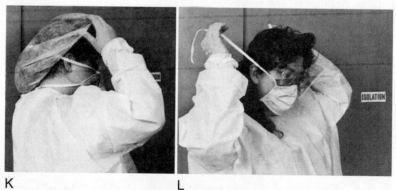

K   L

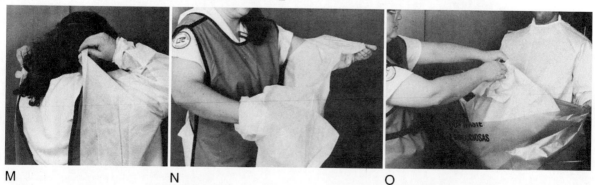

M   N   O

FIG. 16–8, cont'd *F,* Put on nonsterile gloves. *G,* Position the bagged cassette beneath the patient. *H,* Fold the protective bag, never touching the inside while an assistant removes the cassette without touching the outside of the bag. *I,* Untie the gown at waist. *J,* Remove the gloves, turning them inside out. *K,* Remove the cap. *L,* Remove the mask by holding only the ties. *M,* Untie the neck of the gown. *N,* Turn the gown inside out without touching the outside of the gown. *O,* Place the gown in the appropriate receptacle.

contaminated invasive diagnostic and therapeutic devices, and opportunistic microorganisms that are constituents of the normal flora.

The human body has mechanical, cellular, and chemical mechanisms that it uses to fight infection. The presence of the microorganisms included in the normal flora inhibits the attachment and colonization of new microbes. Chemotherapy and immunization have aided in the reduction and eradication of many infectious diseases.

Through asepsis, environmental control of infection is simple. Various chemical and physical methods can be used to achieve surgical or medical asepsis. The use of the medically aseptic hand-washing technique, standard precautions, and transmission-based precautions has contributed significantly in reducing the probability of spreading infectious diseases.

Recommendations and guidelines are issued by the HHS and the CDC. In turn, these guidelines are enforced by OSHA, part of the U.S. Department of Labor. All rules and regulations are strictly enforced and reviewed to ensure the safety of every patient and health care provider within the clinical setting.

Students and practicing technologists are continuously challenged both physically and mentally by the microbial world. In this world of newly found, life-threatening diseases, education has become the key to survival. Each health care provider must make a personal commitment to infection control so that, by collective effort, diseases can be conquered.

BIBLIOGRAPHY

Balows A: *Manual of clinical microbiology,* ed 5, Washington, DC, 1991, American Society for Microbiology.

Benson HJ: *Microbiological applications: a laboratory manual in general microbiology,* ed 5, Dubuque, Iowa, 1990, William C Brown.

Borton, D: Isolation precautions. Clearing up the confusion, *Nursing* 27:49, 1997 Jan.

Madigan MT, Martinko J: *Brock biology of microorganisms,* ed 11, Englewood Cliffs, NJ, 2005, Prentice-Hall.

Gorbach SL, Bartlett JG, Blacklow NR: *Infectious diseases,* ed 3, Philadelphia, 2003, WB Saunders.

Lennette EH, Halonen P, Murphy FA: *Laboratory diagnosis of infectious diseases: principles and practice,* ed 3, vol 2, New York, 1999, Springer-Verlag.

Linne JJ, Ringsrud KM: *Clinical laboratory science: the basics and routine techniques,* ed 4, St Louis, 1999, Mosby–Year Book.

National Safety Council: *Bloodborne pathogens training manual,* Boston, 1992, Jones and Bartlett.

Prendergraph GE, Pendergraph CB: *Handbook of phlebotomy and patient service techniques,* ed 4, Philadelphia, 1998, Lea & Febiger.

Schaechter M, Medoff G, Schlessinger D: *Mechanisms of microbial disease,* ed 3, Baltimore, 1998, Williams & Wilkins.

Volk W et al: *Essentials of medical microbiology,* ed 5, Philadelphia, 1996, JB Lippincott.

Walter JB: *An introduction to the principles of disease,* ed 3, Philadelphia, 1998, WB Saunders.

17

Aseptic Techniques

Steven B. Dowd, EdD, RT(R), (QM), (MR), (M) (CT)

Soap and water and common sense are the best disinfectants.

Sir William Osler (1849-1919)

OBJECTIVES

On completion of this chapter, the student will be able to:

1. Describe the use of a sterile drape to establish a sterile field.

2. List the steps in a surgical scrub.

3. Describe the procedures for gowning and gloving.

4. List the basic principles of sterile technique.

5. Describe the procedure for changing a dressing.

6. Provide care to a patient with a tracheostomy.

7. Provide care to a patient with chest tubes.

8. Describe the care of a patient with a urinary catheter.

9. Contrast intravenous and intraarterial lines.

10. Assist the physician in pacemaker insertion.

Angiography: roentgenographic visualization of blood vessels following the introduction of contrast material; used as a diagnostic aid in conditions such as cerebrovascular attacks (strokes) and myocardial infarctions

Arthrography: roentgenography of a joint after the injection of opaque contrast material

Atelectasis: collapse of a lung

Auscultation: act of listening for sounds within the body, chiefly for ascertaining the condition of the lungs, heart, pleura, abdomen, and other organs and for detecting pregnancy

Foley Catheter: indwelling catheter retained in the bladder by a balloon inflated with air or fluid

Lithotomy Position: patient in the dorsal decubitus position with the hips and knees flexed and the thighs abducted and externally rotated; also called dorsosacral position

Microorganisms: microscopic organisms; those of medical interest include bacteria, viruses, fungi, and protozoa

Pneumothorax: accumulation of air or gas in the pleural space, which may occur spontaneously or as a result of trauma or a pathologic process or which may be introduced deliberately

Purulent: consisting of or containing pus; associated with the formulation of or caused by pus

Serous: resembling serum, having a thin watery constitution

Sterile: aseptic; free of living microorganisms

Tracheostomy: surgical creation of an opening into the trachea through the neck; also used to refer to the creation of an opening in the anterior trachea for insertion of a tube to relieve upper-airway obstruction and to facilitate ventilation

Trendelenburg Position: position in which the patient is supine on the table or bed, the head of which is tilted downward 30 to 40 degrees, and the table or bed is angled beneath the knees

Urinary Meatus: external urethral orifice; the opening of the urethra on the body surface through which urine is discharged

Voiding Cystourethrography: radiography of the bladder and urethra in which radiographs are performed before, during, and after voiding

---

Understanding aseptic (sterile) techniques is an important part of the professional practice of the radiologic technologist. Hand washing is recognized as the first priority for proper sterile technique. The concept of asepsis was discussed in Chapter 16. Along with knowledge of asepsis, the radiologic technologist must never let his or her attitude toward asepsis become too casual. As in radiation protection, the radiologic technologist may become so familiar with equipment and procedures that some steps seem easier to omit. Sloppy aseptic technique can never be tolerated. The purpose of aseptic technique is to reduce the number of harmful **microorganisms.** Surgical asepsis is protection against infection before, during, and after surgery by using sterile technique. Medical asepsis is the removal or destruction of infected material.

Among the numerous radiologic procedures that require sterile technique are angiography, arthrography, hysterosalpingography, and radiography in the surgical environment. Other procedures described here require aseptic technique on the part of the technologist or an understanding of how aseptic technique was used for the specific procedure to improve care for patients.

STERILE DRAPING

A **sterile** field is a microorganism-free area that can receive sterile supplies. In most instances, a sterile field is established using a sterile drape. The first step in using a sterile drape is confirming that the package is sterile. If a package is not clean and dry, it is considered unsterile. If it appears to have been previously opened or the expiration date has passed, it is also considered unsterile. The procedure for opening a sterile package (e.g., one prepared in the hospital) containing a sterile drape on a surface such as a table is as follows (Fig. 17–1):

1. Place the package on the center of the surface with the top flap of the wrapper set to open away from the person opening the package.
2. Pinch the first flap on the outside of the wrapper between the thumb and index finger by reaching around (not over) the package. Some packages require that the uppermost flap at each corner be grasped. The flap should be pulled open and laid flat on the far surface.

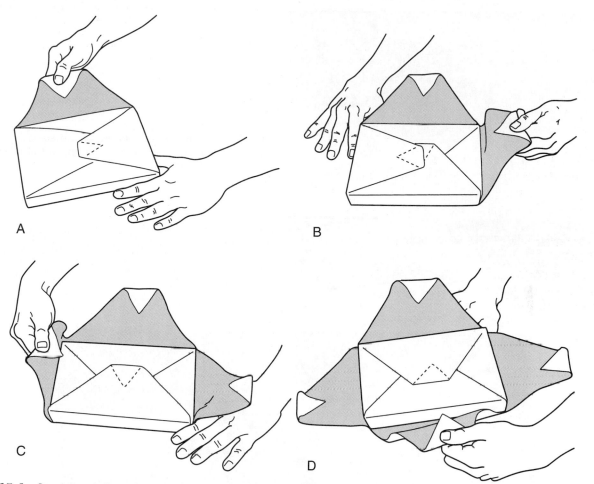

FIG. 17–1 Opening a sterile package. *A,* Opening the first flap. *B* and *C,* Opening the side flaps. *D,* Pulling the last flap by grasping the corner.

3. Use the right hand to open the right flap and the left hand to open the left flap.
4. Grasping the turned-down corner, pull the fourth and final flap. If the inner surface of any of the package touches an unsterile object, such as a sleeve, the entire pack and contents are considered unsterile and must be replaced.

A sterile package may also be opened as follows:

1. Hold the package in one hand with the top flap opening away from the person opening the package.
2. Pull the top flap well back, and hold it away from both the contents of the package and the sterile field. Using the free hand to hold the flap against the wrist of the hand holding the package is an effective technique.
3. Drop the contents gently onto the sterile field from approximately 6 inches above the field and at a slight

angle. These techniques help ensure that the package wrapping does not touch the sterile field at any time (Fig. 17–2).

Commercial packages usually have specific directions written on the package for opening. In general, available packages include those with partially sealed *corners,* in which the container is held in one hand and the flap is pulled back with the other, and those with partially sealed *edges,* in which both sides of the edge are grasped, one with each hand, and gently pulled apart (Fig. 17–3).

To establish a sterile field, the drape is plucked with one hand by the corner and opened. This corner is used to fold back the top. Then the drape is lifted out of the cover and allowed to open freely without touching anything. Another corner of the drape then is picked up carefully and laid on a clean, dry surface with the bottom farthest from the person establishing the field (Fig. 17–4).

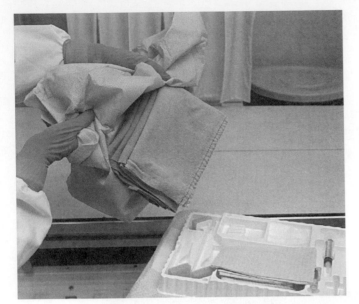

FIG. 17–2 Dropping sterile towels onto a sterile field while keeping the nonsterile wrapping well away from the sterile field.

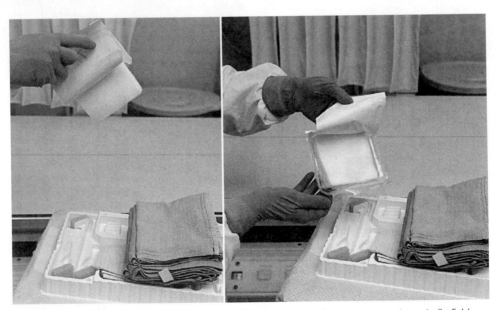

FIG. 17–3 Opening commercially prepared sterile packs to drop sponges onto a sterile field.

Necessary sterile supplies can be added to the field using the proper package-opening techniques.

Finally, sterile solutions are frequently poured into a metal or other container within the sterile field. Bottles containing sterile solutions usually are considered sterile on the inside but contaminated on the outside; thus special care is needed in pouring these solutions. Always try to use the exact amount of solution. Once opened,

the solution can be considered sterile only if it is used immediately. Once the container has been set down, it is no longer considered sterile, and a new container must be opened. Always confirm the name of the solution and its strength by checking three times. When possible, show the name to another person.

The procedure for pouring sterile solutions is as follows:

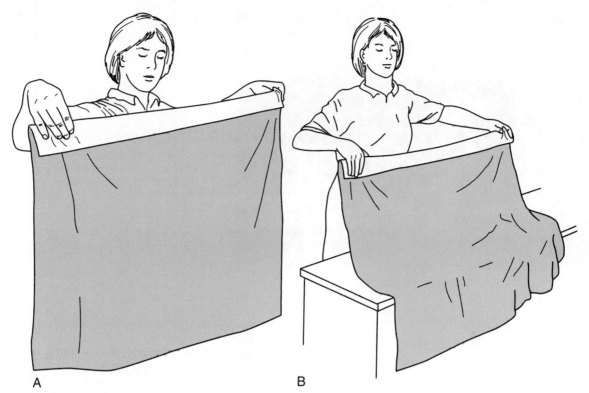

FIG. 17–4 Establishing a sterile field. *A,* Holding the drape with one hand by the corner. *B,* Folding back the top to lift the cover and laying the drape on a clean, dry surface with the bottom farthest from the person establishing the field.

1. Remove the lid or cap from the bottle; place it on an unsterile surface with the topside down immediately to ensure the sterility of the inner surface.
2. Hold the bottle with the label uppermost so that poured solution cannot stain and obscure the label.
3. With as little of the bottle as possible over the field, hold it at a height of approximately 6 inches over the bowl (Fig. 17–5).
4. Pour the solution gently so that no splashing occurs. Splashing of liquids can destroy a sterile field by allowing microorganisms to move from the unsterile tabletop through the wet drape that forms the bottom of the sterile field.

STERILE PACKS

Commonly used sterile packs include myelography, minor procedure, and various special procedure packs used for procedures such as venograms, angiograms, and lymphangiograms. Items in the typical myelography pack are shown in Fig. 17–6 and often include the following:

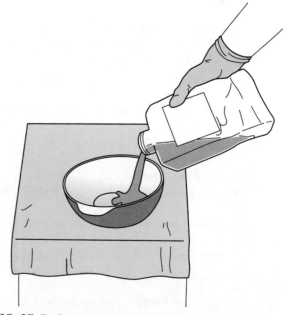

FIG. 17–5 Pouring a sterile solution into a sterile bowl on a sterile field.

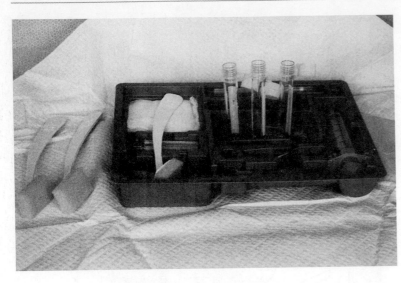

FIG. 17–6 A typical myelography pack.

- Injectable local anesthetic
- Syringes and needles of various sizes
- Sterile drape
- Collection tubes (for spinal fluid)

A minor procedure pack, used for **arthrography** and biopsies, usually contains all of the preceding items, as well as a sterile gown. Although commercially prepared **angiography** packs are available, many hospitals prefer to make up their own trays. Typical supplies might include the following:

- Needles, including three 18-gauge, one 20-gauge, one 22-gauge, and one 25-gauge (the larger gauge needles are used to inject local anesthetic)
- Plastic connector for test injections of contrast material
- One manifold (three stopcocks) for the contrast test, heparin drip, or saline flush
- Scalpel handle and no. 10 scalpel blade used for arterial cutdown techniques
- Large number of gauze pads or topper sponges
- Up to five 10-, 20-, or 30-ml Luer-Lok syringes for saline flush
- Three 10-ml Luer-Lok syringes, two for contrast tests, one for local anesthetic
- Forceps for sponges
- Six sponges for preparation of the puncture site with anesthetic
- Three stainless steel basins—one for saline solution, one for antiseptic, and one used as a waste basin—and one emesis basin

- Straight and curved clamps for arterial cutdown techniques
- Clamp to keep guidewire wrapped
- Sterile screwdriver for tightening screws on manifolds

SURGICAL SCRUBBING

Although persons performing aseptic procedures wear gloves, the skin of their hands and forearms should be cleaned routinely to reduce the number of microorganisms in case a glove tears. A surgical scrub is required before participation in many interventional studies. The purpose of the surgical hand scrub is (1) to remove debris and transient microorganisms from the hands, nails, and forearms; (2) to reduce the resident microbial count to a minimum; and (3) to inhibit rapid rebound growth of microorganisms.

The sterile scrub consists of scrubbing with soap and water and a nailbrush and often an immersion in a mild germicidal solution. Surgical scrubbing involves two basic methods: (1) the *numbered stroke method,* in which a certain number of brush strokes are used for each finger, palm, back of the hand, and the arm; and (2) the *timed scrub.* Although exact procedures and times for the scrub vary among different settings and institutions, the following can serve as a guideline for the timed scrub:

1. Be sure that scrub brushes, antiseptic soap, and nail cleaners are available.
2. Remove all jewelry, including watches.
3. Wash hands and arms with antiseptic soap.
4. Clean subungual areas with nail file.

5. Scrub the sides of each finger, between the fingers, and the back and front of the hand for 2 minutes.
6. Scrub the arm with the hands higher than the elbows. Each side of the arm is washed to 3 inches above the elbow for 1 minute.
7. Repeat the process for the other hand and arm. The hands remain above the elbows at all times.
8. Dry the hands as shown in Fig. 17–7.

STERILE GOWNING AND GLOVING

Gowns and gloves are put on after the surgical scrub. Gowning can be done in two ways: (1) self-gowning and (2) gowning another person. Sterile gowning differs from gowning for isolation in that the focus is on surgical rather than medical asepsis. Gloving can also be done in two ways: (1) self-gloving and (2) gloving another person. A sterile surface is always required for sterile gloving. Gloves have two surfaces: an inside and an outside. Before the gloves are touched, the entire glove is sterile; however, once gloving has started, the inside surface is considered nonsterile. Gloves are packaged in a paper wrapper with the palms of the gloves facing upward and the top of the glove folded over to form a 2- to 3-inch cuff. The exposed cuff is part of the inside of the glove and is therefore part of the nonsterile side.

Self-Gowning (Fig. 17–8)

1. Standing approximately 12 inches from the sterile area, pick up the gown by the folded edges and lift it directly up from the package. The gown is folded so that the outside faces away.
2. Stepping back from the table, make sure no objects are near the gown. Holding the gown at the shoulders, allow it to unfold gently. Do not shake the gown.
3. Place the hands inside the armholes and guide each arm through the sleeves by raising and spreading the arms.
4. An unsterile assistant can adjust the gown by standing behind and reaching inside the sleeves, grasping them, and pulling gently.
5. For the open gloving technique, pull the sleeves over the hands. For the closed gloving technique, keep the hands and fingers covered by the sterile gown.
6. An assistant fastens the back and waistband of the gown.

After the gown is on, only the sleeves and front of the gown down to the waist are considered sterile. To main-

tain sterile technique once in sterile gown and gloves, persons must pass each other back to back.

Self-Gloving

Self-gloving can be done using a closed or an open gloving technique. It is performed after gowning or, in the case of the open gloving technique, may be used during sterile procedures that do not require donning a sterile gown. All jewelry should have been removed. The glove package should be opened facing the person who is going to wear the gloves with the right glove on the right side.

CLOSED TECHNIQUE (Fig. 17–9)

1. After donning a sterile gown with the fingers still inside the cuff of the gown, pick up the glove and lay it palm-down over the cuff of the gown. The fingers of the glove should face toward you.
2. Working through the gown sleeve, grasp the cuff of the glove and bring it over the open cuff of the sleeve.
3. Unroll the glove cuff so that it covers the sleeve cuff.
4. Pull the glove on by grasping the glove cuff and advancing the hand into the glove.
5. Proceed with the opposite hand, using the same technique. Never allow the bare hand to contact the gown cuff edge or outside of glove.
6. The fingers are adjusted until comfortable.

OPEN TECHNIQUE (Fig. 17–10)

1. Pick up the glove by its inside cuff with one hand. Do not touch the outside surface of the glove or the glove wrapper.
2. Slide the glove onto the opposite bare hand leaving the cuff down.
3. With the gloved (and now sterile) hand, pick up the other glove by reaching under the cuff. Touch only the outside surface of the glove with the sterile gloved hand.
4. The glove is then pulled onto the hand without touching the inside surface of the glove, which is actually the outside surface of the folded cuff.

Gowning Another Person (Fig. 17–11)

1. The sterile person picks up the gown by the neckband, holds it at arm's length, and allows it to unfold.
2. The gown is held by the shoulder seams with the outside facing the sterile person.

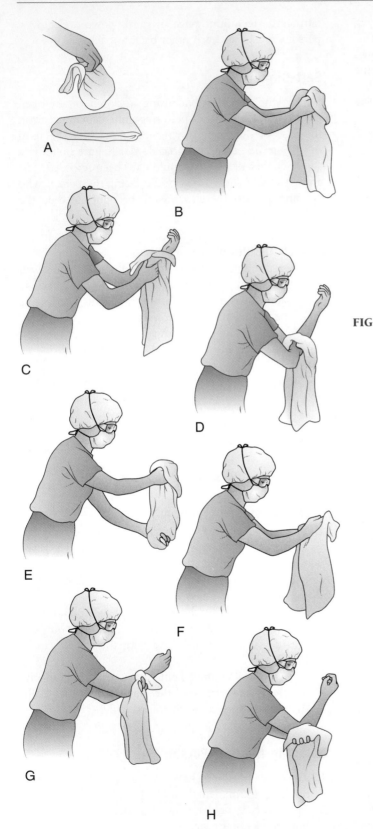

FIG. 17–7 Drying the hands and arms after a surgical scrub. *A,* Pick up a sterile towel from the table, being careful not to drip water on the gown beneath it. *B,* Fold the towel lengthwise. *C,* Use one end of the towel only to dry one hand. *D,* Rotate the arm as you proceed to dry it, working from the wrist to the elbow. Do not allow the towel to contact the scrub suit. *E* and *F,* After the arm is dried, bring the dry hand to the opposite end of the towel and begin drying the other hand. *G,* Dry the arm using the blotting rotating motion. *H,* Proceed to the elbow. The towel must be discarded in the linen hamper or kick bucket. (From Fuller JR: *Surgical technology: principles and practice,* ed 4, Philadelphia, 2005, Elsevier Saunders, p 153.)

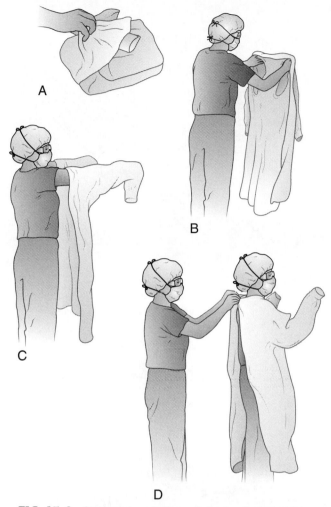

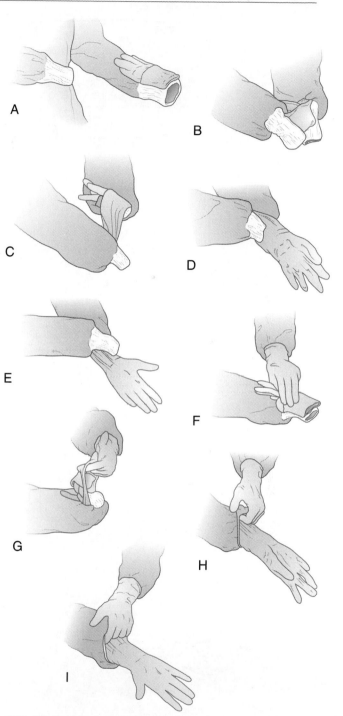

FIG. 17–8 Self-gowning. *A,* Grasp the gown firmly and bring it away from the table. It has been folded so that the outside faces away. *B,* Holding the gown at the shoulders, allow it to unfold gently. Do not shake the gown. *C,* Place hands inside the armholes and guide each arm through the sleeves by raising and spreading the arms. Do not allow hands to slide outside cuff of gown. *D,* The circulator assists by pulling the gown over the shoulders and tying it. (From Fuller JR: *Surgical technology: principles and practice,* ed 4, Philadelphia, 2005, Elsevier Saunders, p 154.)

FIG. 17–9 Self-gloving, closed technique. *A,* Lay the glove palm-down over the cuff of the gown. The fingers of the glove face toward you. *B* and *C,* Working through the gown sleeve, grasp the cuff of the glove and bring it over the open cuff of the sleeve. *D* and *E,* Unroll the glove cuff so that it covers the sleeve cuff. *F* through *I,* Proceed with the opposite hand, using the same technique. Never allow the bare hand to contact the gown cuff edge or outside of glove. (From Fuller JR: *Surgical technology: principles and practice,* ed 4, Philadelphia, 2005, Elsevier Saunders, p 155.)

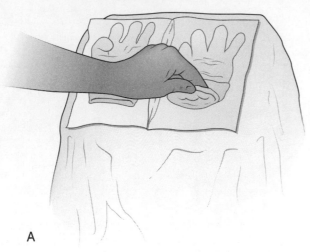

A

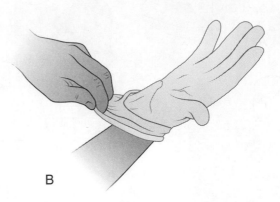

B

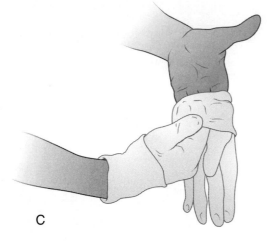

C

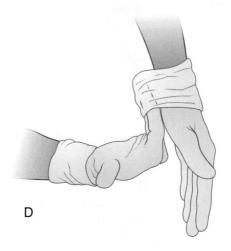

D

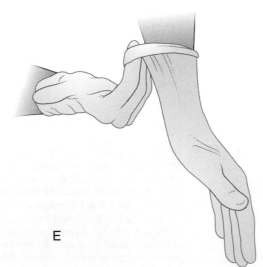

E

FIG. 17–10 Self-gloving, open technique. *A,* Pick up the glove by its inside cuff with one hand. Do not touch the glove wrapper with the bare hand. *B,* Slide the glove onto the opposite hand. Leave the cuff down. *C,* Using the partially gloved hand, slide the fingers into the outer side of the opposite glove cuff. *D,* Slide the hand into the glove and unroll the cuff. *E,* With the gloved hand, slide the fingers under the outer edge of the opposite cuff and unroll it gently, using the same technique. (From Fuller JR: *Surgical technology: principles and practice,* ed 4, Philadelphia, 2005, Elsevier Saunders, p 156.)

3. The sterile gloves are protected by placing both hands under the back panel of the gown's shoulder.
4. The arms are slipped into the sleeves in a downward motion, sliding the gown up to the mid upper arms.
5. A nonsterile circulator pulls the gown up and fastens the back and waistband of the gown.
6. Gently pull the cuff back over the person's hands being careful that your gloved hands do not touch the bare hands.

Gloving Another Person (Fig. 17–12)

1. The sterile person opens the package and picks up the right glove and places the palm away from him or herself. Slide the fingers under the glove cuff and spread them so that a wide opening is created. Keep the thumbs under the cuff.
2. The person thrusts his or her hand into the glove. Having an extremely good grasp on the cuff is important because considerable force is exerted when the hand is pushed down into the tight glove.
3. Gently release the cuff while rolling it over the wrist.
4. Proceed with the left glove using the same technique.

The procedure for removing gloves aseptically is also important to avoid contamination. The procedure to avoid touching the outside portion of the glove is shown in Fig. 17–13.

STERILE PROCEDURES

Box 17-1 lists the basic principles of sterile technique. The field includes the patient, the table and other furniture covered with sterile drapes, and the personnel wearing sterile attire.

Dressing Changes

Dressings are best changed in a team setting with another technologist or health care worker. The physician is responsible for ordering dressing changes and reapplication. Be sure to secure privacy, explain the procedure to the patient, and secure consent before beginning the procedure. The equipment needed is as follows:

STERILE
Disposable gloves
Pack containing scissors, forceps, sterile towel, dressings, cotton-tipped swabs, and solution cup
Antiseptic solution and sterile saline

BOX 17-1 Basic Principles of Sterile Technique

Only sterile items are used in sterile fields.

If in doubt about the sterility of an object, then consider it unsterile. An unsterile object should be removed, covered, or replaced.

A sterile field must be continually monitored to be considered sterile.

Create sterile fields as close to the time of use as possible.

Sterile persons should avoid unsterile areas.

Anything below the level of the table or the level of the waist, as well as the undersurface of the drape, is considered unsterile. Any item that falls below this area is considered contaminated.

Gowns are considered sterile on the sleeves and the front from the waist up. The back of the gown and the area below the waist are considered unsterile.

Persons in sterile gown and gloves must pass each other back to back.

A sterile person may touch only what is sterile.

Unsterile persons cannot reach above or over a sterile field.

Sterile materials must be kept dry. Moisture permits contamination. Packages that become wet must be resterilized or discarded.

If a solution soaks through a sterile field to a nonsterile field, then the wet area may be redraped.

Sterile gloves must be kept in sight and above waist level.

UNSTERILE
Plastic bag for discarded dressings
Properly sized adhesive
Pads to protect surrounding area from secretions

Gowns are recommended by many texts if the wound is **purulent**; in a standard precautions environment, gowns are required at all times.

All dressings are treated as though they are infected. Do not touch a dressing with bare hands. The procedure for changing a dressing is as follows:

1. The hands are washed, and patient privacy and consent are obtained. The adhesive tape surrounding the dressing must be removed. This procedure is often painful, and a solvent such as baby oil might

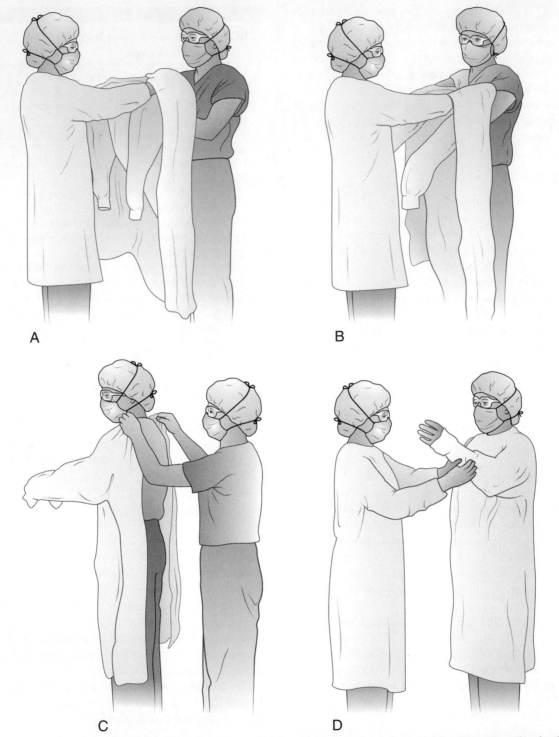

FIG. 17–11 Gowning another person. *A,* Grasp the gown so that the outside faces toward you. Holding the gown at the shoulders, cuff your hands under the gown's shoulders. *B,* The person steps forward and places his or her arms in the sleeves. Slide the gown up to the mid upper arms. *C,* The circulator assists in pulling the gown up and tying it. *D,* Gently pull the cuffs back over the person's hands. Be careful that your gloved hands do not touch his or her bare hands. (From Fuller JR: *Surgical technology: principles and practice,* ed 4, Philadelphia, 2005, Elsevier Saunders, p 157.)

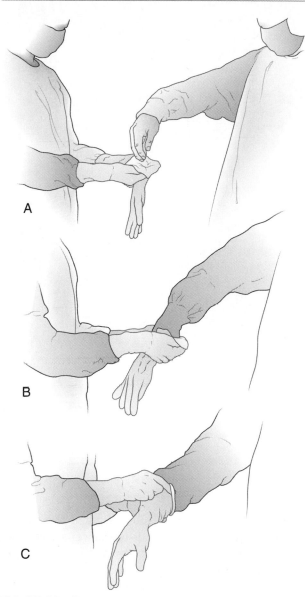

FIG. 17–12 Gloving another person. *A,* Pick up the right glove and place the palm away from you. Slide the fingers under the glove cuff and spread them so a wide opening is created. Keep thumbs under the cuff. *B,* The person thrusts his or her hands into the glove. Do not release the glove yet. *C,* Gently release the cuff (do not let the cuff snap sharply) while unrolling it over the wrist. Proceed with the left glove, using the same technique. (From Fuller JR: *Surgical technology: principles and practice,* ed 4, Philadelphia, 2005, Elsevier Saunders, p 158.)

be needed to loosen the tape. The amount of solvent should be limited to avoid contaminating the wound.

2. The dressing is removed with forceps or gloved hands, wrapped, and placed in the plastic bag. If the dressing does not come off easily, then an appropriate person (e.g., department nurse, department supervisor, physician) should be contacted for additional instructions or to remove the dressing.

3. For reapplication, sterile technique is followed. The hands are washed, and the sterile towel is opened to use as a sterile field on which to place sterile dressings. The dressings are opened and placed on the sterile towel.

4. The tape is cut into the lengths that will be needed. Because the tape is not sterile, it is placed near but not on the sterile field.

5. Gloves are put on and the dressing is applied. The gloves are removed and the dressing is secured with the adhesive tape. The hands are washed again, the patient is covered again, and the waste is discarded according to the institutional policy.

Tracheostomies

A **tracheostomy** is an operation performed under sterile technique that involves incising the skin over the trachea and then making a surgical wound in the trachea. This procedure provides for an airway during upper-airway obstruction. It is used in emergency situations and to replace the airway provided by an endotracheal tube that has been in place for several weeks. To prevent skin breakdown, tracheostomies are always covered with a dressing.

If at all possible, the first task in providing care to a patient with a tracheostomy is to establish communication. This provision usually consists of yes and no questions, hand signals, and simple sign language. Written communication methods are used less often than verbal methods. Because these patients are often extremely ill, they have difficulty in using written communication and little need for complicated messages. In some cases, after a few days, the tracheostomy may be changed to the *talking type,* which will allow for speech.

The technologist caring for the tracheostomy patient must also be sensitive to unmet and inexpressible needs and the need to keep the patient's anxiety level low. Thus these patients often have a great need to have procedures explained and repeated. A technologist may take a lot of time to explain a portable chest radiograph to a patient the

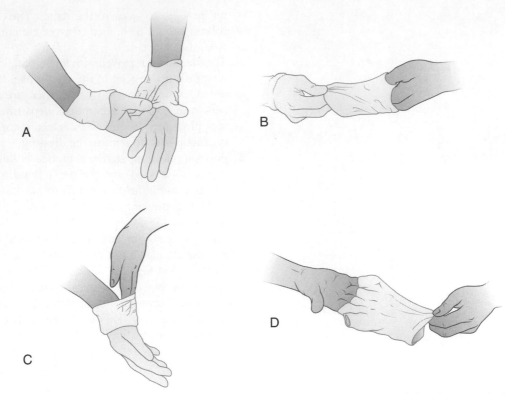

FIG. 17–13 Removing contaminated gloves aseptically. *A*, Grasp the edge of the glove. *B*, Unroll the glove over the hand. Discard the glove (not shown). *C*, With the bare hand, grasp the opposite glove cuff on its inside surface. *D*, Remove the glove by inverting it over the hand. Discard the glove (not shown). (From Fuller JR: *Surgical technology: principles and practice*, ed 4, Philadelphia, 2005, Elsevier Saunders, p 160.)

first time and then slip into a routine of "We're going to take your chest x-ray now" each subsequent morning. The patient may have forgotten, in the midst of all the other procedures performed, exactly what that means and then may consciously or unconsciously resist the procedure.

To minimize the possibility of infection, the technologist should not touch a tracheostomy except under conditions of sterile technique. A tracheostomy must be suctioned often to remove secretions. This task is usually the responsibility of the respiratory therapist or nurse taking care of the patient, although in certain situations (i.e., emergencies), this responsibility may become the technologist's. The patient must be well aerated with 5 to 10 breaths of oxygen before suctioning, which can be accomplished using an Ambu bag hooked to an oxygen source. In addition, before suctioning, the patency of the suction catheter must be tested by aspirating normal saline through the catheter. The procedure for suctioning is as follows:

1. Insert the catheter in the stoma without suction until the patient coughs or until resistance is met. Then withdraw the catheter approximately 1 cm before beginning suctioning.
2. Apply suction intermittently and withdraw the catheter in a rotating motion. Activate suctioning by placing the thumb over the hole in the suction line to cause the suction to pull from the end of the tube where it is placed in the patient's body (Fig. 17–14).
3. Assess the airway by **auscultation** of the lungs. Use a stethoscope to listen to the sounds of inspiration and expiration over the chest wall. Breath sounds are the result of free movement of air into and out of the bronchial tree. The duration, pitch, and intensity of sounds indicate whether breathing is normal or abnormal.
4. Repeat the procedure until the airway is clear. Never suction for longer than 15 seconds, and allow the patient to rest in between.

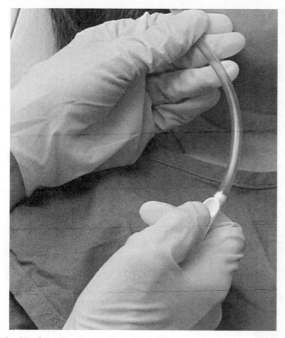

FIG. 17–14 Suction tube shows thumbhole for activation of suctioning.

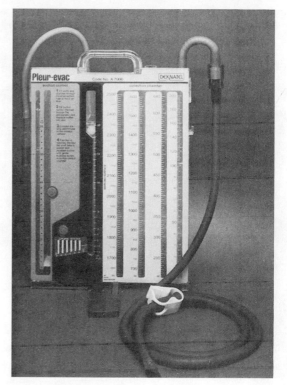

FIG. 17–15 Chest drainage systems.

In some patients, the distance between the skin and trachea is too great to be safely bridged by the standard tracheostomy tube (e.g., obese patients). In such instances, an extra-long tube may be used. It is a single-lumen tube and does not have an inner cannula to remove for cleaning. Given that the tube is of a variable length, its position may be checked radiographically to avoid main-stem ventilation.

Chest Tubes

Chest tubes are used to remove fluid, blood, and air from the pleural cavity. They assist in reinflating collapsed lungs (**atelectasis**) and alleviating **pneumothorax** (i.e., air in the thoracic cavity). They are also used in cases of thoracotomy and open-heart surgery. Normally, the pleural cavity contains no air or blood, containing instead a thin layer of lubricant that allows the pleurae to slide and move over one another without friction.

Chest drainage systems have three compartments to which chest tubes are attached (Fig. 17–15). The first compartment is the collection chamber, which collects any fluid leaving the lung. The second compartment is the water seal chamber, which contains water and prevents air from the atmosphere from entering the cavity through the chest tube. The concept is similar to that of a drinking straw through which air can be blown (e.g., into a glass of water), but none can return. The third compartment is the suction control chamber, which also contains water, the amount of which regulates the amount of suction. This suction removes unwanted air or fluid from the pleural cavity. Some units have an additional fourth chamber, a water seal vented to the atmosphere to prevent potential pressure buildup.

Radiographers often perform chest radiography, especially portable procedures, before and after the insertion of chest tubes to ensure proper placement. Fig. 17–16 shows proper placement of chest tubes on a portable chest radiograph. Radiographers also make chest films to confirm that the tubes can be removed; these are sometimes taken in the radiology department. An initial radiograph confirms full lung expansion; a second is performed 2 hours after clamping to verify continued expansion. A third film is often obtained

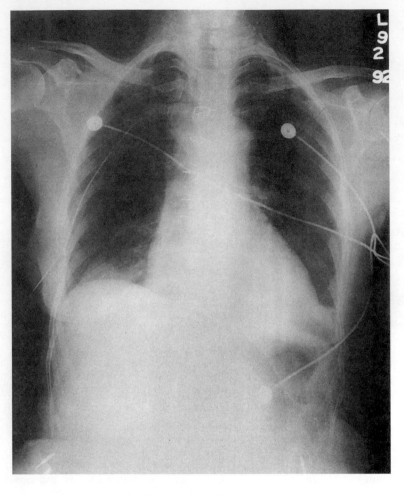

FIG. 17–16   Radiograph verifying proper placement of chest tube in the right upper lobe of the lung. (Courtesy University of Alabama at Birmingham Hospital, Birmingham, Alabama.)

after removal of chest tubes again to confirm full lung expansion.

Radiographers must be careful when entering and leaving the patient's room after the tubes have been inserted; the tubes can be pulled from the body if caught by a mobile x-ray unit or tugged roughly during handling of the patient or cassette. Patients also may come to the radiology department by stretcher or wheelchair if they have had the chest tubes in place for a long time. *The exterior assembly of the chest tubes must always remain lower than the patient's chest.* Caution is necessary when moving and positioning the patient to prevent compromising the integrity of the tubes. In addition, if the patient is in the department for a longer period (greater than 1 hour), then drainage of excess in 100 cc per hour should be reported, as well as any change from a **serous** fluid to a darker red color.

Urinary Catheters

Urinary catheterization is the insertion of a tube into the bladder using aseptic technique. The two main types of urinary catheters are the **Foley catheter** (a retention balloon type) and the straight type catheter (Fig. 17–17). On insertion of the Foley catheter, the balloon is filled with sterile water to hold the catheter in place. Any catheter that remains in place is also called an *indwelling catheter.* Urinary catheters can be used to do the following:

- Empty the bladder (e.g., before surgery, radiologic or other examinations, or childbirth)
- Relieve retention of urine or bypass obstruction
- Irrigate the bladder or introduce drugs
- Permit accurate measuring of urine output
- Relieve incontinence

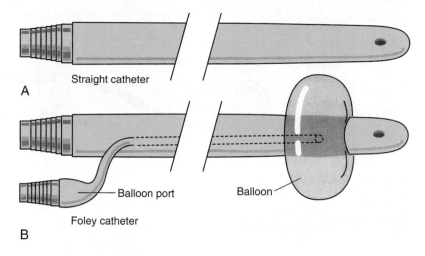

FIG. 17–17 The two main types of urinary catheters: straight *(A)*, Foley *(B)*.

Sizes of catheters range from 8 to 18 in even numbers based on the French system. This system indicates the outer diameter of the catheter. Each unit on this scale is 0.33 mm; thus catheters range in diameter from approximately 2.6 to 5.9 mm. Choose a larger size when possible.

Because a urinary catheter can interrupt the body's defense mechanism against disease, a variety of catheters are available. Plastic catheters, for example, are suitable for short-term use only. Latex catheters can be used for 2 to 3 weeks and polyvinyl chloride catheters for 4 to 6 weeks, whereas the expensive pure silicone catheters are used only for long-term catheterization of 2 to 3 months.

The urine collection bag should be kept low (below the level of the bladder) to prevent reflux of urine back into the bladder. Failure to do so can lead to infection. Keeping the collection bag low also facilitates drainage from the bladder by gravity. Bags should never drag on the floor. When transferring patients by wheelchair or stretcher, ensure that the drainage bag and tubing do not become entangled in wheels or caught on passing objects.

If the technologist empties the urine collection bag, then output must be measured and recorded, unless otherwise noted. Do not forget to reclamp the stopcock after the bag has been emptied. In many cases, the patient's intake of fluids is also being recorded; if the patient is given a drink of water or any other fluid, then it should be recorded in the patient chart along with the recorded output. Always check with the nursing unit whenever a question of recording intake and output exists.

In most instances, technologists do not catheterize patients, although this practice varies depending on the setting. In some institutions, the radiographer might be responsible for catheterizing a patient undergoing a voiding cystogram as an outpatient. The equipment needed to perform urinary catheterization consists of a sterile catheter, a sterile collecting bag, a syringe with sterile water or saline, and a catheterization kit or the following supplies:

- Sterile gloves
- Antiseptic solution
- Sterile cotton balls and sterile forceps
- Lubricant (water-soluble jelly)
- Container to receive urine
- Sterile drape for sterile field

The procedure for performing urinary catheterization is as follows:

1. Wash hands, provide for patient privacy, explain the procedure, and secure consent.
2. Place female patients in the **lithotomy position;** position male patients supine and expose the genitalia.
3. Open the kit and put on the gloves, which will remain sterile during the entire procedure.
4. Place the sterile drape around the penis for a male patient or under the buttocks for a female patient.
5. If a Foley catheter is being used, test-inflate the balloon by injecting a small amount (approximately 1 ml) of sterile water into the balloon port of the catheter. If the balloon holds, then deflate it. If it fails to hold, then obtain a new Foley catheter.
6. Pour antiseptic over the cotton balls.
7. Coat the catheter tip with sterile lubricant.
8. Expose the **urinary meatus** using the nondominant hand. This hand is no longer considered sterile.

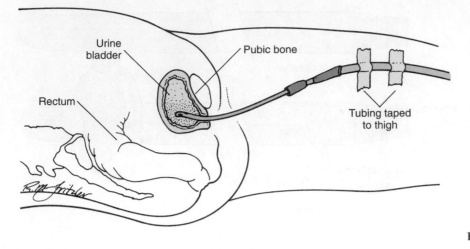

FIG. 17–18 Proper placement of a urinary catheter in a female patient. (Modified from Craig M: *Essentials of sonography and patient care,* ed 2, Philadelphia, 2006, Elsevier Saunders.)

9. With female patients, separate the labia majora and minora. For male patients, hold the penis with the foreskin retracted.

10. Clean the urinary meatus with a cotton ball held by forceps. For men, circle the urinary meatus once and repeat. For women, wipe the labia minora from top to bottom, discard the cotton, and then clean the urinary meatus from top to bottom. The labia or foreskin must not contaminate the meatus before or after cleansing.

11. Insert the catheter slowly with the dominant hand until urine flows. For women, this distance is approximately 0.5 inch (Fig. 17–18); for men,

it is approximately 8 inches (Fig. 17–19). Always apply gentle pressure, and never force a catheter.

12. Reattach the syringe to the balloon port and fill the balloon. A light tug on the catheter ensures that the balloon is holding the catheter in place.

The radiologic technologist is often responsible for removing a urinary catheter after procedures such as **voiding cystourethrograms.** The materials needed to remove an indwelling catheter are a basin, such as an emesis basin, scissors, and several paper towels. The procedure is as follows:

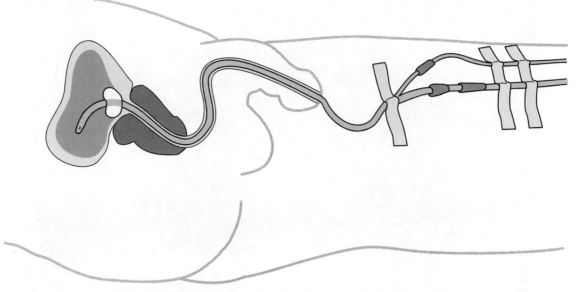

FIG. 17–19   Proper placement of a urinary catheter in a male patient.

1. Wash hands, provide for privacy, explain the procedure to the patient, and secure consent.
2. Uncover the patient and place the basin under the catheter valve. Cut the tip of the balloon valve with the scissors, and allow the water from the balloon to drain into the basin.
3. Once the flow of water has ceased, place the towels under the catheter and pull gently. Stop and notify a physician or nurse if any resistance is noted.
4. When the catheter has been completely removed, wrap it in the towels, cover the patient, and discard the catheter.

Another type of urinary catheter is the *suprapubic catheter,* a closed drainage system inserted approximately 1 inch above the symphysis pubis into the distended bladder. The procedure is performed with the patient under general anesthesia. If the catheter is to be retained in place, then it is sutured to the skin of the abdomen. Reasons for inserting a suprapubic catheter include the need for long-term catheterization, urethral injury or obstruction, and following some gynecologic surgeries.

Male patients may also have a condom catheter, a specially designed condom with a catheter at the end attached to a collecting bag. This device allows an incontinent male patient the use of a catheter without the permanence or inconvenience of a Foley or straight catheter. This type of catheter is susceptible to infection at the tip of the penis and requires regular cleaning, care, and changing of the condom sleeve.

Intravenous and Intraarterial Lines

Sterile technique is required for the insertion of lines (catheters) into veins and arteries. These lines are also called *central venous and arterial lines.* Intravenous lines are inserted for a variety of reasons, including the introduction of medications and intravenous fluids and the measurement of central venous pressure. The Swan-Ganz catheter, a specific type of intravenous catheter, is used to measure the pumping ability of the heart and other heart parameters. Other types of venous lines include the Intracath, Hickman, Broviac, and Arrow-Howes triple lumen. Arterial lines include the radial arterial and femoral arterial. These lines are typically used for drawing blood and measuring blood pressure.

When performing special radiologic procedures, the radiologic technologist may encounter patients with arterial and venous lines in place. In addition, fluoroscopy and portable chest radiography are often used to verify placement of the lines. The portable chest radiograph is also used to assess for pneumothorax. Gloves, masks, and gowns are typically worn. The patient is usually in the **Trendelenburg position** when the line is placed. Fig. 17–20 demonstrates correct placement of a Swan-Ganz catheter.

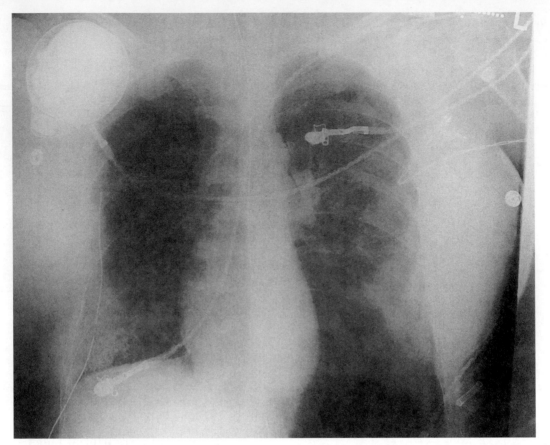

FIG. 17–20 Radiograph verifying proper placement of a Swan-Ganz line. (Also note pacemaker and chest tube.) (Courtesy University of Alabama at Birmingham Hospital, Birmingham, Alabama.)

Pacemakers

Permanent pacemakers are electromechanical devices inserted under the patient's skin to regulate the heart rate. Patients with symptomatic bradycardia (a slow heart rate) are the most likely candidates for permanent pacemakers. A pacemaker can prevent bradycardia by sensing the heartbeats of a patient and pacing the heart when it does not initiate a heartbeat on its own.

Pacemaker units are approximately 1 inch wide, in diameter and thickness, weighing just a little over 1 ounce. The unit consists of a pulse generator and accompanying circuitry and is connected to a lead. The tip of the lead contains a metal electrode that is put into contact with the heart. The electrode senses heartbeats and can also produce an electrical impulse to make the heart contract.

Using aseptic technique, the surgeon makes an incision at the level of the pectoral fascia, secures percuta-

neous access to a vein, and forms a pocket for the pulse generator. Before inserting the pacing lead, a needle and syringe are inserted into the subclavian vein for verification. Then a guidewire is inserted through the needle to establish a pathway through the vein. The role of the radiographer is to assist the physician in placement through fluoroscopy. The position of the guidewire is verified under fluoroscopy. Then an introducer sheath is used to place the pacing lead into the subclavian vein. Under fluoroscopy, the lead is advanced into the right atrium, the introducer sheath is withdrawn, and the lead is positioned in the apex of the right ventricle. At this point, the radiographer's role in the procedure is usually complete.

Temporary pacemakers are also usually connected to a transvenous pacing electrode, but the pacemaker is external to the patient's body. The fluoroscopic technique is similar to the permanent pacemaker insertion.

The patient with a pacemaker may be scheduled for magnetic resonance imaging, and this is possible so long as special care procedures are followed. Special care is also needed for the patient with a pacemaker undergoing radiation therapy; the pacemaker must be shielded from the radiation field, otherwise damage to the circuit may occur.

Portable and Surgical Radiography

Radiography in the surgical environment requires strict attention to sterile technique. Specific guidelines are difficult to give because procedures vary greatly between surgeons and facilities. The one constant is the existence of a *sterile corridor,* the area between the patient drape and the instrument table. Radiographic cassettes are sometimes positioned under the table through a tunnel device; in other cases, they are enclosed in sterile covers and positioned by the physician.

In most cases, especially at first, the radiography student observes procedures performed in surgery. In some cases, the machinery is left outside the room until right before the procedure; in other cases, the surgeon or procedure demands that a setup occur before the operation begins.

NEONATAL PORTABLE RADIOGRAPHY. For radiography of the neonate, two methods of gonadal shielding are accepted: (1) *contact,* which places lead directly on the infant's gonads, and (2) *shadow,* which hangs a piece of lead in the beam (or places a piece of lead on the isolette), casting a shadow in the collimator light. Each method has advantages and disadvantages. Shadow shielding, for example, requires low levels of ambient lighting for proper use. Contact shielding has the greatest potential for cross-infection.

Why is the potential for cross-infection so important? Sepsis and nosocomial infections are recognized as major threats that result in significant morbidity and mortality each year in the neonatal unit. Thus, in neonatal radiography, maintaining asepsis as much as possible is important. The problem of cross-infection might be handled by keeping multiple pieces of lead in the wards and sterilizing after use, covering the lead with a pillow case or other protective covering or assigning a piece of lead to each crib and cleaning after each patient. Each institution will probably decide, based on a number of factors, which method it finds to be the most usable.

USE OF THE C-ARM IN SURGERY. The use of the C-arm in surgery requires increased attention to maintaining a sterile field. Basically, three approaches can be used to maintaining a sterile field, according to Bontrager (2001).

The most common approach is draping the image intensifier and C-arm with what is known as a *snap cover.* A tension band is *snapped* in place when the image intensifier and C-arm are covered with a sterile cloth or bags. This approach allows the physician to manipulate the C-arm while maintaining a sterile field.

Hip pinnings or femur roddings may use an approach known as the *shower curtain* approach. On the patient's affected side, a sterile clear plastic sheet is suspended from a long horizontal metal bar attached to two vertical suspending rods. An opening is located in the middle of the sheet, which is attached using a special adhesive to the patient, allowing access to the surgical site.

A third but less common approach is to drape the site with an additional sterile cloth. The C-arm then is brought over the anatomic area of interest. When the C-arm is no longer needed, it is removed, as is the cloth. This approach is a *stop-gap* measure in many cases and is useful only when the physician does not need to manipulate the C-arm.

SUMMARY

The purpose of aseptic technique is to reduce the number of harmful microorganisms. Surgical asepsis is protection against infection before, during, and after surgery by using sterile technique. Medical asepsis is the removal or destruction of infected material. A variety of radiologic procedures require sterile technique.

A sterile field is a microorganism-free area that can receive sterile supplies. The patient is the center of the sterile field. The field includes the patient, the table and other furniture covered with sterile drapes, and the personnel wearing sterile attire.

Commonly used sterile packs include myelography, minor procedure, and special procedure packs. Minor procedure packs are used for arthrography and biopsy.

The purpose of the surgical hand scrub is to remove debris and transient microorganisms from the hands, nails, and forearms; to reduce the resident microbial count to a minimum; and to inhibit rapid rebound growth of microorganisms.

Gowns and gloves are put on after the surgical scrub. Gowning can be done in two ways: self-gowning and gowning another person. Sterile gowning differs from gowning for isolation in that the focus is on surgical rather than medical asepsis. Gloving can also be done in two ways: self-gloving and gloving another person.

All dressings are treated as though they are infected and are not touched with bare hands. Dressings are best changed with an assistant.

A tracheostomy involves incising the skin over the trachea and then making a surgical wound in the trachea. This procedure provides for an airway during tracheal obstruction. If at all possible, the first task in providing care to a patient with a tracheostomy is to establish communication.

Chest tubes are used to remove fluid, blood, and air from the pleural cavity. Special caution is needed when dealing with a patient with chest tubes to keep the drainage system below the chest and to maintain the integrity of the tube.

Urinary catheterization is the insertion of a tube into the bladder using aseptic technique. The two main types of catheters are the Foley catheter (a retention balloon type) and the straight type catheter.

Intravenous and intraarterial lines are inserted for a variety of reasons, including the introduction of medications and pressure measurements. The radiographer may assist the physician in determining the placement of the line with fluoroscopy or a portable chest radiograph.

Pacemakers are electromechanical devices inserted under the patient's skin to regulate the heart rate. Pacemakers are further subdivided into permanent, which are inserted in a pocket of skin, and temporary, which are placed outside the patient's body. Both types use a transvenous-pacing electrode that is monitored on fluoroscopy for proper placement.

Surgical radiography procedures vary greatly between surgeons and institutions. The one consistency is existence of a sterile corridor, the area between the patient drape and the instrument table.

BIBLIOGRAPHY

American Thoracic Society: Tracheostomy, 2002. Available at *http://www.thoracic.org*.

Askin DF: Bacterial and fungal infections in the neonate, J Obstet Gynecol Neonatal Nurs 24:635, 1995.

Ballinger P, Frank ED: Merrill's atlas of radiographic positions and radiologic procedures, ed 1, vol 1, St Louis, 2003, Mosby.

Bontrager KL, Lampignano JP: Textbook of radiographic positioning and related anatomy, ed 6, St Louis, 2005, Mosby.

Craig M: Introduction to ultrasonography and patient care, Philadelphia, 1993, WB Saunders.

Donowitz LG: Nosocomial infection in neonatal intensive care units, Am J Infect Control 17:250, 1989.

Dugan L: What you need to know about permanent pacemakers, Nursing 21(6):46, 1991.

Ehrlich RA, McCloskey ED, Daly J: Patient care in radiography, ed 6, St Louis, 2004, Mosby.

Fuller JR: Surgical technology: principles and practice, Philadelphia, 1981, WB Saunders.

Goodman LR, Putnam CE, eds: Intensive care radiology: imaging of the critically ill, St Louis, 1978, Mosby.

Kirkwood P: Ask the experts—care of chest tubes. Critical Care Nurse, August 2002. Available at *http://www.findarticles.com*.

Kozier B, Erb G, Olivieri R: Fundamentals of nursing: concepts, process, and practice, ed 4, Menlo Park, Calif, 1991, Addison-Wesley.

Levitsky MG, Cairo JM, Hall SM: Introduction to respiratory care, Philadelphia, 1990, WB Saunders.

Marlowe JE: Surgical radiography, Baltimore, 1983, University Park Press.

Rees-Williams C, Meyrick M, Jones M: Making sense of urinary catheters, Nurs Times 84:46, 1988.

Snopek AM: Fundamentals of special radiographic procedures, ed 4, Philadelphia, 1999, WB Saunders.

Strodtbeck F: Viral infections of the newborn, J Obstet Gynecol Neonatal Nurs 24:659, 1995.

Torres LS: Basic medical techniques and patient care for radiologic technologists, ed 6, Philadelphia, 2003, JB Lippincott.

18

Nonaseptic Techniques

Steven B. Dowd, EdD, RT(R), (QM), (MR), (M), (CT)

As it takes two to make a quarrel, so it takes two to make a disease, the microbe and its host.

Charles Chapin
The Principles of Epidemiology

OBJECTIVES

On completion of this chapter, the student will be able to:

1. Describe the insertion, care, and removal of nasogastric tubes.

2. Assist a patient with the use of the male urinal.

3. Assist a patient with a bedpan.

4. Describe the common types of enemas.

5. Describe the procedure for a cleansing enema.

6. State the need for patient teaching regarding the barium enema—preparation, procedural, and postprocedural.

7. Differentiate between the single-contrast and double-contrast barium enemas.

8. Describe the procedure for a colostomy barium enema.

9. State the needs of a colostomy patient undergoing a barium enema.

GLOSSARY

Barium: bulky, fine white powder, without odor or taste and free from grittiness; used as a contrast medium in roentgenography of the digestive tract

Bedpan: vessel for receiving the urinary and fecal discharges of a patient unable to leave his or her bed

Colostomy: surgical creation of an opening between the colon and the surface of the body; also used to refer to the opening, or stoma, so created

Defecation: evacuation of fecal material from the intestines

Emesis Basin: kidney-shaped vessel for the collection of vomitus

Enema: a liquid injected or to be injected into the rectum

Enterostomal Therapist: health professional (usually a nurse) with special training and certification in the care of ostomies and related concerns

Flatus: gas or air evacuated through the anus

Fowler's Position: position in which the patient's head is raised 18 or 20 inches above the flat position; the knees are also raised

Low-Residue Diet: diet that gives the least possible fecal residue, such as gelatin, sucrose, dextrose, broth, and rice

Lumen: cavity or channel within a tube or tubular organ (plural, lumina)

Nasogastric (NG) Tube: tube of soft rubber or plastic inserted through a nostril and into the stomach; for instilling liquid foods or other substances or for withdrawing gastric contents

Ostomate: one who has undergone enterostomy or ureterostomy

Perineum: region between the thighs, bound in the male by the scrotum and anus and in the female by the vulva and anus

Purgation: catharsis; relief of fecal matter affected by a cathartic

Sims' Position: position in which the patient lies on the left side with the right knee and thigh flexed and the left arm parallel along the back

Stoma: opening established in the abdominal wall by colostomy, ileostomy, and so forth

Urinal: vessel or other receptacle for urine

Viscosity: physical property of liquids that determines the internal resistance to shear forces

---

Understanding nonaseptic techniques (the use of nasogastric tubes, male urinals, bedpans, enemas, and colostomies) is important to the professional practice of the radiologic technologist. Most of these techniques are performed with patients who are very sick or in great discomfort. The radiologic technologist functions in this area in a variety of roles—patient teacher, patient advocate, nurse, and physician extender, to name but a few. In a health care environment that often seems impersonal and overly concerned with procedures than with the patients receiving them, technologists need to develop abilities of compassion, caring, and competency to be the excellent practitioner that we all strive to be. Adlai Stevenson once said that understanding human needs was one half the job of meeting them. Students need to develop the competencies for patient care in nonaseptic techniques, as well as sensitivity to patient needs.

NASOGASTRIC TUBES

Nasogastric (NG) tubes are plastic or rubber tubes inserted through the nasopharynx into the stomach. The primary use of an NG tube is for decompression or removal of **flatus** and fluids from the stomach. They may also be used for feeding, and in these cases, the tube is often connected to an electronic pump that can control and measure the beneficiary's intake and signal any interruption in the feeding.

The two most common NG tubes used for gastric decompression are the Levin tube and the Salem-sump tube (Fig. 18–1). The Levin tube is a single-**lumen** tube with several holes near its tip. The Salem-sump tube is a radiopaque double-lumen tube. One of the lumina provides an air vent; the other is for removing gastric contents. Other types of NG tubes include the Cantor, Keofeed, Miller-Abbott, and Sengstaken-Blakemore.

A patient with an NG tube in place usually suffers from discomfort. The discomfort of an NG tube often exceeds that of the surgical procedure that accompanies it. Keeping the patient reassured and informed is of the utmost importance in ensuring that the procedure is therapeutic and in securing patient cooperation. Care must be taken to prevent accidental withdrawal of the tube after it has been inserted.

Insertion

In most instances, a physician or nurse is responsible for inserting an NG tube. The following materials are needed for passage of an NG tube:

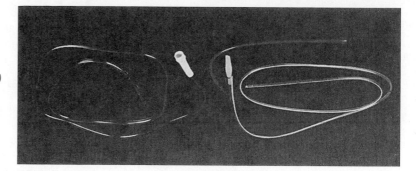

FIG. 18–1 Levin *(left)* and Salem-sump *(right)* nasogastric tubes.

- Rubber or plastic tube, usually a 14- to 18-French (4.7- to 5.3-mm) lumen for an adult patient
- A basin of ice to make the rubber tube more rigid, facilitating passage
- **Emesis basin**
- Clean, disposable gloves
- Towel
- Glass of water with a drinking straw
- 20- to 50-ml aspirating or bulb syringe
- Water-soluble lubricating jelly
- Tape to hold the tube in place at the nose (butterfly tape or 1-inch hypoallergenic tape)
- Stethoscope
- Clamp, drainage bag, or a suction machine if suction is to be used
- Facial tissues

The procedure for inserting an NG tube is as follows:

1. Identify the patient and explain the procedure. Make sure consent for the procedure has been obtained.
2. Place the patient in a high Fowler's position with pillows supporting the head and shoulders. The tissues and the emesis basin should be close for patient use. The procedure is begun by externally measuring the distance from the nose to the stomach. Levin tubes have black markings on them that indicate how far the tube has been inserted.
3. Lubricate the tube at the distal end with the water-soluble lubricating jelly just before insertion. Instruct the patient to swallow water through a straw as the procedure begins. If the patient is unable to take fluids, then air can be swallowed through the straw. The tube should go down easily with little force. The patient should be encouraged to swallow. The proper position is shown in Fig. 18–2.

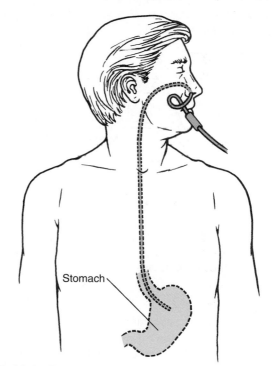

Stomach

FIG. 18–2 Proper nasogastric tube position. (From Craig M: *Essentials of sonography and patient care*, ed 2, Philadelphia, 2006, Elsevier Saunders, p 89.)

Tube placement can be verified by a variety of means, including fluoroscopy. In most instances, a syringe is attached to the end of the tube, and the diaphragm of the stethoscope is placed over the upper left quadrant of the abdomen just below the costal margin. Ten to 20 ml of air is injected while the abdomen is auscultated. A *whooshing* sound indicates that the tube is in the stomach. As a further check, the syringe can be gently aspirated

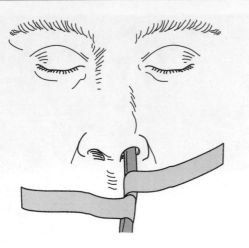

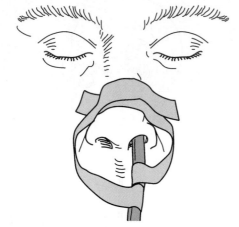

FIG. 18–3   Taping nasogastric tube properly with 1 inch of hypoallergenic tape.

back to obtain gastric contents, which should appear greenish.

The tube is usually secured using the butterfly method (Fig. 18–3):

1. Cut two pieces of tape approximately 2 inches long and tear one lengthwise. Leave the other piece intact.
2. Wrap the intact piece of tape around the tubing.
3. Crisscross the two pieces of tape at the front of the tubing, and place them over the bridge of the nose. A second piece of tape may be placed over the first two to hold them in place.

Levin tubes must be secured so that they are not accidentally withdrawn. No pulling pressure should be present on the tube. Eating or drinking after the insertion of a gastric tube is not allowed unless specifically ordered by the physician. Patients are sometimes allowed to chew gum or suck on small ice chips to increase irrigation and to relieve dryness of the throat.

Removal

The following items are needed to remove an NG tube:

- Emesis basin
- Tissues and several thicknesses of paper toweling
- Impermeable bag for disposal
- Clean, disposable gloves

The procedure for removing an NG tube is as follows:

1. Identify the patient and explain the procedure. Make sure that consent has been secured.
2. Wash hands, and then turn off and disconnect the suction apparatus if one is in place.
3. Gently remove the tape from the patient's nose, and make certain that the tubing is free from the patient's facial skin.
4. Put on clean gloves and ask the patient to take in a deep breath as the tube is gently withdrawn. Wrap the tube in the paper toweling, and place it in the disposal bag. If any resistance occurs, stop the procedure and ask for assistance in the tube withdrawal from an appropriate individual, usually a supervisor or the department nurse.

Transferring a Patient with a Nasogastric Tube

When NG tubes are used for gastric decompression, they are usually connected to an intermittent gastric suctioning device. If a patient is to be transferred, then the radiologic technologist must first confirm that the physician has given an order allowing the transfer and interruption of the suction. The length of time that suction can be interrupted safely also must be known. If it is for only a short time, suction must be reestablished in the radiology department. This task can be accomplished either by taking the patient's portable suction machine to the radiology department or by using suction available in the department (Fig. 18–4). Before transferring the patient, the amount of suction pressure required must be determined. The amount of pressure ordered varies, and the correct level can be determined by reading the physician's orders or by asking the nurse in charge of the patient.

In discontinuing suction on a single-lumen tube, the following materials are needed:

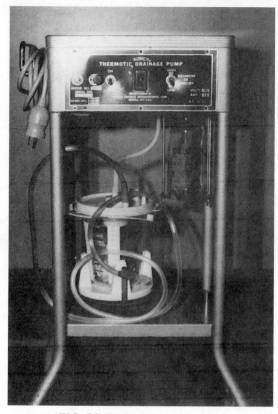

FIG. 18–4 Portable suction unit.

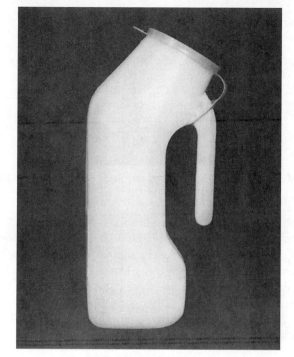

FIG. 18–5 Male urinal.

- Pair of clean, disposable gloves
- Clamping device
- Package of sterile gauze sponges
- Two rubber bands

The procedure for discontinuing suction is as follows:

1. Explain the procedure to the patient, making sure that consent has been given.
2. Wash hands.
3. Open the package of sponges and put on the gloves.
4. Turn off the suction.
5. Clamp or plug the gastric tube with the clamp or stopper, place one gauze pad over the end of the tube, and secure it with a rubber band.
6. Cover the connecting end of the suction tubing or the adapter with the other sponge, and secure it with a rubber band. This gauze covering will keep both ends of the tubing clean while not in use.
7. Secure the suction tubing on the machine so that it will not fall onto the floor, and make certain the NG tube will not be dislodged during the transfer.

If the suction is to be restarted in the radiology department on arrival, set the suction pressure gauge, turn on the suction, and reattach it to the tubing. This procedure is repeated when transferring the patient to the nursing unit.

A double-lumen tube must never be clamped closed with a hemostat or regular clamping device because to do so might cause the lumina to adhere to each other and destroy the double-lumen effect. To prevent leakage from this type of tube, the barrel of a pistonlike syringe may be inserted into the suction-drainage lumen, and it is then pinned to the patient's gown with the barrel upward.

URINALS

The male **urinal** (Fig. 18–5) is made of plastic or metal and is shaped so that it can be used by a patient who is supine, lying on his right or left side, or in **Fowler's position.** The urinal may be offered to the male patient who is not ambulatory—that is, one who is confined to a stretcher or wheelchair or is unable to walk.

If the patient is able to help himself, the radiographer simply hands him an aseptic urinal and allows him to use it, providing privacy whenever possible. When he has finished, the radiographer should put on clean, disposable gloves, remove the urinal, empty it, and rinse it with cold

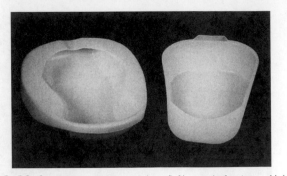

FIG. 18–6 Standard, or regular *(left)*, and fracture *(right)* bedpans.

water. The urinal is then placed with the soiled supplies to be resterilized. The patient should be offered a washcloth with which to wash his hands. The radiographer should then remove the gloves and wash his or her hands.

Some patients require assistance in using a urinal. The radiographer would then proceed as follows:

1. Put on clean, disposable gloves, and raise the cover sheet sufficiently to permit adequate visibility while being careful not to expose the patient excessively.
2. Spread the patient's legs and place the urinal between them. Place the penis into the urinal far enough so that it does not slip out, and hold the urinal in place by the handle until the patient finishes voiding. Remove the urinal, empty it, remove the gloves, and wash your hands.

BEDPANS

The patient who is not ambulatory must be offered a **bedpan** for **defecation;** a nonambulatory female patient requires a bedpan for both defecation and urination. In the radiology department, clean bedpans are stored in a specific area. If not disposable, bedpans must be sterilized between uses.

Bedpans are available in two types (Fig. 18–6). The standard bedpan is made of metal or, more often today, because of concerns over infectious diseases, plastic and is approximately 2 inches high. If a patient has a fracture or another disability that makes using a pan of this height impossible, then a fracture pan is used. It has a shallow upper end approximately $1/2$ inch deep.

Hand washing is important and should be performed both before and after assisting the patient with a bedpan. If the pan is cold, run warm water over it, then dry it. Patient privacy must be secured and respected. Always

place a sheet over the patient. The procedure for assisting a patient with a bedpan is as follows:

1. Remove the bedpan cover and place it at the end of the table. In some instances, having a chair nearby on which to place the pan is best.
2. If the patient is able to move, place one hand under the lower back, asking the patient to raise his or her hips. Place the pan under the hips. Be sure the patient is covered with a sheet.
3. If the patient is able to sit up, then this position is ideal. If possible, the patient's head should be elevated 60 degrees.
4. Because a patient's balance is poor while on a bedpan, do not leave the patient alone for long. In most cases, leaving the patient alone is necessary, but be sure to indicate how help may be summoned.
5. When the patient has finished using the bedpan, put on clean, disposable gloves. Have the patient lie back, place one hand under the lumbar area, and instruct the patient to raise up at the hips.
6. Then remove the pan, cover it, and empty it in the designated area. Plastic bedpans are discarded, and metallic ones are rinsed with cold water and returned to the area where used equipment is placed. Offer the patient a wet paper towel or washcloth to wash hands and a paper towel to dry them. Remove the gloves and wash your hands.

When a patient requires more assistance with a bedpan than can be provided by one person, it becomes necessary to have an assistant. The procedure is as shown in Fig. 18–7:

1. Both persons put on nonsterile gloves.
2. The assistant should stand at the opposite side of the table.
3. Turn the patient to a lateral position.
4. Place the pan against the patient's hips, and then turn the patient back to a supine position while holding the pan in place. Be certain that the hips are in good alignment on the pan. Place pillows under the patient's shoulders and head, and remain nearby in case assistance is needed.
5. When the patient has finished, put on clean gloves and reverse the procedure to remove the pan.

The patient may require assistance in cleaning the **perineum.** Clean, disposable, nonsterile gloves must be worn. Several thicknesses of tissue should be folded into a pad. Wipe the patient's perineum clean and dry. For

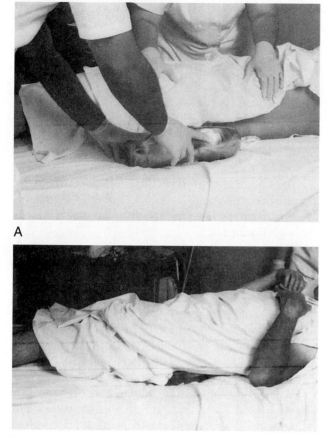

FIG. 18–7 Two-person method of bedpan placement with helpers wearing gloves. *A,* Turn the patient onto side and position bedpan. *B,* Turn the patient onto back.

Tap water (hypotonic)—Plain tap water may be used to cleanse the colon but should not be repeated because of the potential development of water toxicity or circulatory overload.

Hypertonic solution—This solution is often used when the patient cannot tolerate large amounts of fluid. It pulls fluid from the interstitial spaces around the colon. A small amount (120 to 180 ml; 4 to 6 oz) is usually effective. Hypertonic solution is available commercially under the name Fleet Enema.

Saline—Physiologic (normal) saline is the safest, especially for infants, children, and older patients because the fluid is of the same osmolarity as the interstitial spaces of the colon. One teaspoon of salt can be combined with 500 ml (1 pint) of water to prepare this solution.

Soapsuds solution—Pure castile soap may be added to either tap water or normal saline, depending on both patient condition and frequency of administration. Soap should be added to the enema bag after water is in place. Soapsuds enemas promote peristalsis and defecation but produce mild irritation of the bowel.

Oil retention—This method uses an oil-based solution and permits administration of a small volume (120 to 140 ml) to be absorbed by the stool. It should be retained, if possible, for 1 hour. The absorption of oil softens stool for easier evacuation.

In some departments, radiographers administer cleansing enemas to patients the morning of the examination to ensure a good preparation. In fact, some people believe that only radiographers and radiologists have a full understanding of the need for a clean colon and the way in which fecal matter will interfere with the examination. Gelfand and colleagues (1991) note that, in relation to the cleansing enema, "nursing personnel or busy hospital orderlies usually cannot be depended on to perform this task with the necessary diligence" (p. 612). The radiographer may also be responsible for instructing the patient in proper preparation for examinations that require bowel preparation.

In any case, an understanding of the cleansing enema procedure facilitates an understanding of the barium enema procedure, which is standard practice of the radiographer. The materials needed for administering a cleansing enema to an adult patient are as follows:

- Plastic container that holds 1000 to 1500 ml of fluid. This container may be a bucket or a plastic bag with attached tubing. (Fig. 18–8 illustrates popular types of empty enema sets.)

female patients, be sure to wipe from the mons pubis toward the rectal area to avoid contaminating the genital area. Cover the pan, empty it, and place it in the soiled equipment area for resterilization. Remove the gloves and wash your hands.

ENEMAS

Cleansing Enema

A cleansing **enema** is used to promote defecation. For an examination such as a barium enema, to demonstrate a pathologic abnormality or to verify normal structures and function, the bowel should be clear and free of fecal material. The fluid instilled in a cleansing enema breaks up the fecal mass, stretches the rectal wall, and initiates a defecation reflex. The types of enemas are as follows:

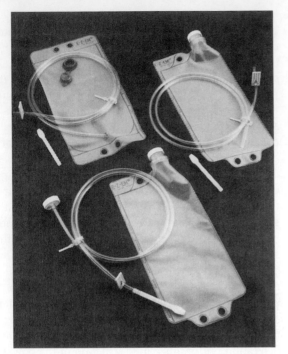

FIG. 18–8 Empty barium enema sets. (Courtesy E-Z-EM, Inc., Lake Success, New York.)

- Plastic tubing with a 22 or 26 French (7.3 to 8.7 mm) lumen approximately 4 feet long with a smooth, perforated tip and a clamping device
- Liquid castile soap (5 to 30 ml)
- Water-soluble lubricant
- Paper or cloth pad to place under the patient's hips, paper towels to receive the enema tip, and a towel to protect the table
- Bedpan
- Clean, disposable gloves
- Drape sheet to cover the patient

The procedure for administering a cleansing enema to an adult patient is as follows:

1. Make sure that the examination has been ordered and that consent has been secured.
2. Inform the patient that a cleansing enema has been ordered and why it has been ordered, and explain the procedure.
3. Attach the tubing to the container if this has not been done, and close the clamp.
4. Prepare the enema solution at a sink capable of providing hot and cold water. The water used should be warmed to approximately 105°F (41°C). Fill the

container with 1000 ml of water. If a soapsuds enema has been ordered, place the soap in the container and mix it.

5. Open the clamp, allowing some of the fluid to run through the tubing into the sink. This action displaces the air so that it will not run into the colon and ensures proper functioning of the set.
6. Drape the patient with the drape sheet and position the patient in a left **Sims' position** (left anterior oblique). Arrange the drape sheet so that only the area of the buttocks that must be exposed for insertion of the enema tip is visible. Place a towel under the patient's hips to protect the table.
7. Put on gloves. Lubricate the tip of the tube if it is not prelubricated.
8. Tell the patient when the tube is about to be inserted.
9. Lift the patient's right buttock with the heel of the hand to expose the anus (Fig. 18–9, A).
10. Ask the patient to exhale slowly and gently insert the enema tip into the rectum toward the umbilicus (anteriorly and superiorly) no more than 3 to 4 inches (Fig. 18–9, B). Make certain that the anus is visualized as the tip is inserted to prevent injury to the patient. Forceful application of the tube may damage the mucous membranes. If problems are encountered in inserting the tip, then a qualified professional such as another radiographer, a supervisor, or the department nurse should be asked to attempt the insertion. The patient may also assist.
11. Explain to the patient that the enema is about to begin. Let the patient know that some cramping may occur as the fluid runs in. Cramping often occurs when the sigmoid colon has been filled (usually after administration of 200 to 400 ml of fluid). Let the patient also know that the enema will be stopped until the cramping stops. The patient should be instructed to breathe through the mouth rapidly. Also inform the patient that the fluid should be retained as long as possible. A stepping stool should also be positioned to assist the patient off the table, and the patient should be told of its presence.
12. When the tip is inserted, hold it in place with the nondominant hand and release the tube clamp with the other hand. Then raise the container of fluid 18 inches above the table.
13. Allow the fluid to run in slowly. Approximately 10 minutes should be required for all the fluid to be used. The patient is asked to lie supine and then turn onto the right side to cleanse the transverse and ascending colon. The quantity of fluid that a patient can retain will vary, but if possible, at least 500 ml of

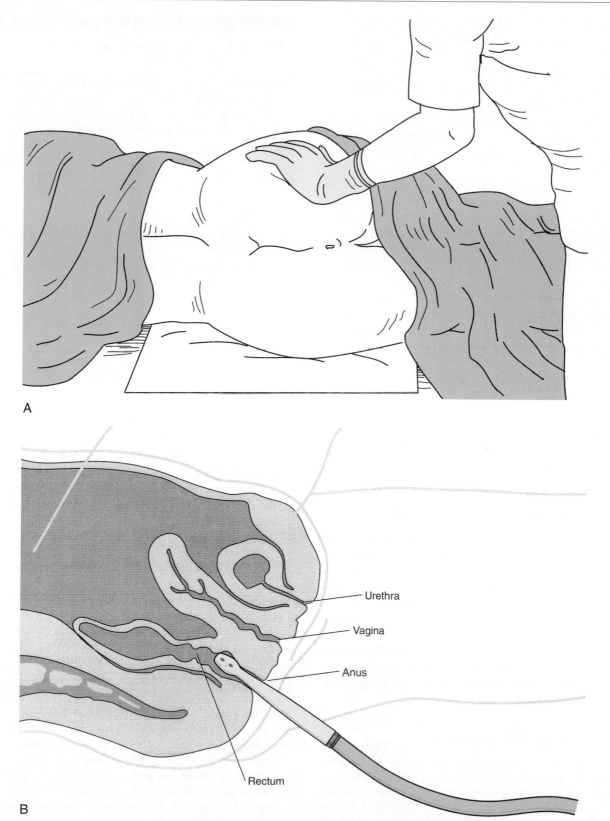

A

B

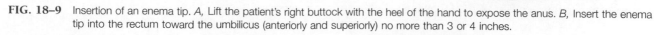

FIG. 18–9 Insertion of an enema tip. *A,* Lift the patient's right buttock with the heel of the hand to expose the anus. *B,* Insert the enema tip into the rectum toward the umbilicus (anteriorly and superiorly) no more than 3 or 4 inches.

fluid should be used. If less than 400 ml of fluid has been used in an adult patient, then it is fairly certain that any feelings of fullness reported by the patient are caused by cramping.

14. Do not allow air to enter the rectum. Clamp off the tube before this can occur.
15. Gently remove the enema tip, wrap it in a paper towel, and place it in the enema container. Dispose of the set in the appropriate receptacle, and remove the gloves.
16. The patient should rest quietly on the table for at least 10 minutes before going to the toilet to expel the enema. Stay close by to assist the patient. If the patient cannot make it to the toilet, a bedpan may be used; be sure to follow proper procedure in using a bedpan (outlined earlier).

In some departments, the patient is told not to flush the toilet until the expelled material has been assessed. Other departments allow the patient to report the color, quantity, and consistency of the fecal material. Preparation for some studies requires that a second or even a third enema be administered so that the bowel is thoroughly cleansed. This process is called giving enemas *until clear* and means that the enema fluid returns with no fecal matter present. This procedure is not usually repeated more than three times because the patient's fluid balance may be jeopardized.

Self-Administered Cleansing Enema

The radiographer may be required to instruct the patient in personal preparation for large bowel cleansing. In most cases, the physician ordering the examination will have provided the patient with instructions relative to preparation. If this provision is not the case, the radiology department will have specific routine instructions, based on the radiologist's order, to be provided to the patient. Patients vary in their understanding of and willingness to accept procedures and preparations; in some cases, referring the patient to a supervisor or back to the personal physician may be necessary.

Other Aspects of Preparation

Bowel preparation is the least standardized aspect of barium enema examinations, but it is also one of the most important. See Boxes 18-1 and 18-2 for some representative preparations.

Most preparations consist of the following:

BOX 18-1 Sample Inpatient Bowel Preparation

1. Consume a clear-liquid diet for the 24 hours before the examination; milk or milk products are restricted.
2. Push fluids, with the patient drinking one full glass of water every hour, if possible. Chart fluid consumption.
3. One hour after lunch, and 3 hours before bisacodyl is given, give 3 oz of milk of magnesia with water.
4. Consume 25 mg of bisacodyl 3 hours after milk of magnesia.
5. Consume nothing by mouth after midnight.
6. Perform a Fleet enema at 6:00 AM the day of examination.
7. Postprocedural: Push fluids and give 2 oz of milk of magnesia to facilitate passage of barium.

Dietary restrictions, usually in the form of a minimal- or **low-residue diet.** This diet severely restricts the patient's intake of milk, overcooked meat, and eggs, and it restricts fruit and vegetables.

Purgation using a variety of laxatives, including castor oil, bisacodyl, or magnesium citrate

Overhydration. A clear liquid diet is often prescribed for the 24-hour period before a barium examination. This diet includes carbonated beverages, clear gelatin, clear broth, and coffee and tea with sugar. Whole-grain cereals, bread, vegetables, fried foods, and milk would be excluded.

Cleansing water enema as previously described

Patients with diabetes require special preparation. Diabetic low-calorie drinks may be added to the standard regimen, and patients with insulin-dependent diabetes often forgo their normal morning insulin dose until after the examination has been completed.

Also noted is that, as a group, older patients (particularly frail older adults) probably require increased education and counseling for preparation for barium enemas (Gurwitz et al, 1992; Grad et al, 1991). Typically, this circumstance occurs not because these patients are, as is stereotypically presented, *senile;* however, their familiarity with, and ability to perform, certain portions of the preparation may be compromised. If assessment indicates that the patient will not or may not be able to perform certain aspects of the preparation, then contacting the radiologist or the patient's referring physician may be necessary.

BOX 18-2 Sample Outpatient Bowel Preparation

Brown Method
On the day before barium enema:

1. Clear fluids only from noon
2. One full glass of water every hour until 10 PM
3. 300 ml of cold magnesium citrate at 4 PM
4. 5 mg of bisacodyl at 6 PM
5. Nothing by mouth after midnight

Picolax Method
On the day before barium enema:

1. Before breakfast: one packet of Picolax; be sure to drink plenty of fluids throughout the day
2. Breakfast: one boiled egg, slice of white bread with honey, one cup of tea or coffee (milk allowed)
3. Lunch: grilled or poached fish or chicken, small portion of cooked rice, plain yogurt, one cup of tea or coffee (may be sweetened; no milk); no potatoes, vegetables other than the rice, and no fruit
4. Take the second packet of Picolax at 4 PM.
5. Take a late supper (7-9 PM) of clear broth.
6. Consume clear fluids only after supper.

Standard Bowman Gray Preparation
(Originators of this method report a 97% success rate in patient preparation)

1. Clear liquid diet 24 hours before examination
2. 8 oz of water each hour day before examination
3. 300 ml of magnesium citrate solution, 4 PM day before examination
4. 60 ml of castor oil 8 PM day before examination
5. Day of examination: 1500 ml cleansing enema in radiology department. Waiting times after cleansing: 30 minutes for single-contrast examination; 60 minutes for double-contrast

Also important to note is that *bowel* preparations and *people* preparations exist. That is, viewing the patient as a bowel rather than a person may lead to a substandard examination because of the lack of patient understanding and cooperation. If, in patient instruction, the radiographer focuses on reciting facts rather than ensuring that the patient understands the preparation, then the examination may be less than adequate as a result of poor preparation.

One good technique to ensure understanding is to have the patient repeat the instructions. Do not fall into the trap of thinking that a simple *yes* really means that the patient understands. Be sure that he or she knows and understands the words, as well as the meaning, of the procedures. For example, patients commonly arrive for a barium enema and exclaim, "What! Another enema! I had three last night!" not knowing that these initial enemas were preparations for the morning examination.

BARIUM ENEMA. The **barium** enema is given in an examination used to diagnose pathologic conditions of the colon or lower gastrointestinal tract. Because of advances in technology, other forms of diagnosis are now often preferred or are even the norm, such as colonoscopy, computed tomographic colonoscopy, and magnetic resonance imaging. A much larger catheter is required than is used for cleansing enemas to allow the barium, which is of greater **viscosity,** to be instilled into the lower bowel. The catheter may have a plain tip or an inflatable cuff attached (Fig. 18–10). The cuff is inflated after the tip is inserted to hold the catheter in place and to prevent involuntary expulsion of barium.

Facilities and physicians vary widely in their use of inflatable cuffs (balloon catheters). Some physicians do so routinely, always inflating the cuff, whereas others always use the cuff but inflate only out of necessity. Still others believe inflatable cuffs should be used only when absolutely necessary. Damage to the rectal wall from improper use of balloon catheters is the most common complication of a barium enema. Balloons should never be overinflated (the amount recommended varies from 30 to 90 ml of air) and are contraindicated in cases of rectal narrowing. Other complications include breaks in the gastrointestinal mucosa caused by trauma or disease, which permit barium to enter the peritoneal cavity or bloodstream. Disease conditions such as ulcers, cancer, and diverticulitis can create minute asymptomatic perforations that can blow out under pressure. Then peritonitis or venous emboli may cause serious complications, including death, as well as fibrosis or barium granuloma. In addition, allergic reactions to latex tips and cuffs have also been reported, which has led to the use of alternate materials.

Barium solution is usually available in a prepared, prepackaged powder, which must be mixed with water, or suspension (Fig. 18–11). Barium suspensions and solutions should have the following characteristics:

Allow rapid flow
Allow good adhesion to the mucosa
Provide adequate radiographic density in a thin layer
Have even, plastic coating
Lack foam or artifacts

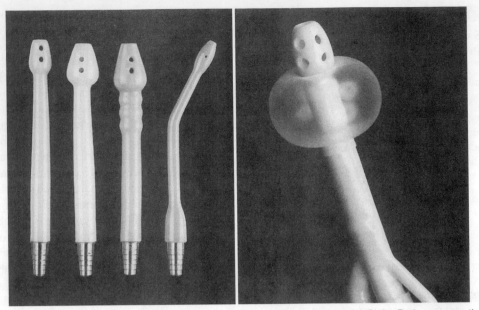

FIG. 18–10 *Left,* Plain barium enema tip. (Courtesy E-Z-EM, Inc., Lake Success, New York.) *Right,* Barium enema tip with an inflatable cuff.

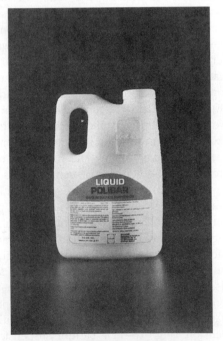

FIG. 18–11 Commercial barium suspension. (Courtesy E-Z-EM, Inc., Lake Success, New York.)

The quantity of barium solution prepared is large. Most bags hold 3000 ml; the actual amount prepared varies. The barium solution may be prepared using warm or cold water. Advocates of the use of cold water hold that this method will reduce irritation to the colon and helps the patient *hold* the enema. Some people also advocate the use of salt (2 teaspoons per 1000 ml of water) to prevent fluid overload. Because of radiologist preferences in terms of viscosity and density, no one correct way exists to mix barium. Let the patient know that the entire 3000 ml in the bag may not be administered.

Because greater pressure is required to secure an adequate flow rate, the bag is usually suspended at a greater distance (up to 30 inches) above the table. Excessive height may cause severe abdominal cramping and rupture of diverticula in the colon as a result of excessive fluid pressure. The initial portion of the procedure is much the same as for the cleansing enema.

Follow the same instructions for inserting the tip as were given in the section on the cleansing enema. The patient may lie in a supine position while waiting for the radiologist.

Patient instruction and reassurance are of utmost importance. Patients must know that they will receive a variety of instructions and also that the radiologist will give a variety of instructions to the radiographer that the patient may ignore. In addition, patients may not understand the difference between the cleansing enemas they have received and the barium enema.

The patient must understand the need to (1) keep the tip firmly in the rectum, (2) relax the abdominal muscles to reduce intraabdominal pressure, and (3) use deep oral breathing to prevent spasms and cramps. As with the cleansing enema, the patient must know that the procedure will be suspended if cramping occurs. Some researchers (Grigoleit and Grigoleit, 2005) have advocated the use of peppermint oil as an anticramping agent.

Student radiographers should carefully observe the interactions among radiographers, radiologists, and patients to develop their own style of patient instruction during the procedure. Although the basic information is consistent from patient to patient, the way it is communicated may vary according to special needs.

Double-Contrast Barium Enemas. In almost all facilities, the double-contrast barium enema (the addition of air or carbon dioxide to provide for two contrasts—barium and the air) has become routine. This type of enema is especially indicated in diarrhea and high-risk cases, for example, the patient with polyps, a family history of colorectal cancer, or a personal history of cancer or rectal bleeding. The patient often receives an injection of a smooth-muscle relaxant such as glucagon immediately before the examination to relieve bowel spasm.

A typical routine for a double-contrast barium enema begins with the patient in a prone position and the table tilted slightly head-down. Barium (approximately 300 ml) is instilled into the splenic flexure, and air is then insufflated (added). This action pushes the barium to fill the transverse colon. The bag is lowered, and the head of the table is raised to drain the rectum, which also traps barium in the transverse colon. The patient may be turned to the right side and more air added to bring barium around the hepatic flexure. The patient then is turned prone to bring the barium to the cecum. Once the colon is filled with barium and distended with air, various radiographic views are taken.

Other means of performing double-contrast examinations described in the literature include Miller's seven-pump method; Pochazevsky and Sherman's single-stage, closed system; and Welin's double-stage or Malmo technique, in which the barium is added, the patient evacuates the barium, and air is added. Various radiologists also have their own routines.

Single-Contrast Barium Enemas. Although double-contrast examinations are now the norm, single-contrast barium enemas may be indicated in certain situations:

- When colon configuration is of prime importance
- When only gross pathologic conditions must be shown
- When fistulas are thought to be present
- When acute appendicitis or diverticulitis is thought to be present
- In children, especially when an intussusception is to be reduced
- When a volvulus or acute obstruction is to be evaluated
- When the patient is not movable or cooperative or is extremely debilitated

In a typical single-contrast barium enema, the suspension is run in slowly with compression applied to the abdomen. Approximately 1500 ml of barium is required for the average adult barium enema. Spot views of the cecum, flexures, and the sigmoid colon are taken. A variety of views of the abdomen (typically anteroposterior, posteroanterior, and decubitus), a 30-degree caudal angulation of the sigmoid colon, and a lateral rectal view are taken. The excess barium is drained back into the bag, the tip is removed, and the patient is sent to the toilet to evacuate as much of the barium as possible. A postevacuation image is taken, usually with the patient in the prone position.

When removing a rectal catheter that has an inflatable cuff attached, the cuff must be deflated before the catheter is removed. The barium is sometimes removed by gravity flow before the catheter tip is removed, and air is then permitted to escape from the cuff. After this activity is complete, the catheter is gently removed. If any resistance occurs, summoning another individual (another radiographer, a supervisor, the department nurse, or in extreme cases the radiologist) may be necessary to remove it.

When perforation of the bowel is thought to exist, water-soluble iodine compounds are the only acceptable contrast media (rather than barium). These compounds, such as Gastrografin, also are used in a variety of other cases in which administration of barium sulfate can prove hazardous. These situations would include delineation of an anastomosis in the immediate preoperative period, outlining of the distal colon and rectum in cases of megacolon and Hirschsprung disease, and when the risk of barium impaction is high. Water-soluble contrast agents are hypertonic, which means they draw fluid into the bowel. A hypertonic agent can cause diarrhea and a sudden reduction in blood volume and is particularly dangerous in neonates and in patients with Hirschsprung disease.

The patient is assisted to the toilet after barium enemas. Patients are often dehydrated as a result of the preparation for a barium enema. Dehydration can lead to a postural drop in blood pressure, which might cause the patient to become dizzy and fall. Allowing the patient to evacuate some of the barium into a bedpan before moving may be necessary.

Postprocedural Instructions

Postprocedural instruction to the patient is necessary after a barium enema because barium retention can cause fecal impaction or intestinal obstruction. Barium has hydroscopic qualities, which means that it will absorb fluid from the bowel. Extreme dehydration as a result of preparation for the examination is another possible postprocedural complication. In older adult patients, fluid imbalance may lead to altered mental status.

Stools are often white or light-colored until all of the barium is expelled. Some physicians regularly prescribe a laxative medication or an enema after barium studies. In any case, the lack of a bowel movement within 24 hours indicates that the personal physician should be contacted. The importance of eliminating the barium cannot be stressed enough to the patient.

The patient should increase fluid intake and dietary fiber for several days unless medically contraindicated and should be instructed to rest after the examination. The personal physician should be contacted immediately if any of the following occur:

Weakness or fainting
Abdominal pain, constipation, or rectal bleeding
Not passing flatus
Polyuria, nocturia, or abdominal distention

COLOSTOMIES

Because of trauma or pathologic condition such as cancer, diverticulitis, and ulcerative colitis, formation of a **stoma** (mouth) from the bowel to the outside of the body may be necessary. Permanent **colostomies** are performed when a portion of bowel is removed. A temporary colostomy is performed to heal or rest a diseased portion of bowel.

Several types of colostomies have been developed. A *descending* or *sigmoid* colostomy is a permanent colostomy in which the diseased portion of the colon or rectum is removed. A *transverse* colostomy has a portion of the transverse colon removed. In a *double-barrel* colostomy, two stomas are formed: the proximal delivers stool, and the distal produces mucus. The longer a colostomy has been in place, the greater will the consistency of stool be.

The radiographer must recognize that an ostomy produces a major change in a patient's body image and that many persons with new colostomies go through the grieving process. The loss of a bowel can be viewed in the same light as any other loss, including death. That is, patients typically pass through various stages, including denial, anger, bargaining, depression, and finally acceptance.

Caring for a patient with a new ostomy requires sensitivity and a matter-of-fact attitude, two seemingly separate entities, both of which must be reconciled for effective care of the ostomy patient. Barbara Mullen, author of *The Ostomy Book* and an **ostomate,** has said that she appreciated plain speaking over half-hearted platitudes after her own ostomy. The patient can negatively interpret even a hint of revulsion or hesitancy. The radiography student who has never seen an ostomy should observe routines until technical competency, a matter-of-fact attitude (plain speaking), and sensitivity can be combined.

A patient with a colostomy needs special instructions for adequate preparation. In most patients, the stoma is irrigated the night before and the morning of the examination. Irrigation is a type of *enema* for the colostomy that should prevent the expulsion of feces for 24 hours. Dietary and laxative preparations also vary depending on the ostomy. The ostomate must be instructed, for example, not to take bismuth subgallate tablets—as he or she may normally do to control odor—because these are radiopaque. If available, an **enterostomal therapist** instructs the patient in preparation. Patients with an ostomy should be instructed to bring an extra pouch with them if they are coming from outside the hospital.

Administering a Barium Enema to a Patient with a Colostomy

Most colostomies are performed because of cancer. Approximately 10% of patients have their bowels removed because of cancer recurrences, which necessitate follow-up studies.

This examination is often called a *loopogram* and evaluates small or large bowel that has been connected to the skin surface with an ostomy. Obstruction, inflammatory bowel disease, and lesions of the bowel wall such as diverticula, polyps, or certain types of cancer may be the focus of the study; in cases of temporary ostomy placement, looking at the bowel before reconnection may also be done, with subsequent ostomy removal.

The patient with a colostomy will have a dressing or drainage pouch in place over the area of the stoma. The

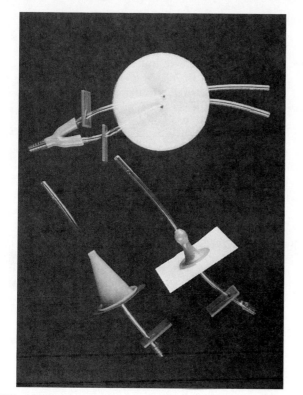

FIG. 18–12 A variety of colostomy tips. (Courtesy E-Z-EM, Inc., Lake Success, New York.)

dressing must be removed by a radiographer wearing clean gloves and then placed in a plastic bag and discarded in a receptacle intended for contaminated waste. The gloves are then removed, and the hands are washed. A drainage pouch should be removed and put aside in a safe place to be reused. Gloves are put on again. The patient may want to perform this action or provide direction for the procedure. The pouch must be kept clean and dry.

The procedure for administering a barium enema to a patient with a colostomy differs somewhat from that for the regular examination because of the lack of a sphincter. The main problem with barium administration through a colostomy is trying to prevent leakage without damaging the colostomy. A cone-shaped tip with a long drainage bag that attaches to it is frequently the tip of choice. Nipple colostomy tips and double-barrel (dual tubing that allows for simultaneous study of the proximal and distal colonic loops) colostomy tips are also available (Fig. 18–12). In some instances, a small catheter with an inflatable cuff is used. If the patient has had the ostomy for some time, self-insertion of the tip may be preferred.

The radiographer typically lubricates the tip of the cone and hands it to the patient for insertion. If the patient is unable to do so, the radiologist, who also tapes the device in place, performs the task. Clean, disposable gloves should be put on. A much smaller amount of barium solution is often needed, especially when the study is done for the distal portion of the remaining colon.

Once the cone or catheter has been inserted, the diagnostic procedure is similar to that for other patients. An intravenous smooth-muscle relaxant is usually necessary to prevent peristalsis, which continually empties the colon. Approximately 250 ml of barium is usually used. Care must be taken, if air insufflation is used, not to overdistend the colon. So as not to traumatize the stoma site, prone views are not performed.

When the procedure is completed, the drainage bag can be attached to the cone and the barium drained. When the drainage is complete, the ambulatory patient can be escorted to the toilet with the drainage bag still in place to be cleaned; the ostomy pouch is then replaced.

Ostomates are often independent if they have had the ostomy for a long time. The patient must be allowed a certain degree of self-control in addition to the direction given to the patient by the radiographer and the physician.

SUMMARY

NG tubes, male urinals, bedpans, enemas, and colostomies are a part of the daily practice of a radiographer. The detailed routines are described here as they are commonly performed in hospitals and other health care facilities; the actual routine at any given institution may vary slightly.

The radiographer is most likely to encounter the Levin tubes and Salem-sump NG tubes. Patients with NG tubes in place usually suffer from discomfort and require a good deal of assurance. The radiographer may assist in inserting NG tubes and is sometimes responsible for their removal. Before moving a patient with an NG tube, the radiographer must be sure of the length of time that suction may be discontinued.

Urinals are used by male patients who are unable to walk or stand for urination. These urinals must be rinsed between uses by the same patient and sterilized after each patient. Bedpans are used by female patients for urination and defecation and by male patients for defecation only. The two basic types are the standard bedpan and the fracture bedpan. Maintaining a patient's sense of dignity and privacy is important when using a bedpan.

In some departments, radiographers or other workers in the department are responsible for administering cleansing enemas as a means of bowel preparation. The five basic types of cleansing enemas are tap water (hypotonic), hypertonic solution, physiologic (normal saline), soapsuds, and oil retention. Radiographers function as patient educators in informing patients of the standardized bowel preparation used at their institution. These preparations usually include dietary restrictions, purgation, overhydration, and cleansing enemas. The professional radiographer focuses on patient understanding of the procedure rather than simply reciting facts to the patient.

The barium enema is given in an examination to diagnose potential pathologic conditions of the colon. The barium used is more viscous than water and is administered differently from the water enema. Patient instructions before, during, and after the procedure are necessary to ensure a diagnostic outcome without postprocedural complications. The two main types of barium enemas are the single-contrast examination, in which only barium is used, and the double-contrast examination, in which both barium and air are used to outline the colon.

Colostomies are formed by bringing a portion of the colon to the outside in the form of a stoma or mouth. Patients with ostomies require special care that often comes only through observation and experience. Allowing as much patient control as possible while maintaining control over the examination, as well as not showing signs of revulsion or hesitancy, is important. Administration of a barium enema in a patient with a colostomy is different from that in a regular patient because of the lack of a sphincter and the sensitivity of the stoma site.

BIBLIOGRAPHY

The perils of a barium blowout when contrast medium escapes from the GI tract, *Emerg Med* 16:57, 1984.

Ballinger P, Frank ED: *Merrill's atlas of radiographic positions and radiologic procedures,* ed 10, vol 1, St Louis, 2003, Mosby.

Bartram CI: The large bowel. In Whitehouse GH, Worthington BS, eds: *Techniques in diagnostic imaging,* ed 2, Boston, 1990, Blackwell Scientific Publications.

Craig M: *Introduction to ultrasonography and patient care,* Philadelphia, 1993, WB Saunders.

Ehrlich RA, McCloskey ED, Daly J: *Patient care in radiography,* ed 6, St Louis, 2004, Mosby.

Gelfand DW, Chen DYM, Ott DJ: Preparing the colon for the barium enema examination, *Radiology* 178:609, 1991.

Grad RM et al: Adequacy of preparation for barium enema among elderly outpatients, *Can Med Assoc J* 144:1257, 1991.

Grigoleit HG, Grigoleit P: Gastrointestinal clinical pharmacology of peppermint oil, *Phytomedicine* 12:607, 2005.

Gurwitz JH et al: Barium enemas in the frail elderly, *Am J Med* 92:41, 1992.

Metheny N, Titler M: Assessing placement of feeding tubes, *Am J Nurs* 101:36, 2001.

Miller RE: Barium pneumocolon: technologist-performed "7-pump" method, *AJR Am J Roentgenol* 139:1230, 1982.

Mullen BD, McGinn KA: *The ostomy book,* Palo Alto, Calif, 1992, Bull.

Pochazevsky R, Sherman S: A new technique for roentgenologic examination of the colon, *AJR Am J Roentgenol* 89:787, 1963.

Robinson SB, Demuth PL: Diagnostic studies for the aged: What are the dangers? *J Gerontol Nurs* 11:6, 1985.

Rockey DC et al: Analysis of air contrast barium enema, computed tomographic colonography, and colonoscopy: prospective comparison, *Lancet* 365(9456):305, 2005.

Torres LS: *Basic medical techniques and patient care for radiologic technologists,* ed 6, Philadelphia, 2003, JB Lippincott.

Troupin RH: *Diagnostic radiology in clinical medicine,* Chicago, 1985, Year Book.

19

Medical Emergencies

Joanne S. Greathouse, EdS, RT(R), FASRT, FAERS

Important to proper evaluation of the critically ill patient is a spirit of cooperation and ongoing communication.

Lawrence Goodman and Charles Putman
Intensive Care Radiology, 1978

OBJECTIVES

On completion of this chapter, the student will be able to:

1. Define terms related to medical emergencies.

2. List the objectives of first aid.

3. List general priorities in working with patients in acute situations.

4. Explain the purpose of an emergency cart and its contents.

5. Differentiate between the two primary types of external cardiac defibrillators.

6. Explain the four levels of consciousness.

OBJECTIVES—Cont'd

7. Describe the signs and symptoms of various medical emergencies.

8. Discuss methods of avoiding the factors that contribute to shock.

9. Discuss factors that contribute to the development of hypoglycemia.

10. Describe the appropriate procedure for handling patients with various medical emergencies.

11. Describe the correct procedure for administration of cardiopulmonary resuscitation.

12. Describe the general procedure for the use of an automatic external cardiac defibrillator.

13. Demonstrate appropriate principles of cardiopulmonary resuscitation.

GLOSSARY

Aura: subjective sensation or motor phenomenon that precedes and marks the onset of a paroxysmal attack, such as an epileptic attack

Automatic External Defibrillation (AED): application of external electrical shock to restore normal cardiac rhythm and rate

Cardiac arrest: sudden stoppage of cardiac output and effective circulation

Cardiopulmonary Resuscitation (CPR): artificial substitution of heart and lung action as indicated for cardiac arrest or apparent sudden death resulting from electric shock, drowning, respiratory arrest, and other causes

Cerebrovascular Accident (Stroke or Brain Attack): condition with sudden onset caused by acute vascular lesions of the brain; it is often followed by permanent neurologic damage

Emergency: unexpected or sudden occasion; an urgent or pressing need

Epistaxis: nosebleed; hemorrhage from the nose

Hemorrhage: escape of blood from the vessels; bleeding

Hyperglycemia: abnormally increased concentration of glucose in the blood

Hypoglycemia: abnormally diminished concentration of glucose in the blood

Lethargy: abnormal drowsiness or stupor; a condition of indifference

Nausea: unpleasant sensation, vaguely referred to the epigastrium and abdomen and often culminating in vomiting

Pallor: paleness; absence of skin coloration

Shock: condition of profound hemodynamic and metabolic disturbance characterized by failure of the circulatory system to maintain adequate perfusion of vital organs

Syncope: temporary suspension of consciousness as a result of generalized cerebral ischemia; faint or swoon

Urticaria: vascular reaction, usually transient, involving the upper dermis, representing localized edema caused by dilatation and increased permeability of the capillaries and marked by the development of wheals; also called hives

Ventricular Fibrillation: disorganized cardiac rhythm

Vertigo: illusion of movement; sensation as if the external world were revolving around the patient or as if the patient were revolving in space

Vomiting: forcible expulsion of the contents of the stomach through the mouth

Wound: bodily injury caused by physical means with disruption of the normal continuity of structures

Wound Dehiscence: separation of the layers of a surgical wound; may be partial, or superficial only, or complete, with disruption of all layers

MEDICAL EMERGENCY

Definition and Objectives of First Aid

An **emergency** is a situation in which the condition of a patient or a sudden change in medical status requires immediate action. Emergency actions on the part of the radiologic technologist generally have the objectives of preserving life, avoiding further harm to the patient, and obtaining appropriate medical assistance as quickly as possible. Although instances in which a radiologic technologist is required to initiate emergency measures are infrequent, the technologist must be able to recognize emergency situations, maintain a calm and confident presence, and take appropriate action. The recognition of need for assistance is a critical first step; the technologist must be able to recognize when such assistance might be warranted.

General Priorities

Although most patients are sent to the radiology department only after they have been stabilized, some patients are not stable, and the status of others may change while they are in the department. Radiologic technologists should never underestimate their ability to contribute to a patient's survival and well being through quick thinking and appropriate action. The technologist should keep in mind the following priorities when working with patients in emergency situations:

1. Ensure an open airway.
2. Control bleeding.
3. Take measures to prevent or treat shock.
4. Attend to wounds or fractures.
5. Provide emotional support.
6. Continually reevaluate and follow up appropriately.

Emergency Cart

Familiarity with the location of emergency equipment in the radiology department is an important part of being able to respond appropriately. Most radiology departments have at least one emergency cart (often referred to as a *crash cart*). This cart is a wheeled container of equipment and drugs typically required in emergency situations (Fig. 19–1).

The cart itself and its contents—drugs and equipment needed to handle typical life-threatening emergencies—are similar from one institution to another (Box 19-1). The ready availability of emergency equipment and drugs reduces the time required to respond to medical crises. A radiologic technologist's orientation to a department should include learning the location of emergency carts and a familiarity with the contents and organization of the carts at that particular institution.

Automatic External Defibrillator

Increasingly, radiology departments and other public places have automatic external defibrillators available. This movement has been identified as public access defibrillation (PAD) and has resulted in significant reduc-

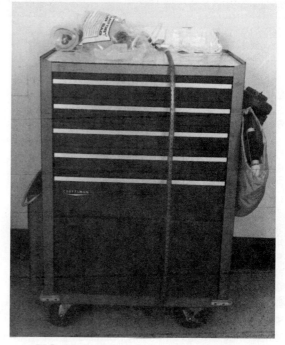

FIG. 19–1 A typical emergency *crash cart.*

tion in mortality from cardiac arrhythmia. External defibrillators come in two primary types:

1. *Fully automatic,* which analyze the patient's cardiac rhythm, determine whether defibrillation is necessary, and, if necessary, deliver a shock
2. *Semiautomatic,* which analyze the patient's cardiac rhythm, determine whether defibrillation is necessary, and, if needed, advise the operator to deliver a shock by pushing a button

If such devices are available in the hospital, the technologist should become familiar with the type and specific model, given that each operates somewhat differently.

HEAD INJURIES

Victims of head trauma are often seen in the radiology department. Although diagnosing head injuries is not the responsibility of the radiologic technologist, having knowledge of categorization is useful so that a basic assessment can be made and changes in a patient's status noted. Of the several ways to categorize head injuries, the simplest form of classification is by level of consciousness.

BOX 19-1 Equipment and Drugs Typically Found on an Emergency Cart

Standard Equipment

Backboard	Tracheal tubes
Stethoscope	Cut-down tray
Blood pressure cuff	Suction bottle
Ambu bag	Hemostat
Laryngoscope	Scissors
Flashlight	Surgeon's gloves, various
Batteries	sizes
Extension cord	Syringes, various sizes
Oxygen flow meter	Needles, various sizes
Tourniquet	Stopcocks and connectors
Airways	Tongue blades
Endotracheal tubes	Sterile gauze
Nasopharyngeal tubes	Adhesive and paper tape
Suction catheters	Alcohol swabs
Levine tubing	Surgical lubricant
Jelco cannulas	Blood collection tubes

Emergency Drugs Commonly Found on a Crash Cart

Medication	*Indication*
Adenocard	Arrhythmias
Atropine	Bradycardia
Benadryl	Allergic reaction
Cordarone	Arrhythmias
Decadron	Allergic reaction
Dilantin	Seizures
Dobutrex	Shock
Epinephrine	Cardiac arrest, anaphylaxis
Intropin	Shock
Isoptin	Arrhythmias
Lasix	Edema
Levophed	Shock
Pronestyl	Arrhythmias
Sodium bicarbonate	Metabolic acidosis
Xylocaine	Arrhythmias

Levels of Consciousness

The patient with the least severe injury is classified as alert and conscious. In most instances, this patient can respond fully to questions and other stimuli. A more seriously injured patient is drowsy but can be roused to response with loud speaking or gentle physical contact. Even more serious injury produces a patient who is unconscious and reacts only to painful stimuli. These patients typically do not respond to verbal stimuli but react to stimuli such as pinches and pinpricks. The most serious condition is that of a patient who is comatose and unresponsive to virtually all stimuli.

Indications of Deteriorating Situations

The technologist should quickly assess a patient when the procedure is begun so that it is readily noticeable if the patient deteriorates from one level of consciousness to another. Findings in an alert or drowsy patient that can signify a deteriorating head injury include irritability, **lethargy**, slowing pulse rate, and slowing respiratory rate.

When working with an intoxicated patient with a head injury, the technologist is cautioned against assuming that the patient has passed out merely from inebriation. If any doubt exists about the cause of the patient's loss of consciousness, then assuming a more serious head injury and obtaining medical assistance is far better than for a patient to suffer further deterioration needlessly.

Response to Deteriorating Situations

If the radiologic technologist recognizes a deteriorating head injury, the first priority is maintaining an open airway while moving the patient as little as possible. The procedure should be stopped and medical assistance obtained quickly. Obtaining vital signs while waiting for help to arrive is also helpful.

SHOCK

Definition and Types

Another situation typically encountered with emergency patients is shock. **Shock** is a general term that indicates a failure of the circulatory system to support vital body functions. Several types of shock can occur:

Hypovolemic caused by loss of blood or tissue fluid
Cardiogenic caused by a variety of cardiac disorders, including myocardial infarction
Neurogenic caused by spinal anesthesia or damage to the upper spinal cord
Vasogenic caused by sepsis, deep anesthesia, or anaphylaxis

The technologist is most likely to encounter hypovolemic shock or anaphylactic shock, a special type of vasogenic shock, as a result of reaction to contrast media administered in the course of a procedure.

Prevention

Several factors can contribute to the likelihood that a patient will experience shock or to the degree of shock experienced. Any sudden change in body temperature is one such factor. This change illustrates the importance of keeping patients covered to maintain normal body temperature; to avoid overheating the patient is equally important.

Pain, stress, and anxiety also contribute to the development of shock. Handling patients gently during a procedure is not only an important aspect of good psychologic care, but it also can be a factor in the patient's physical condition. The technologist should also work calmly and confidently, even in a situation of maximum stress; this demeanor helps reassure emergency patients and can contribute to their overall physiologic well being.

Signs and Symptoms

Signs and symptoms that a patient might be going into shock include restlessness, apprehension or general anxiety, tachycardia, decreasing blood pressure, cold and clammy skin, and **pallor.** If the radiologic technologist believes that such a situation is developing, then he or she should stop the procedure, ensure maintenance of the patient's body temperature, call for medical assistance, and measure the patient's vital signs while awaiting assistance.

Contrast Media Reactions (Anaphylactic Shock)

Anaphylactic shock is a type of vasogenic shock and is most commonly encountered in the radiology department in connection with the administration of iodinated contrast media. Although a great deal of debate exists about the nature of contrast media reactions, at least some agreement has been found that these reactions have an element of an allergic reaction. Although such reactions are not common, neither are they so rare as to warrant complacency on the part of the technologist. Reaction to contrast media can range from mild to severe. Because the most severe reaction can result in death from cardiac arrest, contrast media should not be administered without first taking an adequate history.

In general, the longer it takes for a reaction to develop, the less severe it is. Accordingly, the most severe reactions typically arise very quickly. A possibility exists, however, for a severe delayed reaction to occur. Thus, constantly monitoring patients who have had contrast media injections is important.

Mild reactions are similar to other allergic reactions. Patients develop localized itching and **urticaria** (hives) and may experience nausea and vomiting. Generalized itching and hives are indicative of a systemic reaction, which is generally more serious than most mild reactions. Although none of these reactions are serious in and of themselves, they may signal the onset of a more serious reaction. The physician should be notified immediately in the event of any reaction. In most instances, a mild antihistamine is administered to counter the allergic reaction.

The most serious reactions might include laryngeal edema, shock, and cardiac arrest. All of these conditions are life threatening and should be handled accordingly. The physician must be notified at once and vital signs taken. Patients who suffer cardiac arrest should be treated with cardiopulmonary resuscitation.

DIABETIC CRISES

Many patients who undergo radiologic procedures are required to have had gastrointestinal preparation, which might include a special diet or fasting. Most patients can tolerate this preparation fairly easily (if not necessarily comfortably), but such alterations in dietary patterns can be particularly troublesome for patients with diabetes.

In the healthy patient, the body adjusts its insulin production and excretion to meet the demands made on it by the body's intake of carbohydrate. In some patients with diabetes (type 1, typically juvenile onset), however, the insulin is given exogenously, and the patient must adjust dietary intake to balance the insulin taken. The gastrointestinal preparation can create havoc with this balance.

Hypoglycemia

Hypoglycemia is a condition in which excessive insulin is present. This excess insulin can be the result of a patient's taking the usual dose of insulin before a gastrointestinal study and then not having a normal breakfast. The brain requires glucose for normal metabolism. If no food is eaten, then the administered insulin depletes the body's energy store, leading fairly quickly to insulin shock (sometimes called an *insulin reaction*). Patients who are experiencing this condition are intensely hungry, weak, and shaky and may sweat excessively. They also may become confused and irritable, sometimes to the point of aggression and mild hostility. Most patients, especially those who have lived with the condition for a time, recognize the condition before it becomes serious. The patient needs a quick form of carbohydrate. Some patients carry glucose tablets with them.

If these tablets are not available, then any form of carbohydrate should be administered as long as the patient is conscious. Orange juice sweetened with sugar, a sugared soft drink, a candy bar, or any form of carbohydrate can be consumed. Because physical activity continues to deplete the patient's energy stores, the patient should be encouraged to sit quietly until the food has had a chance to take effect, usually 10 to 15 minutes. No food or fluid should be given to an unconscious patient. If a patient with hypoglycemia becomes unconscious, then immediate medical attention is required.

Hyperglycemia

Hyperglycemia is a condition of excessive sugar in the blood and is the characteristic typically associated with diabetes. This condition develops gradually, generally over a period of hours or days, so it is not likely to be noticed by a technologist. These patients exhibit excessive thirst and urination, dry mucosa, rapid and deep breathing, and drowsiness and confusion. The condition leads to diabetic coma if left untreated. The patient needs insulin; therefore, if this condition is believed to be present, the technologist should get medical help.

RESPIRATORY DISTRESS AND RESPIRATORY ARREST

Asthma

Another medical crisis that occasionally occurs in the radiology department is respiratory distress. Patients with asthma seem to react in particularly stressful situations, such as they might experience in a radiology department. A patient in respiratory distress generally exhibits wheezing, a result of dilatation of bronchi on inspiration and collapse on exhalation. Because asthma is a chronic condition, many patients carry an aerosol inhaler or other form of bronchodilator. The radiologic technologist should stop the procedure, assist the patient to a sitting position to support easier respiration, and attempt to reassure the patient. If the patient has medications available, then the technologist should allow the patient to use them. If not, then medical assistance should be obtained.

A calm, confident manner is important when faced with a patient having an asthmatic attack. When the patient begins to exhibit respiratory distress, the anxiety is likely to increase, which further interferes with respiratory function. Thus the technologist's calm handling of the situation not only comforts the patient, but it may also be a factor in limiting the severity of the problem.

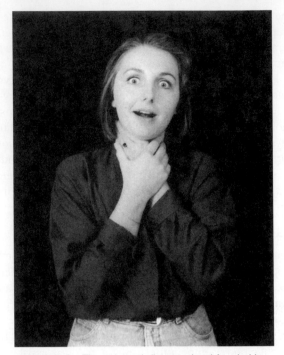

FIG. 19–2   The universal distress signal for choking.

Choking

Radiologic technologists should also be familiar with the Heimlich maneuver. This maneuver is used in situations in which a person appears to be choking. The technologist should first ascertain that the patient is choking by asking the question, "Can you speak?" Patients with partial obstruction can verbalize their problem, but complete obstruction prevents the patient from speaking. A person who is choking and cannot verbalize a response generally clutches the throat with both hands and becomes red in the face. This signal is the universal distress signal for choking (Fig. 19–2). In cases of either partial or complete obstruction, the patient should be encouraged to cough. If coughing is unsuccessful in dislodging the obstruction, the Heimlich maneuver should be used.

Heimlich Maneuver

The purpose of the Heimlich maneuver is to increase intrathoracic pressure sufficiently to propel the lodged object out of the throat. To apply, the rescuer stands behind the victim and wraps both arms around him or her, clutching one fist with the other hand. The thumb side of the fist is placed in the midline of the victim's

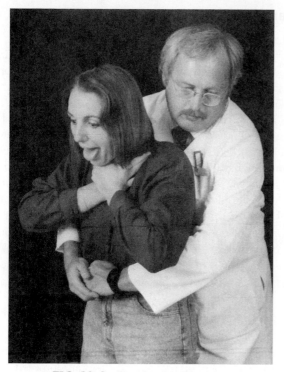

FIG. 19–3   The Heimlich maneuver.

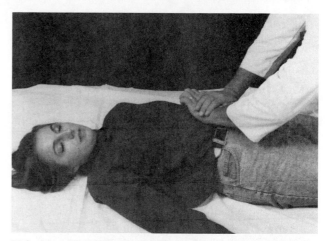

FIG. 19–4   The Heimlich maneuver on an unconscious victim.

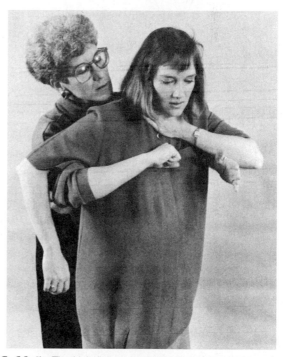

FIG. 19–5   The Heimlich maneuver adapted for a woman in an advanced stage of pregnancy. (Courtesy George Greathouse.)

abdomen, above the navel and well below the sternum. With the rescuer's elbows held out from the victim, pressure is exerted inward and upward (Fig. 19–3). Although each thrust should be administered separately, the procedure may be repeated quickly 6 to 10 times or until the obstructing object is expelled.

An unconscious patient should be placed in the supine position. The rescuer kneels astride the victim and places the heel of one hand as described previously. The second hand is placed directly on top of the first, and pressure is applied in a quick upward thrust (Fig. 19–4).

These maneuvers should not be used with women in advanced stages of pregnancy or with infants or small children. Variations of the Heimlich maneuver have been developed for these situations.

MODIFICATION FOR PREGNANT PATIENTS. Because abdominal thrusts can be dangerous for women in late stages of pregnancy, chest thrusts are used instead. The rescuer again stands behind the patient but places his or her arms under the victim's armpits and around the victim's chest. The thumb side of the fist is placed in the center of the sternum, the second hand is placed over the fist, and backward thrusts are given (Fig. 19–5).

MODIFICATION FOR INFANTS. In infants younger than 1 year, a combination of back blows and chest thrusts is recommended. The infant is held by the rescuer along his or her arm with the head lower than the trunk and supported by holding the victim's jaw. With the arm holding the infant resting on the rescuer's thigh, the rescuer uses the heel of the hand to deliver four back blows between

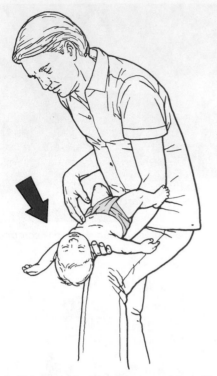

FIG. 19–6   The Heimlich maneuver on an infant. Position the infant face up over the forearm. Use two or three fingers to perform the *abdominal* thrust. (From Craig M: *Essentials of sonography and patient care,* ed 2, Philadelphia, 2006, Elsevier Saunders.)

the infant's scapulae. While continuing to support the head and neck, the infant is turned over, and four chest thrusts are given with two or three fingers (Fig. 19–6). To determine the location of the hand for chest thrusts, the index finger is placed on the sternum just below the intermammary line. Two or three fingers are used to perform the chest thrusts.

CARDIAC ARREST

Signs and Symptoms

Cardiac arrest is the sudden stoppage of cardiac output and leads to permanent organ damage or death if not treated. Death from cardiac arrest has been reduced significantly since the advent of **cardiopulmonary resuscitation (CPR)** and the more recent availability of **automatic external defibrillators (AEDs).** Patients who are experiencing cardiac arrest generally complain of crushing chest pain, often described as feeling as though an elephant is standing on the victim's chest. The pain may also radiate down the left arm.

Cardiopulmonary Resuscitation

The radiologic technologist should be familiar with an institution's protocol for cardiac emergencies. On realization that a patient has suffered cardiac arrest, the appropriate alert should be initiated before the beginning of CPR.

Because cerebral function is generally impaired if the brain is deprived of oxygen for more than 4 to 6 minutes, CPR must be initiated immediately on verifying that cardiopulmonary distress exists, but these procedures absolutely must be performed only after determining that true cardiopulmonary distress exists. CPR provides external support for circulation and respiration and consists of three primary aspects—the ABCs: *a*irway, *b*reathing, and *c*irculation. The following abbreviated protocol is based on the standards and guidelines of the American Medical Association.

ONE-PERSON RESCUE

1. *Establish unresponsiveness* by gently shaking and shouting at the victim (Fig. 19–7, *A*). If these actions fail to rouse the person, then call for help and proceed with CPR.
2. *Position the patient* on his or her back on a hard surface to facilitate CPR. A radiographic table is suitable. If the patient is lying on a stretcher, then the backboard from the emergency cart should be used.
3. *Open the airway* by tilting the head back, which helps prevent the tongue from falling back and obstructing the airway. Place one hand on the victim's forehead and apply firm backward pressure while placing the fingers of the other hand beneath the bony part of the chin and lifting upward (Fig. 19–7, *B*). The lips should be close together, but the mouth should not be completely closed.
4. *Establish breathlessness* by placing an ear over the patient's nose and mouth and looking toward the patient's chest (Fig. 19–7, *C*). In this position, listen for breath sounds, look for any rise and fall in the chest, and feel for flow of air from the victim's nose. If no breath is apparent, then proceed with rescue breathing.
5. *Perform rescue breathing* by putting the palm of the hand on the victim's forehead and using the thumb and fingers to pinch shut the victim's nostrils. Take a deep breath, and seal your lips around those of the victim or place a facemask tightly over the nose and mouth (Fig. 19–7, *D*). Initially, blow two deep breaths, each of 1-second duration, into the patient's mouth or into the mask, while watching to determine

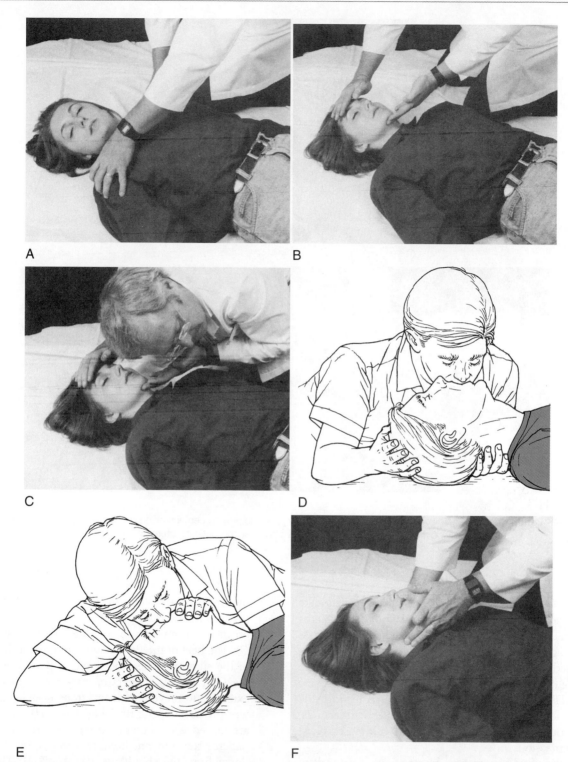

FIG. 19-7 Cardiopulmonary resuscitation: one-person rescue. *A,* Establishing unresponsiveness of victim. *B,* Head tilt–chin lift maneuver. *C,* Proper position for establishing breathlessness. *D,* Mouth-to-mouth rescue breathing. *E,* Mouth-to-nose rescue breathing. (*D* and *E* from Craig M: *Essentials of sonography and patient care,* ed 2, Philadelphia, 2006, Elsevier Saunders.) *F,* Establishing circulatory inadequacy by palpating the carotid artery.

(*Continued on next page*)

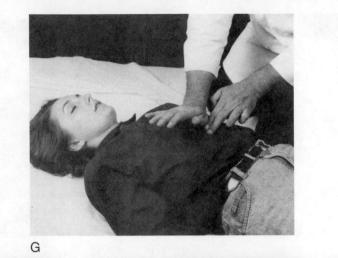

G

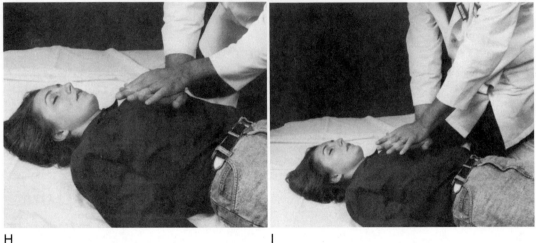

H   I

FIG. 19–7, cont'd *G,* Correct placement of hand along sternum. *H,* Correct placement of hands for external chest compressions. *I,* Locked elbows with the arms extended directly over the patient's sternum to apply compression straight down from the shoulders.

whether the chest is rising and falling. Then take another breath between the ventilations. The breaths should not be rapid or forceful. If the mouth is damaged or clogged, then sealing the victim's mouth closed and sealing your lips or the mask around the nose of the victim is possible (Fig. 19–7, *E*).

6. *Establish circulatory inadequacy* by palpating the carotid artery (Fig. 19–7, *F*). If, after 5 to 10 seconds, the pulse is absent, then proceed with closed chest compressions.

7. *Perform chest compressions* by positioning yourself to one side of the patient and placing the hands properly. This action is done by using the hand to find the lower edge of the rib cage and running the middle and index fingers along the lower edge to the point where the ribs meet the sternum. Place the middle finger at this notch, and then place the heel of the other hand on the sternum next to the index finger (Fig. 19–7, *G*). The heel of the hand should rest along the length of the sternum. The other hand is placed on top of the first, and the fingers of both are interlaced and extended to prevent their tips from applying inadvertent pressure on the ribs (Fig. 19–7, *H*). The elbows are locked with the arms extended directly over the patient's sternum, and compression is applied straight down from the shoulders (Fig. 19–7, I). The force applied should be sufficient to depress the sternum $1\frac{1}{2}$ to 2 inches in an adult. Pressure should be released after each compression to allow the sternum to return to its original position, but the hands should

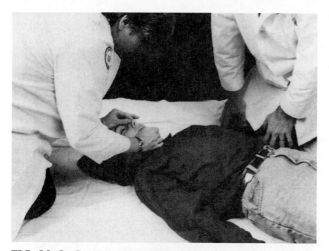

FIG. 19–8 Position of two rescuers for two-person cardiopulmonary resuscitation.

not be lifted from the sternum. Thirty compressions should be alternated with two ventilations; the compressions are given at a rate of approximately 100 per minute.

8. *Reassess*, after four complete cycles of compressions and ventilations (15 : 2 ratio), by taking no more than 7 seconds to reevaluate the patient. If breathing and pulse are still absent, then continue CPR, checking every few minutes for the return of pulse and breathing.

TWO-PERSON RESCUE. The protocol for CPR with two rescuers is similar, but each rescuer independently performs compressions or ventilations with periodic switches of position. One rescuer is at the victim's side and performs chest compressions. The second rescuer is at the victim's head and maintains the open airway and provides breathing, usually mouth to mask (Fig. 19–8).

Compressions are delivered at the rate of approximately 100 per minute, with cycles of 30 compressions and 2 breaths. The breaths are given during pauses in compression and should be of approximately 1-second duration. When rescuers become fatigued, an organized switch of positions should take place.

INFANT RESCUE. The CPR procedure for infants and children is basically the same as that for adults, with adjustments made in the volume of air delivered during artificial breathing and the placement of the hands and the depth of depression of the sternum during external chest compressions. When breathing for a pediatric victim, the volume of air should be just enough to cause the rise and fall of the chest.

When performing chest compressions on infants, the index finger should be placed on the sternum just under the point where it intersects with the intermammary line. Using the second, third, and fourth (or only the third and fourth) fingers, compress the sternum to a depth of $1/2$ to 1 inch at a rate of 100 per minute. In infants and children, two ventilations are given after 15 compressions. For a child up to 8 years of age, the hand placement is the same as for an adult. The chest, however, is compressed with only one hand to a depth of only 1 to $1^{1}/_{2}$ inches.

CONSIDERATIONS. CPR is not indicated in all situations of cardiac arrest. If any doubt exists as to its appropriateness, then it should be initiated. CPR is clearly *not* indicated in instances in which the patient, the patient's family, or the patient's physician has specifically requested that resuscitation not be done. In these cases, a *do not resuscitate (DNR)* order should be clearly indicated on the patient's chart.

Once begun, basic life support should (and for legal reasons, must) be continued until the victim resumes spontaneous respiration and circulation, a physician or other responsible health care professional calls a halt, or the rescuer is too exhausted to continue.

Improperly performed CPR can be not only ineffective, but it can also be hazardous. Possible complications from CPR include rib fractures, fractured sternum, pneumothorax, lacerated liver and spleen, and fat emboli. The incidence of complications can be reduced (but not eliminated) by adherence to guidelines.

The American Medical Association recommends that health professionals be taught all CPR skills, including single-rescuer, two-rescuer, and infant rescue. The professional technologist is encouraged to become familiar with all required skills and to achieve certification in all CPR procedures.

Automatic External Defibrillation

Ventricular fibrillation is a fluttering or ineffective cardiac rhythm that results in the heart's inability to pump blood. Effective ventricular rhythm must be restored within a few minutes to preserve life. The use of AEDs is one of the few times CPR can be interrupted. One of the most important elements of defibrillation is time; performing it in less than 5 minutes is considered critical to survival.

Because each type of external defibrillator operates somewhat differently, the following guidelines are very general. The reader is encouraged to become familiar with any defibrillator in his or her institution. The goal of AED is to determine the need for electric shock and, when necessary, to deliver it.

1. *Determine* that the patient is in cardiac arrest.
2. *Turn on* the defibrillator and prepare the equipment, reading the instructions as necessary.
3. *Attach* the defibrillator cables to the pads if not already connected, and place the pads on the patient. One pad should be placed below the right clavicle on the lateral border of the sternum. The second pad should be placed 2 to 3 inches below the left axilla.
4. *Initiate rhythm analysis,* usually by pressing the ANALYZE button.
5. If indicated, *deliver the shock.* The need to do so may be indicated by a written message, an audio alarm, a synthesized voice announcement, or a combination of these. After the first shock, press the ANALYZE button again to begin another analysis. Following a third shock, CPR should be performed for 1 minute, at which point check again for a pulse and continue as appropriate.
6. If no shock is indicated, continue CPR.

CEREBROVASCULAR ACCIDENT

A **cerebrovascular accident (stroke or brain attack)** may occur in patients in the radiology department. Strokes are more likely to occur in older patients (over 75 years of age) but can occur in any adult. The onset of a stroke may be sudden or may develop gradually over a period of several hours. Warning signs include paralysis on one or both sides, slurred speech or complete loss of speech, extreme dizziness, loss of vision (particularly if only in one eye), and complete loss of consciousness. The symptoms are sometimes only temporary.

If the radiologic technologist observes any of these signs or symptoms, even if they are only temporary, they should be reported to a nurse or physician. Because the potential for paralysis or loss of consciousness is present, the patient should not stand or be moved before further medical assessment can be made. If the patient loses consciousness, CPR may be required and should proceed as described.

MINOR MEDICAL EMERGENCIES

Nausea and Vomiting

Other minor incidents may happen in the radiology department that, although not threatening serious injury,

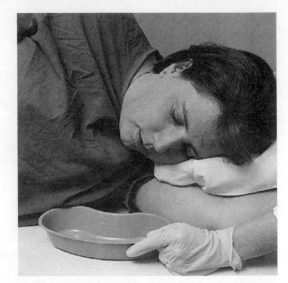

FIG. 19–9 Lateral decubitus position to prevent aspiration of vomitus.

should nevertheless be handled expeditiously. **Nausea** and **vomiting** are frequent occurrences. Nausea tends to be both a psychologic and a physiologic reaction. Patients who feel nauseous often report the feeling to the health care worker. Patients who follow instructions to breathe slowly and deeply through their mouths often become calmer, and nausea and vomiting are avoided.

If the technique does not work and vomiting does occur, then the patient should be in a position in which aspiration of vomitus into the lungs is not likely. Recumbent patients should be helped into a lateral decubitus position if possible (Fig. 19–9). If such movement of the patient is contraindicated (e.g., in a patient with a fracture of an arm or leg), then the patient should be assisted in turning his or her head to the side. All patients should be provided with an emesis basin and moist cloths.

Epistaxis

Epistaxis, or nosebleed, is another common occurrence. Again, this event is seldom life threatening. Patients should lean forward and pinch the affected nostril against the midline nasal cartilage with digital pressure (with the fingers). Patients should not be put in a recumbent position or instructed to tilt the head backward because this action allows the blood to flow down the throat, resulting in the patient's swallowing it. If gentle pressure fails to stop the blood flow, then a moist compress also may be applied, which will stop most nosebleeds. If these actions are not effective within 15 minutes, then medical assistance should be obtained.

Vertigo and Syncope

Many otherwise healthy patients who have been bedridden or who have had limited mobility for a period often experience **vertigo** (dizziness) or **syncope** (fainting). Vertigo is also often a precursor to syncope. A patient who experiences vertigo should be assisted to a seated or recumbent position, which prevents injury from falling as a result of problems with equilibrium. Patients who arise from a radiographic table often experience vertigo as a result of orthostatic hypotension; therefore care should be exercised not to rush these patients, letting them sit on the side of the table for a few minutes before they are escorted from the radiography room.

Syncope is a self-correcting, temporary state of shock and the result of lack of blood flow to the brain. Treatment is aimed at increasing blood flow to the head. The patient should be assisted to a recumbent position, with the feet elevated. Any tight clothing should be loosened. These actions assist in increasing overall blood flow. A moist cloth may be applied to the forehead. Patients should remain recumbent until they feel strong enough to undergo the remainder of the procedure or return to their rooms.

Seizures

A seizure by a patient is one of the most frightening events a radiologic technologist might experience. Seizures are caused by a variety of factors, few of which are clearly understood, and may range from mild to severe. A patient who undergoes a mild seizure may experience a brief loss of consciousness or may stare into space for a brief time. This patient may be only slightly confused and weak after such an episode, but the procedure should nevertheless be postponed until another time.

Severe seizures are characterized by involuntary contraction of muscles on either one or both sides of the body. They may last for only a minute or up to several minutes. The patient may drool from his or her mouth because of loss of control. The goal is to prevent the patient from injuring him or herself to the extent possible. No attempt should be made to restrain the patient because the involuntary movements make this not only ineffective, but also dangerous. Similarly, no health care worker should ever place his or her hand in a patient's mouth to prevent a backward tongue drop.

Patients who are about to have a seizure often experience an **aura**, a physical or mental warning of an impending seizure. The aura is unique for each individual but can be an important help to both the patient and the health care professional. If sufficient warning is given, the patient should be moved to the floor away from objects against which he or she might hit his or her head. A pillow should be placed under the head so it is not banged against the floor. The same precautions should be taken with all patients who experience a seizure, although the absence of a warning aura requires the technologist to be more creative in minimizing the potential for patient harm.

After a seizure, the technologist should be sure that the patient has an open airway, clearing mucus from the mouth as necessary. The patient typically is weak and perhaps disoriented and generally has no memory of the seizure.

Although these experiences are often startling, noting a few things about the seizure itself is helpful to the patient's caregiver. First, make note of where the seizure began, whether it was one-sided or two-sided, and its length. These pieces of information are often important clues in determining the nature of the seizure and may prove helpful in later management and treatment.

Falls

Despite appropriate assistance and care, a patient occasionally falls while in the radiology department. In such a situation, the technologist should attempt to minimize the physical impact of the fall to the extent possible and then proceed with appropriate emergency action as indicated by the patient's condition.

WOUNDS

Hemorrhage

Some patients come to the radiology department with **wounds** sustained previously or during surgery. Such wounds may **hemorrhage** (i.e., bleed outside a vessel). The technologist should always make note of the condition of dressings. If they are clean at the outset of a procedure but become saturated, then attention is needed. The saturated dressing should not be removed. Pressure should be applied directly over the saturated dressing, preferably with an additional sterile bandage pressed against it. Because clotting can take up to 10 minutes, the pressure may need to be maintained for some time. Once the bleeding appears to be under control, the bandage should be tied or taped into place.

When a bleeding wound is on an extremity, the affected extremity may be placed above the level of the heart unless other problems that would contraindicate such a procedure exist. This action slows the blood flow to the extremity and results in less blood loss.

Burns

The radiologic technologist may be required to perform radiologic procedures on patients with burns. Because a burn injury disrupts the normal protective function of the skin, maintaining sterile precautions is imperative. Burns are typically extremely painful injuries; therefore extra gentle care in handling is also indicated.

Dehiscence

Wound dehiscence is uncommon but may happen. Dehiscence refers to a situation in which a patient's sutures separate, allowing abdominal contents to spill out of the peritoneal cavity. No attempt should be made to replace tissues inside the wound, but a sterile dressing should be used to cover the area. The patient should be placed in a seated position, somewhat bent forward to relieve any additional pressure on the wound. Medical attention should be obtained quickly.

SUMMARY

The thought of some of these medical emergencies may be somewhat frightening, but most of them are uncommon. They do occur with enough regularity, however, that the technologist must be aware of typical signs and symptoms associated with the various conditions. The radiologic technologist should be prepared to deal with major medical emergencies, including head injuries, shock, diabetic crises, respiratory distress or arrest, and cardiac arrest. Minor emergencies that may be encountered include nausea and vomiting, epistaxis, syncope and vertigo, seizures, falls, and problems with wounds. An alert technologist who obtains medical assistance quickly may significantly reduce a patient's morbidity and may also play a role in saving a life.

In addition to the technical knowledge necessary, responding to all of these situations in a calm, confident manner is also important for the radiologic technologist. Thinking and acting appropriately in such periods of stress is difficult, but being able to do so is important to the overall outcome. Moving too quickly and risking a mistake is not worth the potential harm that might result.

BIBLIOGRAPHY

Adult basic life support, *Circulation* 112(Suppl I):III-5, 2005.
Defibrillation, *Circulation* 112(Suppl I):III-60, 2005.
Pediatric basic and advanced life support, *Circulation* 112 (Suppl I):III-17, 2005.
American Medical Association: Standards and guidelines for cardiopulmonary resuscitation (CPR) and emergency cardiac care (ECE), *JAMA* 255:2905, 1986.
Copass MKet al: *EMT manual,* ed 3, Philadelphia, 1998, WB Saunders.
Judd RL, Ponsell DD: *Mosby's first responder,* ed 7, St Louis, 1995, Mosby.
Limmer D, Elling B, O'Keefe MP: *Essentials of emergency care,* ed 3, Upper Saddle River, NJ, 2002, Prentice Hall.
Limmer D et al: *Emergency care,* ed 10, Los Angeles, 2004, Pearson Education.
Shade BR et al: *EMT-intermediate textbook,* St Louis, 2002, Mosby.
Thompson JM et al: *Mosby's clinical nursing,* ed 5, St Louis, 2002, Mosby.

20

Pharmacology

Samuel L. Gurevitz, RPh, PharmD
Marcia S. Mulcahey, MSN, RN, NP

It depends only upon the dose whether a poison is poison or not . . . a lot kills, a little cures.

Paracelsus
Grandfather of Pharmacology, 16th c.

OBJECTIVES   *On completion of this chapter, the student will be able to:*

1. Recognize common definitions and nomenclature associated with pharmacology.

2. Recognize the various classifications of drugs.

3. Describe the actions, indications, and precautions related to various drugs.

4. List the *five rights* of drug administration.

5. List the methods of drug administration.

6. Prepare intravenous drugs for injection.

7. Perform venipuncture using appropriate universal precautions.

8. Describe documentation procedures related to drug administration.

GLOSSARY

Ampule: small sealed glass container that holds a single dose of parenteral solution in a sterile condition

Analgesic: drug that relieves pain without causing a loss of consciousness

Anaphylaxis: condition of shock caused by hypersensitivity to a drug or other substance that results in life-threatening respiratory distress and vascular collapse

Anesthetic: drug that produces a loss of feeling or sensation

Angina Pectoris: severe constricting pain in the chest, often radiating to the shoulder and down the arm, caused by ischemia (obstruction of blood supply) of the heart muscle usually caused by coronary disease

Anticholinergic: drug that blocks the passage of impulses through the parasympathetic nerves

Arrhythmia: any variation from the normal rhythm of the heartbeat

Atherosclerosis: condition in which thickening of the wall of a blood vessel occurs caused by the deposit of plaque (atheroma)

Bolus: concentrated mass of pharmaceutical preparation

Bronchodilator: drug that causes expansion of the lumina of the air passages of the lungs

Coagulation: process of clot formation

Contraindication: any condition that renders the administration of some drug or some particular line of treatment improper or undesirable

Diabetes Mellitus: primarily a disorder of carbohydrate, protein, and fat metabolism secondary to insufficient secretion of insulin or insulin resistance

Diabetic Gastroparesis: form of nerve damage that affects the stomach; food does not move through the stomach in a normal way, resulting in vomiting, nausea, or bloating

Diuretic: drug that promotes the excretion of urine

Drug: any substance that, when taken into a living organism, may modify one or more of its functions.

Edema: presence of abnormally large amounts of fluid in the tissues of the body

Extravasation: discharge or escape of fluid from a vessel into the surrounding tissue that can cause localized vasoconstriction, resulting in sloughing of tissue and tissue necrosis if not reversed with an antidote

Gastroesophageal Reflux Disease (GERD): inflammation of the lower esophagus from regurgitation of acid gastric contents; symptoms include heartburn

Generic Name: drug name that is usually descriptive of its chemical structure but is not protected as is a trademark

Hematoma: localized collection of blood in the tissue resulting from a break in the wall of the blood vessel

Hyperlipidemia: elevations of plasma lipid concentration

Hypertension: persistently high arterial blood pressure, usually exceeding 140 mm Hg systolic and 90 mm Hg diastolic

Idiosyncratic Reaction: unusual response to a drug that is peculiar to the individual

Infiltration: diffusion of fluid into a tissue; often used interchangeably with *extravasation*

Intramuscular: within the muscle tissue

Intravenous: within a vein

Laxative: agent that promotes evacuation of the bowel

Metabolic Acidosis: condition resulting from accumulation of acid or depletion of alkaline reserves (bicarbonate in the blood and body tissues)

Microorganism: microscopic organism such as a bacterium or a virus that is too small to be seen without a microscope

Opioid: any drug, natural or synthetic, that has activity similar to those of morphine

Parenteral: not through the gastrointestinal tract but by injection through some other route

GLOSSARY—Cont'd

Peristalsis: waves of contraction that propel contents through the gastrointestinal tract

Pharmacokinetics: study of the metabolism and action of drugs with particular emphasis on the time required for absorption, duration of action, distribution in the body, and method of excretion

Pharmacist: person who is licensed to prepare and dispense drugs

Pharmacology: study of drugs and their origin, nature, properties, and effects on living organisms

Physical Dependence: state of adaptation exhibited by a withdrawal syndrome specific to a class of drugs and that may be produced by abrupt cessation, rapid dose reduction, or administration of an antagonist

Schizophrenia: chronic mental disorder characterized by periods of withdrawn or bizarre behavior

Shock: condition characterized by profound hypotension and reduced tissue perfusion

Side Effect: consequence other than the one for which a drug is used

Subcutaneous: beneath the skin

Sublingual: beneath the tongue

Therapeutic: pertaining to the art of healing

Thromboembolic Disorders: conditions involving the partial or complete obstruction of a blood vessel

Tolerance: state of adaptation in response to drug exposure that results in a decrease of one or more of the drug's effects over time

Topical: applied to a certain area of the skin and affecting only the area to which it is applied

Transdermal: entering through the skin

Vasoconstrictor: drug that causes constriction of the blood vessels

Vasodilator: drug that causes dilatation of the blood vessels

Venipuncture: puncture of a vein

Vial: small glass bottle containing multiple doses of a drug

INTRODUCTION TO PHARMACOLOGY

The preparation of drugs is often a responsibility of radiologic technologists. Under the direction of a licensed practitioner, usually a radiologist, the technologist is frequently required to administer drugs in the radiology department. Increasingly, the radiologic technologist is expected to have broad knowledge of drugs, including their classification, actions, interactions, reactions, and principles and methods of administration, as well as the skills necessary to assist with drug administration in many different clinical situations. This knowledge is essential to good patient care and competent professional practice. As the role and responsibilities of the radiologic technologist continue to expand in the area of drug administration, the information presented in this chapter will provide a fundamental theoretical framework within which the level of knowledge may increase.

A **drug** is any chemical substance that produces a biologic response in a living system. More specifically, a drug is a substance used as medicine to aid in the diagnosis, treatment, or prevention of disease. The science concerned with the origin, nature, effects, and uses of drugs is called **pharmacology.**

Drug Nomenclature

A *nomenclature* is a classified system of names. In pharmacology, drugs are classified in many different ways. For example, a drug may be classified by its name, its action, or its method of legal purchase. When drugs are classified by name, knowing which kind of name is being used is important because the same drug has at least three different names: (1) a chemical name, (2) a generic name, and (3) a trade name.

CLASSIFICATION BY NAME. The first name that is likely to be applied to a drug is the *chemical name,* which identifies the actual chemical structure of the drug. The chemical name is often complex and is seldom of practical importance to the technologist.

The **generic name** is the name given to the drug when it becomes commercially available. The generic name is a simpler name derived from the more complex chemical name. It is usually easier to pronounce than the chemical and is never capitalized; it is also called the *nonproprietary* name. Some drugs are best known by their generic name.

A *brand name* is the name given to a drug manufactured by a specific company. It is usually short and easy to remember. It may or may not reflect any characteristic of the chemical structure of the drug. Because the same drug is manufactured by more than one company, each company selects its own brand name or trademark for the drug. *Trademark, brand name, trade name,* and *proprietary name* are all terms used interchangeably to indicate a specific generic drug manufactured by several different companies. An example of the names currently used for a single drug follows:

Chemical name—7-chloro-1,3-dihydro-1-methyl-5-phenyl-2H-1,4-benzodiazepin-2-one
Generic name—diazepam
Brand name—Valium

Confusion occurs when some physicians use generic names and others use trade names when requesting drugs. Therefore the radiologic technologist should be aware of drug information resources that are available. One such source is the *Physicians' Desk Reference,* or *PDR,* as it is frequently called. The *PDR* is an annual publication that contains current product information. The pages are color coded for easy reference, and the *PDR* lists drugs by both their generic and their brand names. The *PDR* gives the accepted uses, side effects, **contraindications**, and doses for available drugs. If a *PDR* is not readily available in the radiology department, then the next best source of drug information is the hospital pharmacist.

CLASSIFICATION BY ACTION. Drugs are also classified according to action or function. Drugs that have similar chemical actions are grouped into categories called *drug families.* For example, drugs that relieve pain are classified as **analgesics,** drugs used to treat high blood pressure are classified as *antihypertensives,* and drugs used to fight inflammation are classified as *antiinflammatories.* Although this system is a convenient way to classify drugs for study purposes, it is not totally reliable or exclusive because one drug may have several different physiologic effects on the body, which means it would be listed under more than one category.

LEGAL CLASSIFICATION. According to federal laws, drugs are classified legally as either prescription or nonprescription. Prescription drugs require an order by a legally authorized health practitioner who is usually, but not always, a physician. The prescription is the documentation that specifies precisely the name of the patient, the name of the drug, and the dosage regimen to be followed. Prescription drugs are usually dispensed by a licensed **pharmacist**, although some physicians supply prescription drugs to their patients. Nonprescription drugs, better known as *over-the-counter drugs,* can be obtained legally without a prescription. Another group of substances that can be obtained without a prescription are called *dietary supplements.* Vitamins, supplements, and herbal remedies are classified as dietary supplements and by law are not classified as drugs and are therefore not controlled by the U.S. Food and Drug Administration (FDA). This classification means that herbal remedies can be sold without proof of safety or efficacy. The radiologic technologist should be aware that many over-the-counter products and herbal remedies are capable of producing toxic effects if they are misused or used in combination with other drugs. For example, St. John's wort interacts with dozens of prescription medications.

Dose Forms

The *dose form* of a drug refers to the type of preparation or the manner in which the chemical agent is transported into the human body. A single drug may be available in many different forms to facilitate the administration and action of the drug under a variety of conditions. The dose form may determine the speed, or onset, of the drug's therapeutic effect. Some of the common dose forms include tablets, capsules, suppositories, solutions, suspensions, and transdermal patches.

TABLET. *Tablets* are the most common oral dose form and one of the easiest to administer. A tablet is a granulated drug that has been compressed into a solid hard disc. Tablets are single-dose units that may be scored to facilitate division into halves or quarters. A tablet that is not scored should not be broken into smaller parts. Some tablets are coated with a substance that delays the dissolution of the tablet until it is in the small intestines rather than in the stomach, where it is normally dissolved. These so-called *enteric-coated* tablets are used for drugs that might irritate the stomach (such as aspirin) or for drugs destroyed by the acid in the stomach.

CAPSULE. A *capsule* is a dose form in which a powdered or liquid drug is contained in a gelatin shell. The gelatin shell dissolves in the stomach and releases its contents.

INHALANT. The *inhalation* route of administration may be used for either local or systemic effects (general anesthetics). Inhalants are used for their local effects in the treatment of asthma or chronic obstructive pulmonary disease (COPD). After inhalation, high drug concentrations are deposited to the respiratory mucosa and exert action by producing bronchodilation or reducing inflammation. Local therapeutic effects are optimized, and systemic side effects are minimized.

SUPPOSITORY. A *suppository* is a dose form shaped for insertion into a body orifice such as the rectum, vagina, or urethra. Once inserted, the suppository dissolves and releases the drug. It may have a local or systemic effect.

SOLUTION. A *solution* is a dose form in which one or more drugs are dissolved in a liquid carrier. Solutions are usually rapidly absorbed and may be administered orally or parenterally. **Parenteral** administration includes any injection of the drug with a needle and syringe beneath the surface of the skin.

SUSPENSION. A *suspension* is a dose form in which one or more drugs in small particles are suspended in a liquid carrier. Most suspensions are administered orally and should be shaken thoroughly just before administration. Suspensions should never be administered intravenously.

TRANSDERMAL PATCH. A *transdermal patch* is a dose form that permits a drug to be applied on the skin surface, where it is absorbed into the bloodstream. The patchlike device containing the drug is applied to the skin with a water-resistant covering. The patch releases the drug gradually over time.

CLASSIFICATION OF DRUGS

For easy reference, Table 20-1 lists commonly used drugs alphabetically by the trade name. Table 20-2 provides a cross-reference by generic name, and Table 20-3 provides a classification by drug action. The dietary supplements and herbal remedies commonly used are listed alphabetically in Table 20-4 along with the potential interactions that may occur with prescription and nonprescription drugs. The drugs commonly found on a crash cart for emergency situations are listed alphabetically by trade name in Box 20-1.

Actions, Indications, and Precautions

ANALGESICS. *Analgesics* are drugs that relieve pain without causing loss of consciousness. Analgesics can be divided into two groups: the nonopioids (nonnarcotic) and the **opioids** (narcotic). Health professionals are encouraged to use the word *opioid* or *opioids* rather than *narcotic* or *narcotics*. The term opioid is less likely than a narcotic to carry a stigma of drug of abuse. Opioids such

BOX 20-1	Emergency Drugs Commonly Found on a Crash Cart	
Medication	**Indication**
Adenocard	Arrhythmias
Atropine	Bradycardia
Benadryl	Allergic reaction
Cordarone	Arrhythmias
Decadron	Allergic reaction
Dilantin	Seizures
Dobutrex	Shock, hypotension
Epinephrine	Cardiac arrest, anaphylaxis
Intropin	Shock
Isoptin	Arrhythmias
Lasix	Edema
Levophed	Shock
Pronestyl	Arrhythmias
Sodium bicarbonate	Metabolic acidosis
Xylocaine	Arrhythmias

as morphine and oxycodone (OxyContin) are used in the treatment of moderate to severe pain. Whereas **physical dependence** and **tolerance** is common with long-term opioid use, addiction is not. *Addiction* is a chronic neurobiologic disease characterized by one or more of the following behaviors: impaired control over drug use, compulsive use, continued use despite harm, inappropriate use, and craving. Adverse side effects such as nausea, vomiting, and constipation are frequently associated with the administration of opioid analgesics. Nonopioid analgesics such as acetaminophen (N-acetyl-para-amino-phenol [APAP]; Tylenol) are relatively safe drugs used in the treatment of mild to moderate pain. They do not cause physiologic dependency.

ANESTHETICS. Anesthetics are agents that act on the central nervous system (CNS) to produce a loss of sensation. Two types of anesthetic agents are general anesthetics and local anesthetics. General anesthetics can be divided into inhalation agents such as sevoflurane (Ultane) or intravenous agents such as propofol (Diprivan). They act as CNS depressants by producing muscle relaxation and loss of consciousness. General anesthesia is commonly used on patients undergoing major surgical procedures. Local anesthetics such as mepivacaine (Carbocaine) block nerve conduction from an area of the body to the CNS. The extent of their action depends on the area to which they are applied.

Text continued on p. 298

TABLE 20-1 Commonly Used Drugs by Brand Name

BRAND NAME	GENERIC NAME	ROUTE(S)	CLASSIFICATION
Activase	Alteplase	Parenteral	Thrombolytic
Actos	Pioglitazone	Oral	Antidiabetic
Adderall	Amphetamine salts	Oral	Stimulant
Adenocard	Adenosine	Parenteral	Antiarrhythmic
Advair	Salmeterol/fluticasone	Inhalation	Bronchodilator/corticosteroid
Adrenalin	Epinephrine	Parenteral	Stimulant
Allegra	Fexofenadine	Oral	Antihistamine
Amaryl	Glimepiride	Oral	Antidiabetic
Ambien	Zolpidem	Oral	Hypnotic
Amoxil	Amoxicillin	Oral	Antibiotic
Aricept	Donepezil	Oral	Cholinesterase inhibitor
Aspirin	Aspirin	Oral	Analgesic/antiplatelet
Ativan	Lorazepam	Oral/parenteral	Antianxiety
Atropine	Atropine	Oral/parenteral	Anticholinergic
Atrovent	Ipratropium	Inhalation	Bronchodilator
Avandia	Rosiglitazone	Oral	Antidiabetic
Benadryl	Diphenhydramine	Oral/parenteral	Antihistamine
Biaxin	Clarithromycin	Oral	Antibiotic
Bumex	Bumetanide	Oral/parenteral	Diuretic
Carbocaine	Mepivicaine	Parenteral	Local anesthetic
Cardura	Doxazosin	Oral	Antihypertensive
Catapres	Clonidine	Oral/transdermal	Antihypertensive
Celebrex	Celecoxib	Oral	Antiinflammatory
Celexa	Citalopram	Oral	Antidepressant
Claritin	Loratadine	Oral	Antihistamine
Chloral hydrate	Chloral hydrate	Oral	Sedative
Cipro	Ciprofloxacin	Oral/parenteral	Antibiotic
Compazine	Prochlorperazine	Oral/parenteral	Antiemetic
Cordarone	Amiodarone	Oral/parenteral	Antiarrhythmic
Coumadin	Warfarin	Oral/parenteral	Anticoagulant
Cozaar	Losartan	Oral	Antihypertensive
Darvocet N	Propoxyphene/APAP	Oral	Analgesic
Decadron	Dexamethasone	Oral/parenteral	Corticosteroid
Deltasone	Prednisone	Oral	Corticosteroid
Depakote	Valproate	Oral/parenteral	Antiepileptic
Depo-Medrol	Methylprednisolone	Parenteral	Corticosteroid
Detrol LA	Tolterodine	Oral	Anticholinergic
Diflucan	Fluconazole	Oral/parenteral	Antifungal
Dilantin	Phenytoin	Oral/parenteral	Antiepileptic
Diovan	Valsartan	Oral	Antihypertensive
Diprivan	Propofol	Parenteral	Anesthetic
Ditropan XL	Oxybutynin	Oral/transdermal	Anticholinergic
Dobutrex	Dobutamine	Parenteral	Stimulant
Dulcolax	Bisacodyl	Oral	Laxative
Duragesic	Fentanyl	Parenteral/transdermal	Analgesic
Epivir	Lamivudine	Oral	Antiviral
Erythromycin	Erythromycin	Oral/parenteral	Antibiotic
Flovent	Fluticasone	Inhalation	Corticosteroid
Fungizone	Amphotericin B	Parenteral	Antifungal
Glucophage	Metformin	Oral	Antidiabetic
Glucotrol	Glipizide	Oral	Antidiabetic
Haldol	Haloperidol	Oral/parenteral	Antipsychotic
Heparin	Heparin	Parenteral	Anticoagulant
Hydrochlorothiazide	Hydrochlorothiazide	Oral	Diuretic
Intropin	Dopamine	Parenteral	Stimulant
Keflex	Cephalexin	Oral	Antibiotic
Klonopin	Clonazepam	Oral	Antiepileptic/antianxiety
Lanoxin	Digoxin	Oral/parenteral	Antiarrhythmic

TABLE 20-1 **Commonly Used Drugs by Brand Name—cont'd**

BRAND NAME	GENERIC NAME	ROUTE(S)	CLASSIFICATION
Lasix	Furosemide	Oral/parenteral	Diuretic
Levophed	Norepinephrine	Parenteral	Vasoconstrictor
Lipitor	Atorvastatin	Oral	Antihyperlipidemic
Lithium	Lithium	Oral	Mood stabilizer
Lopid	Gemfibrozil	Oral	Antihyperlipidemic
Lopressor	Metoprolol	Oral/parenteral	Antihypertensive
Lotensin	Benazepril	Oral	Antihypertensive
Lovenox	Enoxaparin	Parenteral	Anticoagulant
Mephyton	Phytonadione	Oral/parenteral	Coagulant
Micronase	Glyburide	Oral	Antidiabetic
Monopril	Fosinopril	Oral	Antihypertensive
Morphine	Morphine	Oral/parenteral	Analgesic
Motrin	Ibuprofen	Oral	Antiinflammatory
Naprosyn	Naproxen	Oral	Antiinflammatory
Neurontin	Gabapentin	Oral	Antiepileptic
Nitroglycerin	Nitroglycerin	Oral/parenteral/transdermal	Vasodilator
Nitropress	Nitroprusside	Parenteral	Vasodilator
Norvasc	Amlodipine	Oral	Antihypertensive
OxyContin	Oxycodone	Oral	Analgesic
Paxil	Paroxetine	Oral	Antidepressant
Pepcid	Famotidine	Oral/parenteral	Antiulcer
Percocet	Oxycodone/APAP	Oral	Analgesic
Plavix	Clopidogrel	Oral	Antiplatelet
Premarin	Conjugated estrogen	Oral	Female hormone
Prevacid	Lansoprazole	Oral/parenteral	Antiulcer
Prilosec	Omeprazole	Oral	Antiulcer
Proventil	Albuterol	Oral/inhalation	Bronchodilator
Prozac	Fluoxetine	Oral	Antidepressant
Reglan	Metoclopramide	Oral/parenteral	Antiemetic
ReoPro	Abciximab	Parenteral	Antiplatelet
Restoril	Temazepam	Oral	Hypnotic
Retavase	Reteplase	Parenteral	Thrombolytic
Risperdal	Risperidone	Oral/parenteral	Antipsychotic
Ritalin	Methylphenidate	Oral	Stimulant
Rocephin	Ceftriaxone	Parenteral	Antibiotic
Serevent	Salmeterol	Inhalation	Bronchodilator
Solu-Cortef	Hydrocortisone	Parenteral	Corticosteroid
Spiriva	Tiotropium	Inhalation	Bronchodilator
Tenormin	Atenolol	Oral	Antihypertensive
Topamax	Topiramate	Oral	Antiepileptic
Tylenol	Acetaminophen	Oral	Analgesic
Ultane	Sevoflurane	Inhalation	Anesthetic
Ultram	Tramadol	Oral	Analgesic
Valium	Diazepam	Oral/parenteral	Antianxiety
Vasotec	Enalapril	Oral/parenteral	Antihypertensive
Verapamil	Verapamil	Oral/parenteral	Antiarrhythmic
Versed	Midazolam	Oral/parenteral	Antianxiety
Vicodin	Hydrocodone/APAP	Oral	Analgesic
Vistaril	Hydroxyzine	Oral/parenteral	Sedative
Wellbutrin	Bupropion	Oral	Antidepressant
Xanax	Alprazolam	Oral	Antianxiety
Xylocaine	Lidocaine	Parenteral	Antiarrhythmic/local anesthetic
Zantac	Ranitidine	Oral/parenteral	Antiulcer
Zestril	Lisinopril	Oral	Antihypertensive
Zithromax	Azithromycin	Oral/parenteral	Antibiotic
Zocor	Simvastatin	Oral	Antihyperlipidemic
Zofran	Ondansetron	Oral/parenteral	Antiemetic
Zoloft	Sertraline	Oral	Antidepressant
Zovirax	Acyclovir	Oral/parenteral	Antiviral
Zyprexa	Olanzapine	Oral/parenteral	Antipsychotic

TABLE 20-2 Commonly Used Drugs by Generic Name

GENERIC NAME	BRAND NAME	ROUTE(S)	CLASSIFICATION
Abciximab	ReoPro	Parenteral	Antiplatelet
Acetaminophen	Tylenol	Oral	Analgesic
Adenosine	Adenocard	Parenteral	Antiarrhythmic
Albuterol	Proventil	Oral/inhalation	Bronchodilator
Alprazolam	Xanax	Oral	Antianxiety
Alteplase	Activase	Parenteral	Thrombolytic
Acyclovir	Zovirax	Oral/parenteral	Antiviral
Amiodarone	Cordarone	Oral/parenteral	Antiarrhythmic
Amlodipine	Norvasc	Oral	Antihypertensive
Amoxicillin	Amoxil	Oral	Antibiotic
Amphetamine salts	Adderall	Oral	Stimulant
Amphotericin B	Fungizone	Parenteral	Antifungal
Aspirin	Aspirin	Oral	Analgesic/antiplatelet
Atenolol	Tenormin	Oral	Antihypertensive
Atorvastatin	Lipitor	Oral	Antihyperlipidemic
Atropine	Atropine	Oral/parenteral	Anticholinergic
Azithromycin	Zithromax	Oral/parenteral	Antibiotic
Benazepril	Lotensin	Oral	Antihypertensive
Bisacodyl	Dulcolax	Oral	Laxative
Bumetanide	Bumex	Oral/parenteral	Diuretic
Bupropion	Wellbutrin	Oral	Antidepressant
Celecoxib	Celebrex	Oral	Antiinflammatory
Cephalexin	Keflex	Oral	Antibiotic
Chloral hydrate	Chloral hydrate	Oral	Sedative
Chlorpromazine	Thorazine	Oral/parenteral	Antipsychotic
Ciprofloxacin	Cipro	Oral/parenteral	Antibiotic
Citalopram	Celexa	Oral	Antidepressant
Clarithromycin	Biaxin	Oral	Antibiotic
Clonazepam	Klonopin	Oral	Antiepileptic
Clonidine	Catapres	Oral/transdermal	Antihypertensive
Clopidogrel	Plavix	Oral	Antiplatelet
Conjugated estrogens	Premarin	Oral	Female hormone
Dexamethasone	Decadron	Oral/parenteral	Corticosteroid
Diazepam	Valium	Oral/parenteral	Antianxiety
Digoxin	Lanoxin	Oral/parenteral	Antiarrhythmic
Diphenhydramine	Benadryl	Oral/parenteral	Antihistamine
Dobutamine	Dobutrex	Parenteral	Stimulant
Donepezil	Aricept	Oral	Cholinesterase inhibitor
Dopamine	Intropin	Parenteral	Stimulant
Doxazosin	Cardura	Oral	Antihypertensive
Enalapril	Vasotec	Oral/parenteral	Antihypertensive
Enoxaparin	Lovenox	Parenteral	Anticoagulant
Epinephrine	Adrenalin	Parenteral	Stimulant
Erythromycin	Erythromycin	Oral/parenteral	Antibiotic
Famotidine	Pepcid	Oral	Antiulcer
Fentanyl	Duragesic	Parenteral/transdermal	Analgesic
Fexofenadine	Allegra	Oral	Antihistamine
Fluconazole	Diflucan	Oral/parenteral	Antifungal
Gabapentin	Neurontin	Oral	Antiepileptic
Gemfibrozil	Lopid	Oral	Antihyperlipidemic
Glimepiride	Amaryl	Oral	Antidiabetic

TABLE 20-2 Commonly Used Drugs by Generic Name—cont'd

GENERIC NAME	BRAND NAME	ROUTE(S)	CLASSIFICATION
Glipizide	Glucotrol	Oral	Antidiabetic
Glyburide	Micronase	Oral	Antidiabetic
Fluoxetine	Prozac	Oral	Antidepressant
Fluticasone	Flovent	Inhalation	Corticosteroid
Fosinopril	Monopril	Oral	Antihypertensive
Furosemide	Lasix	Oral/parenteral	Diuretic
Haloperidol	Haldol	Oral/parenteral	Antipsychotic
Heparin	Heparin	Parenteral	Anticoagulant
Hydrochlorothiazide	Hydrochlorothiazide	Oral/parenteral	Diuretic
Hydrocodone/APAP	Vicodin	Oral	Analgesic
Hydrocortisone	Solu-Cortef	Parenteral	Corticosteroid
Hydroxyzine	Vistaril	Oral/parenteral	Sedative
Ibuprofen	Motrin	Oral	Antiinflammatory
Ipratropium	Atrovent	Inhalation	Bronchodilator
Lamivudine	Epivir	Oral	Antiviral
Lansoprazole	Prevacid	Oral/parenteral	Antiulcer
Lidocaine	Xylocaine	Parenteral	Antiarrhythmic/local anesthetic
Lisinopril	Zestril	Oral	Antihypertensive
Lithium	Lithium	Oral	Mood stabilizer
Loratadine	Claritin	Oral	Antihistamine
Lorazepam	Ativan	Oral/parenteral	Antianxiety
Losartan	Cozaar	Oral	Antihypertensive
Mepivicaine	Carbocaine	Parenteral	Local anesthetic
Metformin	Glucophage	Oral	Antidiabetic
Methylphenidate	Ritalin	Oral	Stimulant
Methylprednisolone	Depo-Medrol	Parenteral	Corticosteroid
Metoclopramide	Reglan	Oral/parenteral	Antiemetic
Metoprolol	Lopressor	Oral/parenteral	Antihypertensive
Midazolam	Versed	Oral/parenteral	Antianxiety
Morphine	Morphine	Oral/parenteral	Analgesic
Naproxen	Naprosyn	Oral	Antiinflammatory
Nitroglycerin	Nitroglycerin	Oral/parenteral/transdermal	Vasodilator
Nitroprusside	Nitropress	Parenteral	Vasodilator
Norepinephrine	Levophed	Parenteral	Vasoconstrictor
Olanzapine	Zyprexa	Oral/parenteral	Antipsychotic
Omeprazole	Prilosec	Oral	Antiulcer
Ondansetron	Zofran	Oral/parenteral	Antiemetic
Oxybutynin	Ditropan XL	Oral/transdermal	Anticholinergic
Oxycodone	OxyContin	Oral	Analgesic
Oxycodone/APAP	Percocet	Oral	Analgesic
Paroxetine	Paxil	Oral	Antidepressant
Phenytoin	Dilantin	Oral/parenteral	Antiepileptic
Phytonadione	Mephyton	Oral/parenteral	Coagulant
Pioglitazone	Actos	Oral	Antidiabetic
Prednisone	Deltasone	Oral	Corticosteroid
Prochlorperazine	Compazine	Oral/parenteral	Antiemetic
Propofol	Diprivan	Parenteral	Anesthetic
Propoxyphene/APAP	Darvocet-N	Oral	Analgesic
Ranitidine	Zantac	Oral/parenteral	Antiulcer
Reteplase	Retavase	Parenteral	Thrombolytic
Risperidone	Risperdal	Oral/parenteral	Antipsychotic
Rosiglitazone	Avandia	Oral	Antidiabetic

Continued

TABLE 20-2 Commonly Used Drugs by Generic Name—cont'd

GENERIC NAME	BRAND NAME	ROUTE(S)	CLASSIFICATION
Salmeterol	Serevent	Inhalation	Bronchodilator
Salmeterol/fluticasone	Advair	Inhalation	Bronchodilator/corticosteroid
Sertraline	Zoloft	Oral	Antidepressant
Sevoflurane	Ultane	Inhalation	Anesthetic
Simvastatin	Zocor	Oral	Antihyperlipidemic
Temazepam	Restoril	Oral	Hypnotic
Tolterodine	Detrol LA	Oral	Anticholinergic
Topiramate	Topamax	Oral	Antiepileptic
Tramadol	Ultram	Oral	Analgesic
Valproate	Depakote	Oral/parenteral	Antiepileptic/mood stabilizer
Valsartan	Diovan	Oral	Antihypertensive
Verapamil	Verapamil	Oral/parenteral	Antiarrhythmic
Warfarin	Coumadin	Oral/parenteral	Anticoagulant
Zidovudine (AZT)	Retrovir	Oral/parenteral	Antiviral
Zolpidem	Ambien	Oral	Hypnotic

APAP, N-acetyl-para-amino-phenol (acetaminophen).

ANTIANXIETY AGENTS. *Antianxiety agents,* or anxiolytics, are drugs used in the treatment of anxiety. They act on the CNS to calm or relax the anxious patient. Diazepam (Valium) and lorazepam (Ativan) are benzodiazepines that are prescribed for the treatment of anxiety, muscle spasms, and seizures. Benzodiazepines are often used as a preoperative drug for various procedures performed in the radiology department. Another benzodiazepine, Midazolam (Versed), is also used as a preoperative drug. Benzodiazepines can be abused, and physical dependence has been documented.

ANTIARRHYTHMICS. *Antiarrhythmics* are drugs used to treat **arrhythmias,** which are any variation from the normal rhythm of the heartbeat. The abnormal rhythm may occur in the *atria* (the upper chambers of the heart) or in the *ventricles* (the lower chambers of the heart). The antiarrhythmic agent used depends on the type of arrhythmia to be treated. Amiodarone (Cordarone) is used for ventricular arrhythmias.

ANTIBIOTICS. *Antibiotics* or *antimicrobials* are drugs used to kill or inhibit the growth of **microorganisms.** An antibiotic that is effective against a large number of microorganisms is termed a *broad-spectrum antibiotic;* if it is effective against only a few, it is termed a *narrow-spectrum antibiotic.* Ciprofloxacin (Cipro), a fluoroquinolone, is a broad-spectrum antibiotic, and erythromycin (Erythrocin), a macrolide, is a narrow-spectrum antibiotic used primarily for treating respiratory tract infections. Allergic reactions to antibiotics are common and range from mild to severe or even fatal.

ANTICHOLINERGICS. Anticholinergics, or antimuscarinics, are drugs that reduce smooth muscle tone, motility of the gastrointestinal tract, and secretions from respiratory tract and secretory glands. Oxybutynin (Ditropan XL) and tolterodine (Detrol La) are two commonly used anticholinergics in the treatment of overactive bladder. *Atropine* is used preoperatively to inhibit the secretions that can be stimulated by general anesthetics and to prevent bradycardia (slowing of the heart) that may result from general anesthesia. The most common side effect of an anticholinergic agent is a dry mouth, but high doses of these drugs can produce serious side effects such as delirium, rapid heartbeat, and coma.

ANTICOAGULANTS. *Anticoagulants* are drugs that inhibit clotting of the blood or increase the **coagulation** time. They are used primarily to prevent or treat **thromboembolic disorders.** Heparin and enoxaparin (Lovenox) are commonly used parenteral anticoagulants. Heparin and enoxaparin are not effective when administered orally because they are not absorbed from the gastrointestinal tract and should not be administered intramuscularly because they may cause a **hematoma.** Warfarin

Text continued on p. 302

TABLE 20-3 Commonly Used Drugs by Classification

CLASSIFICATION/BRAND NAME	GENERIC NAME	ROUTE(S)
Analgesics		
Aspirin	Aspirin	Oral
Darvocet-N	Propoxyphene/APAP	Oral
Duragesic	Fentanyl	Parenteral/Transdermal
Morphine	Morphine	Oral/parenteral
OxyContin	Oxycodone	Oral
Percocet	Oxycodone/APAP	Oral
Tylenol	Acetaminophen (APAP)	Oral
Ultram	Tramadol	Oral
Vicodin	Hydrocodone/APAP	Oral
Anesthetics		
Carbocaine	Mepivacalne	Parenteral
Diprivan	Propofol	Parenteral
Ultane	Sevoflurane	Inhalation
Antianxiety		
Ativan	Lorazepam	Oral/parenteral
Valium	Diazepam	Oral/parenteral
Versed	Midazolam	Oral/Parenteral
Xanax	Alprazolam	Oral
Antiarrhythmics		
Adenocard	Adenosine	Parenteral
Cordarone	Amiodarone	Oral/parenteral
Lanoxln	Digoxin	Oral/parenteral
Verapamil	Verapamil	Oral/parenteral
Xylocalne	Lidocaine	Parenteral
Antibiotics		
Amoxil	Amoxicillin	Oral
Biaxin	Clarithromycin	Oral
Cipro	Ciprofloxacin	Oral/parenteral
Erythromycin	Erythromycin	Oral/parenteral
Rocephin	Ceftriaxone	Parenteral
Zithromax	Azithromycin	Oral/parenteral
Anticholinergics		
Atropine	Atropine	Oral/parenteral
Detrol LA	Tolterodine	Oral
Ditropan XL	Oxybutynin	Oral/transdermal
Anticoagulants		
Coumadin	Warfarin	Oral/parenteral
Heparin	Heparin	Parenteral
Lovenox	Enoxaparin	Parenteral
Antidepressants		
Celexa	Citalopram	Oral
Lexapro	Escitalopram	Oral
Paxil	Paroxetine	Oral
Prozac	Fluoxetine	Oral
Wellbutrin	Bupropion	Oral
Zoloft	Sertraline	Oral
Antidiabetics		
Actos	Pioglitazone	Oral
Amaryl	Glimepiride	Oral
Avandia	Rosiglitazone	Oral
Glucophage	Metformin	Oral
Glucotrol	Glipizide	Oral
Micronase	Glyburide	Oral

Continued

TABLE 20-3 Commonly Used Drugs by Classification—cont'd

CLASSIFICATION/BRAND NAME	GENERIC NAME	ROUTE(S)
Antiemetics		
Compazine	Prochlorperazine	Oral/parenteral
Reglan	Metoclopramide	Oral/parenteral
Zofran	Ondansetron	Oral/parenteral
Antiepileptics		
Depakote	Valproate	Oral/parenteral
Dilantin	Phenytoin	Oral/parenteral
Klonopin	Clonazepam	Oral
Neurontin	Gabapentin	Oral
Topamax	Topiramate	Oral
Antifungals		
Diflucan	Fluconazole	Oral/parenteral
Fungizone	Amphotericin B	Parenteral
Antihistamines		
Allegra	Fexofenadine	Oral
Benadryl	Diphenhydramine	Oral/parenteral
Claritin	Loratadine	Oral
Antihyperlipidemics		
Lipitor	Atorvastatin	Oral
Lopid	Gemfibrozil	Oral
Zocor	Simvastatin	Oral
Antihypertensives		
Cardura	Doxazosin	Oral
Catapres	Clonidine	Oral/transdermal
Cozaar	Losartan	Oral
Diovan	Valsartan	Oral
Lopressor	Metoprolol	Oral/parenteral
Lotensin	Benazepril	Oral
Monopril	Fosinopril	Oral
Norvasc	Amlodipine	Oral
Tenormin	Atenolol	Oral/parenteral
Vasotec	Enalapril	Oral/parenteral
Zestril	Lisinopril	Oral
Antiplatelets		
Aspirin	Aspirin	Oral
Plavix	Clopidogrel	Oral
ReoPro	Abciximab	Parenteral
Antipsychotics		
Haldol	Haloperidol	Oral/parenteral
Risperdal	Risperidone	Oral/parenteral
Zyprexa	Olanzapine	Oral/parenteral
Antiulcer		
Pepcid	Famotidine	Oral/parenteral
Prevacid	Lansoprazole	Oral/parenteral
Prilosec	Omeprazole	Oral
Zantac	Ranitidine	Oral/parenteral
Antivirals		
Epivir	Lamivudine	Oral
Retrovir	Zidovudine (AZT)	Oral/parenteral
Zovirax	Acyclovir	Oral/parenteral/topical
Bronchodilators		
Adrenalin	Epinephrine	Inhalation/parenteral
Atrovent	Ipratropium	Inhalation

TABLE 20-3 Commonly Used Drugs by Classification—cont'd

CLASSIFICATION/BRAND NAME	GENERIC NAME	ROUTE(S)
Proventil	Albuterol	Oral/inhalation
Serevent	Salmeterol	Inhalation
Spiriva	Tiotropium	Inhalation
Cholinesterase Inhibitor		
Aricept	Donepezil	Oral
Coagulant		
Mephyton	Phytonadione	Oral/parenteral
Corticosteroids		
Decadron	Dexamethasone	Oral/parenteral
Deltasone	Prednisone	Oral
Depo-Medrol	Methylprednisolone	Parenteral
Flovent	Fluticasone	Inhalation
Solu-Cortef	Hydrocortisone	Parenteral
Diuretics		
Bumex	Bumetanide	Oral/parenteral
Hydrochlorothiazide	Hydrochlorothiazide	Oral/parenteral
Lasix	Furosemide	Oral/parenteral
Hormones		
Premarin	Conjugated estrogens	Female hormone
Synthroid	Levothyroxine	Thyroid hormone
Laxative		
Dulcolax	Bisacodyl	Oral
Hypnotics		
Ambien	Zolpidem	Oral
Restoril	Temazepam	Oral
Mood Stabilizer		
Lithium	Lithium	Oral
Nonsteroidal Antiinflammatories		
Celebrex	Celecoxib	Oral
Motrin	Ibuprofen	Oral
Naprosyn	Naproxen	Oral
Sedatives		
Chloral hydrate	Chloral hydrate	Oral
Vistaril	Hydroxyzine	Oral/parenteral
Stimulants		
Adderall	Amphetamine salts	Oral
Dobutrex	Dobutamine	Parenteral
Intropin	Dopamine	Parenteral
Ritalin	Methylphenidate	Oral
Thrombolytics		
Activase	Alteplase (tPA)	Parenteral
Retavase	Reteplase	Parenteral
Vasoconstrictor		
Levophed	Norepinephrine	Parenteral
Vasodilators		
Nitroglycerin	Nitroglycerin	Oral/parenteral/transdermal
Nitropress	Nitroprusside	Parenteral

APAP, N-acetyl-para-amino-phenol (acetaminophen); *AZT,* azidothymidine.

TABLE 20-4 Herbals

COMMON NAME	ACTION/PROPERTIES	ADVERSE EFFECTS	POTENTIAL INTERACTION
Echinacea	Stimulates immune system	Hypersensitivity	Acetaminophen (liver toxicity)
Fever few	Antiinflammatory, migraine headache	Bleeding, flushing	Aspirin, clopidogrel, warfarin
Garlic	Cholesterol reduction, lowers blood pressure	Bleeding, heartburn	Aspirin, clopidogrel, warfarin
Ginger	Antiemetic	Bleeding	Aspirin, clopidogrel, warfarin
Ginseng	Maintain normal function in time of stress	Insomnia	Digoxin
Ginkgo biloba	Stimulates circulation, increases mental alertness	Bleeding	Aspirin, clopidogrel, warfarin
Kava	Antianxiety, promotes sleep	Liver toxicity	Alprazolam, epinephrine
Saw palmetto	Promotes prostate health	Headache, diarrhea	Oral contraceptives
St. John's wort	Depression	Photosensitivity	Digoxin, antidepressants
Valerian	Promotes sleep	Headache, drowsiness	Benzodiazepams (e.g., lorazepam)

(Coumadin) is an oral anticoagulant. Patients undergoing interventional procedures in the radiology department are often receiving these drugs and should be monitored closely to prevent massive hemorrhage, which can occur with overdose.

ANTICONVULSANTS. *Anticonvulsants* or *antiepileptic drugs* are drugs used to prevent or control the occurrence of seizures. These drugs do not treat the cause of seizures; they reduce or eliminate seizure activity. Although divalproex (valproate; Depakote) is an effective oral antiepileptic, it is also used to treat bipolar disease and for the prophylaxis of migraine headaches. It is also available in a parenteral form. Depakote has been associated with liver toxicity, thrombocytopenia (a decrease in the number of platelets), and pancreatitis. Phenytoin (Dilantin) is another effective antiepileptic that is available in oral or parenteral form.

ANTIDEPRESSANTS. *Antidepressants* are drugs used in the treatment of depression. These drugs often require several weeks of administration to achieve their maximal **therapeutic** effect. Withdrawal effects (called discontinuation syndrome) after abrupt discontinuation have been reported. The selective serotonin reuptake inhibitors (SSRIs) fluoxetine (Prozac), sertraline (Zoloft), paroxetine (Paxil), citalopram (Celexa), and escitalopram (Lexapro) are considered the drugs of choice in treating clinical depression. The SSRIs are also used in the treatment of anxiety disorders. Nausea, vomiting, and diarrhea are common side effects. Drug interactions can occur in patients receiving other drugs in combination with antidepressants.

ANTIDIABETIC AGENTS. **Diabetes mellitus** (DM) affects approximately 18.2 million Americans (6.3% of the U.S. population). DM is currently classified as *type 1,* in which insulin is absent, and *type 2,* in which insulin deficiency and insulin resistance exist. Insulin is the only treatment used to treat type 1 diabetes but is also used in the treatment for type 2 diabetes. Glyburide (Micronase), glipizide (Glucotrol), glimepiride (Amaryl), metformin (Glucophage), and Pioglitazone (Actos) are commonly used for type 2 diabetes. Hypoglycemic (low glucose) reactions are the most common complication of antidiabetic agents. The major concern with metformin is lactic acidosis. Although lactic acidosis is rare, it has a mortality rate of approximately 50%. Recommendation are that metformin be temporarily discontinued before the use of radiographic contrast agents.

ANTIEMETICS. *Antiemetics* are drugs used to prevent and treat nausea and vomiting. In general, these agents are more effective in preventing nausea and vomiting than they are in treating the symptoms once they have developed. Thus they are most effective when given before the onset of symptoms. Prochlorperazine (Compazine) and ondansetron (Zofran) are two commonly used antiemetic agents and are available in both oral and parenteral form.

ANTIFUNGAL AGENTS. *Antifungal agents* are substances that destroy or suppress the growth or multiplication of fungi. Fungal infections are more likely to occur in patients who are immunocompromised. Fungal infections can be divided into two major groups: (1) those that affect the skin or mucosa and (2) those that affect the whole body *(systemic).* Fungizone (amphotericin B) is usually the drug of choice for treating most serious systemic infections. It must be administered intravenously because it is poorly absorbed from the gastrointestinal tract. Fungizone can cause a variety of adverse effects, such as chills, fever, and kidney damage. Fluconazole (Diflucan), which is available in oral and parenteral form, is effective in serious systemic infections and vaginal fungal infections. It is generally well tolerated.

ANTIHISTAMINES. *Antihistamines* are drugs used primarily to treat allergic disorders, both acute and chronic. They are also used to treat the symptoms (e.g., runny nose) of upper respiratory tract infections and the common cold, both of which are viral infections. Antihistamines fall into two major groups: (1) those that are *sedating* (first generation) and (2) those that are *nonsedating* (second generation). Diphenhydramine (Benadryl) is a sedating antihistamine and is available in oral and parenteral form. It is administered intramuscularly for moderately severe allergic reactions. Loratadine (Claritin) is a nonsedating antihistamine that is administered orally.

ANTIHYPERLIPIDEMIC AGENTS. **Hyperlipidemia** is associated with the development of **atherosclerosis** that leads to coronary heart disease (CHD). CHD remains the single largest killer of American men and women. Large, randomized, controlled clinical trials have demonstrated that cholesterol lowering significantly reduces CHD mortality and reduces the risk of having a stroke. Drugs called *statins* are usually the drugs of choice in the management of hyperlipidemia. Two common statins, atorvastatin (Lipitor) and simvastatin (Zocor), are used to treat hyperlipidemia. Liver abnormalities and muscle pain can occur, but these agents are generally well tolerated. Gemfibrozil (Lopid), niacin (Niaspan ER), and ezetimibe (Zetia) are other hyperlipidemic agents.

ANTIHYPERTENSIVES. *Antihypertensives* are drugs used to treat **hypertension** (high blood pressure). Hypertension is a common disorder that affects approximately 60 million Americans. If left untreated or improperly treated, then hypertension can lead to heart disease, kidney disease, strokes, and blindness. The Seventh Report of the Joint National Committee on Prevention, Detection, Evaluation, and Treatment of High Blood Pressure (the JNC 7 report), the American Diabetes Association (ADA), and the National Kidney Foundation recommend a blood pressure less than 140/90 mm Hg in the general population and less than 130/80 mm Hg in patients with chronic kidney disease or diabetes. Many different drugs are used

to treat hypertension because high blood pressure can be caused by many factors. Up to four different antihypertensive agents may be required to control hypertension. Besides lowering blood pressure, many antihypertensive agents are used in the management of other cardiovascular diseases. Angiotensin-converting enzyme inhibitors such as lisinopril (Zestril) and beta-blockers such as metoprolol (Lopressor, Toprol XL) are used in the management of heart failure. Calcium channel blockers such as amlodipine (Norvasc) are used in the management of **angina pectoris.**

ANTIPLATELETS. *Antiplatelet drugs* inhibit platelet aggregation. Antiplatelet drugs are indicated in the prevention of myocardial infarction (MI), stroke, and transient ischemic attacks (TIAs). Aspirin, clopidogrel (Plavix), and abciximab (Repro) are frequently used agents. Aspirin and clopidogrel are administered orally, and abciximab is administered parenterally. The major complication for these drugs is bleeding.

ANTIPSYCHOTICS. *Antipsychotic drugs* (neuroleptics) are used to treat psychiatric disorders such as **schizophrenia,** delusional disorders, acute mania, and agitated states. The antipsychotics agents are divided into two major groups: (1) traditional antipsychotics and (2) atypical (novel) antipsychotics. A well-known traditional antipsychotic is haloperidol (Haldol). It is available in both oral and parenteral form. Olanzapine (Zyprexa) is a commonly used atypical antipsychotic. It is also available in oral and parenteral form. A wide variety of adverse side effects, including sedation and orthostatic hypotension, may be associated with both types of antipsychotic agents.

ANTIULCER AGENTS. *Antiulcer agents* are used to treat peptic ulcers, both gastric and duodenal, and **gastroesophageal reflux disease (GERD).** GERD is caused by the reflux of acid from the stomach into the esophagus. The most common symptom is heartburn. GERD can cause chest pain, which can be mistaken as a heart attack and trigger an emergency room visit. Ranitidine (Zantac), famotidine (Pepcid), lansoprazole (Prevacid), and omeprazole (Prilosec) reduce the production of acid within the stomach. They are effective in the management of peptic ulcers and GERD. Metoclopramide (Reglan), available in oral and parenteral form, increases **peristalsis** and accelerates gastric emptying without increasing gastric secretions. Reglan is indicated for the relief of symptoms associated with **diabetic gastroparesis** and for short-term therapy for GERD. It is also used as an antiemetic. Reglan can cause parkinson-like symptoms (e.g., tremors, rigidity).

ANTIVIRAL AGENTS. *Antiviral agents* are substances that destroy or suppress the growth or multiplication of viruses. Antiviral agents are used to treat herpes simplex, chicken pox, shingles, influenza (flu), and infection with the human immunodeficiency virus (HIV). Acyclovir (Zovirax) is used in the treatment of genital herpes, chicken pox, and shingles and is available in oral, topical, and parenteral form. Zidovudine (Retrovir), also known as azidothymidine (AZT), is used in the treatment of HIV infections. It is available in both an oral and a parenteral form.

BRONCHODILATORS. **Bronchodilators** are drugs used in the treatment of asthma and COPD. These drugs relax bronchial smooth muscles and dilate the respiratory passages. They can be classified as short-acting and long-acting bronchodilators. Albuterol (Proventil) is the most commonly used fast-acting bronchodilator. It is generally administered by inhalation but can be administered orally. Most common side effects are tremors, nervousness, and increased heart rate (tachycardia). Tiotropium (Spiriva) is a long-acting bronchodilator, administered by inhalation. The most common side effect is dry mouth.

CHOLINESTERASE INHIBITORS. *Cholinesterase inhibitors* increase the levels of acetylcholine, a major neurotransmitter in the CNS. In Alzheimer's disease (AD), concentrations of acetylcholine are reduced by 90%. Cholinesterase inhibitors such as donepezil (Aricept) are used in the management of AD. Approximately 4.5 million Americans have AD. The most common side effects are nausea, vomiting, and diarrhea. Cholinesterase inhibitors may exaggerate muscle relaxation under general anesthesia.

COAGULANTS. *Coagulants* are drugs used to control hemorrhage or to speed up coagulation. Most coagulants are commercial preparations of vitamin K, a fat-soluble vitamin needed for normal blood coagulation. Phytonadione (Mephyton) is a coagulant available in both oral and parenteral form.

CORTICOSTEROIDS. *Corticosteroids* are drugs used to reduce the symptoms associated with chronic inflammatory disorders or for the short-term treatment of acute inflammatory conditions. Dexamethasone (Decadron) and hydrocortisone (Solu-Cortef) are steroidal drugs used systemically, whereas methylprednisolone (Depo-Medrol)

is generally injected locally at the inflammatory site, such as a joint or bursa. Fluticasone (Flovent) is administered by inhalation to decrease inflammation in the lungs. Prolonged use of corticosteroids can cause a variety of adverse side effects.

DIURETICS. **Diuretics** are drugs that increase the amount of urine excreted by the kidneys, thus removing sodium and water from the body. Furosemide (Lasix) is a potent diuretic often used to treat the **edema** associated with congestive heart failure. Diuretics are often used in conjunction with antihypertensive drugs for the treatment of high blood pressure. Patients receiving diuretics should be monitored for excessive fluid loss, which might result in an electrolyte imbalance.

HORMONES. *Hormones* are drugs that affect the endocrine system. The most important clinical application of these drugs is their use in replacement therapy, such as hypothyroidism. Levothyroxine (Synthroid) is used in the management of hypothyroidism. Conjugated estrogen (Premarin) is a female hormone used in treating moderate to severe vasomotor symptoms (e.g., night sweats, hot flashes) associated with menopause and to prevent osteoporosis. Other agents that affect sex hormones may inhibit the actions of naturally occurring sex hormones. Tamoxifen (Nolvadex) is an antiestrogen used to prevent and treat *breast cancer.*

LAXATIVES. **Laxatives** are drugs that act to promote the passage and elimination of feces from the large intestines. Laxatives are frequently used in radiology to prepare patients for both gastrointestinal procedures and urinary tract procedures. Bisacodyl (Dulcolax) is a stimulant laxative that increases the motility of the gastrointestinal tract and tends to produce a loose, watery stool.

MOOD-STABILIZING DRUGS. *Mood-stabilizing drugs* prevent mood swings in patients with manic-depressive (bipolar) disorder. Lithium is one agent used in treating bipolar disorder. It is orally administered. Polyuria (large volume of urine), tremor, and hypothyroidism (deficiency of thyroid function) are potential adverse effects.

NONSTEROIDAL ANTIINFLAMMATORY DRUGS. *Nonsteroidal antiinflammatory drugs* (NSAIDs) have analgesic, antipyretic (reduces fever), and antiinflammatory actions. Ibuprofen (Motrin) is an example of a traditional NSAID commonly used to treat inflammatory conditions, mild to moderate pain, and fever. Traditional NSAIDs can cause gastrointestinal irritation, gastric ulcers, bleeding, and acute renal failure. When the cyclooxygenase 2 (COX-2) inhibitors, celecoxib (Celebrex), valdecoxib (Bextra), and rofecoxib (Vioxx), were first introduced, they were promoted as pain relievers and inflammation reducers and were less likely to cause adverse gastrointestinal effects compared with traditional NSAIDs. However, concerns about their cardiovascular safety have been increasing and led to the removal of Vioxx and Bextra.

SEDATIVES OR HYPNOTICS. *Sedatives* or *hypnotics* can produce varying degrees of CNS depression ranging from a mild sedation to inducing sleep. Zolpidem (Ambien) is a commonly used hypnotic. Extended use of these drugs can lead to physical dependence. Chloral hydrate syrup is often used as an effective sedative for children undergoing difficult procedures.

STIMULANTS. *Stimulants* are drugs that increase activity. CNS stimulants increase the activity of the brain and spinal cord. Amphetamine salts (Adderall) and methylphenidate (Ritalin) are examples of CNS stimulants used to treat attention deficit hyperactivity disorder (ADHD). Dobutamine (Dobutrex) and dopamine (Intropin) stimulate the myocardium of the heart and are administered parenterally to treat conditions such as hypotension and **shock.**

THROMBOLYTICS. *Thrombolytics* are drugs that dissolve thrombi (clots) that have already formed. Alteplase (tPA, Activase) and reteplase (Retavase) are common thrombolytics. They are administered parenterally in cases of acute MI and stroke. The major adverse effect is bleeding complications.

VASOCONSTRICTORS. **Vasoconstrictors** are drugs that cause blood vessels to constrict, thus increasing heart action and raising blood pressure. Norepinephrine (Levophed) is a potent vasoconstrictor administered parenterally in the treatment of shock. This drug should be injected intravenously only because **infiltration** can cause tissue necrosis.

VASODILATORS. **Vasodilators** are drugs that cause blood vessels to dilate. They are useful in treating vascular disease, particularly angina. Nitroglycerin is an effective coronary vasodilator administered sublingually, orally, topically, or parenterally. Nitroprusside (Nitropress) is a peripheral vasodilator that is effective when used in a hypertensive crisis or in treating heart failure.

Response Factors

The study of how a drug is absorbed into the body, circulates within the body, is changed by the body, and leaves the body is called **pharmacokinetics.** Four basic factors influence the movement of a drug:

- Absorption is defined as the movement of a drug from its site of administration into the blood.
- Distribution is defined as drug movement from the blood to various tissues and organs of the body.
- Metabolism is defined as the chemical alteration of various substances (drugs). The liver is the main organ involved in drug metabolism, taking a drug that is fat soluble and turning it into a water-soluble substance so it can be eliminated from the body.
- Excretion is the movement of drugs out of the body. The kidney is the most important organ for drug excretion.

Many factors can affect the pharmacokinetics of drugs and therefore affect the intended drug response. The older adult patient (65 years or older) may respond differently to drugs than younger patients because of decreased absorption, metabolism, and excretion. They generally require a reduction in dose. Additionally, children, especially in their first year of life, because of reduced capacity for the metabolism and excretion of drugs, will generally need a reduction in dose. The presence of diseases may decrease the function of vital organs. Liver or kidney disease can influence the metabolism and excretion of drugs, potentially leading to a greater incidence of adverse effects. A drug's effect that can be modified by previous or concomitant administration of another drug or food is referred to as a drug interaction. Other factors that can affect the intended drug effect are sex, genetics, weight, and route and time of administration.

Drugs have a variety of effects in the human body: the clinically desirable actions and the undesirable effects. These adverse drug effects include side effects, toxic effects, allergic reactions, and idiosyncratic reactions. An **idiosyncratic reaction** is an abnormal response to a drug caused by individual genetic differences. **Side effects** result from the drug acting on tissues other than those intended, which causes a response unrelated to the intended action. For example, an antihistamine is intended to counteract an allergic condition, but one of the side effects commonly produced by the drug is drowsiness, which is caused by the drug's unintended effect on the CNS. Toxic effects are adverse drug effects related to the dose of drug administered. Most drugs are capable of producing toxic effects if the therapeutic dose is greatly exceeded. Allergic reactions occur when the body's immunologic system is hypersensitive to the presence of the drug. Allergic reactions can occur only after repeated exposure to the specific drug or a chemically related compound; however, the radiologic technologist must remember that prior sensitization to the drug may have taken place without the knowledge of the patient. An allergic reaction may take one of two forms: immediate or delayed. Immediate reactions may range from a mild response such as hives to a severe life-threatening response such as **anaphylaxis**, which may include respiratory or circulatory collapse. Delayed reactions are usually less severe than immediate reactions and may not become evident for hours or even days after the drug is administered.

In radiology, drugs are often administered to patients, particularly pediatric patients, to sedate them during a lengthy or difficult procedure. The American Society of Anesthesiologists has developed a continuum to describe the various levels of sedation. The sedation levels are:

- Minimal sedation (anxiolysis)
- Moderate sedation or analgesia (conscious sedation)
- Deep sedation or analgesia
- General anesthesia

Minimal sedation is a drug-induced state during which patients will respond normally to verbal commands. Cognitive function and coordination may be affected, but ventilation and cardiovascular function are unaffected. With moderate sedation, a drug-induced depression of consciousness occurs, but patients respond purposefully to verbal commands. This term has replaced the term *conscious sedation*. Ventilation is adequate and cardiovascular function is usually maintained. With deep sedation, a drug-induced depression of consciousness occurs during which patients cannot be easily aroused. They can respond purposefully after repeated or painful stimuli. Ventilation may be inadequate but cardiovascular function is usually maintained. General anesthesia is a drug-induced loss of consciousness during which patients are not arousable even to painful stimuli. Ventilation is frequently inadequate, and cardiovascular function may be impaired. Because levels of sedation are along a continuum, predicting how a patient will respond is not always possible. Children, in particular, are prone to slip from one state to another without much warning.

BOX 20-2 Five Rights of Drug Administration

Right drug
Right amount
Right patient
Right time
Right route

PRINCIPLES OF ADMINISTRATION

In preparing to administer drugs, the radiologic technologist should always follow the golden rules of drug administration, or what are commonly referred to as the *five rights* of drug administration (Box 20-2).

The *right drug* must be given. To ensure that the right drug is administered, always check the label on the container three times: once when the container is removed from the shelf, again when the drug is removed from the container, and a third time when the container is replaced. Remember that the names of different drugs sometimes sound similar. *Check the name carefully.* Never use a drug that is unlabeled, and always check labels for the expiration date. A person should never administer a drug that someone else has prepared. If you are asked to prepare a drug for another health professional to administer, always show the container to the person who will administer the drug before you give him or her the dose.

The *right amount* of the drug must be used. To ensure that the right amount of the drug is used, it must be measured carefully and accurately. When preparing to administer an injectable drug, selecting the right size and type of syringe and needle is important.

The *right patient* must be given the drug. To ensure that you are administering the drug to the right patient, check the patient's armband for proper identification, and ask the patient to state his or her name. In addition, many hospitals are now asking the patient his or her date of birth. If the patient is too young to speak or is unable to speak, ask a parent or someone else present to identify the patient. Last, address the patient by name before administering the drug.

The drug must be administered at the *right time*. The physician or practitioner responsible for ordering the drug usually determines the right time for the administration of the drug. As a general rule, the radiologic technologist does not determine the time but should administer the drug at the time specified.

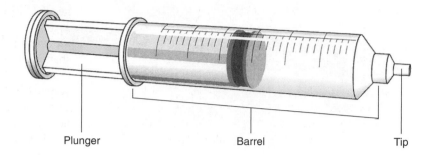

FIG. 20–1 Parts of a syringe.

Plunger   Barrel   Tip

The *right route* must be used. Make certain that the drug is administered by the correct route. The physician usually specifies the route by which the drug should be administered. The radiologic technologist must be familiar with the terminology associated with the most common routes.

Routes

Drugs are administered in a variety of ways, including oral, sublingual, topical, and parenteral. General principles associated with each route of administration are discussed herein.

ORAL. The oral route is the most common method of drug administration. The drug is taken by mouth and swallowed; it is absorbed from the gastrointestinal tract. When receiving drugs by the oral route, the patient must be conscious, and the head should be elevated to aid in swallowing.

SUBLINGUAL. Administration by the **sublingual** route means that the drug is placed under the tongue and allowed to dissolve. Drugs intended to be administered sublingually should not be swallowed. One drug commonly given by the sublingual route is nitroglycerin.

TOPICAL. The **topical** route of drug administration involves the application of a drug directly onto the skin. The drug is diffused through the skin and absorbed into the bloodstream. Topical drugs can be applied as lotions or ointments. Drugs for topical application have become available in a unit-dose device called a **transdermal** patch. The patch is applied to the skin and provides a precise dose of drug released over a specified time.

PARENTERAL. The term *parenteral* means administered by injection or by a route other than the gastrointestinal tract. Strict aseptic technique and standard precautions should always be used when drugs are administered with a needle. Infection control is of paramount importance in parenteral therapy. The Occupational Safety and Health Administration (OSHA) issued standards on blood-borne pathogens, mandating the use of *Universal Precautions* and the *Needlestick Safety Prevention* program. If a drug is injected incorrectly, it may cause nerve damage, or it may introduce microorganisms into the patient's system. The three most common routes by which drugs are administered parenterally are **intramuscular, subcutaneous,** and **intravenous.**

Supplies

Drugs are injected into the body with a plastic syringe. Plastic syringes are disposed of after being used only once. A syringe has three parts: (1) the *tip,* where the needle attaches, (2) the *barrel,* where the calibration scales are printed, and (3) the *plunger,* the inside part that fits into the barrel. The parts of a syringe are shown in Fig. 20–1. Several different kinds of syringes have been produced, and they vary in size and shape. The tuberculin and insulin syringes are designed for situations that require the precise measurement of a small volume of drug. The general-purpose syringe comes in a variety of sizes, including 2, 2.5, 3, 5, 10, 20, and 50 ml. Some syringes, such as Luer-Lok syringes, have a locking device on the tip that holds the needle firmly in place. An eccentric tip syringe is one that has the tip located to the side rather than in the center.

Most hospitals are now using needleless systems for intravenous administration of drugs. Many companies are making these systems, and many different varieties are available. All of these different systems have a few features in common. All needleless hep-locks have a white ring on the port shown in Fig. 20–2. This feature identifies the lock as a needleless system, and needles should not be used.

Needles used for injection are made of stainless steel and may or may not be disposable. The needle has three

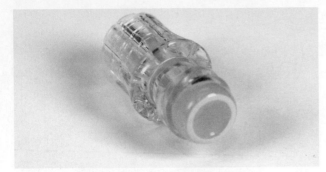

FIG. 20–2 A needleless injection system (Courtesy of Baxter Healthcare Corporation, Deerfield, Illinois.)

parts: (1) the *hub,* which is the part that attaches to the syringe, (2) the *cannula* or *shaft,* which is the length of the metal part, and (3) the *bevel,* which is the slanted part at the tip of the needle. The parts of a needle are shown in Fig. 20–3. Needles are sized according to length and gauge. The *gauge* refers to the thickness or diameter of the needle. The *length* refers to the measurement in inches of the shaft portion. The length will vary from 0.25 to 5 inches, the gauge from 14 to 28. As a general rule, shorter needles are used for subcutaneous injections, and longer

needles are used for intramuscular injections. Needles 1- to $1\frac{1}{2}$-inch in length are most commonly used for intravenous injections. The smaller the diameter of the shaft or the finer the needle is, the larger the gauge number will be. For example, a 25-gauge needle has a very small diameter, and an 18-gauge needle has a large diameter. Subcutaneous injections often use a 25-gauge needle, and an intravenous injection generally uses a 20- or 21-gauge needle. A large-diameter needle such as an 18-gauge needle is often used to draw a drug or solution into the syringe but is seldom used to inject the drug into the patient. The package label indicates both the length and the gauge of the needle. Two examples of prepackaged needles are shown in Fig. 20–4. Thus a package labeled *20 g/1½* indicates that the needle is 20 gauge and $1\frac{1}{2}$ inches in long. The bevel of the needle may also vary from long to short. Fig. 20–5 illustrates the difference

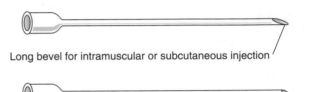

Long bevel for intramuscular or subcutaneous injection

Short bevel for intravenous injection

FIG. 20–5 Needle bevels. Long or regular bevels are usually used for intramuscular or subcutaneous injections. Short bevels are commonly used for intravenous injections.

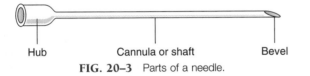

Hub   Cannula or shaft   Bevel

FIG. 20–3 Parts of a needle.

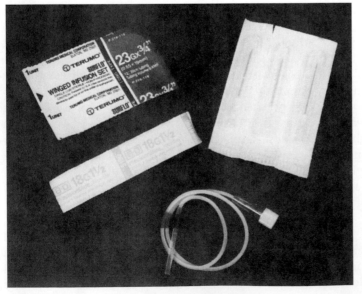

FIG. 20–4 Prepacked needles and winged/butterfly infusion sets showing the gauge and length of needle.

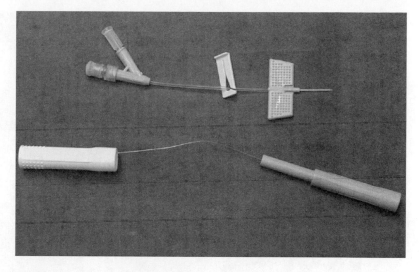

FIG. 20–6 Angiocath venipuncture set. *Top,* Set ready for use. *Bottom,* Set after use with catheter on left and needle sheath on right. The needle is pulled inside the protective sheath at the top so it cannot accidentally stick anyone.

between a long-bevel needle and a short-bevel needle. Long bevels are generally used for subcutaneous and intramuscular injections, and short bevels are used for intravenous injections.

An *angiocath* is a safer device compared with other systems to use when performing venipuncture (Fig. 20–6). An angiocath is used the same as any other needle to puncture the vein. It differs from other systems in that, after venipuncture, the user pulls on a sheath, which extracts the needle up through a catheter and into the protective sheath, where it cannot accidentally puncture anyone (Fig. 20–7).

Drugs intended for use by parenteral administration are packaged in two different kinds of containers: ampules and vials. An **ampule** is a sealed glass container designed to hold a single dose of a drug and intended for use only once. It is made of clear glass and has a shape with a scored constricted neck that is weakened so that it breaks more easily than other parts of the glass structure. If the neck is not scored, then it must be filed with a small metal file before it is broken. To prepare the ampule, it should be held upright and the top of the neck flicked with a finger until all the drug is in the bottom part of the ampule (Fig. 20–8). Then a dry gauze pad is wrapped around the neck of the ampule and the top snapped off (see Fig. 20–8, B and C). Care should be taken to avoid contaminating the needle by touching the outer broken edge of the ampule with the shaft of the needle when inserting it to draw out the contents. This task is best accomplished by letting the tip of the needle rest on the inside of the ampule (see Fig. 20–8, D). The

procedure is most easily performed when one person opens and holds the ampule while a second person withdraws the drug. When drawing medication from a glass ampule, you must use a filter needle, then change the needle before injecting.

A **vial** is a small glass bottle with a sealed rubber cap. Vials are manufactured in different sizes and may contain multiple doses of a drug. To prepare the vial, the metal cap is removed without breaking the outside metal seal, and the exposed rubber stopper is wiped with an alcohol sponge. After a syringe package has been opened, the syringe plunger is pulled back to pull air into the syringe equal to the amount of drug that will be withdrawn from the vial. After the needle package is open, the needle is inserted on the end of the syringe without letting the end of the syringe or the end of the needle touch anything but each other. The vial is held securely in the nondominant hand and the vial inverted and, using the dominant hand, the needle can be inserted without letting the tip of the needle touch anything but the rubber stopper of the vial. With the tip of the needle in the fluid, air is injected equal to the volume of drug to be removed.

If the needle is above the fluid level in the vial, then air, instead of solution, will be drawn into the syringe. After pulling back on the plunger until the correct amount of drug has been drawn into the syringe, the needle can be removed and the syringe held with the needle pointing up while the technologist is tapping it with his or her finger to move any air bubble toward the hub, where it can be expelled by gently pushing on the plunger of the syringe. After use, the entire syringe and

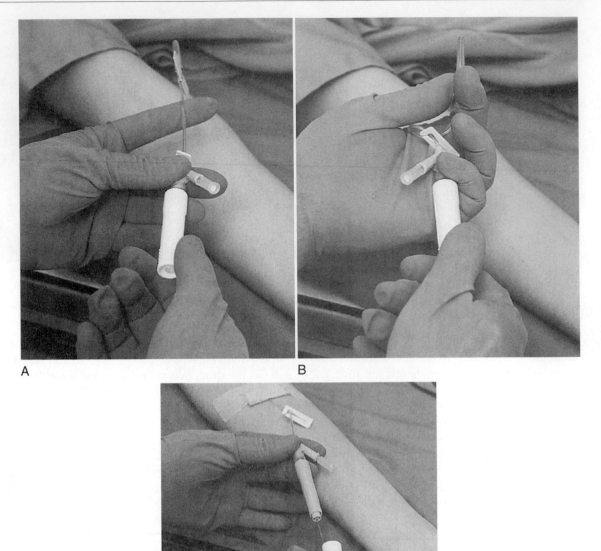

A

B

C

FIG. 20–7 Using an angiocath venipuncture set. *A,* Perform normal venipuncture. *B,* After successful venipuncture, pull sheath away gently. This pulls the needle up the catheter and into the protective sheath. *C,* Continue pulling the sheath until it separates from the catheter, leaving the catheter in place inside the vein while the needle is safely encased in the protective sheath.

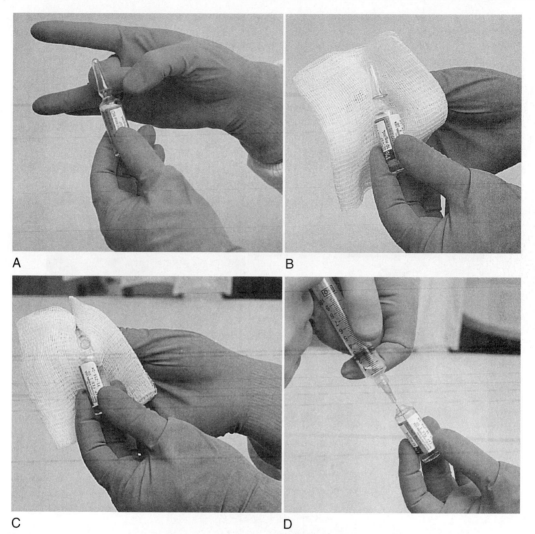

FIG. 20–8 Withdrawing a drug from a glass ampule. *A,* Flick the top of the neck until all liquid is in the bottom of the container. *B* and *C,* With a gauze pad, snap off the top. *D,* Withdraw the contents, being careful not to let the shaft of the needle touch the broken edge of the ampule. One person opens and holds the ampule while a second person withdraws the drug.

needle *must* be discarded into an acceptable *sharps* biohazard container. Fig. 20–9 illustrates the entire procedure.

METHODS OF ADMINISTRATION

Oral

Oral administration is a safe and convenient method of drug administration if a few simple rules are followed (Box 20-3). Remember to always wash your hands thoroughly before preparing or administering an oral

---

BOX 20-3 Rules for Oral Drug Administration

1. Wash hands thoroughly.
2. Place drug directly into a medicine cup or on a clean paper towel. Do not touch the drug with your hands.
3. Read the label three times.
4. Check the patient's identification.
5. Explain the procedure to the patient.
6. Elevate the patient's head.
7. Provide water or liquid to aid in swallowing.
8. Chart all relevant information.

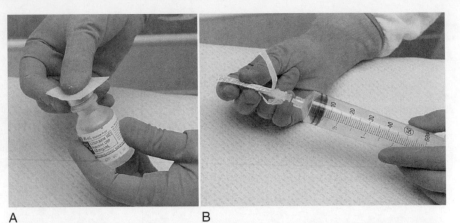

A   B

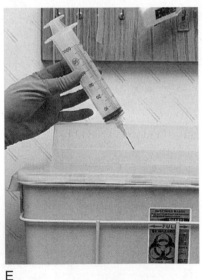

C   D

E

FIG. 20–9 Withdrawing a drug from a vial. *A,* Break the seal, expose the rubber stopper, and wipe the stopper with an alcohol swab. *B,* Open a syringe package and pull back the syringe plunger to pull air into the syringe equal to the amount of drug that will be withdrawn from the vial. Open a needle package, and insert the needle on the end of the syringe without letting the end of the syringe or the end of the needle touch anything but each other. *C,* Invert the vial, and with the dominant hand, insert the needle without letting the tip of the needle touch anything but the rubber stopper of the vial. With the tip of the needle in the fluid, inject air equal to the volume of drug to be removed. Pull back on the plunger until the correct amount of drug has been drawn into the syringe. *D,* Remove the needle and hold the syringe with the needle pointing up while tapping it with your finger to move any air bubble toward the hub, where it can be expelled by gently pushing on the plunger of the syringe. *E,* After use, dispose of the entire syringe and needle into an acceptable *sharps* biohazard container.

medication. Avoid touching tablets or capsules with your hands. Transfer tablets, capsules, or liquid from the container directly into a medication cup or clean paper towel. When pouring liquids, pour away from the label, and wipe the neck of the bottle with a clean, damp cloth before replacing the cap. Always follow the golden rules of medication administration. Never chart that a medication has been given until the patient takes the medication. At completion of the procedure, chart the drug and all pertinent information with regard to the administration. In preparing a drug for the sublingual route of administration, follow the same rules as indicated for oral administration.

Topical

Drugs applied topically include tinctures, ointments, lotions, and sprays. To administer a topical drug to the skin properly, follow the steps outlined in Box 20-4. Drugs administered by this route should not be applied with the bare hand. Following topical administration, the skin area must be monitored for any signs of local irritation.

Parenteral

Drugs that are injected have a rapid onset of action because they are absorbed directly into the bloodstream. All forms of parenteral administration require the use of a needle, syringe, and container. Because this method of administration involves penetrating the protective layer of the skin, strict aseptic technique and standard precautions should be followed when preparing and administering the drug. Selecting the proper equipment and supplies for parenteral administration depends on the specific injection route, as well as the kind and amount of drug to be administered. Each parenteral route of injection is discussed separately.

Recommendations are that radiographic contrast media be stored in a warming unit to bring the drug to body temperature before injection (Fig. 20–10).

SUBCUTANEOUS INJECTION. When administering a subcutaneous injection, the drug is placed under the skin into the subcutaneous tissue that lies under the epidermal layers. The thickness of the subcutaneous tissue

---

BOX 20-4 Rules for Topical Drug Administration

1. Wash hands thoroughly.
2. Put on disposable gloves.
3. Read the label three times.
4. Check the patient's identification.
5. Explain the procedure to the patient.
6. Apply the amount of drug prescribed.
7. Chart all relevant information.

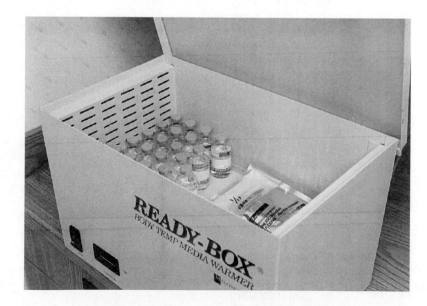

FIG. 20–10 Contrast media warmer.

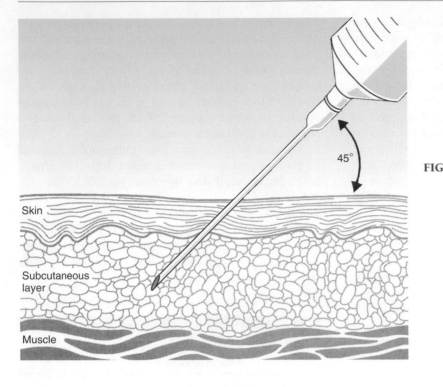

Skin

Subcutaneous
layer

Muscle

45°

FIG. 20–11 Proper needle placement for injection into the subcutaneous tissue. The needle is inserted at a 45-degree angle.

depends on whether the patient is obese and, if so, to what degree. The most commonly used subcutaneous sites include the anterior thigh, upper back, outer surface of the upper arm, and lower abdomen. The needle length and angle of insertion depend on the thickness of the subcutaneous tissue. Fig. 20–11 illustrates the proper placement of the needle for a subcutaneous injection. For average-size patients, a 25-gauge, $^5/_8$-inch needle at a 45-degree angle of insertion is generally used. For above-average-size patients, a 25-gauge, $^1/_2$-inch needle at a 90-degree angle of insertion is generally used. Box 20-5 lists the steps involved in subcutaneous injection.

INTRAMUSCULAR INJECTION. For an intramuscular injection, the drug is placed into muscle tissue that lies under the subcutaneous tissue layer. The most commonly used intramuscular injection sites include the deltoid muscle in the upper arm, the vastus lateralis muscle in the lateral thigh, and the gluteus maximus muscles in the buttocks. In general, a needle length is 1 to 3 inches and 19 to 25 gauge, depending on the viscosity of the drug to be injected. Fig. 20–12 demonstrates the proper placement of the needle for an intramuscular injection. A 90-degree angle of insertion is used for intramuscular injections. Box 20-6 lists the steps involved in intramuscular injection.

BOX 20-5 Steps Involved in Subcutaneous Drug Injection

1. Wash hands thoroughly.
2. Put on disposable gloves.
3. Check the patient's identification.
4. Explain the procedure to the patient.
5. Prepare the site by cleansing it with an alcohol swab using a circular motion and moving from the center to the outside.
6. With your free hand, pinch the skin gently together, and insert the needle quickly at the appropriate angle for the patient's size.
7. Release the skin and pull back on the syringe plunger to make certain the needle is not in a blood vessel.
8. Inject drug slowly, and quickly withdraw the needle at the same angle used for insertion.
9. Massage the site with an alcohol swab while applying gentle pressure. If heparin is injected, then do not massage the site.
10. Dispose of the syringe and needle properly.
11. Chart all relevant information.

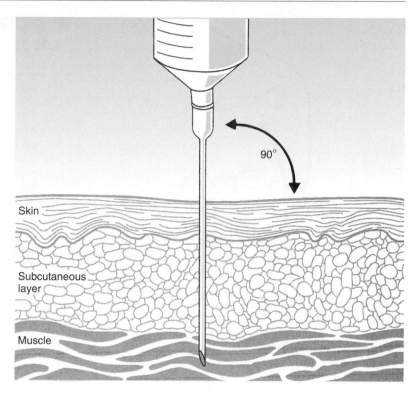

Skin

Subcutaneous
layer

Muscle

FIG. 20–12 Proper needle placement for injection into the muscle tissue. The needle is inserted at a 90-degree angle.

BOX 20-6 Steps Involved in Intramuscular Drug Injection

1. Wash hands thoroughly.
2. Put on disposable gloves.
3. Check the patient's identification.
4. Explain the procedure to the patient.
5. Prepare the site by cleansing the skin with an alcohol swab using a circular motion and moving from the center to the outside.
6. With your free hand, retract the skin approximately 1 inch to either side of the site and hold it firmly.
7. Dart the needle in a 90-degree angle of insertion.
8. Continue to hold the skin while you gently pull back on the plunger to make certain needle is not in a blood vessel.
9. If blood does appear in the syringe, then remove the needle and prepare another site for injection. If no blood appears in the syringe, then slowly inject the drug.
10. Withdraw the needle while releasing the tension on the skin.
11. Apply gentle pressure to the site with an alcohol swab.
12. Unless contraindicated, massage the injection site.
13. Dispose of the syringe and needle properly.
14. Chart all relevant information.

INTRAVENOUS INJECTION. When administering an intravenous injection, the drug is placed directly into a vein. The most commonly used intravenous injection sites include the cephalic vein on the lateral side and the basilic vein on the medial side of the anterior surface of the forearm and elbow or the cephalic and basilic veins on the posterior surface of the hand. Fig. 20–13 shows the sites commonly used for **venipuncture**. The needle length and gauge depend on the viscosity of the drug, the site selected, and the specific method of injection.

One of the most commonly used intravenous needles is the winged-tip or butterfly needle, which is manufactured in lengths of $1/4$ to $1 1/4$ inches and 18 to 25 gauge. It has tubing 3 to 12 inches long that extends from the needle to the hub. A butterfly needle is shown in Fig. 20–4. Box 20-7 identifies the steps involved in venipuncture and intravenous injection. While injecting a drug into the vein, observing the site closely for any signs of **extravasation** or infiltration is important. If extravasation occurs, then the first step is to remove the needle, apply pressure to the injection site, and apply warm moist heat to relieve the discomfort. If the extravasation involves a corrosive drug, then immediate attention is needed to prevent tissue necrosis. When a corrosive drug infiltrates the tissue, a cold compress rather than heat should be applied to the site, and the physician and

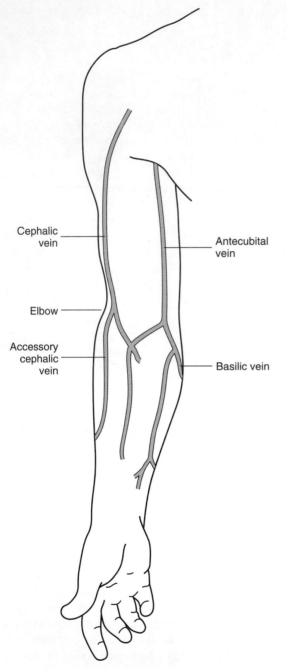

Cephalic
vein

Antecubital
vein

Elbow

Accessory
cephalic
vein

Basilic vein

FIG. 20–13   Sites commonly used for venipuncture.

BOX 20-7 Steps Involved in Venipuncture and Intravenous Drug Injection

1. Wash hands thoroughly.
2. Check the patient's identification.
3. Explain the procedure to the patient.
4. Assemble all needed supplies, and prepare the drug for administration.
5. Put on disposable gloves.
6. Once an appropriate site for venipuncture has been selected, clean it with an alcohol swab using a circular motion while moving from the center to the outside.
7. Apply a tourniquet above the site using sufficient tension to impede the flow of blood in the vein. Ask the patient to open and close the fist to distend the vein fully. When the vein has been identified, ask the patient to hold the fist in a clenched position.
8. To stabilize the vein, place your thumb on the tissue just below the site and gently pull the skin and vein toward the patient's hand.
9. Hold the needle with the bevel facing upward. When using a butterfly needle, pinch the wings together tightly.
10. Insert the needle next to the vein at a 15-degree angle and gently advance it into the vein. Blood flows back into the tubing when the needle is correctly positioned.
11. If the tubing of the butterfly needle has not previously been filled with solution, then allow the blood to flow from the hub before attaching the syringe to ensure that no air bubbles are contained in the system.
12. Remove the tourniquet and inject the drug.
13. Unless otherwise instructed, remove the needle and apply gentle pressure to the site with an alcohol swab.
14. Dispose of the syringe and needle properly.
15. Chart all relevant information.

pharmacy are notified. An antidote may exist for the particular drug.

DRIP INFUSION. Drugs that are administered by the intravenous route may be injected using one of three methods. One method involves a single administration in which the drug is injected slowly. A second method involves the administration of a drug by intravenous bolus or intravenous push. The term **bolus** refers to the amount of fluid injected, and *intravenous push* refers to a rapid injection. This method is generally used in an emergency when immediate drug action is required. The third method of administration involves the intravenous infusion of a large volume of fluid. This method is sometimes called a *drip infusion,* and it requires some additional equipment to ensure accurate delivery of the intravenous solution.

An administration set for infusion of the solution and an intravenous pole are needed. Box 20-8 outlines the

BOX 20-8 Steps Involved in Intravenous or Drip Infusion Drug Administration

1. Wash hands thoroughly.
2. Check patient's identification.
3. Explain the procedure to the patient.
4. Assemble all needed supplies.
5. Remove the administration set from the box, and straighten the tubing while checking for any cracks or holes.
6. Slide the clamp up to the drip chamber and close it.
7. If the intravenous (IV) solution to be infused is contained in a bottle, then place the bottle on a hard surface and remove the metal cap and rubber diaphragm that covers the rubber stopper. Wipe the rubber stopper with an alcohol sponge. Remove the protective cap from the spike on the drip chamber, and firmly insert the spike into the center of the bottle's rubber stopper. Check to make certain the clamp is closed and invert the bottle. Hang the bottle on the IV pole, and squeeze the drip chamber until it is one half full.
8. If the IV solution to be infused is contained in a plastic bag rather than a bottle, then place the bag on a hard surface, remove the protective cap from the tubing insertion port on the bag, and wipe it with an alcohol sponge. Remove the protective cap from the spike on the drip chamber of the tubing, and insert the spike into the port. Check again to make certain the clamp is closed, hang the bag on the IV pole 18 to 24 inches above the site, and squeeze the drip chamber until it is one half full.
9. Prime all tubing before using the IV setup by removing the protective cap from the end of the tubing and holding it over a sink or wastebasket. Take care to preserve the sterility of the cap and end of the tubing.
10. Release the clamp and allow the solution to run freely until all air bubbles are cleared from the tubing.
11. Reclamp the tubing to stop the flow and replace the protective cap over the end of the tubing.
12. Loop the tubing over the IV pole until the injection site has been selected and the venipuncture is complete.
13. Chart all relevant information.

steps involved in preparing for drip infusion. The proper procedure for setting up drip infusion solutions is demonstrated in Fig. 20–14.

When a standard administration set is used, adjusting the clamp below the drip chamber controls the flow rate or drip rate. Unless otherwise instructed by a physician, 10 to 20 drops per minute is an acceptable flow rate. Patients receiving intravenous infusion should be monitored closely. If the flow stops, then the site of injection should be checked for signs of infiltration. If evidence such as swelling and pain around the injection site exists, then the infusion must be stopped immediately, the needle removed, and a warm cloth applied to the area.

Patients receiving medication by the intravenous infusion method may come to the radiology department with additional equipment attached to the administration set. An intravenous pump and controller are devices used to regulate the flow rate electronically (Fig. 20–15). A controller regulates the flow rate by counting the drops and compressing the intravenous tubing to adjust the flow. A pump propels the solution through the tubing at the desired rate under pressure. The pump is more accurate than the controller. Both devices have alarms that sound a beep or flash a light when the infusion fails to flow at the prescribed flow rate.

CHARTING DRUG INFORMATION

Any time a drug is administered to a patient, relevant information must be recorded on the patient's chart to document the event. The necessary information includes the name and dose of the drug, the route of administration, the date, and the time. If the drug is administered parenterally, then the site of injection should be included.

Legal Considerations

Increasingly, radiologic technologists are expected to chart a drug that they administered or helped to administer. The technologist must follow the proper precautions and make certain that all information is documented on the patient's chart. If an error occurs in the administration of a drug, or if the patient experiences any adverse effects from the drug, make certain to document the details of the incident thoroughly. Both students and radiologic technologists must follow these simple rules. Errors associated with drug administration are among the most common legal problems in which radiologic technologists are involved.

Common Abbreviations

Health care professionals who order, dispense, or administer drugs often use abbreviations. Becoming thoroughly familiar with the common abbreviations that are used is important to ensure the safe and accurate administration

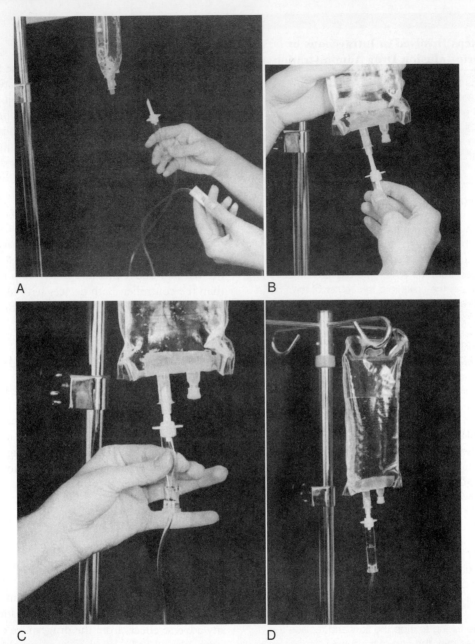

FIG. 20–14 Drip infusion setup. *A,* Remove the administration set from the box, straighten the tubing while checking for any cracks or holes, and slide the clamp up to the drip chamber and close it. *B,* Place the bag on a hard surface, remove the protective cap from the tubing insertion port on the bag, and wipe it with an alcohol sponge. Remove the protective cap from the spike on the drip chamber of the tubing, and insert the spike into the port. *C,* Check again to make certain the clamp is closed, hang the bag on the intravenous (IV) pole, and squeeze the drip chamber until it is one half full. *D,* Prime the IV setup by removing the protective cap from the end of the tubing and holding it over a sink or wastebasket. Taking care to preserve the sterility of the cap and end of the tubing, release the clamp and allow the solution to run freely until all air bubbles are cleared from the tubing. Reclamp the tubing to stop the flow and replace the protective cap over the end of the tubing.

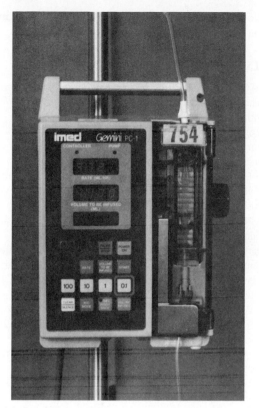

FIG. 20–15 A typical intravenous pump and controller device.

TABLE 20-5 Common Abbreviations

ABBREVIATION	MEANING
ac	Before meals
bid	Twice a day
c̄	With
et	And
g	Gram
gtt(s)	Drop(s)
h	Hour
hs	At bedtime
Hypo	Hypodermic(ally)
IM	Intramuscular(ly)
IV	Intravenous(ly)
mg	Milligram
ml	Milliliter
mm	Millimeter
od	In the right eye
os	In the left eye
pc	After meals
po	By mouth
prn	As needed
qh	Every hour
q2h	Every 2 hours
q3h	Every 3 hours
qid	Four times a day
s̄	Without
SC	Subcutaneous
Stat	Immediately
tid	Three times a day

of drugs. The list of abbreviations found in Table 20-5 includes those that are frequently encountered when administering drugs. The Joint Commission on Accreditation of Healthcare Organizations (JCAHO) has published a *DO NOT USE* list of abbreviations. A current list can be found on their website at *http://www.jcaho.org*. For example, the abbreviation *U* meaning *unit* has been mistaken for a *0* (zero), the number *4* (four) or *cc* and *IU*, which stands for International Unit, has been mistaken for *IV*, which means intravenous or the number *10* (ten). Another common abbreviation, *cc* for *cubic centimeter,* has been mistaken for *u* or *units,* and, as a result, recommendations are that *ml* or *milliliter* be used in its place. In addition to the JCAHO, the Institute for Safe Medication Practices (ISMP) has also published a list of error-prone abbreviations, symbols, and dose designations that can be found on their website at *http://www.ismp.org*. Organizations are expected to standardize the abbreviations, acronyms, and symbols that will be used and have a list of abbreviations, acronyms, and symbols that should not be used.

SUMMARY

Pharmacology is the scientific study of drugs, including the origin, nature, effects, and uses of drugs. The radiologic technologist is expected to have a basic knowledge of pharmacology to prepare and administer drugs under the supervision of a licensed practitioner.

Drugs are classified in a variety of ways. A drug may be classified by name, action, or method of purchase. When drugs are classified by name, a single drug has a chemical name that represents its actual chemical structure; a generic name, which is a simplified version that reflects the chemical structure but is easier to pronounce; and the brand name, which is unique to the company that manufactures the drug. The *PDR* is a reference, usually found in the radiology department, that lists drugs by both generic and trade names. Drugs also are classified according to action, with drugs that have similar chemical actions grouped together. When drugs are classified according to the method of purchase, they are divided into two groups: prescription drugs and non-prescription drugs.

The dose form indicates the type of preparation for drug administration. Some common dose forms include tablets, capsules, suppositories, solutions, suspensions, and transdermal patches.

The radiologic technologist should be familiar with the actions and precautions associated with commonly used drugs. A listing of commonly used drugs arranged alphabetically by trade name and a list of drugs most often found on an emergency cart are provided in this chapter for easy reference. An additional list arranged alphabetically by generic name is also provided.

The golden rules of drug administration should always be followed when preparing to administer or when assisting with drug administration. Simply stated, the rules remind us to check for the right drug, right amount, right patient, right time, and right route. Drugs can be administered by the following routes: oral, sublingual, topical, and parenteral. When a drug is administered parenterally, it may be injected under the skin (subcutaneously), into the muscle (intramuscularly), or into the vein (intravenously). In all three methods of injection, strict aseptic technique should be followed when preparing and administering the drug.

Syringes and needles are manufactured in a variety of shapes and sizes. Selecting the proper needle and syringe is important when preparing drugs. Angiocaths are recommended to avoid accidents. Drugs that are to be injected come in two different kinds of containers. One type is an ampule, which usually holds a single dose, and the other is a vial, a small bottle that holds multiple doses.

Numerous factors affect the patient's response to a drug, which may be undesirable. Adverse effects include side effects, toxic effects, allergic reactions, and idiosyncratic reactions. Following drug administration by any route, the patient should be monitored closely for any signs of adverse effects.

Guidelines for oral, topical, and parenteral administration are included in this chapter. Detailed instructions are provided for subcutaneous injections, intramuscular injections, and intravenous injections. Following administration, relevant information should be recorded on the patient's chart.

BIBLIOGRAPHY

Albers GW et al: Antithrombotic and thrombolytic therapy for ischemic stroke: the Seventh ACCP Conference on Antithrombotic and Thrombolytic Therapy, *Chest* 126:483S, 2004.

Argonin ME: *Dementia: practical guides in psychiatry,* Philadelphia, 2004, Lippincott Williams & Williams.

Basch E, Ulbricht C: *Natural standard herb and supplement handbook: the clinical bottom line,* St Louis, 2005, Elsevier Mosby.

Carey KW, Goldberg KE: *Medications and IVs: clinical pocket manual.* Springhouse, Pa, 1987, Springhouse.

Chobanian AV et al: The seventh report of the Joint National Committee on Prevention, Detection, Evaluation, and Treatment of High Blood Pressure: the JNC 7 report, *JAMA* 289:2460, 2003.

Gotto AM Jr, Pownall HJL: *Manual of lipid disorders: reducing the risk for coronary heart disease,* ed 3, Philadelphia, 2003, Lippincott Williams & Wilkins.

Katzung BG: *Basic and clinical pharmacology,* ed 9, New York, 2004, McGraw-Hill.

Koda-Kimble MA et al: *Applied therapeutics: the clinical use of drugs,* ed 8, Baltimore, 2005, Lippincott Williams & Wilkins.

Lehne RA et al: *Pharmacology for nursing care,* ed 3, Philadelphia, 1998, WB Saunders.

Mangoni AA, Jackson SHD: Age-related changes in pharmacokinetics and pharmacodynamics: basic principles and practical applications, *Br J Clin Pharmacol* 57:6, 2003.

Nasrallah, HA, Smeltzer DJ: *Contemporary diagnosis and management of the patient with schizophrenia,* Newton, Pa, 2003, Handbooks in Health Care.

Physicians' desk reference, Montvale, NJ, 2005, Thompson PDR.

Phillips LD: *Manual of IV therapy,* ed 3, Philadelphia, 2001, FA Davis.

Shargel L, Wu-Pong S, Yu ABC: *Applied biopharmaceutics and pharmacokinetics,* ed 5, New York, 2005, McGraw-Hill Companies.

Stedman's medical dictionary for the health profession and nursing, Baltimore, 2005, Lippincott Williams & Wilkins.

Steele J: *Practical IV therapy,* ed 2, Springhouse, Pa, 1996, Springhouse.

Contrast Media and Introduction to Radiopharmaceuticals

Audrey Harris, MAEd, RT(R) (CT) (M) (QM)
Norman E. Bolus, MPH, CNMT

To array a person's will against their sickness is the supreme art of medicine.

Henry Ward Beecher

OBJECTIVES

On completion of this chapter, the student will be able to:

1. State the purpose of contrast media.

2. Differentiate between low and high subject contrast.

3. Compare negative and positive contrast agents.

4. Name the general types of contrast media used for specific radiographic procedures.

5. List the serious complications of the administration of barium sulfate.

OBJECTIVES—Cont'd

6. Match specific procedures to particular patient instructions.

7. Explain the importance of osmosis as it relates to various effects of iodinated ionic contrast media.

8. Discuss the advantages of nonionic iodinated contrast media.

9. Differentiate among the major adverse effects of various contrast agents.

10. Recognize clinical symptoms of adverse reactions to iodinated contrast media to the level of treatment required.

11. Relate the patient history to the possibility of adverse reactions.

12. Introduce the concept of radiopharmaceuticals.

GLOSSARY

Acid Group: contains carbon double bonded to an oxygen, single bonded to another oxygen, and has a negative charge at the pH of the body

Amine Group: contains nitrogen bonded to two hydrogen atoms

Anaphylactoid: resembling an immune system response to foreign material (antigen)

Atomic Number: number of protons in the nuclei of the different elements

Bond: interactions between electrons of atoms that hold the atoms together in a stable group; line drawn between atoms indicates a bond: H-O-H

Bronchospasm: involuntary constriction of the bronchial tubes usually resulting from an immune system reaction to a foreign particle or molecule

Compound: substance composed of two or more elements combined in definite ratios that give the substance specific properties

Contraindications: factors of a patient's history or present status that indicate that a medical procedure should not be performed or that a medication should not be given

Creatinine: nitrogen-containing waste products of metabolism excreted by the kidney's filtration system; high blood plasma levels indicate poor filtration by the kidney

Dimer: compound formed by bonding of two identical simpler molecules

Ester: group of organic compounds formed when alcohols and acids are combined chemically

Ethyl Group: two carbon atoms linked to each other and to hydrogen atoms

Extravasation: leakage from a vessel into the tissue

Fatty Acid: long chains of carbon atoms linked to each other and to hydrogen atoms; at one end of the chain is an acid group that contains two oxygen atoms and a hydrogen atom arranged in a particular way

Flocculation: formation of flaky masses resulting from precipitation or coming out of a suspension or solution

Histamine: molecular substance containing an amine group; causes bronchial constriction and a decrease in blood pressure

Hydroxyl: common chemical group, part of the water molecule, containing one atom of hydrogen and one atom of oxygen; carries a negative charge (anion) when not a part of a molecule

Ion: atom or molecule having a negative charge (anion) or positive charge (cation)

Methyl Group: common biochemical group containing one carbon atom and three hydrogen atoms

Molecule: stable group of bonded atoms having specific chemical properties

Monomer: simple molecule of a compound of relatively low molecular weight

Osmolality: measurement of the number of particles (molecules or ions or cations) that can crowd out water molecules in a measured mass (kilogram) of water

Osmosis: movement of water from an area of high concentration to an area of low concentration through a semipermeable membrane such as blood vessel walls and cell membranes

pH: relative acidity or basicity (alkalinity) of a solution; pH below 7.0 is acidic and has more hydrogen cations than hydroxyl anions, whereas a pH above 7.0 is alkaline and has more hydroxyl anions than hydrogen cations

Radiopharmaceutical: pharmaceutical compound that is attached to a radioisotope

Shock: inadequate blood flow within the body with resulting loss of oxygen and therefore energy

Solution: uniform mixture of two or more substances composed of molecule-sized particles that do not react together chemically

Suspension: nonuniform mixture of two or more substances, one of which is composed of larger-than-molecule-size particles that have a tendency to cluster together

INTRODUCTION TO CONTRAST MEDIA

Historical Aspects of Contrast Agents

Air, a negative contrast medium, was used initially in 1918 by Walter Dandy, a neurosurgeon who did injections of air to study the cerebral ventricles of children with hydrocephalus. Dandy's published articles initiated the use of air to localize tumors within the brain and spinal cord. Later, carbon dioxide, nitrous oxide, and oxygen came into use.

Immediately after Roentgen's discovery of x-rays, physiologists realized that the functions of the digestive system could be monitored by giving animals food mixed with compounds of high atomic number and watching the mixture's passage by way of a fluorescent screen. In 1896, lead subacetate was used to study the digestive system of the guinea pig. It later proved to be toxic, however. In the same year, Walter Cannon, then a Harvard medical student, began a series of experiments to study the digestive system using bismuth subnitrate. His subjects included geese, cats, and a 7-year-old girl. Although bismuth subnitrate eventually proved to be toxic, Cannon is credited with awakening the medical profession to the realization that diseases of the gastrointestinal (GI) tract could be studied by watching the movement of radiopaque media through the tract.

Toxicity remained a problem with many of the high–atomic-number compounds in these early years. In fact, Thorotrast, which incorporated thorium, proved to be radioactive. By 1910, articles about the advantages of the inert and insoluble compound barium sulfate began to appear in the medical literature. Its use increased rapidly because of its lack of toxicity, its low cost, and its availability.

Water-soluble iodinated contrast media were introduced by Egas Moniz in 1927 when he injected sodium iodide into the cerebrovascular circulation by way of the carotid arteries. Sodium iodide proved to be a blood vessel irritant.

During the 1930s, chemical methods improved. Atoms with high atomic numbers, such as iodine, could be placed on nontoxic water-soluble carrier **molecules.** Eventually, more iodine atoms per molecule were added, which increased visualization of the vascular and urinary systems. The 1950s saw the beginning of the use of three iodine atoms per carrier molecule. These triiodinated molecules are the basic chemical structures from which both ionic and nonionic water-soluble iodine contrast media originate.

Purpose of Contrast Media

To visualize anatomic detail, the area of interest must differ in radiographic density from its surrounding tissue. The ability to distinguish between radiographic densities enables differences in anatomic tissues to be visualized. Factors that affect the degree of radiographic density differences include absorption characteristics of the tissues that comprise the anatomic part, technical factors used, characteristics of the image receptor, automatic image processing, and the use of contrast media agents.

The body absorbs x-ray photons according to the various tissue **atomic numbers** and the amount of matter per volume of tissue. Higher–atomic-number tissues absorb more x-ray photons than low–atomic-number tissues. For example, increased absorption of x-ray photons occurs with bone because calcium has a high atomic number, whereas soft tissues transmit or scatter x-ray photons more easily, resulting in decreased x-ray absorption.

Radiographic images of anatomic areas classified as low in subject contrast result in few density differences and are difficult to visualize. Instilling a contrast medium into the area of interest will change the absorption characteristics of the anatomic area and alter its subject contrast and the radiographic density differences. Enhancing the density differences within the area of interest will improve visualization of the anatomic detail.

Contrast media are diagnostic agents that are instilled into body orifices or injected into the vascular system, joints, and ducts to enhance subject contrast in anatomic areas where low subject contrast exists. The ability of the contrast media used in radiographic procedures to enhance subject contrast depends greatly on the atomic number of the element used in a particular medium and the concentration of atoms of the element per volume of the medium.

Contrast media are generally classified as negative or positive contrast agents. Negative contrast agents decrease attenuation of the x-ray beam and produce areas of increased density on the radiograph, whereas positive contrast agents increase the attenuation of the x-ray beam and produce areas of decreased density on the radiograph.

General Types of Contrast Agents

RADIOLUCENT (NEGATIVE). X-ray photons are easily transmitted or scattered through radiolucent contrast media. As the name implies, these media are relatively lucent to x-rays. Because the anatomic areas filled by

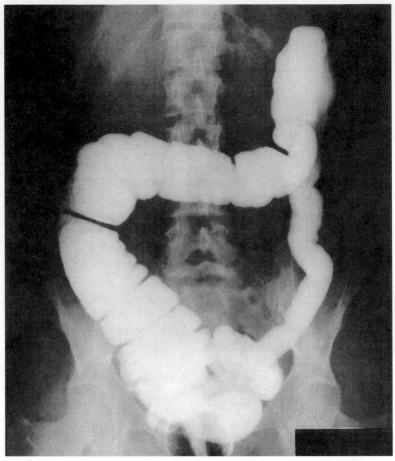

FIG. 21–1 *A,* Radiopaque barium sulfate fills the colon in a lower gastrointestinal study. (Courtesy Margaret Weaver, RT[R].)

A

these agents appear dark (increased density) on radiographs, they are also called *negative contrast agents.* These media are composed of elements with low atomic numbers.

RADIOPAQUE (POSITIVE). X-ray photons are absorbed by radiopaque contrast media because these media are opaque to x-rays. Because the anatomic areas filled by these agents appear light (decreased density) on radiographs, they are also called *positive contrast agents.* These media are composed of elements with high atomic numbers.

In some instances, negative and positive agents are used together so that the lumen of organs, such as the colon (Fig. 21-1), can be visualized or so that anatomic structures within a space, such as the menisci of the knee, can be visualized.

SPECIALTY CONTRAST AGENTS. Contrast agents of varying types are also being used in other modalities,

such as magnetic resonance imaging (MRI) and diagnostic medical sonography. A common intravenous contrast agent used in MRI studies is gadolinium diethylenetri-aminepenta-acetic acid (gadolinium-DTPA). This contrast agent is a metallic and magnetic agent that will affect the signal intensity used to image the anatomic area of interest. Ultrasound contrast agents are generally gas-filled microbubbles that affect the sound wave to enhance ultrasound contrast. Although not the focus of this chapter, these agents have a purpose similar to that of radiographic contrast agents, that is, of enhancing the subject contrast of the area of interest.

NEGATIVE CONTRAST MEDIA

Physical Properties

Negative contrast media are composed of low–atomic-number elements and are administered as gas (air) or gas-producing tablets, crystals, or soda water (carbon

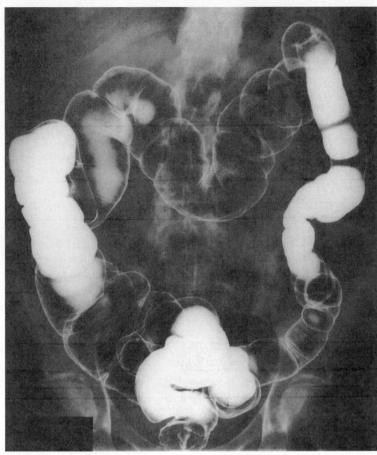

FIG. 21–1, cont'd *B,* Barium sulfate and air are used together to visualize the lumen of the colon.

B

dioxide). Because cells absorb oxygen quickly, this gas is rarely used alone as a contrast agent.

Specific Procedures

Air alone provides negative contrast for laryngopharyngography because upper respiratory structures contain air naturally. Otherwise, radiolucent contrast media are used in combination with radiopaque media to outline the lumens of, or spaces within, body structures. Table 21-1 lists common double-contrast studies, contrast media used, method of administration, patient preparations, instructions, and patient care.

Adverse Reactions

Generally, complications from the administration of negative contrast agents are minimal, although air can cause emboli. These small air masses can enter the circulatory system and become lodged in blood vessels, causing pain and loss of oxygen to the area. Patients who receive barium sulfate with air should be instructed to drink plenty of fluids after the procedure to dilute and eliminate the barium sulfate. Administration of water-soluble iodine contrast media along with air in the joint spaces usually does not result in complications.

POSITIVE CONTRAST MEDIA

Barium Sulfate Contrast Media

PHYSICAL PROPERTIES. The element barium has an atomic number of 56; thus it is radiopaque. Barium sulfate is an inert powder composed of crystals that is used for examining the digestive system. The chemical formula is $BaSO_4$, which indicates a ratio of one atom of barium to one atom of sulfur to four atoms of oxygen; thus it is a **compound.** Because barium sulfate is not

TABLE 21-1 Common Double-contrast Studies

AREA	CONTRAST AGENT	METHOD OF ADMINISTRATION	PATIENT PREPARATIONS	PATIENT INSTRUCTIONS/CARE DURING PROCEDURE
Stomach	Barium sulfate Carbon dioxide as tablets, crystals, or soda water	Oral	Nothing to eat or drink after midnight before examination	Patient should not belch after carbon dioxide is given so that the lumen of the stomach can be seen.
Large intestine	Barium sulfate Air	Rectal	Large amount of fluid before examination or fluid diet Nothing to eat or drink after midnight before examination Cleansing enema before examination	Provide supportive communication so that the patient does not lose control.
Arthrography: shoulder, knee, wrist, hip	Water-soluble iodine media Air	Injection into joint space	None	Provide supportive communication because stress views performed during procedure can be painful.

Reprinted with permission of the American College of Radiology. No other representation of this article is authorized without express, written permission of the American College of Radiology.

soluble in water, it must be mixed or shaken into a **suspension** in water. Depending on the environment of the barium sulfate, such as acid within the stomach, the powder has a tendency to clump and come out of suspension. This action is called **flocculation.** Stabilizing agents such as sodium carbonate or sodium citrate are usually used to prevent flocculation. These ingredients are listed as suspending agents on the container labels. Other ingredients used in orally administered barium sulfate include vegetable gums, flavoring, and sweeteners to increase palatability. Barium sulfate suspensions must be concentrated enough so that x-rays are absorbed. These suspensions must flow easily and yet coat the lining of organs.

For studies of the small intestine, oral formulations of barium sulfate and methylcellulose, a nondigestible starch, have been introduced. These preparations are designed to give a *see-through* effect to better diagnose small lesions.

For lower GI studies, general recommendations are that barium sulfate be mixed with *cold* tap water to reduce irritation to the colon and to aid the patient in holding the enema during the examination. The cold tap water reduces spasm and cramping, although mixing the barium sulfate with room temperature water has also been recommended for maximal patient comfort.

A primary function of the colon is to absorb water from waste; however, increased water absorption by the colon can result in excess fluid entering the circulatory system (hypervolemia), a serious, sometimes fatal, complication. The addition of 2 teaspoons of table salt per liter of water used in the enema preparation reduces the risk of hypervolemia. Following the manufacturer's directions is critical when mixing barium sulfate suspensions so that diagnostic radiographs will be obtained. Figure 21-2 shows various barium sulfate preparations, carbon dioxide crystals used for double-contrast studies, and enema tips used for lower GI studies.

SPECIFIC PROCEDURES. The administration of barium sulfate can result in complications, generally as a result of preexisting patient disease or status. If a patient is thought to have a perforation in the digestive tract, then barium sulfate is contraindicated because the body does not absorb barium sulfate naturally. If it enters the peritoneal or pelvic cavity, barium sulfate can cause peritonitis and must be surgically removed. In place of barium sulfate, a water-soluble iodine contrast agent is recommended. The body is capable of absorbing this type of agent.

In certain patients, the administration of barium sulfate can result in trauma such as perforation of the colon. The radiologic technologist must obtain a detailed patient history to give appropriate patient care. Table 21-2 outlines patient history factors that should be considered before administering barium sulfate. Table 21-3 lists the specific procedures that use a barium sulfate suspension.

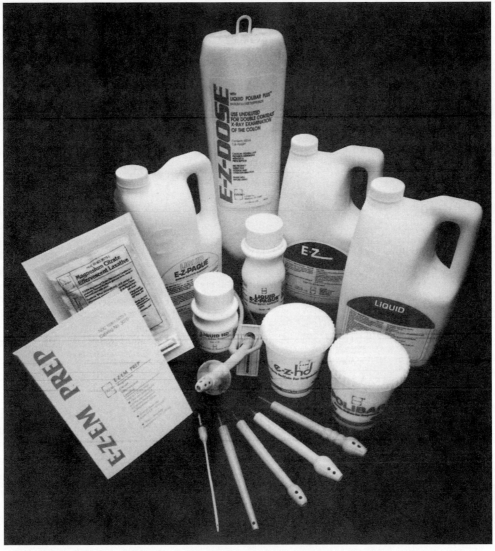

FIG. 21–2 Various barium preparations and supplies. (Courtesy E-Z-EM, Inc., Lake Success, NY.)

TABLE 21-2 Patient History Factors in Barium Sulfate Examinations

FACTOR	IMPORTANCE
Age	Ability to communicate, hear, and follow directions
	↑ Risk of colon perforation caused by loss of tissue tone
Diverticulitis or ulcerative colitis	↑ Difficulty in holding an enema
	↑ Risk of colon perforation
Long-term steroid therapy	↑ Risk of colon perforation
Colon biopsy within previous 2 wks	Lower gastrointestinal series contraindicated
Pregnancy	Inform radiologist before proceeding with examination
Mental retardation, confusion, or dizziness	↑ Risk of aspiration during upper gastrointestinal series
Recent onset of constipation or diarrhea	↑ Risk of colon perforation or tumor rupture
Nausea and vomiting	↑ Risk of aspiration during upper gastrointestinal series

↑, Increased.
Reprinted with permission of the American College of Radiology. No other representation of this article is authorized without express, written permission of the American College of Radiology.

TABLE 21-3 Common Procedures for Which Barium Sulfate Suspensions Are Used

AREA	CONCENTRATION (WT/VOL %)	METHOD OF ADMINISTRATION	PATIENT PREPARATION	PATIENT INSTRUCTIONS/CARE DURING PROCEDURE
Esophagus: esophagram	30-50	Oral	None	Provide supportive communication. For esophageal varices, the patient should exhale, swallow barium, and then hold his or her breath on that exhalation for that exposure.
Stomach: upper gastrointestinal series	30-50	Oral	Nothing to eat or drink after midnight before examination	Provide supportive communication. Provide explanation of reasons for various positions.
Small intestine: small bowel series	40-60 if included with stomach examination	Oral	If included with a stomach examination, low-residue diet eaten for 2 days before examination	Provide supportive communication. Provide explanation for length of procedure. *Note:* In most patients, the transit time of the barium sulfate suspension through the small intestine is approximately 1 hr.
Large intestine: colon or barium enema	12-25	Rectal	Large amount of fluid or fluid diet day before examination. Nothing to eat or drink after midnight before examination. Cleansing enema before examination	Provide supportive communication so that the patient does not lose control. Watch patient for changes in mental status that may indicate fluid overload.
Stomach: computed tomography*	12-25	Oral	Nothing to eat or drink after midnight before examination	Provide supportive communication. The patient should believe that the radiographer is constantly watching the procedure.

*Generally used to accent contrast in the abdomen.

ADVERSE REACTIONS. As previously mentioned, patients should be instructed to drink plenty of fluids after receiving barium sulfate. All barium sulfate suspensions transit the colon. Because one function of the colon is to absorb water from waste, barium sulfate residue within the colon can dry and cause an obstruction. The major symptom of obstruction is constipation.

A complication related to the administration of barium sulfate during a lower GI examination is perforation of the colon with **extravasation** (leakage through a duct or vessel) into the abdominal cavity. Extravasation results in inflammation of the abdominal cavity, called *barium peritonitis*. Older adult patients or persons receiving long-term steroid medication are at increased risk for colon perforation because their tissues have become *atrophic* (lost elasticity and muscle tone). Also at risk are patients with diverticulitis and ulcerative colitis because these diseases result in inflammation and degradation of the colon tissues. Patients with toxic megacolon should not have lower GI procedures because this serious complication of ulcerative colitis results in a dilated colon that can rupture. Recent biopsy of the colon is a contraindication to a lower GI series until the area heals. The barium retention catheter can be a source of colon perforation. The radiologic technologist should use one or two gentle squeezes to inflate the retention cuff.

Vaginal rupture, a rare complication of barium sulfate administration, is due to misplacement of the catheter before lower GI examinations. Knowing the anatomy of the female pelvis in the anteroposterior and lateral configurations is critical. Female patients should be asked whether they can feel the enema tip in the rectum.

Water absorption from the colon is a serious complication of lower GI administration of barium sulfate suspensions. Water from the cleansing enema and the barium enema can be shifted from the colon into the circulatory system with a resulting increase in blood volume. Consequences of this fluid overload are pulmonary edema (fluid in the lungs), seizures, coma, and death. The table salt **solution** previously discussed reduces the possibility of hypervolemia. The radiologic technologist must observe patients for changes in mental status, such as apathy and drowsiness, that would indicate onset of hypervolemia. Symptoms of fluid overload are masked in sedated patients; therefore sedative premedication is contraindicated for lower GI examinations.

Sedated patients should not undergo upper GI examinations because the swallowing reflex is diminished, which greatly increases the risk of aspiration (inhalation) of the barium sulfate suspension with resultant barium pneumonia. Aspiration is also a risk for mentally handicapped patients and persons with altered mental status because of age or disease.

A few allergic type reactions have been noted, but these may have been caused by preservatives in the particular barium sulfate preparation or to latex used in barium enema retention catheters. Occasionally, barium sulfate has collected within the appendix. No directly related complications have resulted from this occurrence.

Water-Soluble Iodine Contrast Media

PHYSICAL PROPERTIES

Ionic Iodine Contrast Media. The element iodine has an atomic number of 53, making it relatively radiopaque. Ionic media dissociate into two molecular particles in water or blood plasma just as table salt does. These media are **ionic** because one particle has a negative charge called an *anion,* and the other particle has a positive charge called a *cation.* The anion part of the molecule begins with a six-carbon bonded hexagon called *benzene.* A carbon atom is located at each corner of the hexagon but is not usually drawn because the molecular diagram would appear cluttered. Every other carbon **bond** site of the benzene is bonded to an iodine atom; therefore each anion portion contains three iodine atoms and is therefore triiodinated. Of the three remaining carbon bond sites, one is occupied by an **acid group.** The acid group carries the negative charge at physiologic **pH.**

At the acid group, the anion and cation dissociate on injection. The other two carbon bond sites are occupied by chemical structures that increase the solubility or the excretion rate of the contrast by the body. These two carbon bond sites result in the different classes of ionic media: *diatrizoate, metrizoate,* and *iothalamate* (Fig. 21-3). The cation part of the molecule is either a sodium atom or a more complex structure, methylglucamine. Its rather long name describes its structure. The six carbons bonded to each other in a straight line and bonded to oxygens and hydrogens (**hydroxyl** groups) come from glucose, a common biologic sugar. The hydroxyl groups increase solubility. The nitrogen on the left is part of an **amine group.** (Amines are found in amino acids, and ammonia contains nitrogen.) Finally, a one-carbon, three-hydrogen group is attached to a nitrogen on the left. These one-carbon, three-hydrogen **methyl groups** are extremely common.

Methylglucamine is sometimes identified as *meglumine* on package inserts. Most ionic iodine contrast media are identified as *higher-osmolality contrast media* because of their osmotic effects. **Osmolality** is a measure of the total number of particles in solution per kilogram of water. The osmolality of contrast media is of great biologic significance. Most adverse reactions to contrast media have been related to the osmolality of the media because the osmolality of a solution determines osmotic pressure, which controls the movement of water in the body. High-osmolality contrast media have an increased number of particles in solution, such as blood plasma, which pull water toward them.

Nonionic Iodine Contrast Media. Efforts to decrease the many side effects of ionic iodine contrast media resulted in the development of molecules that do not dissociate into anions and cations (nonionics) or that are ionic but too big to have osmotic effects, such as ioxaglate (Hexabrix). These agents are identified as *lower-osmolality contrast media.*

Ioxaglate is an ionic molecule composed of two connected benzene hexagons, one that carries an acid group that dissociates on injection. This contrast agent is a **dimer** because it is composed of two identical simpler molecules. Ioxaglate carries six iodine atoms per molecule. It is ionic because it dissociates into two particles in blood plasma. Most ionic iodine contrast media are **monomers,** or simple molecules of relatively low molecular weight. Because dimers are large molecules, their osmotic effects are low. Because of their high molecular weights, they are viscous.

Recently, a nonionic dimer, iodixanol (Visipaque), was introduced. Iodixanol is made to be isomolal (same number of particles) to blood plasma by the addition of electrolytes, small anions, and cations, which are

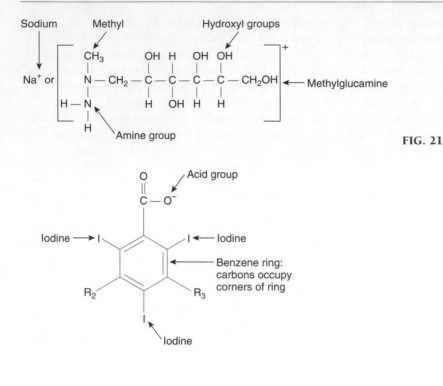

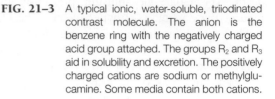

FIG. 21–3 A typical ionic, water-soluble, triiodinated contrast molecule. The anion is the benzene ring with the negatively charged acid group attached. The groups R_2 and R_3 aid in solubility and excretion. The positively charged cations are sodium or methylglucamine. Some media contain both cations.

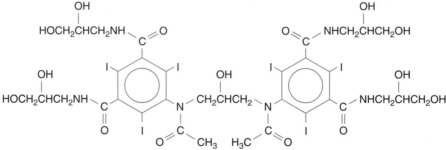

FIG. 21–4 The nonionic, water-soluble dimer iodixanol (Visipaque). (Courtesy Nycomed, Inc.)

normally present in blood plasma. Figure 21-4 shows the molecular structure of the nonionic dimer iodixanol.

An additional advantage of the lower-osmolality contrast media is that they are more hydrophilic (water soluble) than the higher-osmolality contrast media. As a result, they may be less likely to be reactive with the cells that can trigger allergic effects. Figure 21-5 shows the molecular structure of one of the water-soluble nonionic iodine contrast agents, ioversol (Optiray). It is a triiodinated benzene ring and does *not* carry an acid group. Many oxygen-hydrogen hydroxyl groups surround the benzene ring. These groups increase the solubility of the media in blood plasma. Figure 21-6 shows radiographs

of some procedures performed using water-soluble nonionic iodine contrast agents.

Figure 21-7 shows a photograph of another nonionic agent, iopamidol (Isovue). Iodine in its elemental form is chemically reactive and can be toxic in the body. Consequently, both ionic and nonionic agents contain additives such as citrate and calcium disodium edetate. These compounds prevent iodine atoms from being removed from the contrast molecules.

General Effects. Water-soluble iodine contrast media have known physiologic effects. High osmolality and the aspects of chemical structure are the major characteristics of the water-soluble media that are responsible for these effects. Although both ionic and nonionic iodine media have physiologic effects on the body, most ionic agents are higher-osmolality contrast media and therefore have shown greater effects and adverse reactions. Viscosity, or *friction,* of the media is influenced by the concentration and size of the molecule. It affects the injectability, or delivery, of the media. Heating the media to body temperature significantly reduces the viscosity and facilitates the ability for rapid injection. Heating is commonly accomplished through the use of a *contrast warmer.*

Osmotic Effects. Because ionic media dissociate in water, their injection into the blood plasma results in a great increase in the number of particles present in the plasma, which has the effect of displacing water. Water moves from an area of high concentration to an area of low concentration; the process is called **osmosis.** When the plasma water is displaced by contrast particles, water from body cells moves into the vascular system. This movement results in hypervolemia and blood vessel dilatation, producing pain and discomfort. Blood pressure may decrease because of vessel dilatation, or it may increase as a result of hypervolemia and the effects of hormones in the kidneys.

When higher-osmolality contrast media are given for imaging of the intestinal tract, fluid from cells is drawn into these areas. This osmotic effect can aid in reducing obstructions because the increase in fluid increases peristalsis. In dehydrated patients, however, the osmotic effect further reduces body cell volume and can result in **shock.** Consequently, obtaining a patient history and conveying any **contraindications** to the radiologist or other physician are important. The number of molecular particles of a particular contrast medium is shown on the package insert in units of milliosmoles per kilogram of water at 37°C. The higher the number is, the greater the number of particles that can produce osmotic effects will be. As an example, the osmolality of iodixanol at 300 mg of iodine per milliliter in milliosmoles per kilogram is 290, equal to that of blood plasma.

Allergic-Like Effects (Anaphylactoid). Allergic reactions to water-soluble iodinated contrast media resemble allergic reactions to foreign substances, such as pollen grains. Reactions of typical allergic patients may be minor, such as urticaria (hives). Some patients, however, experience wheezing and edema in the throat and lungs, with accompanying **bronchospasm.** Other anaphylactoid effects of water-soluble iodinated contrast media are nausea and vomiting. These reactions are thought to be

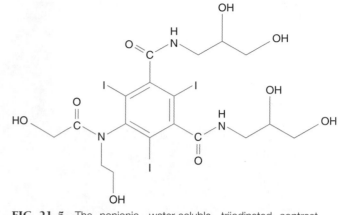

FIG. 21–5 The nonionic, water-soluble, triiodinated contrast molecule ioversol (Optiray). (Courtesy Amersham Health.)

caused by the release of a substance called **histamine** from certain cells found in the lungs, stomach, and lining of blood vessels. Although some radiologists believe that the allergic-like effects are due to extreme anxiety, the radiologic technologist should consider these effects as serious. Premedication with steroids and antihistamines (to prevent the release of histamine) can reduce or eliminate allergic effects.

Renal Effects. High-osmolality contrast media can cause the arteries of the kidneys to expand as a result of the osmotic effect. Arterial expansion results in the release of vasoconstrictors. These substances cause constriction of the renal arteries. Therefore injection of the contrast media results in dilatation and then constriction of the renal arteries. The end result is diminished blood supply to the kidneys.

Osmotic effects are also presumed to cause an increase in the amount of molecular substances that cannot be reabsorbed by the renal tubules. This increase results in *osmotic diuresis* (increased secretion of urine) and dehydration. An increased blood urea nitrogen (BUN) and **creatinine** (waste product of metabolism) level indicates that the patient may have renal disease and is a good indicator for possible contrast media–induced renal effects. Patients with renal disease or diabetes and older patients are at increased risk for these complications. Intravenous fluid given before and during procedures can reduce the severity of renal effects. Theophylline, a substance found in tea, is currently being investigated as a preventative of toxic renal effects by increasing the filtering action of the kidneys.

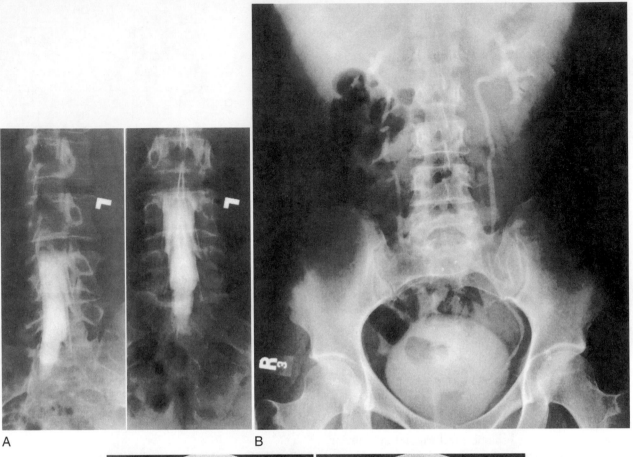

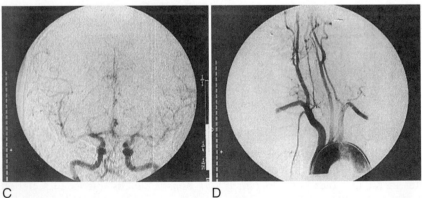

FIG. 21–6 *A,* Posteroanterior (PA) and oblique views of a lumbar myelogram. *B,* PA view of an excretory urogram. (*A* and *B* courtesy Margaret Weaver, RT[R].) *C,* Digital cerebral angiogram. Vessels appear dark because of computer manipulation. *D,* Digital angiogram of the thoracic aorta and the main arteries it supplies (four-vessel study). Vessels appear dark because of computer manipulation. (*C* and *D* courtesy David Skarbek, RT[R].)

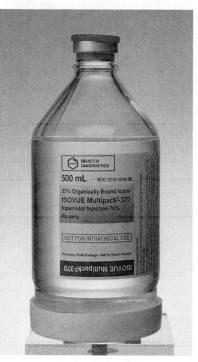

FIG. 21–7 Iopamidol (Isovue) shown in the type of bottle used for injections into the arterial or venous system. (Courtesy Bracco Diagnostics, Inc.)

Other Effects. Carotid artery injection of water-soluble iodine contrast media can alter the blood-brain barrier (separation between brain capillaries and support cells for the neurons) by causing the capillary cells to shrivel because of water loss. Some of these media can stimulate areas in the carotid artery that help control heart rate and blood pressure. Clinical symptoms of these effects include increased blood pressure, bradycardia (slow heartbeat), and tachycardia (fast heartbeat).

In patients with sickle cell anemia and those who carry the trait but who are asymptomatic, injection of high-osmolality contrast media can cause the red blood cells to shrink and to *sickle* (assume an elongated shape). These sickled cells may be trapped in small-diameter blood vessels and capillaries, causing pain and blood clots. A common effect is a sensation of warmth and pain on injection into the arterial vessels. Theories suggest that this effect is due to dissociation of the contrast media into anions and cations.

In helical computed tomographic (CT) procedures, a large amount of contrast material is injected at a rate of at least 2.5 ml per second. This amount increases the probability of nausea and vomiting and extravasation of the contrast with patient motion as a result.

Drug Interactions and Considerations. One class of drugs used to treat hypertension is the β-adrenergic blockers. These drugs reduce cardiac output, but they also reduce dilatation of bronchial smooth muscle and block the effect of epinephrine. Patients who take these drugs are at an increased risk for anaphylactoid reactions during procedures in which water-soluble iodine contrast media are used.

Calcium-channel blockers reduce hypertension by relaxing electrical conduction of cell membranes in arterioles (small arteries) and in heart muscle. Patients who take these drugs are at risk for heart block and abrupt decrease in blood pressure if ionic contrast media are used during cardiac catheterization.

Metformin (Glucophage) is a new type of drug used to treat non–insulin-dependent diabetes. Metformin should be discontinued for 48 hours before and 48 hours after the use of iodine contrast media. Although metformin does not interact with the iodine contrast agents, if renal failure should occur as an effect of iodine contrast administration, then drug levels of metformin would accumulate in the patient and lactic acidosis might develop. (Metformin increases the uptake of glucose in body cells. One end product of glucose metabolism is lactic acid. Consequently, increased levels of metformin will increase lactic acid production and decrease the pH in body cells: acidosis.)

Considerations in the Use of Nonionic Contrast Media. Most adverse reactions associated with water-soluble ionic iodine contrast media are significantly decreased with the use of the nonionic media. This decrease is attributed to the decreased osmolality of the nonionic media. In addition, the injection of nonionics during angiography is much less painful compared with injection of ionic media; however, kidney toxicity has not been reduced. Including the patient's BUN and creatinine level in the history is therefore important. Nonionic iodine contrast media cost two to three times more than ionic media. Therefore decisions about which patients will receive nonionic media are controversial. Some institutions have decided to use low-osmolality contrast media on all patients regardless of cost. Other institutions have established a selective use of these agents.

Sample criteria for the use of low-osmolality (nonionic) contrast media might include the following:

- Patients with histories of adverse reactions to contrast media, excluding mild reactions such as the sensation of heat or flushing
- Patients with a history of asthma or allergies

- Patients with known cardiac problems
- Patients with generalized severe debilitating conditions
- Patients who will undergo helical CT procedures

These criteria include patients with diabetes mellitus, renal disease or elevated creatinine levels, or sickle cell disease.

SPECIFIC PROCEDURES. A wide variety of radiologic procedures use water-soluble iodine contrast media. These agents are important in visualizing the urinary and cardiovascular systems in particular. They are also commonly used in CT studies of the brain, chest, and abdomen. Table 21-4 provides a list of the common procedures that use water-soluble iodine contrast agents.

The most important patient care aspect before administering water-soluble iodine contrast media is the patient history. The possibility of patient reaction is closely related to the patient's disease state or age. Moreover, the chemical nature of these contrast media can provoke severe reactions. The radiologic technologist is responsible for observation of patient well being. Table 21-5 lists some patient history factors to consider before administering water-soluble iodine contrast media.

ADVERSE REACTIONS. As discussed in the section on the general effects of water-soluble iodine contrast media, these media have physiologic effects that may result in adverse reactions. The responsibility of the radiologic technologist in patient surveillance is critical in assessing the severity of these effects. Box 21-1 lists adverse reactions divided into three categories: mild, moderate, and severe. A discussion of treatment is also provided. Box 21-2 details the management of patients with acute reactions. Although adverse reactions can occur when using low-osmolality (nonionic) contrast media, they are most often associated with the higher-osmolality (ionic) contrast media.

Oil-Based Iodine Contrast Media

PHYSICAL PROPERTIES. Oil-based iodine contrast media are made from **fatty acids** commonly found in plants and animals. A two-carbon atom chemical group called an **ethyl group** takes the place of the alcohol chemical group usually found in fatty acids. These chemical manipulations change the fatty acids into **esters.** Then iodine atoms are added at certain areas of the ester molecules.

The result is the description seen on the package inserts: iodinated ethyl esters of fatty acids.

Oil-based media are insoluble in water and do not flow easily because they are relatively viscous. When these esters are exposed to light, heat, or air, they decompose. Consequently, these media should be stored in a cool, dark area. Do not use any media that have darkened from their original pale yellow or pale amber color because the dark color indicates that they have decomposed. Plastic syringes should not be used for injection of oil-based iodine contrast media because toxic substances from the plastic can dissolve into the media. The main disadvantage of oil-based iodine contrast media is that they persist in the body because they are insoluble in water.

SPECIFIC PROCEDURES. Oil-based iodine contrast media are used for a select number of procedures that are generally performed infrequently. These procedures include bronchography, dacryocystography, sialography, and lymphography and are outlined in Table 21-6. Before the introduction of nonionic contrast media, myelography was a common procedure that used an oil-based medium.

As with all radiologic procedures, obtaining a complete patient history is important. In particular, the preexisting patient history factors outlined in Table 21-7 may present complications during or after bronchography and lymphography.

ADVERSE REACTIONS. Any iodine-containing contrast agent may provoke an **anaphylactoid** (allergic-like) reaction, although this is rare with the use of oil-based media. The persistence of these media in the body generally does not pose problems unless preexisting disease involves the areas examined.

Some adverse reactions are associated with specific examinations that use oil-based media. During bronchography, pulmonary function is temporarily reduced. Therefore, after the procedure, the patient should be encouraged to cough up the contrast media. Nausea, vomiting, and headache also can occur. During dacryocystography and sialography, very small ducts are dilated. Therefore contrast media may be extravasated if an accidental tear occurs. In some patients, iodine contrast injected into the parotid salivary gland causes inflammation of the gland, iodine parotitis. During lymphography, extravasation may also occur. Itchy skin rashes, temporary lymphedema, and thrombophlebitis have been reported, although these reactions are infrequent.

TABLE 21-4 Some Procedures for Which Water-Soluble Iodine Contrast Media Are Used

AREA	CONTRAST AGENT	METHOD OF ADMINISTRATION	PATIENT PREPARATION	PATIENT INSTRUCTIONS/CARE DURING PROCEDURE
Brain: cerebral angiography, computed tomography	Usually nonionic	Injection into vein or artery	Usually liquid diet to minimize nausea Premedication for sedation Intravenous fluids to aid hydration	Provide supportive communication. Tell the patient that he or she may feel warm and sense a metallic taste on injection. Explain what is being done as it is being done. Watch the patient for adverse reactions. Apply pressure to injection site after procedure is completed.
Thorax: thoracic angiography or four-vessel study	Usually nonionic	Injection into vein or artery	Usually liquid diet to minimize nausea Premedication for sedation Intravenous fluids to aid hydration	Provide supportive communication. Tell the patient that he or she may feel warmth and sense a metallic taste on injection. Explain what is being done as it is being done. Watch the patient for adverse reactions. Apply pressure to injection site after procedure is completed.
Lower limbs: venography	Usually nonionic	Injection into vein	Sometimes premedication for sedation Intravenous fluids for hydration	Provide supportive communication. Tell the patient that he or she may feel warmth and sense a metallic taste on injection. Explain what is being done as it is being done; some pain may be present. Watch the patient for adverse reactions. Apply pressure to injection site after procedure is completed.
Spinal canal: myelography	Only nonionic	Injection into subarachnoid space	Usually liquid diet Usually premedication for sedation	Provide supportive communication. Explain the use of shoulder braces and that the table will be tilted but the patient's head must be kept in extension. Explain what is being done as it is being done. Watch the patient for adverse reactions. Advise nursing staff and patient that patient should remain in bed with the head up for 24 hr to prevent headache and nausea.
Kidneys, ureters, and bladder: excretory urography, renal angiography, cystography	Usually nonionic	Injection into vein or artery For cystography, usually through catheter in urinary bladder	Liquid diet day before examination to reduce gas formation Laxatives or a cleansing enema may be given Bladder should be emptied before the examination begins	Provide supportive communication. Tell the patient that he or she may feel warmth and sense a metallic taste during and just after injections; several injections may be performed. Explain the timing of the radiographs and the x-ray tube movement if tomography is done. Watch the patient for adverse reactions. Angiography: apply pressure to the injection site after procedure is completed.

Continued

TABLE 21-4 Some Procedures for Which Water-Soluble Iodine Contrast Media Are Used—cont'd

AREA	CONTRAST AGENT	METHOD OF ADMINISTRATION	PATIENT PREPARATION	PATIENT INSTRUCTIONS/CARE DURING PROCEDURE
Heart and coronary arteries: cardiac catheterization	Usually nonionic	Usually through catheter	Liquid or low-residue diet usually ordered the evening before the procedure Antibiotics usually ordered Premedication for sedation Intravenous fluids for hydration Blood clotting (prothrombin) time must be within a range acceptable to the physician Catheter may be inserted in femoral artery; therefore strength of dorsal pedal pulses is evaluated	Provide supportive communication. Tell the patient that he or she may feel warmth and sense a metallic taste on injection. Explain what is being done as it is being done. The patient may be apprehensive about the movements of the x-ray tube around the body or the use of two x-ray tubes. Lead glass shielding should be explained. Nursing procedures: monitoring of peripheral pulses and blood pressure. Watch the patient for adverse reactions. Advise nursing staff that temperature may be elevated after procedure.

TABLE 21-5 Patient History Factors in Water-Soluble Iodine Contrast Examinations

FACTORS	IMPORTANCE
Age	↑ Risk with increased age
Allergies or asthma	↑ Risk of allergic-like reactions
Diabetes	Insulin usually given before procedure; these patients should be scheduled before others
Coronary artery disease	↑ Risk of tachycardia, bradycardia, hypertension, myocardial infarction (heart attack)
Hypertension	Hypertension with tachycardia
Renal disease	Inform radiologist if creatinine level is above 1.4 mg/dl
Multiple myeloma	Abnormal protein binds with contrast and can cause renal failure Patients must be hydrated
Confusion or dizziness	Blood-brain barrier effects
Sickle cell anemia or family history of chronic obstructive pulmonary disease	↑ Risk of blood clots ↑ Risk of dyspnea (difficulty in breathing)
Previous iodine contrast examinations	Did the patient have difficulties with procedure?
Pregnancy	Inform radiologists before proceeding
History of blood clots	↑ Risk of blood clots
Use of beta blockers	↑ Risk of anaphylactoid reactions
Use of calcium channel blockers	↑ Risk of heart block
Use of metformin (Glucophage)	↑ Risk of lactic acidosis if renal failure occurs

↑, Increased.

BOX 21-1 Categories of Reactions

Mild

Nausea, vomiting
Altered taste
Sweats
Cough
Itching
Rash, hives
Warmth
Pallor
Nasal stuffiness
Dizziness
Flushing
Swelling: eyes, face
Shaking
Chills
Anxiety

Signs and symptoms appear self-limited without evidence of progression (e.g., limited urticaria with mild pruritus, transient nausea, one episode of emesis).

Treatment: Requires observation to confirm resolution and/or lack of progression but usually no treatment. Patient reassurance is usually helpful.

Moderate

Moderate degree of clinically evident focal or systemic signs or symptoms including:

Tachycardia/bradycardia
Hypotension
Bronchospasm, wheezing
Hypertension
Dyspnea
Laryngeal edema
Pronounced cutaneous reaction

Treatment: Clinical findings should be considered as indications for immediate treatment. These situations require close, careful observation for possible progression to a life-threatening event.

Severe

Life-threatening with more severe signs or symptoms, including:

Laryngeal edema
Profound hypotension
Unresponsiveness
Convulsions
Clinically manifest arrhythmias
Cardiopulmonary arrest

Treatment: Requires *prompt* recognition and treatment; almost always requires hospitalization.

From Version 5.0 of the *ACR Manual on Contrast Media*, with permission of the American College of Radiology. No other representation of this article is authorized without express, written permission from the American College of Radiology.

RADIOPHARMACEUTICALS

General Characteristics

A radiopharmaceutical is not a contrast agent. A **radiopharmaceutical** is a radionuclide that is attached (chemically bound) to a pharmaceutical that has a specific biodistribution in the human body. This biodistribution is dependent on many factors, such as route of administration; gas, liquid, or solid state of the radiopharmaceutical; and sensitivity, as well as specificity, of the pharmaceutical in the body as it is taken up. The radioisotope attached to the pharmaceutical is imaged using a gamma camera, which *sees* or detects where the radiopharmaceutical is in the body and forms an image of more or less concentration of the radiopharmaceutical.

Physicians read the images knowing the normal biodistribution patterns and look for pathologic conditions within the body based on where the radiopharmaceuticals concentrate. The functionality of this procedure lies in the ability of many radiopharmaceuticals to be taken up by an organ of interest and then metabolized and used or to begin the process of elimination in the body. A prime example would be renal imaging whereby the radiopharmaceutical is taken up by the kidneys, metabolized into urine, and collected in the bladder. If a patient has a kidney stone that is blocking the path of urine in one of the ureters, then this stone would show up while performing the study. Physicians can also determine the rate of uptake and elimination of the radiopharmaceutical in the kidneys and determine if it is functioning normally or not. This method is how an

BOX 21-2 Management of Acute Reactions in Adults

Urticaria

1. Discontinue injection if not completed
2. No treatment needed in most cases
3. Give H_1-receptor blocker: Diphenhydramine (Benadryl) PO/IM/IV 25-50 mg. If severe or widely disseminate: Alpha-agonist (arteriolar and venous constriction) Epinephrine SC (1 : 1,000) 0.1-0.3 ml (=0.1-0.3 mg) (if no cardiac contraindications)

Facial or Laryngeal Edema

1. Give alpha-agonist (arteriolar and venous constriction): epinephrine SC or IM (1 : 1000) 0.1-0.3 ml (=0.1-0.3 mg) or, if hypotension is evident, Epinephrine (1 : 10,000) slowly IV 1 ml (=0.1 mg). Repeat as needed up to a maximum of 1 mg
2. Give O_2 6-10 L/min (via mask). If not responsive to therapy, or if there is obvious acute laryngeal edema, seek appropriate assistance (e.g., cardiopulmonary arrest response team)

Bronchospasm

1. Give O_2 6-10 L/min (via mask). Monitor: electrocardiogram, O_2 saturation (pulse oximeter), and blood pressure
2. Give beta-agonist inhaler (bronchiolar dilators, such as metaproternol [Alupent], terbutaline [Brethaire], or albuterol [Proventil, Ventolin]) 2 to 3 puffs; repeat prn. If unresponsive to inhalers, use SC, IM or IV epinephrine
3. Give epinephrine SC or IM (1 : 1,000) 0.1-0.3 ml (=0.1-0.3 mg) or, if hypotension evident, epinephrine (1 : 10,000) slowly IV 1 ml (=0.1 mg). Repeat as needed up to a maximum of 1 mg

   Alternatively: Give aminophylline: 6 mg/kg IV in D5W over 10-20 minutes (loading dose), then 0.4-1 mg/kg/hr, as needed (caution: hypotension).

   Call for assistance (e.g., cardiopulmonary arrest response team) for severe bronchospasm or if O_2 saturation <88% persists.

Hypotension with Tachycardia

1. Elevate legs 60° or more (preferred) or Trendelenburg position
2. Monitor: electrocardiogram, pulse oximeter, blood pressure
3. Give O_2 6-10 L/min (via mask)
4. Rapid IV administration of large volumes of isotonic Ringer's lactate or normal saline.

   If poorly responsive: Epinephrine (1 : 10,000 slowly IV 1 ml (=0.1 mg) (if no cardiac contraindications). Repeat as needed up to a maximum of 1 mg. If still poorly responsive, seek appropriate assistance (e.g., cardiopulmonary arrest response team).

Hypotension with Bradycardia (Vagal Reaction)

1. Monitor vital signs
2. Elevate legs 60° or more (preferred) or Trendelenburg position
3. Secure airway: give O_2 6-10 L/min (via mask)
4. Secure IV access: rapid fluid replacement with Ringer's lactate or normal saline
5. Give atropine 0.6-1.0 mg IV slowly if patient does not respond quickly to steps 2-4
6. Repeat atropine up to a total dose of 0.04 mg/kg (2-3 mg) in adult
7. Ensure complete resolution of hypotension and bradycardia prior to discharge

Hypertension, Severe

1. Give O_2 6-10 L/min (via mask)
2. Monitor: electrocardiogram, pulse oximeter, blood pressure
3. Give nitroglycerine 0.4-mg tablet, sublingual (may repeat ×3); *or,* topically 2% ointment, apply 1-in strip
4. Transfer to intensive care unit or emergency department
5. For pheochromocytoma: phentolamine 5 mg IV

Seizures or Convulsions

1. Give O_2 6-10 L/min (via mask)
2. Consider diazepam (Valium) 5 mg (or more, as appropriate) or midazolam (Versed) 0.5-1.0 mg IV
3. If longer effect needed, obtain consultation; consider phenytoin (Dilantin) infusion 15-18 mg/kg at 50 mg/min
4. Careful monitoring of vital signs required, particularly of pO_2 because of risk to respiratory depression with benzodiazepine administration
5. Consider using cardiopulmonary arrest response team for intubation if needed

Pulmonary Edema

1. Elevate torso, rotating tourniquets (venous compression)
2. Give O_2 6-10 L/min (via mask)
3. Give diuretics: furosemide (Lasix) 20-40 mg IV, slow push
4. Consider giving morphine (1-3 mg IV)
5. Transfer to intensive care unit or emergency department
6. Corticosteroids optional

D5W, Dextrose 5% in water; *IM,* intramuscular; *IV,* intravenous; *SC,* subcutaneous; *PO,* orally.
From Version 5.0 of the *ACR Manual on Contrast Media,* with permission of the American College of Radiology. No other representation of this article is authorized without express, written permission from the American College of Radiology.

TABLE 21-6 Some Procedures for Which Oil-Based Iodine Contrast Media Are Used

AREA	CONTRAST AGENT	METHOD OF ADMINISTRATION	PATIENT PREPARATION	PATIENT INSTRUCTIONS/CARE DURING PROCEDURE
Lungs*: bronchography (usually imaged now by computed tomography or examined by bronchoscopy)	Iodine compounds suspended in oil such as propyl iodine in peanut oil	Usually through catheter into the bronchus	Nothing to eat or drink after midnight before examination	Provide supportive communication. The patient should avoid coughing. Explain to the patient that he or she is tilted into various angles to spread the contrast throughout the bronchial tubes.
Tear ducts: dacryocystography	Iodinated ethyl esters; low viscosity such as Ethiodol	Usually through catheter into the duct	None	Provide supportive communication. Advise patient that the contrast material will drain through the nose.
Salivary glands: sialography (suspected large masses are usually imaged by computed tomography)	Iodinated ethyl esters; low viscosity such as Ethiodol	Usually through catheter into the duct	None	Provide supportive communication. After injection of contrast, the patient is given gum to chew to increase the flow of saliva; this reason should be explained to the patient.
Lymphatic system: lymphography	Iodinated ethyl esters; low viscosity such as Ethiodol	Through catheter into lymph vessel	None, although the patient should be advised that this procedure may take an hour or more to complete and that 24-hr follow-up images are done to demonstrate the lymph nodes	Advise patient that he or she will have to remain relatively motionless on the x-ray table during the 30-min contrast injection and for a time after the injection. A pad should be placed on the table for patient comfort. Consistently reassure the patient that the examination is going well. If patient complains of pain at or above injection site, inform the radiologist; injection pressure may be too high.

*Some of these procedures have been superseded by other imaging methods.

TABLE 21-7 Patient History Factors in Bronchography and Lymphography

FACTOR	IMPORTANCE
Age	Ability to communicate, hear, and follow instructions
Lower back problems	Lymphography requires the patient to lie supine for a long period
Chronic obstructive pulmonary disease	Procedures are contraindicated
Radiation therapy to the lungs	Procedures are contraindicated
Suspected spread of malignancy to the lymphatic system	Inform the radiologist before proceeding
Surgery involving part of the lymphatic system (most common is breast cancer surgery)	Inform the radiologist before proceeding

TABLE 21-8 Selected Radiopharmaceuticals

RADIONUCLIDE	PHARMACEUTICAL	MAIN ENERGY	HALF-LIFE	MAIN ORGAN OF INTEREST
^{99m}Tc	Medronate	140 keV	6.02 hr	Bone
^{99m}Tc	Mertiatide	140 keV	6.02 hr	Kidneys
^{99m}Tc	Sulfur colloid	140 keV	6.02 hr	Liver/spleen
^{99m}Tc	Mebrofenin	140 keV	6.02 hr	Hepatobiliary
^{99m}Tc	Albumin aggregated	140 keV	6.02 hr	Lung perfusion
^{99m}Tc	Tetrofosmin	140 keV	6.02 hr	Myocardial perfusion
^{99m}Tc	Fanolesomab	140 keV	6.02 hr	Appendix
^{201}Tl	Thallous chloride	68-80 keV	3.04 days	Myocardial perfusion
^{131}I	Sodium iodide	364 keV/gamma Beta used for therapy	8.02 days	Thyroid imaging or therapy ablation
^{67}Ga	Citrate	412 keV	3.26 days	Inflammation
^{133}Xe	Xenon gas	81 keV	5.243 days	Lung ventilation

TABLE 21-9 Selected PET Agents

RADIONUCLIDE	PHARMACEUTICAL	MAIN ENERGY	HALF-LIFE	MAIN ORGAN OF INTEREST
^{18}F	Flurodeoxyglucose	511 keV	109.71 min	Brain/heart/tumors
^{11}C	Raclopride	511 keV	20.3 min	Neurologic and psychiatric disorders/Parkinson's disease
^{15}O	Saline	511 keV	122 sec	Myocardial and cerebral perfusion
^{13}N	Acidic saline	511 keV	9.97 min	Myocardial and cerebral perfusion

effective renal plasma flow is determined. Table 21-8 lists several radionuclides, their characteristics, and associated pharmaceuticals for some typical nuclear medicine studies.

Positron Emission Tomography Agents

A positron is a positive electron, which is also known as antimatter. Antimatter cannot exist for long because when it comes into contact with a negative electron, it annihilates itself into two 511 keV photons of energy that are approximately 180 degrees apart from each other. Positron emission tomographic (PET) imaging takes advantage of these two 511 keV nearly 180 degrees opposite each other to do coincidence imaging whereby the gamma camera accepts only two 180-degree opposing events to form an image. Positron emitters are formed in a cyclotron and often have very short half-lives. Table 21-9 lists several different PET agents and their clinical use.

Special Considerations When Working with Unsealed Radiation Sources

The primary concern when working with short-lived (small half-lives of hours, minutes, or seconds) unsealed radiation sources is contamination that can occur on patients, personnel, floors, tables, or imaging equipment that might be misconstrued as part of the image produced for physicians to read. These artifacts may not be easily ascertained and might be misinterpreted by a physician as a pathologic abnormality in a patient when reading a study. Another concern with contamination of unsealed sources is increased radiation exposure to personnel and patients that might occur. This contamination might be in the form of external or internal contamination. External contamination would be dropped, splashed, or spilled unsealed sources deposited on someone or something. Internal contamination might occur if these dropped, splashed, or spilled unsealed sources are internalized via inhalation, absorption, or ingestion. Unsealed sources must be contained as much as possible before, during, and after their use. This contamination is why nuclear medicine personnel recap needles on a syringe, whereas all other medical personnel do not.

HEALTH PROFESSIONAL RESPONSIBILITIES

Qualifications of Personnel

The supervising physician should be a licensed physician with the following qualifications:

1. Certification in radiology or radiation oncology by the American Board of Radiology, the American Osteopathic Board of Radiology, the Royal College of Physicians, or Surgeons of Canada
2. A minimum of 6 months documented formal dedicated training in the interpretation and formal reporting of general radiographs or whose residency or fellowship that did not include formal training in the interpretation and formal reporting of general radiographs but can demonstrate sufficient knowledge of the pharmacology, indications, contraindications, safe administration, and the ability to initiate treatment in the event of adverse reactions
3. Be familiar with the various risk factors, premedication strategies, and preprocedural screening
4. Must be immediately available to respond in the event of an adverse reaction
5. Must have appropriate alternate imaging methods knowledge
6. Must be aware of the signs and symptoms of adverse reactions and how to monitor the patient having a contrast reaction

The technologist has the responsibility of patient comfort throughout the duration of the procedure, as well as being able to identify the signs and symptoms of adverse reactions and adequate knowledge of how to treat any adverse reaction.

Patient Selection and Preparation

The general considerations for the patient have two aims: (1) contrast media reaction prevention and (2) preparedness in the event of an adverse reaction. The prevention of contrast media reactions depends on obtaining a thorough patient history that can indicate contrast media contraindications or an increased likelihood of adverse reactions, patient preprocedural preparations and instructions to include adequate hydration and appropriate premedication when indicated, and adequate knowledge in the treatment and use of emergency equipment in cases of adverse reactions.

Sources of Information

In almost no other medical specialty do practitioners inject, or have the patient ingest, such large amounts of nonbiologic substances over a short time as in radiology. Obviously, the chemical structures of these agents greatly influence the (1) ability of the agents to enhance subject contrast, (2) types of agents used for specific procedures, and (3) reasons for adverse reactions that can occur in patients.

The discussion presented in this chapter about the physical properties of contrast media aids in reading the package inserts. The technologist must look at the chemical structure presented and locate the common chemical groups discussed. Then the radiologic technologist can consider other information in the package inserts about specific procedures, doses, and adverse reactions.

Technical representatives from pharmaceutical companies that supply contrast agents can also supply journal articles as important sources of information. Problems arising from specific contrast media examinations should be discussed with the radiologist. Valuable insights for effective patient care are gained in this manner.

Patient Care and Surveillance

The setup for any contrast media procedure, patient positioning, and radiographic technique are important professional responsibilities. The patient must remain the focus of the procedure, however. The patient is usually anxious about the procedure and the reasons that made the procedure necessary. In many instances, the patient has an empty stomach; therefore he or she may be irritable. These feelings combined with the reasons for the adverse reactions from contrast media may result in an increased possibility of these reactions.

Owing to an increase in outpatient procedures that use water-soluble iodine contrast media, reported instances of adverse reactions occur hours later. These reactions have been poorly communicated to radiologists because of a lack of patient knowledge. The radiographer might develop an instruction sheet about mild adverse reactions and discuss these issues with the patient after the procedure is complete but before the patient leaves. Such instructions might include calling the department (direct telephone number) if any of the following occurs within 24 hours: hives, flushing, chills, nasal stuffiness, swelling of the eyes or face, or wheezing.

A calm, supportive manner on the part of the radiologic technologist is a necessity. Continued communication, with questions regarding patient comfort, allows observation of the patient's physical and emotional status. A professional demeanor can increase the well being of the patient and thereby reduce the possibility of adverse reactions.

Many procedures require patient preparation at home, such as enemas before lower GI procedures and fasting after midnight before some procedures. The diagnostic quality of procedures that require patient preparation is diminished by patient failure to follow instructions. Before beginning the examination, the radiologic technologist must ask the patient if he or she followed the instructions for it. Some patients comply with some but not all the instructions. Therefore the radiologic technologist must also find out *to what extent* the patient complied. This information can usually be obtained by one question, "What did you do at home to prepare for your x-ray today?" If the patient forgets an aspect of the instructions, then the radiologic technologist should use prompts such as, "What about the pills, Mr. Jones?"

Many referring physicians do not tell their patients what to expect during contrast media procedures. Additionally, many people have only a rudimentary knowledge of body functions. Explaining to the patients, in simple terms, what will be done is the radiologic technologist's responsibility. The radiologic technologist must also convey to the patient *a sense of being cared for* and *a sense of being safe* during the procedure. These subjective qualities can be communicated by addressing the patient by name (e.g., Mr. Jones, Mrs. Green), by using blankets or sheets for warmth and modesty, by using pillows when possible, and by asking questions such as, "Are you warm enough?" Many patients exhibit reduced anxiety if the radiologic technologist explains the procedure as it is performed. Finally, a universal form of supportive communication is touch.

SUMMARY

Radiographic contrast media are used to visualize areas within the body that otherwise might not be seen well. These agents are not drugs; however, they can affect the physiologic status of patients.

Radiolucent contrast media transmit x-rays and are usually used with radiopaque contrast media to visualize the lumens of organs and joint spaces. Radiopaque contrast media absorb x-rays and are used to demonstrate the gastrointestinal, biliary, urinary, circulatory, lymphatic, and respiratory systems.

Most adverse reactions encountered by patients are associated with the use of radiopaque contrast agents. Serious complications from the administration of barium sulfate include hypervolemia and colon and vaginal rupture. Water-soluble iodine contrast agents can cause allergic-like effects and can increase the severity of sickle cell anemia, renal disease, and diabetes. The patient history obtained by the radiologic technologist gives information about preexisting disease that can increase the possibility of some adverse reactions. Appropriate patient preparation and care can then be given to eliminate or decrease these adverse reactions.

The radiologic technologist should be familiar with the general chemical structure of contrast media and the relationship of the structure to the formal and trade names of the particular medium. The radiologic technologist absolutely must relate the various media to examinations for which they are best suited. Knowledge of specific patient preparations and adverse reactions associated with each agent is imperative.

The radiologic technologist should be aware that radiopharmaceuticals are not contrast agents; and he or she must be aware of the special considerations when using PET agents and any unsealed radiation sources used in a nuclear medicine department.

The manner in which patient care is given can decrease the possibility of adverse reactions and can increase the diagnostic quality of the examination by increasing patient cooperation.

BIBLIOGRAPHY

Ansell G, ed: *Complications in diagnostic radiology*, Philadelphia, 1976, JB Lippincott.

Ballinger P: *Merrill's atlas of radiographic positions and radiologic procedures*, ed 10, St Louis, 2003, Elsevier Mosby.

Benison S, Walter B: *Cannon: the life and times of a young scientist*, Cambridge, Mass, 1987, Harvard University Press.

Bettmann M: Ionic versus nonionic contrast agents for intravenous use: are all the answers in? *Radiology* 175:616, 1990.

Curry N et al: Fatal reactions to intravenous nonionic contrast media, *Radiology* 178:361, 1991.

Jacobson PD: Who decides who gets low-osmolar contrast? *Diagn Image* 13:77, April 1991.

Katayama H et al: Adverse reactions to ionic and nonionic contrast media: a report from the Japanese committee on the safety of contrast media, *Radiology* 175:621, 1990.

Katzburg W, ed: *The contrast media manual,* Baltimore, 1992, Williams & Wilkins.

Kowalsky RJ, Falen SW: *Radiopharmaceuticals in nuclear pharmacy and nuclear medicine,* ed 2, Washington DC, 2004, American Pharmacists Association.

Manual on contrast media, version 5.0, American College of Radiology, Reston, Va.

Martin DW, Rodwell, VW, Mayes PA: *Harper's review of biochemistry,* ed 20, East Norwalk, Conn, 1986, Appleton & Lange.

McClennan B: Ionic and nonionic iodinated contrast media: evolution and strategies for use, *AJR Am J Roentgenol* 155:225, 1990.

Package Insert: Metformin (Glucophage), Bristol-Myers Squibb Company, 1995.

Radioisotope Decay Tables, MDS Nordion Company, 2002.

Saha GB: *Fundamentals of nuclear pharmacy,* ed 5, New York, 2004, Springer-Verlag.

Silverman P: Nonionic contrast use optimizes helical CT, *Diagn Imag* August:67, 1996.

Skucas J: *Radiographic contrast agents,* ed 2, Rockville, Md, 1989, Aspen Publishers.

Torsten A: Relations between chemical structure, animal toxicity and clinical adverse effects of contrast media. In Enge I, Edgren J, eds: *Patient safety and adverse events in contrast medium examinations,* New York, 1989, Elsevier.

Ethical and Legal Issues

Professional Ethics

Robert A. Buerki, PhD, RPh
Louis D. Vottero, MS, RPh

Knowing what's right doesn't mean much unless you do what's right.

Anonymous

OBJECTIVES

On completion of this chapter, the student will be able to:

1. Explain the ethic of the radiologic technology profession.

2. Differentiate the systems of ethics, law, and morals.

3. Explain the four-step problem-solving process of ethical analysis.

4. Explain two sources of moral judgment that underlie ethical decision making.

5. Identify moral dilemmas encountered in patient relationships.

6. Identify moral dilemmas encountered in physician relationships.

7. Identify moral dilemmas encountered in relationships with other health professionals.

8. Recognize values associated with ethical decision making in the practice of radiologic technology.

9. Apply critical analysis to ethical decision making.

GLOSSARY

Autonomy: person's self-reliance, independence, liberty, rights, privacy, individual choice, freedom of the will, and the self-contained ability to decide

Beneficence: doing of good; active promotion of good, kindness, and charity

Caring: to care for; an emotional commitment to and a willingness to act on behalf of a person with whom a caring relationship exists

Codes of Ethics: articulated statement of role morality as seen by the members of a profession

Common Morality: socially approved norms of human conduct that takes its basic premises from the morality shared in common by the members of a society; includes common sense and tradition

Confidentiality: belief that health-related information about individual patients should not be revealed to others; maintaining privacy

Consequentialism: belief that the worth of actions is determined by their ends or consequences; actions are right or wrong according to the balance of their good and bad consequences

Duties: obligations placed on individuals, groups, and institutions by reason of the so-called *moral bond* of our interdependence with others

Ethical Dilemma: situation requiring moral judgment between two or more equally problem-fraught alternatives; two or more competing moral norms are present, creating a challenge about what to do

Ethical Outrage: gross violation of commonly held standards of decency or human rights

Ethical Theories: bodies of systematically related moral principles used to resolve ethical dilemmas

Ethics: systematic study of rightness and wrongness of human conduct and character as known by natural reason

Ethics of Care: ethical reflections that emphasize an intimate personal relationship value system that includes such virtues as sympathy, compassion, fidelity, discernment, and love

Fidelity: strict observance of promises or duties; loyalty and faithfulness to others

Justice: equitable, fair, or just conduct in dealing with others

Laws: regulations established by government and applicable to people within a certain political subdivision

Legal Rights: rights of individuals or groups that are established and guaranteed by law

Liberal Individualism: basis for rights-based ethical theory; each individual is protected and allowed to pursue personal projects

Moral Principles: general, universal guides to action that are derived from so-called basic moral truths that should be respected unless a morally compelling reason exists not to do so; also referred to as *ethical principles*

Moral Rights: rights of individuals or groups that exist separately from governmental or institutional guarantees; usually asserted based on moral principles or rules

Moral Rules: statements of right conduct governing individual actions

Moral Virtue: trait of character that is morally valued; a disposition to act—or a habit of acting—in accordance with moral principles, obligations, or ideals

Morality: widely shared social conventions about right and wrong human conduct, including a conformity to the rules of right conduct; also see *Common Morality*

Morals: generally accepted customs, principles, or habits of right living and conduct in a society and the individual's practice in relation to these

Nonconsequentialism: belief that actions themselves, rather than consequences, determine the worth of actions; actions are right or wrong according to the morality of the acts themselves

Nonmaleficence: ethical principle that places high value on avoiding harm to others

Norm: standard set by individuals or groups of individuals

Principle-Based Ethics: use of moral principles as a basis for defending a chosen path of action in resolving an ethical dilemma; also see *Principlism*

Principlism: belief system based on a set of moral principles that are embedded in a common morality

Professional Ethic: publicly displayed ethical conduct of a profession, usually embedded in a code of ethics; affirms the professional as an independent, autonomous, responsible decision maker

Professional Ethics: internal controls of a profession based on human values or moral principles

Professional Etiquette: manners and attitudes generally accepted by members of a profession

Rights: justified claims that an individual can make on individuals, groups, or society; divided into *legal rights* and *moral rights*

GLOSSARY—Cont'd

Rights-Based Ethics: belief that individual rights provide the vital protection of life, liberty, expression, and property

Social Contract: relationship that exists when two mutually dependent groups in a society recognize certain expectations of one another and conduct their affairs accordingly

Standards of Professional Conduct: practice behaviors that are defined by members of a profession

Values: ideals and customs of a society toward which the members of a group have an affective regard; a value may be a quality desirable as an end in itself

Value System: collection or set of values that an individual or group have as each person's personal guide

Veracity: duty to tell the truth and avoid deception

Virtue: trait of character that is socially valued, such as courage; see also *Moral Virtue*

Virtue-Based Ethics: ethical theory that emphasizes the agents who perform actions and make choices; character and virtue form the framework of this ethical theory

IMPORTANCE OF A PROFESSIONAL ETHIC

Health care professionals often encounter situations in their practices that they find deeply disturbing. These situations, which are usually unrelated to clinical procedures or medical intervention, may involve such basic human rights as the right to privacy and dignity or even the simple right to be told the truth. Professionals may encounter conflicting value or belief systems that can compromise patient care. They also must make difficult choices that depend on their understanding of such moral principles as justice and beneficence, such virtues as compassion and **caring,** and such fundamental duties as honesty and loyalty to both patients and physicians.

All of these situations are generally encompassed under the term **professional ethics.** Principles of professional ethics may be reduced to a written code, but professionals who attempt to apply such unyielding standards to their daily practice often become dismayed and frustrated because the code does not address their specific problems. When faced with an ethical problem or dilemma, many professionals simply obey the rules of their institution, follow the policies of their supervisor, or choose the least objectionable course of action among a bewildering array of choices, each of which may have profound consequences for patient care.

As emerging health care professionals in their own right, radiologic technologists play a critical supportive role between the physician and the patient. They assist in providing valuable information that enables physicians to make accurate diagnoses and establish sound therapeutic plans. As such, radiologic technologists must meet established standards of professional conduct as professional persons, standards that support the emotional and physical needs of the patients with whom they come in contact. Radiologic technologists, as with all health care professionals, believe that their professional conduct is based on their complete, uncompromised devotion to patients as individuals while providing them with the highest possible quality of medical care.

The public expects all professionals to exhibit self-discipline within a system of self-regulation. This sense of self-discipline is particularly important within the health care professions, in which errors in judgment can have serious, even life-threatening, consequences. Furthermore, despite the increasing sophistication among segments of the American public, few individuals are able to judge the quality of the professional services they receive. Patients who submit to radiologic procedures, for example, have no way of determining whether the procedures have been performed properly or even whether they have been injured in the process. As a result, a **professional ethic** is one of several generally accepted criteria that serve to distinguish a profession from other occupations or trades.

State licensing laws reflect the public's demand that it be served by qualified health care practitioners. The professional licensing boards that enforce these and other professional practice laws provide one element of self-regulation. Professionals are given certain prerogatives by society, such as a quasimonopoly to operate in a certain professional arena. In return for granting these prerogatives, society expects professionals to be guided by a standard of conduct beyond mere conformity to law. This

TABLE 22-1 Comparison of Systems of Ethics, Law, and Morals

SYSTEM	APPLICATION	CONTROL	ENABLING SOURCE	SANCTIONS
Ethics	Specific group	Within group	Codes of ethics	Expulsion
Law	Political subdivision	Outside group	Legislation	Fines, prison
Morals	Individuals	Conscience	Religious writing	Shame, guilt

standard of conduct, this common concern for collective self-discipline, this control of the profession from within is known as **ethics.**

In philosophy, *ethics* is often defined as the science of rightness and wrongness of human conduct as known by natural reason. Professional ethics, however, may be defined as rules of conduct or standards by which a particular group regulates its actions and sets standards for its members. The system of ethics is closely related and overlaps two other systems designed to control society: law and morals. **Laws** refer to regulations established by a government applicable to people within a certain political subdivision; **morals** are generally accepted customs of right living and conduct and an individual's practice in relation to these customs. Table 22-1 summarizes these distinctions.

At first glance, the system of laws, with its sanctions of fines and imprisonment for noncompliance, would seem to have the greatest payoff to society. Moreover, the system of laws is dynamic, subject to the ever-changing will of the people and their legislators; however, the system of laws does not cover all areas of professional conduct or potential risks that a professional encounters. No matter how broadly laws and regulations are written or how detailed they may seem, areas still exist that must be covered by a system of voluntary self-discipline, the system of ethics.

Society expects a profession, through its collective members, to generate its own statement of acceptable and unacceptable behavior, usually in the form of a **code of ethics;** practice behaviors that are defined by the members of a profession are **standards of professional conduct.** The code of ethics adopted by the American Registry of Radiologic Technologists (ARRT) is Part A of the ARRT Standards of Ethics and is reproduced in Appendix D; the code comprises ten principles, which are intended to be aspirational. Part B of the Standards contains mandatory rules of acceptable professional conduct for radiologic technologists, and these rules are enforceable through ARRT-prescribed sanctions.

Ideally, all radiologic technologists subscribe to the ethical principles contained in these documents and apply them to problems in their professional practice. These codes serve the profession well by providing the practitioner with a detailed, explicit, operational blueprint of **norms** of professional conduct. Unfortunately, some of these principles are stated in abstract or idealized terms that provide little in the way of concrete guidance for young practitioners. For example, Principle 9 of the ARRT Code of Ethics states that the radiologic technologist "reveals confidential information only as required by law or to protect the welfare of the individual or the community." Under what circumstances, if any, might a patient's right to privacy be infringed? What standards are used to determine when the welfare of the community supersedes the welfare of the individual? What information can be released, to whom, and under what circumstances? The answers to these questions, of course, are not usually found in codes of ethics. Furthermore, you may encounter situations that are not even remotely related to the statements in the codes, reflecting the static nature of any professional code. Finally, do the principles that make up the code take into consideration the role of human **values** and virtues in deciding professional practice behavior? This question suggests that a more serviceable method for determining the correct conduct in professional practice involves something beyond mere reflection on a code of ethics.

ETHICAL EVALUATIONS

Before we can develop our own personal set of internal guidelines for determining what constitutes right conduct in our professional practice, we must clarify a few additional concepts. **Professional etiquette,** the manners and attitudes toward patients generally accepted by practitioners, should not be confused with professional ethics. For example, being rude toward patients or being insensitive to their need for preserving their modesty may violate our sense of professional propriety, but these actions are not considered breaches in professional ethics. We will consider professional ethics as rules of conduct or standards beyond conformance to either law or etiquette, the internal controls of a profession based on human values or moral principles.

Next, we must develop some skill in both recognizing and analyzing **ethical dilemmas.** Although we all may agree on what constitutes patently unethical conduct, the so-called **ethical outrage**, the true ethical dilemma invites a wide range of personal opinion among colleagues in a profession, each of which is based on a highly individualistic, strongly held **value system.** For example, we might agree that refusing to provide services to dirty, unkempt patients or to those infected with the acquired immunodeficiency syndrome (AIDS) virus is unethical, but we might hold a variety of opinions on what degree of loyalty we owe to our fellow workers on the health care team. When does our loyalty to physicians or administrators overshadow our loyalty to our patients? On the other hand, if our loyalty to our patients' autonomy interferes with their decisions to accept needed medical treatment, we may wish to set aside this value temporarily so that a higher human value, the resulting benefit to these patients, is served. To a greater or lesser extent, all professional decisions in radiologic technology and other health care practices involve a consideration of human values. By the same token, every ethical decision also involves human values, values that often conflict and compete for recognition and acceptance among our professional colleagues.

Once we have identified an ethical dilemma and the human values that may be associated with that dilemma, how should we proceed to analyze the situation? The process of ethical analysis generally contains the following four components:

- Identifying the problem
- Developing alternative solutions
- Selecting the best solution
- Defending your selection

Many students encounter difficulty in *identifying the problem* simply because they are eager to proceed with the problem-solving process. Thoroughness in problem identification, that is, looking at every possible twist or nuance in a given situation, is absolutely essential for successful resolution of any ethical dilemma. In *developing alternative solutions,* we attempt to exhaust all possible pathways to a resolution of the dilemma, taking care to view the dilemma from the perspective not only of the patient and the patient's family, but also of the health care

professionals and administrators to whom they entrust their care. The most challenging step in the problem-solving process is *selecting the best solution,* a highly personal activity that involves choosing an alternative not only based on widely held moral standards, but one that is also in full accord with your own individual value system. Finally, by *defending your selection,* you can explain the basis for your ethical decision in terms that you can justify to both colleagues and patients. Although this process may seem difficult or even impossible at first glance, we can approach it with confidence once we have considered the underlying sources of moral judgment that allow us to move beyond feelings, emotions, and intuitions toward more structured foundations for our ethical decision making. These sources of moral judgment are discussed under the general headings of moral rules and ethical theories.

Moral Rules

In making our ethical decisions, we might rely on widely held **moral rules:** The Bible admonishes us to abide by the *golden rule* and to obey the Ten Commandments, our schools teach us that cheating is wrong, and our professional associations promulgate codes of ethics that encourage practitioners to *do no harm.* Many individuals successfully use moral rules to guide their behavior, but this approach has its limitations. The most serious limitation to using moral rules as a primary guide to moral behavior is that most people lack access to a complete set of moral rules or that a complete set of moral rules simply does not exist. As noted, most codes of ethics are incomplete and do not speak to all ethical issues that radiologic technologists and other health care professionals encounter.

Ethical Theories

Another approach to establishing a foundation on which to base ethical decision making involves normative ethical systems, that is, sets of principles that tell us what actions are right or wrong, or **ethical theories.** These systems are usually divided into two groups. **Consequentialism** evaluates the rightness or wrongness of ethical decisions by assessing the consequences of these decisions on the patient—that is, producing a good effect for the patient or at least avoiding some potential harm; **nonconsequentialism** holds that other right-making characteristics of our actions beyond consequences exist that are needed to determine whether a given behavior is right or wrong. For example, persons who use the consequentialist system for ethical decision making may lie to a patient if they believe the lie might ultimately benefit the patient; persons using the nonconsequentialist system would caution against lying to a patient under any circumstances because the act of lying is generally accepted as morally wrong in our society.

Recently, modifications to these ethical theories have been developed, including such concepts as social contracts, the ethics of care, rights-based ethics, principle-based ethics, and virtue-based ethics. These refinements are being used increasingly in medical practices to analyze and defend actions and their outcomes, especially practices that attempt to fulfill the ethical mandates of quality patient care.

Social contract theory attempts to describe the relationship that exists between two mutually dependent persons or groups of persons in a society. Under this theory, these persons or groups—radiologic technologists and patients, in our context—recognize certain expectations of one another and act accordingly. For example, patients expect their radiologic technologist to tell them the truth; by the same token, radiologic technologists expect their patients to tell them the truth. Whereas social contract theory sounds simple and straightforward, social contracts can be perplexing. Unlike legal contracts, with their precise language and implicit sanctions, social contracts are unwritten, leaving the specific duties and actions expected of health care practitioners and their patients to be resolved through a process of reasoning and discernment.

The **ethics of care** cautions that our actions should not be examined as isolated events; instead, our actions should be considered as an integral part of the context of specific situations. For example, lying to a patient is not an isolated event; rather, this act is surrounded by a welter of circumstances—who the patient is, what his or her particular ills might be, how he or she relates to us, what beliefs we have, and so on. Furthermore, a caring ethic requires us to make moral judgments that reflect the values of the communities within which we live. The ethics of care require the decision maker to focus as clearly as possible on such basic moral skills as kindness, sensitivity, attentiveness, tact, patience, and reliability. Indeed, the ethics of care emphasizes the need for an accurate understanding of moral competence, a clear vision of the meaning of a *virtuous person,* and finely honed skills in human relations.

Rights-based ethics, one of the increasingly popular approaches to ethical reasoning, is based on an understanding of *human rights.* Advocates often express their human rights openly and forcefully, claiming a *right to health care.* Advocates who are medical practitioners often champion the *rights of the health professions.* The importance of human rights is reflected in the tenets of **liberal individualism,** a belief that an individual in a democratic society is shielded from undue forces and allowed to enjoy and pursue personal projects; that is, the individual has certain *rights.*

Rights are justified claims that an individual can make on others (individuals or groups) or on society and may be considered as either **legal rights** or **moral rights.** *Legal rights* are claims that have a foundation in legal principles and rules; *moral rights* are claims that are justified by moral principles and rules. Moreover, a right, whether legal or moral, carries with it a corresponding duty that is placed on someone. **Duties** may be considered as obligations placed on individuals, groups, and institutions by reason of the so-called *moral bond* of our interdependence with others. We expect to receive positive responses to our own needs and to be treated humanely. In addition, we form special relationships with our parents, our children, our spouses, our teachers, and our health care professionals. Realizing our duties as radiologic technologists helps us to know to whom and for what we are accountable. For this reason, rights-based ethical reasoning can have great appeal to beginning practitioners; however, radiologic technologists who attempt to apply rights theory to ethical dilemmas must be cautious because they may encounter considerable tension between what they envision as professional duties and what their patients claim as human rights.

Principle-based ethics, or **principlism,** the use of moral principles as a basis for defending a chosen path of action in resolving an ethical dilemma, has been widely accepted by medical communities. **Moral principles** (also referred to as *ethical principles*) are general, universal guides to action that are derived from so-called basic moral truths that should be respected unless a morally compelling reason exists not to do so. Moral principles include not only the two principles traditionally associated with the health care professions, **beneficence** and **nonmaleficence,** but also several newer principles such as **justice, autonomy, veracity,** and **fidelity.** Most professional codes of ethics are based primarily on the principle of *beneficence;* that is, the codes encourage practitioners to engage in actions that ultimately benefit their patients. For example, the Code of Ethics for radiologic technologists states that the ethical radiologic technologist "acts in the best interest of the patient," a clear appeal to beneficence. Although these principles seem forbidding and difficult to grasp, they can be understood with some careful reading and reflection. Table 22-2 provides

TABLE 22-2 **Selected Ethical Principles**

MORAL PRINCIPLE	YOUR ASPIRATION
Beneficence (bringing about good)	Perform actions that benefit others. Decide and act always to benefit the patient.
Nonmaleficence (preventing harm)	Above all, do no harm. Never perform or allow acts that may harm the patient.
Autonomy (acting with personal self-reliance)	Perform actions that respect the independence of other persons. The patient must decide what is done to his or her person.
Veracity (telling the truth)	Being truthful is right. To tell the truth is expected.
Fidelity (being faithful)	Perform acts that observe covenants or promises are right. Be faithful.
Justice (acting with fairness or equity)	Perform acts that ensure the fair distribution of goods and harm are right. Be fair.

some definitions and examples of ethical principles to help clarify these difficult concepts.

Living a good life, becoming a good person, and acquiring certain desirable characteristics (called **virtues**) have been the main goals of ethics during most of its long history. **Virtue-based ethics,** the use of virtues in establishing right reason in action, offers the opportunity to include the character of each participant involved in an ethical dilemma and is an especially important consideration when linked to principlism. Virtues include such character traits as caring, faith, trust, hope, compassion, courage, and fidelity. Principle 2 of the ARRT Code of Ethics emphasizes this call to virtue by pledging the intent of the profession "to provide services to humanity with full respect for the dignity of mankind."

PATIENT CARE AND INTERPROFESSIONAL RELATIONSHIPS

As with members of the other allied health professions, radiologic technologists place a high value on quality patient care and solid interprofessional relationships. This section will help you explore these relationships in the context of ethical dilemmas that you may face in your professional practice. We have also provided several case studies to help you work through the problem-solving approach outlined earlier. We have analyzed the first case for you by way of illustration; the other cases give you an opportunity to practice using the problem-solving approach.

Patient Relationships

Two of the most frequently encountered ethical issues that affect the relationship between radiologic technologists and their patients involve maintaining patient faithfulness (i.e., keeping faith with our patients) and

maintaining patient **confidentiality.** The following cases illustrate the types of problems associated with these ethical issues.

CASE 1: MAINTAINING PATIENT FAITHFULNESS. Radiologic technologists are often confronted by situations that test their ability to deal with sensitive patient care information. In many instances, the duty to respect the patient's confidences is compromised by pressures from authority figures or other persons who may not share the radiologic technologist's value system.

"Do You Think My Doctor Is Doing the Right Thing?"

Mrs. Brown, a 27-year-old patient of Dr. Smith, looks apprehensive as you begin your radiologic procedure. Mrs. Brown has found a lump in her breast and is worried about the possibility of having to endure a mastectomy. Your mammographic examination reveals that Mrs. Brown is probably suffering from a small fibroid cyst. Mrs. Brown confides to you that Dr. Smith has mentioned the possibility of surgery. You are also aware that, given a choice, Dr. Smith nearly always operates. As you conclude your procedure, Mrs. Brown asks you whether surgery is indicated, adding, "Do you think my doctor is doing the right thing?"

Identifying the Problem. In this case, Mrs. Brown is seeking information that you may or may not be at liberty to provide. On one hand, as a health care professional, you sense a duty to provide Mrs. Brown with all the information available to you at this point about her condition. On the other hand, you feel a professional loyalty toward Dr. Smith and all other health professionals involved with Mrs. Brown's case.

Developing Alternative Solutions. You might respond to Mrs. Brown's question truthfully by revealing your understanding of her medical condition and your concerns about Dr. Smith's tendency to use surgery as a primary treatment. Alternatively, you might try to avoid answering her questions directly. Finally, you might refer Mrs. Brown's questions to Dr. Smith or to some other physician in whom you have more confidence.

Selecting the Best Solution. The first alternative forces you to choose between being truthful to Mrs. Brown (veracity), possibly saving her from some harm (nonmaleficence), or maintaining your loyal relationship with Dr. Smith. The second alternative forces you to be evasive (and possibly untruthful) with your answers, thereby compromising your respect for Mrs. Brown's right to make informed decisions about her care (autonomy). The final alternative seems to be the best solution because it not only allows you to include Dr. Smith (or another physician) in Mrs. Brown's decision-making process, but it also places a high value on actions that may ultimately benefit Mrs. Brown (beneficence).

Defending Your Selection. Principle 5 of the ARRT Code of Ethics states that the radiologic technologist "assesses situations; exercises care, discretion and judgment; assumes responsibility for professional decisions; and acts in the best interest of the patient." In this particular case, being completely truthful to Mrs. Brown may create unnecessary anxiety or cause her to question Dr. Smith's competence. By referring Mrs. Brown's questions to Dr. Smith and tactfully suggesting that she may wish to seek a second opinion if she has lingering concerns, we support Dr. Smith's treatment plan while allowing Mrs. Brown to increase her involvement in making decisions affecting her personal health care.

CASE 2: MAINTAINING PATIENT CONFIDENTIALITY. Of the values associated with radiologic practice, patient confidentiality is the most easily identified and the most prevalent. On the surface, it seems that the trust that patients place in their health care providers cannot be compromised. Information obtained directly from the patient, observed, or obtained from other sources should be kept strictly confidential. The radiologic technologist should be alert to situations that may compromise patient confidences.

"Does Mr. Gray Have Cancer?"

The images you took of Mr. Gray do not look good. As a matter of fact, you overheard Dr. Jones mutter about the "advanced stage" of Mr. Gray's condition. The transporting aide wheels Mr. Gray back to his room and returns with your next patient. The patient slips behind a screen to change into an examination gown and is out of earshot. "Mr. Gray seemed real depressed," the aide volunteers. "How did his film look? Does Mr. Gray have cancer?" The aide is a good friend of yours and always has seemed committed to good patient care. How do you respond?

Identifying the Problem. Is Mr. Gray's condition confidential? Is an aide considered a member of the health care team? Does your friendship with the aide (loyalty) play a role in this case?

Developing Alternative Solutions. Would Mr. Gray's confidence be compromised by telling the aide the truth? Should you refer the aide to Mr. Gray or to Mr. Gray's physician? Is Mr. Gray's condition none of the aide's business?

Selecting the Best Solution. What solution would satisfy your professional ethics, the aide's curiosity, and Mr. Gray's right to privacy? Is any possible action possible that would benefit Mr. Gray?

Defending Your Selection. What principles in the ARRT Code of Ethics apply to this case? Is it possible to take an action that will strike a balance between providing a benefit to Mr. Gray and protecting his right to privacy?

Physician Relationships

As a radiologic technologist, your relationships with physicians will be one of the most important aspects of your professional practice. Loyalty, faithfulness, and fairness are virtues all health professionals need to share with one another. Observing professional discretion in your relationships with physicians and recognizing your professional limitations in practice will serve as a firm foundation for maintaining your ethical standards.

CASE 3: OBSERVING PROFESSIONAL DISCRETION. Radiologic technologists see, hear, and experience a wide variety of personal and sensitive patient care activities.

Radiologic technologists must both respect the confidences of their patients and safeguard the knowledge they obtain through their everyday practice activities. Questions concerning the competency or professional judgment of the physicians working with you often raise serious ethical issues and should be handled with professional discretion.

"I Think Dr. Jones Misread the Image."

You have just finished a routine radiologic procedure on Mrs. Green. As you process the image, it becomes clear that Mrs. Green is probably suffering from a rare form of bone disease. Dr. Jones, a young resident, glances at the image and smiles. "I didn't think Mrs. Green had anything to worry about," he says. "That joint pain she was complaining about must be all in her head." Later, you see Dr. Jones talking to Mrs. Green's family. He is smiling and joking with them as he signs Mrs. Green's discharge papers. Shaken, you mutter to yourself, "I think Dr. Jones misread the image." What action, if any, should you take?

Identifying the Problem. Do you have an equal degree of loyalty to both Mrs. Green and Dr. Jones? Are conflicting professional duties present in this case?

Developing Alternative Solutions. Is this situation a personal matter between you and Dr. Jones? Should you discuss the issue with Dr. Jones's chief resident? The medical board? Mrs. Green or her family?

Selecting the Best Solution. Does a radiologic technologist have a professional obligation to point out a physician's possible errors? Does Mrs. Green have a right to know about her possible serious condition?

Defending Your Selection. Principle 6 of the ARRT Code of Ethics states that "interpretation and diagnosis are outside the scope of practice" for radiologic technologists. Does this principle apply in this case?

CASE 4: RECOGNIZING PROFESSIONAL LIMITATIONS. As with other health professionals, radiologic technologists have a specific role to perform on the health care team. Teamwork implies cooperation, as well as a sharing of professional functions. Radiologic technologists should be aware of the limitations of their professional practice.

"In My Opinion, You'll Be Just Fine."

You are assisting Dr. Roe with a particularly complicated radiation treatment. Mr. Black has been on the table for nearly an hour and is clearly exhausted. As Dr. Roe leaves the area to respond to a page, Mr. Black groans as you help him off the table into his wheelchair and begins asking questions about his condition. "Is Dr. Roe doing the right thing? I feel terrible. What do you think?" Mr. Black has acquired a reputation of being somewhat of a hypochondriac. You are aware that Mr. Black is being treated for cancer and has a 50/50 chance of remission. Your initial impulse is to reassure him with a smile and say something such as, "In my opinion, you'll be just fine."

Identifying the Problem. How do radiologic technologists identify the boundaries of their professional practice? Does your compassion for Mr. Black supersede your duty to respect your boundary of professional practice?

Developing Alternative Solutions. Do you have a duty to respond to Mr. Black's questions? Should you follow your first impulse and simply reassure Mr. Black? Should you alert Dr. Roe to Mr. Black's concerns?

Selecting the Best Solution. Does Mr. Black share your value system? Do all your alternative solutions respect the values of the individuals associated with this case?

Defending Your Selection. Principle 5 of the ARRT Code of Ethics states that radiologic technologists should always act "in the best interest of the patient." Can your decision be justified by this principle?

Relationships with Other Health Professionals

Although your primary professional responsibilities are to the physicians with whom you work, the radiologic technologist also interacts with a wide range of other health professionals. These relationships often provide a source of satisfaction and support but can be marred by so-called turf battles or role conflicts and unrealistic practice expectations. Although most of us have grown up with a sense of loyalty and a corresponding aversion to report bad behavior in others, health care professionals have a special obligation to place the interests of their patients before such personal loyalty.

CASE 5: REPORTING UNETHICAL CONDUCT IN OTHERS. Radiologic technologists have an ethical obligation to provide *quality patient care* and act *in the best interest of the patient.* Taken to its logical extension, this obligation includes the reporting of unethical conduct in other health professionals.

"Do You Think Nurse Smith Is Abusing Drugs?"

During your lunch break on the night shift, you decide to visit with Miss White, a patient with whom you have developed a friendship. Miss White's room is directly across from the nursing station, and she tells you that she has noticed Nurse Smith slipping medications from the drug cart into her pocket. You recall seeing Nurse Smith occasionally swallowing some pills while on duty, but you had thought little about it up to this point. Because Nurse Smith is the only nurse providing patient care during this shift, you are concerned about the quality of patient care, as well as Nurse Smith's health. Miss White asks, "Do you think Nurse Smith is abusing drugs?" You answer, "I hope not," However, you believe that you must confront Nurse Smith directly. Despite your best efforts to be tactful, Nurse Smith explodes, "What I do on this ward is none of your business!" What do you do next?

Identifying the Problem. You have met the initial obligation to identify unprofessional conduct. Do you have an obligation to carry your complaint to Nurse Smith's superiors? What competing loyalties are involved in this case?

Developing Alternative Solutions. Once you have confronted Nurse Smith, can you let the matter rest? Should Miss White become involved as a witness or complainant? Should you tell Nurse Smith's supervisor? Someone in the hospital administration? Should you call the police?

Selecting the Best Solution. What solution would both best serve Nurse Smith and improve patient care on her ward? Can you choose between your ethical obligation to report unprofessional behavior and good patient care? What balance should exist between *doing no harm* to the patient and loyalty to your colleagues?

Defending Your Selection. Principle 9 of the ARRT Code of Ethics states that the radiologic technologist "respects confidences entrusted in the course of professional prac-

tice." Does this principle apply in this case? Do other personal values that you hold apply?

Dealing with Mistakes

All humans make mistakes, and health care professionals are no exception. Because of the life-and-death nature of medical practice, mistakes made by health care professionals can create considerable, though unintentional, harm to patients. A full response to the human dimensions of health care requires that all persons involved be prepared to act faithfully and honestly when a patient-care mistake has been made. Radiologic technologists will make mistakes because of the lack of attention to detail, preoccupation with other matters, or even a lack of professional commitment. A mistake can place significant emotional, financial, and psychologic burdens on everyone involved in addition to the possible harm caused to the patient.

CASE 6: DEALING WITH MISTAKES. Including patients in the resolution of a practice error also presents an opportunity for them to practice the virtue of forgiveness. Nonetheless, developing safeguards in your practice that will prevent mistakes is far more desirable. Dealing with mistakes openly in such a way that the patient and others involved know all aspects, including your remorse and proposed outcome, tests the mettle of the most experienced radiologic technologist and will require virtuous action, as the following case demonstrates.

"Keep this Matter Between the Two of Us."

Your assigned duties in the radiology department of the 1000-bed medical center in which you are employed are far from routine. The operation of the department is complex and at times hectic. Recently, the department head authorized a *tech check tech* system of work management in response to a shortage of staff and a dwindling budget. This situation resulted in the shifting of greater responsibilities onto your shoulders, including random review of image quality. During a monthly review of patients' examinations, you discover an error was made: A chest procedure was ordered for a patient, but the examination performed was an abdomen that was ordered for a different patient. You immediately pull both patients' records and request a meeting with the department head who, after closely examining both records cautions, "Look, there is no harm done. Keep this matter between the two of us."

Identifying the Problem. A potentially serious error has been made, but by the time it is discovered, it seems clear that no real harm has been done to either patient. The real benefit and harm in this case, however, may not be with the patients involved; rather, others may gain or lose, including the radiologic technologist who made the mistake and even the department head who authorized the management shift. More important, future patients may receive greater benefits if a more rigorous set of controls is instituted.

Developing Alternative Solutions. Agreeing to the suggested silence would be the easiest alternative to follow. Another approach might be to request the department head to expand the meeting to include the two patients, their physicians, and the radiologists and to discuss the situation fully. Finally, you might request that an *incident report* be completed and filed with the medical center administration.

Selecting the Best Solution. Following the advice of the department head seems to ignore certain rights of the patients while at the same time shielding both the radiologic technologist and the department head from possible censure. Informing the medical center administration through an incident report may prompt beneficial management changes. The inclusion of the patients' physicians in the full discussion of the regrettable incident allows for the participation of both the concerned physicians and the radiologic technologists in the resolution of the incident.

Defending Your Solution. As mentioned in an earlier case, Principle 5 of the ARRT Code of Ethics pledges the radiologic technologist to act "in the best interests of the patient." Cases dealing with mistakes often require the balancing of patient interests with the interests of others involved. Patients' interests in this case include not only physical well being, but also certain rights that need to be addressed.

SUMMARY

The profession of radiologic technology shares the ethical concerns of other health professionals toward promoting good patient care. Radiologic technologists have emerged as health care professionals in their own right, as witnessed by their educational programs, licensure requirements, professional associations, journals, and a unique code of ethics that reflects their professional function in the health care arena.

Beyond subscribing to the principles contained in a professional code of ethics, however, radiologic technologists need to reflect on a broader base of moral principles in their ethical decision making.

Moreover, ethical radiologic technologists must possess a keen sense of the role that human values can play in resolving ethical dilemmas that arise in their professional practice, both in their dealings with patients and in their interactions with physicians and other health professionals. By practicing the ethical problem-solving technique of identifying the problem, developing alternative solutions, selecting the best solution, and defending that solution, radiologic technologists not only can improve their professional stature, but they can also enhance the health outcomes of the patients in their care.

BIBLIOGRAPHY

Ashcroft RE, Goddard PR: Ethical issues in teleradiology, *Br J Radiol* 73:578, 2000.

Dowd SB, Durick D: Elder abuse: the R.T.'s role in diagnosis and prevention, *Radiol Tech* 68:23, 1997.

Golden DG: Medical ethics courses for student technologists, *Radiol Tech* 62:452, 1991.

Haddad AM: Teaching ethical analysis in occupational therapy, *Am J Occup Ther* 42:300, 1988.

Lynn SD: Ethics and law for the radiologic technologist, *Radiol Tech* 70:257, 1999.

Maestri WF: *Basic ethics for the health care professional,* Lanham, Md, 1982, University Press of America.

Purtilo R: *Ethical dimensions in the health professions,* ed 2, Philadelphia, 1993, WB Saunders.

Veatch RM, Flack HE: *Case studies in allied health ethics,* Upper Saddle River, NJ, 1997, Prentice-Hall.

Warner SL: Code of ethics: legal implications, *Radiol Tech* 52:485, 1981.

Wright RA: *Human values in health care: the practice of ethics,* New York, 1987, McGraw-Hill.

Health Records and Health Information Management

Margaret A. Skurka, MS, RHIA, CCS

Health information is indeed a strategic resource crucial to the health of individual patients and the population, as well as to the success of the institution or enterprise.

Mervat Abdelhak
Health Information: Management of a Strategic Resource, 2001

OBJECTIVES

On completion of this chapter, the student will be able to:

1. Identify major health information management department functions.

2. List the key components of a patient health record in acute care.

3. List the key components of a patient health record in alternate health care settings, including ambulatory care and long-term care.

4. Describe how health record documentation affects health care facilities and physician reimbursement.

5. Describe the prospective payment system, including diagnosis-related groups and coding and classification systems.

6. Identify coding as it relates to radiologic procedures and the reimbursement impact for health care facilities.

7. Identify components of quality management and the relationship of quality management to all hospital departments.

8. Differentiate between confidential and nonconfidential information.

Objectives—Cont'd

9. Apply the Health Insurance Portability and Accountability Act privacy and security requirements in a radiologic setting.

10. Discuss the procedure for correcting or amending documentation errors in a patient health record.

Glossary

Ambulatory Payment Classifications (APCs): classification system of patients based on the *International Classification of Diseases,* 9th edition, clinical modification codes for diagnoses, current procedural terminology evaluation and management codes, and procedure codes, age, sex, and visit disposition; used for reimbursement to health care provided in the hospital outpatient setting

Current Procedural Terminology (CPT): comprehensive listing of medical terms and codes for the uniform designation of diagnostic and therapeutic procedures; used in the United States for coding for physician reimbursement

Diagnosis-Related Groups (DRGs): system that categorizes into payment groups patients who are medically related with respect to diagnosis and treatment and statistically similar with regard to length of stay

Electronic Health Record (EHR): electronic health record system generally considered as the portal through which clinicians access a patient's health record, order treatments or therapy, and document care delivered to patients; allows providers to gather multiple types of data about a patient (clinical, financial, administrative, and research)

Healthcare Facilities Accreditation Program (HFAP): accreditation program of the American Osteopathic Association that accredits health care facilities in the United States

Health Information Management Practitioner: term used to encompass both the registered health information administrator and the registered health information technician as individuals with either of these credentials who hold a variety of positions within the health information management profession

Health Insurance Portability and Accountability Act of 1996 (HIPAA): federal legislation passed to improve the efficiency and effectiveness of the health care system; components that affect health information include privacy, security, and the establishment of standards and requirements for the electronic transmission of certain health information

Health Record: permanent or long-lasting document of all patient care information that applies to an individual patient

International Classification of Diseases, 9th edition, Clinical Modification (ICD-9-CM): universal statistical classification system used throughout the United States and the world for coding and reporting diagnoses and procedures

Joint Commission on the Accreditation of Healthcare Organizations (JCAHO): organization that accredits hospitals and other health care institutions in the United States

Prospective Payment System (PPS): system for Medicare patients where a predetermined level of reimbursement is established before the services are provided

Quality Management: process that monitors and evaluates the quality of the care and services provided to patients within a health care facility

Registered Health Information Administrator (RHIA): professional who possesses the expertise to develop, implement, and/or manage individual, aggregate, and public health care data in support of patient safety and privacy, as well as the confidentiality and security of health information

Registered Health Information Technician (RHIT): professional who is the technical expert in health data collection, analysis, monitoring, maintenance and reporting activities in accordance with established data quality principles, legal and regulatory standards, and professional best practice guidelines

HEALTH INFORMATION MANAGEMENT AND TECHNOLOGY

Hospitals, ambulatory care facilities, physician practices, emergency and trauma centers, rehabilitation centers, long-term care facilities, and home care programs all maintain **health records** on all persons receiving health care services. Although these settings vary according to the type and range of medical and health-related services they provide, they all have a common need to concentrate, within a single record, either paper based or computer based, all patient care information that applies to an individual patient. Such a concentration promotes effective communication among all the health care professionals involved in the care of the patient, as well as continuity of patient care.

Every health care institution needs a health information management department that has been organized and staffed to provide adequate record management systems and practices. These systems facilitate the use of health records and protect the content of the record against unauthorized disclosure.

The functions of the health information management department are service oriented and support the optimal standards set forth for quality of care and services in the health care institution. Although the functions of the health information management department and specific demands for its services vary according to the type of institution, the common function of all these departments is the maintenance of health information systems in one or more forms to provide storage and ready retrieval of clinical information by patient name or number, physician name or number, diagnosis, procedure, and other subject items deemed necessary.

Health records can be stored as hard copy or in miniaturized form (microfilm), or they can be scanned and stored in computerized form. The health information department's functions support the current and continuing care of patients; the institution's administrative processes; patient billing and accounting processes; medical education programs; health services research; utilization management, risk management, and quality management programs; privacy and security issues related to the **Health Insurance Portability and Accountability Act of 1996 (HIPAA)**; legal requirements; and extraneous patient services.

Because clinical decision making and financial reimbursement depend on the information contained in the health record, maintaining a complete and accurate record is essential. An error in recording the medications administered to a patient, for example, might lead to a life-threatening situation. An error in data reporting might mean a sizable financial loss for the hospital.

Since the implementation by the federal government of the **Prospective Payment System (PPS)** and **diagnosis-related groups (DRGs)** in 1983, the importance of several health information management functions has grown significantly. The coding of inpatient and outpatient diagnoses and procedures is of highest priority. Coding involves converting diagnoses and procedures into a numerical classification system. The numbers are reported to Medicare and other third-party payors, such as insurance companies. Coding must be complete and accurate so that claims can be processed within prescribed time frames. The record has to be designed so that the physician can easily provide complete patient information throughout the stay and provide a comprehensive recording of patient diagnoses and procedures at discharge.

The health record must also be complete and readily accessible to anyone who has a right to the information and the need to use it. The record is used for patient care, for hospital statistics and research, and for activities such as quality management and risk and utilization management. **Health information management practitioners** (that is, **registered health information technicians** and **administrators [RHITs and RHIAs]**) must communicate needed data to departments such as radiology. Radiology may also make requests from health information management departments for data used for administrative, research, and applied health informatics activities. Hospitals and other types of health care facilities need quality health care data for operations. Whether an electronic (or e-health) environment or a more traditional paper system, robust and relevant clinical information supports decision makers and all persons involved in patient care.

PATIENT RECORD IN ACUTE CARE

Standards for the maintenance and the adequacy of health records have been established by accrediting agencies such as the **Joint Commission on the Accreditation of Healthcare Organizations (JCAHO)** or the American Osteopathic Association via its **Healthcare Facilities Accreditation Program (HFAP)** as a part of its information management standards for hospital operations. One of the responsibilities of the health information management practitioner is to keep abreast of the standards for information management published in the latest edition of the accreditation manuals for the appropriate organizations. These organizations are authorized by the Centers for Medicare and Medicaid Services (CMS) to survey hospitals under Medicare. These accrediting agencies are also recognized by state governments, insurance carriers, and managed care organizations.

Health Record Content

Regardless of the method used to record health information, the content of each health record depends on which health care facility department is treating the patient and recording the information. All departments that take part in the care of a patient must document that care in the health record. Documenting in the patient's record, or *charting,* should be done by radiologists and radiographers when a patient receives either diagnostic or therapeutic radiologic services. Charting information about the procedure is appropriate, particularly about contrast media administration, along with the patient's condition during an examination. This charting is routinely done as a part of most special procedures, especially invasive procedures such as angiography and myelography. Any time a patient has an unusual reaction during a procedure, this information should be documented as well.

Neither various accrediting agencies nor the American Hospital Association recommends any specific format or forms for use in hospital health records. Hospitals use forms and establish computerized or **electronic health record (EHR)** systems that best fit their needs; however, the JCAHO accrediting agency, for example, has established standards for health record content. The health record, per JCAHO, must contain sufficient information to identify the patient, support the diagnoses, justify the treatment, document the course and results, and facilitate continuity of care. Briefly, standards for inpatient records require that the records include the following information:

- Patient identification data
- Medical history of the patient, including chief complaint, present illness or injury, relevant family and social histories, and inventory by body system
- Report of relevant physical examination
- Diagnostic and therapeutic orders
- Clinical observations, including results of therapy
- Reports of diagnostic and therapeutic procedures and tests, as well as their results
- Evidence of appropriate informed consent (when consent is not obtainable, the reason should be entered in the record)
- Conclusions at termination of hospitalization or evaluation of treatment, including any pertinent instructions for follow-up care

Radiographers should be familiar with the health record format at their place of employment. Reviewing the chart or accessing the health information system is often necessary for radiographers to gather information, such as laboratory results, about their patients. A radiology department, in addition to using the hospital mainframe or electronic health information system for the master patient index or billing information, may have a department film tracking system. A computerized system tracks film and folders with a bar code system. Film control is a key issue because lost or missing film can have a negative impact on patient care.

The JCAHO standards require that the health record contain evidence of informed consent for procedures and treatment for which hospital policy requires informed consent. The policy on informed consent is typically developed by the medical staff and the hospital governing board, consistent with legal requirements for appropriate informed consent. The term *informed consent* implies that the patient has been informed of the procedures or operation to be performed, of the risks involved, and of the possible consequences. By signing the consent form, the patient or the patient's representative indicates that he or she has been informed of and consents to the procedure or treatment.

An authorization for treatment, signed at the time of admission, is not to be confused with an informed consent. If, for some reason, the informed consent is not filed with the record, the record must then indicate that an informed consent was obtained for a given procedure or treatment and must indicate where the informed consent form is located.

Incident reports contain information relative to patient incidences or occurrences. Incident reports must be completed after an event; however, the reports themselves should not be a part of the patient record. Rather, they are an administrative document and are typically maintained by hospital legal counsel or perhaps the risk management team. The event should be completely documented in the patient health record. This documentation would include the incident itself, patient reaction, notification of health personnel, patient progress, and so on. The incident report, on the other hand, would include information relative to perhaps the actual equipment failure rather than what happened to the patient because of the equipment failure.

Health Record in Radiology

Before a radiologic procedure is performed, a radiology order or request for service is completed. This order

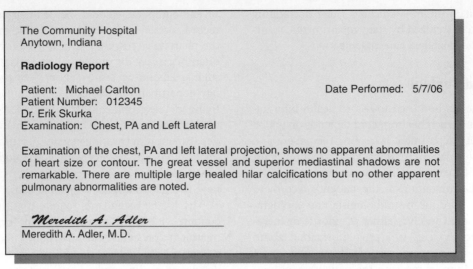

The Community Hospital
Anytown, Indiana

Radiology Report

Patient: Michael Carlton   Date Performed: 5/7/06
Patient Number: 012345
Dr. Erik Skurka
Examination: Chest, PA and Left Lateral

Examination of the chest, PA and left lateral projection, shows no apparent abnormalities of heart size or contour. The great vessel and superior mediastinal shadows are not remarkable. There are multiple large healed hilar calcifications but no other apparent pulmonary abnormalities are noted.

Meredith A. Adler
Meredith A. Adler, M.D.

FIG. 23–1 Sample radiology report for a chest procedure.

includes the patient demographic information (name, health record number, other identifying information) along with the specific procedure being requested. The physician ordering the procedure should also be identified. Typically, these orders are sent to the radiology department by means of the computerized information system within the hospital. For documentation of medical necessity, a diagnosis or sign or symptom for which the test is being performed *must* accompany each request. Failure of the attending physician to report such a diagnosis or sign or symptom will result in a delay of the procedure being performed. Hospital and billing requirements under medical necessity require that the medical necessity be justified before a procedure is performed. This requirement applies to inpatient and outpatient procedures. If Medicare does not cover the procedure, then the patient must be notified and is required to sign an advance beneficiary notice (ABN). The patient then assumes responsibility for payment when Medicare denies the claim.

The results of the procedure are documented on a radiology report (diagnostic, therapeutic, and nuclear medicine). These reports must be included in the patient record to describe the radiologic services that the patient received. A physician, usually a radiologist, writes or dictates and authenticates a description of what is seen on the radiograph and the implications for the patient (Fig. 23–1). A written report must be completed for every service for which a medical claim will be filed. The name of the study must be on the report. With therapeutic radiology, required documentation includes the amount of

the dose of the x-ray or radioactive material administered, as well as the date and time. Again, authentication is required on the report before it becomes a part of the patient's permanent record.

Any special reports documenting evaluation or treatment of a patient must be made a part of the patient's permanent record. The radiology department usually maintains a copy of the information submitted to the patient record with the hard copy images; however, the original document should be placed in the patient's permanent health record. Radiology reports are almost always transcribed, and the radiologist electronically signs or otherwise authenticates the report before permanent placement in the record.

Requirements of Health Record Entries

Federal requirements and accrediting bodies such as the JCAHO require that the medical staff of an institution have bylaws, rules, and regulations that include a provision for accurate and complete medical records with the original copies of documents in the patient record. Medical records must incorporate all significant clinical information regarding a patient. The record is the means of communication between the attending physician and all others rendering patient care.

Various regulations and standards exist throughout federal, state, and accrediting bodies that address signatures in the patient record. The JCAHO, for example, requires that all health record entries be dated, authenticated, and their authors identified. The use of a computer-generated signature is of significance to radiology departments because most radiologists choose this method of authenticating radiology reports. If a hospital allows the radiologist the use of a computer signature or rubber stamp, then a signed statement must be available in the hospital's administrative offices indicating that only the radiologist is in possession of the computer access code or stamp and that he or she is the only one who will use the code or stamp. A computer signature or stamp authorized for one person cannot be used by anyone else. All entries made in a patient health record should be in ink. Pencil documentation is not legal in any state. In the era of the electronic patient record, this point will be moot. Authorized access to the EHR will be the key.

Regulations also address other health record documentation issues such as abbreviations used in the record, timeliness of documentation, record legibility, and correction of errors or omissions. Basically, an abbreviation in the record can be used only if it has been approved by the medical staff and if an abbreviation list is on file that explains the abbreviations. Federal requirements mandate that current and discharged patient records be completed promptly. Record reports such as x-rays should be documented and completed as soon as possible after the procedure takes place.

In a paper record, the person who makes an error in documentation is responsible for correcting the error. The individual should draw a single line through the erroneous documentation, write an explanatory note such as "ERROR" near it, and then document the current information. The note should be dated and signed.

A long-standing basic principle of health record documentation is the adage of *not documented, not done.* This tenet applies to all health care practitioners who make entries in the patient health record. If the record is submitted in court in any type of legal case, then the statement holds true. Without the requisite documentation in the health record of what was done to the patient, the assumption is that the event did not take place.

HEALTH RECORD AND RADIOLOGY IMPLICATIONS IN ANCILLARY HEALTH SYSTEMS

Radiology reports generated by a patient's encounter with health services need to be maintained in the patient's record, whether that be a hospital-based ambulatory care record or a record used in a variety of free-standing facilities. Examples of other health care areas in which radiology reports are often generated include emergency department encounters, ambulatory surgery centers, ambulatory care facilities, physician offices, and urgent care centers. Ambulatory care records have similar requirements to inpatient care records. Federal and state regulations need to be followed, as well as those of any other accrediting body such as HFAP or the JCAHO. The JCAHO, for example, specifies that ambulatory records include items such as patient identification; relevant history of the illness or injury; physical findings; diagnostic and therapeutic orders; clinical observations; reports of tests, procedures, and results; diagnostic impression; patient disposition and pertinent follow-up instructions; immunization records; allergy history; growth charts for pediatric patients; and referral information to and from any other health care facilities.

A long-term care health record is similar to an inpatient record. The long-term care facility can be subject to state, federal, and accreditation agency regulations. In a long-term care facility, radiology services may be provided through a contract with an outside provider. The record must contain a written order for the service and the reason for the service. The actual radiology report should be dated, authenticated, and placed in the patient record. The physician is notified of the results of the diagnostic service.

HEALTH RECORDS IN REIMBURSEMENT

Prospective Payment System

Health record data serve as the basis for hospital reimbursement in the PPS using the DRG system. The concept of the DRG is that patients fall into statistically similar, diagnostically related groups. Therefore the hospital receives payments based on the group into which the patient fits. The health information professional uses the diagnoses and procedure terminology provided by the physician and codes this information into the numbering system of the *International Classification of Diseases,* **9th edition, Clinical Modification (ICD-9-CM).** Using a computer software program called a *grouper,* the health information practitioner computes the patient's DRG. For a Medicare patient, and for some other payors, the hospital hopes to receive, as payment for its services, this DRG amount. The numerical ICD-9-CM codes are the basis for the DRG to which the inpatient is classified. **Current Procedural Terminology (CPT)** codes are used to code procedures for outpatient encounters and coding for ancillary services such as radiology and laboratory.

The coding and classification functions of the health information services department have become complex and significantly increased in importance since the implementation of PPS-based DRGs. The DRG classification is based on an inpatient classification scheme that categorizes patients who are medically related with respect to diagnosis and treatment and who are statistically similar in their lengths of stay. The health information management professional must be knowledgeable in the various case-mix classification systems used to measure the categories of patients and the types of patients treated by a health care institution.

A criticism of DRGs has been that the system does not take into account the severity of a patient's disease. Existing and available severity of illness methodologies go beyond DRGs to classify the extent of a patient's illness. Clinical differences in patients with the same diagnosis can account for varying levels of care rendered and varying amounts of resources used. DRG payment is not currently affected but may be in the future.

The management personnel in a radiology department must understand communication through the diagnostic codes of ICD-9-CM. The correct billing process in a major revenue-producing department of a hospital such as radiology is critical to a hospital's financial solvency. Payors carefully review radiology services for medical necessity. The diagnosis code may be critical to the payment and is the reason to either justify or deny reimbursement. Hospitals may use a computer program called a *chargemaster* to report radiologic procedures. When a radiologic procedure is ordered and performed, the computer automatically assigns the code and applies the charge. Chargemaster codes must be correct to reflect the code and payment for all radiology procedures accurately. Radiology must work with the health information management department and billing in chargemaster updating and maintenance.

Ambulatory patient classifications (APCs) constitute an ambulatory case-mix system used for prospective payment in ambulatory care. The system is a patient-classification scheme that explains the amount and types of resources used in an ambulatory visit. Patients in each APC have similar clinical characteristics, resource use, and costs. ICD-9-CM diagnosis codes and CPT procedure codes drive the procedural and ancillary APCs. Radiologic procedures are all coded via CPT and affect the APC assigned for each patient. Again, accuracy in the documentation of the procedure performed leads to accuracy in the CPT procedure coded and appropriate reimbursement for the outpatient facility.

Coding Function

The ICD-9-CM classification system is used for inpatient reporting. For outpatients, hospitals must report the diagnosis using the ICD-9-CM system and, in most instances, both the CPT and the ICD-9-CM codes for the procedures. The physician's office uses the ICD-9-CM coding system for the diagnosis and the CPT coding system for the procedures. Radiology codes in CPT include diagnostic and therapeutic radiology, nuclear medicine, diagnostic ultrasonography, and radiation oncology. The code numbers range from 70010 to 79999. For example, a chest radiograph, single view, frontal, would be coded as 71010. A magnetic resonance image of the cervical spine with contrast material is coded to 72142.

Radiology departments may use the Index of Radiologic Diagnoses (IRD) of the American College of Radiology to classify radiologic specimens. This information can be used for statistics, for follow-up, or for evaluation of patient care. The JCAHO requires that information about important aspects of diagnostic radiology or therapy services be collected. The IRD consists of a listing of diagnostic code numbers and an alphabetic index. The code number signifies topography and the pathology. For example:

Osteogenic sarcoma of proximal tibia
Code number: 45.321

40.	Indicates extremities
45.	Indicates knee and leg
.300	Indicates neoplasm
.320	Indicates neoplasm, malignant, primary
.321	Indicates osteogenic sarcoma

The health information management department would use an ICD-9-CM code to report this same diagnosis for billing and information management purposes. In this system, the code assigned would be 170.7. This coded indicates a malignant neoplasm of the long bones of the lower limb.

QUALITY MANAGEMENT

Quality management is a process that monitors and evaluates the quality of the care and services provided to patients within a health care facility. The terms *quality assurance* and *quality assessment* are used to encompass all activities related to quality management, including utilization and risk management, infection control, surgical case review, medication usage evaluation, health record review, blood usage review, pharmacy and therapeutic review, and case management. Quality management activities include work performed by various hospital committees and the medical staff, as well as other professional staff from various hospital departments. A separate quality management department exists in many hospitals. In others, a unit or section within the health information management department is responsible for quality management.

The JCAHO standards will be discussed here, but similar standards exist in other accrediting bodies. The JCAHO's standards require that hospitals have a planned, systematic, and hospital-wide approach for monitoring, evaluating, and improving the quality of care and of key governance, managerial, and support activities. The JCAHO's current standards, for example, for improving an organization's performance emphasize the following points:

- Activities are collaborative and interdisciplinary.
- New or modified processes are well designed.
- Data are collected to monitor the stability of existing processes, identify opportunities for improvement, and identify changes that lead to and sustain improvement.
- Data are aggregated and analyzed on an ongoing basis.
- Improved performance is achieved and sustained.

Data are collected in areas such as the following: operative; other invasive and noninvasive procedures that put the patient at risk; processes related to medication and use of blood; the needs, expectations, and satisfactions of patients; and the staff's views regarding performance and improvement opportunities.

The JCAHO's standards also encourage the use of multiple data sources to identify problems and discourage the use of quality management studies for the sole purpose of documenting high-quality care. Examples of quality assurance activities in radiology departments include studying patient waiting times, doing *timely reporting* reviews, and doing equipment quality control.

The JCAHO's 10-step process was created to help organizations make the transition from quality assurance to continuous quality improvement. Facilities who use the 10-step process are required to do the following:

1. Assign responsibility for the department or service's monitoring and evaluation activities.
2. Delineate the scope of care or service that the department provides.
3. Identify the most important aspects of that care or service.

4. Identify indicators of quality and appropriate nature for the recognized important aspects of care.
5. Establish thresholds (levels, patterns, trends) for evaluation (maximum allowable error rates).
6. Collect and organize relevant data, compare the data with preestablished criteria, and analyze the findings.
7. Evaluate care. (Compare actual rate to thresholds.)
8. Take action to improve care and services.
9. Assess the effectiveness of the actions and maintain the gain.
10. Communicate results to affected individuals and groups.

Dimensions of Performance

The JCAHO requires the medical and professional staff to participate in review functions. Many approaches should be used to evaluate performance. The JCAHO has defined various dimensions of performance that need to be addressed in quality management activities in health care organizations. These dimensions include the following:

Efficacy—Have our activities achieved desired outcomes?
Appropriateness—Is the activity relevant to our clinical needs?
Availability—Is intervention available and accessible?
Timeliness—Is activity done at the most beneficial time?
Effectiveness—Do care and resources achieve the desired outcome?
Continuity—How are activities or interventions coordinated among providers and over time?
Safety—What is the degree to which associated risks are minimized?
Efficiency—How do we maximize the relationship between outcomes and resources?
Respect and caring—What is the degree of patient involvement in care decisions and the degree of sensitivity shown for individual needs?

Operation of a Quality Management Program

Each department or service is responsible for documenting the effectiveness of its quality management activities and for reporting such activities to the hospital-wide program. In turn, the staff members who perform the quality management coordinating function should be responsible for demonstrating that the overall hospital program is functional and effective. The data must be consolidated and reported to the medical staff and to the hospital's board of trustees. Such a report might include a description of a process identified for improvement, the method used to identify that process, the department or service involved, the person assigned to perform the study, the data sources used, the cause of any identified variation, any corrective action taken, the person who implemented the action, the timetable for implementation, whether the process was improved, plans for a monitoring procedure, and plans for restudy. The persons involved must remember that quality management activities are confidential matters, and special procedures should be followed to avoid or minimize possible incrimination of the parties involved. The JCAHO uses the evaluation or clinical outcomes as part of the accreditation process. The hospital must work to systematically improve its performance and must take action if it has identified a person with performance problems who is unable or unwilling to improve. This action may mean a modification in a staff member's clinical privileges.

LEGAL ASPECTS OF HEALTH RECORDS

The patient record is an important legal document that the health care institution uses to define what was or was not done to the patient. The record may be submitted as evidence in court cases and used in any litigation in which the institution is involved.

Principles of both common law and statutory law have an impact on the legal aspects of medical records. Federal regulations affect an institution's participation in Medicare and Medicaid programs. Radiographers may be required to give depositions or testimony regarding information in the health record or, in the case of a radiograph, testimony regarding the procedures involved.

Correcting or Amending the Health Record

The proper method for correcting an error that an author makes, as mentioned earlier, is for the author to draw a single line through the error, write "ERROR," and then record the correct information. The individual then should date and authenticate the entry. The patient has the right to amend a record, but the original entry is not altered. The amendment then becomes a permanent part of the patient health record.

Confidentiality of Health Records

Radiographers and students bear the same responsibility as all other hospital personnel to safeguard the confidentiality of health record information. Computerized information systems are a significant part of these

records. Some employers require that any employee or student who has access to the medical record sign a confidentiality statement (Fig. 23–2). Technologists may be asked to release information to patients concerning results of procedures. Informing patients of examination results is the physician's responsibility, and the technologist should refer the patient to his or her physician.

Implications of the Health Insurance Portability and Accountability Act

The HIPAA regulations refocus the health care industry on the need to protect health information from inappropriate access or use. The federal regulations generated by HIPAA support the need for timely access to health information and support the concept that the EHR is needed. The regulations mandate both security of the information and privacy of the information for the patient. The health care facility makes health care information available in an automated form that benefits the facility, without sacrificing the privacy of the patient. The HIPAA regulations require that health care facilities design and maintain systems to protect the security and privacy of electronically transmitted data. The systems must prevent unauthorized individuals from accessing, creating, or modifying information while at the same time allowing authorized users to have access.

Privileged Communication

States can enact statutes specifically recognizing the physician-patient privilege. If this legislation exists, a physician cannot testify in court or in any legal proceeding without the consent of the patient. A patient can waive this privilege through specific actions, such as bringing the subject of the medical condition into evidence.

Consents to Release Information

Consents to release information from the patient record must be in writing and should contain items such as to whom the information is to be released; the patient's name, address, and birth date; the extent of the information to be released; the date; and the signature of the patient or legal representative. Figure 23–3 represents excerpted information from the American Health Information Management Association (AHIMA) regarding disclosure of health information. A department needs to ensure that disclosure of health information is consistent with HIPAA requirements.

FIG. 23–2 Sample confidentiality statement. (From the American Health Information Management Association. Copyright 1997 by the American Health Information Management Association. All rights reserved. No part of this may be reproduced, reprinted, stored in a retrieval system, or transmitted, in any form or by any means, electronic, photocopying, recording, or otherwise, without the prior written permission of the association.)

SAMPLE CONFIDENTIALITY STATEMENT

I understand and agree that in the performance of my duties as an employee of

_____ , I

must hold medical information in confidence. I understand that any violation of the confidentiality of medical information may result in punitive action.

_____   _____
          Date   Signature of Employee

(It is recommended that this form be completed by any employee having access to medical information. It should be used as a part of an institution's orientation to its policies on the confidentiality of medical information.)

Disclosure of Health Information

Background

Complete, accurate health information must be readily available for patient care, but patients must be assured that the information they share with healthcare professionals will remain confidential. Without such assurance, patients may withhold critical information that could affect the quality and outcome of care, as well as the reliability of the information.

Disclosure of Health Information

Health records (regardless of the media on which they are maintained) are the property of the healthcare provider, but the health information contained in the records belongs to the patient. Disclosure of health information must be done prudently to protect the patient's right to privacy.

Each healthcare facility must develop policies and procedures for disclosure of health information in accordance with federal and state laws. To assure consistent compliance with these policies and procedures, disclosure of health information should be made only by those appropriately trained and qualified to do so.

Patient Care

Complete, accurate health information must be readily available for patient care. Information may be disclosed without patient authorization as required for continued care.

Nonpatient Care

Careful consideration must be given to any other disclosure of any health information, even that information generally considered to be nonconfidential. Although healthcare providers have no obligation to disclose this information, it may be disclosed to legitimate requesters on a "need-to-know" basis without the patient's authorization unless otherwise requested by the patient or his legal representative or prohibited by law. When disclosing this information, there should be evidence that the requester has a legitimate right to the information which is not inconsistent with the patient's best interests.

Redisclosure of Health Information

A healthcare provider's records may contain information about a patient from another healthcare provider. Such information is sent with patients who are transferred or referred to a facility for definitive treatment or continuing care. At times, a patient hospitalized and treated in one facility may be referred to another facility for diagnostic testing or therapeutic treatment not available at the first facility. The resultant reports are sent to the referring to be incorporated into the patient's record.

A provider may redisclose health information from another provider facility without authorization from the patient or his legal representative if it is needed urgently for the patient's continuing care. If time permits, authorization from the patient or his legal representative should be obtained prior to redisclosure to a third party.

FIG. 23–3 Excerpted information from a disclosure document.

Facsimile Transmission of Health Information

Transmission of Health Information

The American Health Information Management Association (AHIMA) recommends facsimile transmission of health information only when the original record or mail-delivered copies will not meet the needs of immediate patient care. The sensitive information contained in health records should be transmitted via facsimile only when (1) urgently needed for patient care or (2) required by a third-party payer for ongoing certification of payment for a hospitalized patient. The information transmitted should be limited to that necessary to meet the requester's needs. Routine disclosure of information to insurance companies, attorneys, or other legitimate users should be made through regular mail or messenger service.

Except as required by law, a properly completed and signed authorization should be obtained prior to the release of patient information. An authorization transmitted via facsimile is acceptable. If authorization cannot be obtained in cases of explained medical emergency, information may be released for patient care without authorization from the patient or legal representative.

The cover page accompanying the facsimile transmission should include a confidentiality notice that indicates the information is confidential and limits its use. A sample statement is provided below:

Confidentiality Notice

The documents accompanying this telecopy transmission contain confidential information belonging to the sender, that is legally privileged. This information is intended only for the use of the individual or entity named above. The authorized recipient of this information is prohibited from disclosing this information to any other party and is required to destroy the information after its stated need has been fulfilled.

If you are not the intended recipient, you are hereby notified that any disclosure, copying, distribution, or action taken in reliance on the contents of these documents is strictly prohibited. If you have received this telecopy in error, please notify the sender immediately to arrange for return of these documents.

Reasonable efforts should be made to assure the facsimile transmission is sent to the appropriate destination. Destination numbers should be pre-programmed into the machine, if possible, to eliminate errors in transmission from misdialing.

FIG. 23-4 Sample facsimile transmission of health information.

Facsimile Transmission of Health Information

The use of a facsimile (fax) machine is commonplace in health care communications today. The instant transmission of data enhances patient care but also presents confidentiality issues. The AHIMA has developed a *Practice Brief* detailing an appropriate procedure for faxing (Fig. 23-4).

Information Security

The confidential nature of electronic or paper health records is paramount in this information-driven age. Hospitals and other institutions must protect patient information in the health information system. Figure 23-5 summarizes key points of access to patient information.

Patient Access to the Health Record

The HIPAA regulations mandate the confidentiality of health information. A patient or patient representative should have access, the right of copy, and the right of amendment, or correction of health care information concerning the patient; however, a collection of health information should be restricted to the extent necessary to carry out the legitimate purpose for which it was collected. The HIPAA contains penalties for wrongful disclosure of individually identifiable health information.

Because of federal laws, patients have a right to access their medical records. Hospitals however, have the right to charge a copy fee to the patient for this record. The hospital also has the right to require a properly completed and signed patient authorization. A hospital does have the right to prohibit patient access when the provider reasonably believes that having access is not in the best interest of the patient's health or if the knowledge of the health care information might cause danger to the life or safety of any person. Patients sometimes ask radiographers whether patients can examine their records while in transit, waiting for a procedure, or undergoing an examination. The record information should not be shared with the patient in this fashion because misinterpretation

Information Security: A Checklist for Healthcare Professionals

Access Control

❏ The organization has written policies outlining who may access patient information.

❏ There are mechanisms in place to control access to both paper and computer-based patient records. These mechanisms apply to all settings where records are kept in the organization, including physician offices that may have access to the organization's information system.

❏ There is a written organizational policy prohibiting the disclosure or sharing of passwords, access codes, key cards, or other user identifiers, and the policy is strictly enforced.

❏ Passwords contain at least seven alphanumeric characters to make them more difficult to guess.

❏ Passwords are changed frequently and users are limited to one log-on at a time.

❏ Each user's access is restricted to the information needed to do his/her job.

❏ If a user attempts to access information beyond his/her security clearance with repeated use of an improper code, the system locks the user out or sounds an alarm.

❏ When a user leaves the facility, his/her password and access codes are deactivated immediately.

❏ Access to computer-based records is tracked by individual user to discourage unauthorized viewing.

❏ The information system limits mass copying, printing, or downloading of patient records.

❏ Periodic audits are done to see if the organization's policies are being followed and are still effective.

❏ If inactive paper-based or computer-based records are archived, they are protected from loss, defacement, or unauthorized disclosure.

❏ Access controls are in place for clinical systems such as laboratory, radiology, and nuclear medicine.

❏ Appropriate protections are in place to protect the organization's computer system from remote access risks. (Dial-up access enables outsiders to make repeated attempts to gain access without being visible to the organization using the system.)

Financial Data

❏ There are adequate procedures to protect patient-related financial data that contain diagnostic or procedural codes and other information that may reveal the reason for a patient's treatment.

Information Services

❏ If confidential information is transmitted via the Internet, it is encrypted to protect it during transmission.

FIG. 23–5   Key points of access to patient information.

of information can occur. Again, the technologist should refer the patient to the physician for discussion of record documentation.

According to the Mammography Quality Standards Act, a facility must keep a mammogram in the permanent medical record of the patient for no less than 5 years or no less than 10 years if a patient has had no other mammograms at that facility. A facility must also, on request, transfer the mammogram to another medical institution to a physician or to the patient directly.

Health Record in Court

The health record is a legal document that is admissible as evidence in court. A health information manager may be required to honor a subpoena for the record and take the record to court. The original record is never left in court; rather, a photocopy is used. The original record is then retained in the hospital health information management department. An increasingly common approach is that a copy of the record is sent by certified mail.

SUMMARY

The health information management department is a key hospital department that affects many other departments. Health information management departments do not render patient care but rather are identified as a support service department. Because of the coding function, health information management departments directly affect hospital revenue and therefore hospital operation. The health record is the document that communicates information pertaining to patient care. The record is also a valuable tool in preparing health service statistics; substantiating patient care services and treatment provided; supporting medical education, health services, and clinical research; maintaining quality assessment and risk management; and making financial planning decisions. Health information management professionals manage health data and information resources. The health information management professionals ensure the availability of health information for health care delivery and information for critical decisions across various organizations, settings, and disciplines. The profession serves the health care system, including patient care organizations, payors, research and policy agencies, and other health care–related industries.

The health record is the legal document that attests to the care that was rendered to the patient. The record is a recapitulation of all patient care events. The radiology department contributes to this complete record by thorough documentation of all cases.

BIBLIOGRAPHY

Abdelhak M et al: *Health information: management of a strategic resource,* Philadelphia, 2001, WB Saunders.

Addison K, Braden JH, Cupp JE: Practice brief, guidelines for defining the legal health record for disclosure purposes, *J AHIMA* 76:64A, Sept 2005.

American College of Radiology: *Index for radiologic diagnoses. revised,* ed 4, Chicago, 1992, American College of Radiology.

American Medical Association: *Current procedural terminology,* Chicago, 2005, The Association.

LaTour K, Eichenwald Maki S: *Health information management: concepts, principles, and practice,* Chicago, 2002, American Health Information Management Association.

Joint Commission on Accreditation of Healthcare Organizations: *Accreditation manual for hospitals 2005,* Chicago, 2004, JCAHO.

Shaw P et al: *Quality and performance improvement in healthcare,* ed 2, Chicago, 2003, American Health Information Management Association.

Skurka M: *Health information management: principles and organization for health information services,* Chicago, 2003, AHA Press, Josey-Bass.

U.S. Department of Health and Human Services: *International classification of diseases,* ed 9, Clinical Modification (ICD-9-CM), 2006 Annual Hospital Version, Reno, Nev, 2006, Channel Publishing.

Medical Law

Ann M. Obergfell, JD, RT(R)

The liability of the technologist is not the same as the radiologist involved, but the liability is potentially real.

Albert Bundy, MD, JD, 1988

OBJECTIVES

On completion of this chapter, the student will be able to:

1. Differentiate among the various types of law.

2. Outline how the standard of care is established for radiologic technologists.

3. Discuss the concept of tortious conduct and causes of action that may arise from the behavior of a health care practitioner.

4. Argue the importance of privacy of records and the relationship between privacy of records and patient confidentiality issues.

5. Explain negligence and the four elements necessary to meet the burden of proof in a medical negligence claim.

6. Explain the legal theory of *res ipsa loquitur* and how an attorney may use it in a claim of medical negligence.

7. Illustrate how a hospital may be liable under the doctrine of respondeat superior.

8. Justify the need for informed consent.

9. Outline the information a patient must have before an informed consent may be given.

GLOSSARY

Assault: any willful attempt or threat to inflict injury on the person of another, when coupled with the apparent present ability to do so, and any intentional display of force such as would give the victim reason to fear or expect immediate bodily harm

Battery: any unlawful touching of another that is without justification or excuse

Defamation: holding up a person to ridicule, scorn, or contempt in a respectable and considerable part of the community

False Imprisonment: conscious restraint of the freedom of person without proper authorization, privilege, or consent

Fraud: intentional perversion of truth for the purpose of inducing person to rely on the false information to his or her detriment

Informed Consent: person's agreement to allow something to happen (such as surgery) that is based on a full disclosure of the facts needed to make the decision intelligently—that is, knowledge of risks involved, alternatives, benefits, and other information needed by a reasonable person to make a decision

Negligence: failure to do something that a reasonable person guided by the ordinary considerations that ordinarily regulate human affairs would do or the doing of something a reasonable and prudent person would not do

Res Ipsa Loquitur: meaning *the thing speaks for itself;* legal theory requiring three elements: (1) that the type of injury did not occur except for negligence, (2) that the activity was under the complete control of the defendant, and (3) that the plaintiff did not contribute to his or her own injury in any way

Respondeat Superior: meaning *let the superior respond* or *the master speaks for the servant;* the physician, supervisor, or employer may be liable in certain cases for the wrongful acts of employees or subordinates

Tort: private or civil wrong or injury, other than breach of contract, for which the court provides a remedy in the form of an action for damages

LAW

Today's litigious society requires that all health care professionals, including radiologic technologists, be aware of the areas of the law that may affect the delivery of health care services. A basic principle of the law was defined in *Schloendorf v. Society of New York Hospital* in 1914 and lays a foundation for the relationship between patients and health care practitioners:

> "Every human being of adult years and sound mind has a right to determine what shall be done with his own body, and a surgeon who performs an operation without his patient's consent commits an assault, for which he is liable in damages."

This doctrine serves six functions. It (1) protects individual autonomy, (2) protects the patient's status as a human being, (3) avoids fraud and duress, (4) encourages health care practitioners to consider their decisions carefully, (5) fosters rational decision making by the patient, and (6) involves the public in medicine. Despite this carefully formed doctrine and its well-articulated functions, many members of the health care team take a paternalistic role in their practice and forget the patient's right to be informed of and to make decisions about his or her own health care diagnosis and treatment. This violation of patient rights, as articulated in the American Hospital Association's Patient Care Partnership (Appendix E), not only is improper from a moral and ethical standpoint, but it also may well be construed as improper from a legal perspective. Although health care practitioners clearly need to inspire confidence in their patients, they must remember this fundamental principle underlying the delivery of health care in the United States.

Medicine and the law are sometimes in conflict because each looks at a situation from a different perspective. One entity is looking to see that the patient's physical needs are being met through diagnosis and treatment, whereas the other attempts to control the abuse of patients and to ensure that they are compensated for injuries suffered at the hands of negligent health care practitioners. Both processes are necessary to ensure that the patient receives the best possible care. To gain a better understanding of the relationship between law and the delivery of health care, looking at the law and how it may be applied to everyday situations in radiology is helpful.

TYPES OF LAW

The law is multifaceted and draws its principles from several foundations. The first and probably most important foundation is the Constitution of the United States.

This document, considered as the supreme law of the land, was written to separate powers of the three branches of government: the Executive (the Presidency), the Legislative, and the Judiciary. The separation offers a system of checks and balances that prohibits any one branch from becoming more powerful than another. The Constitution also protects the individual rights of all citizens of the United States. Each state has a constitution that defines its government and articulates the rights of its citizens.

The second form of law is that enacted by legislative bodies or administrative agencies. This system of statutes and regulations is written at local, state, and federal levels and runs the gamut from who will drive cars to how citizens will be taxed. Many areas of health care are defined and regulated by these statutes and regulations. For instance, state legislators may adopt a statute that defines radiation machine operators and may, through statutes, delegate power to an administrative agency, such as a board of health, to establish regulations and guidelines that closely define the practice. Examples of such definitions may include restrictions on who may practice and how ionizing radiation equipment is registered. These statutes and regulations may change from time to time at the discretion of the legislature or agency as needs and scopes of practice change within the profession. Legislators and administrators may also be persuaded to make changes if the profession or others find that the statutes or regulations are too loose or restrictive as written.

The third area of the law is case law, which is derived from the Common Law of England. This type of law is decided on a case-by-case basis by either a judge or a jury. The decisions in these cases may be precedent setting for future cases, but if the factual situation varies enough, the controversy may be decided contrary to what has gone before.

Whereas the Constitution defines individual rights and the statutes define the practice, the case law will dictate the fate of the health care practitioner who has been sued for medical negligence or malpractice. The judge and jury hear the facts as presented by both parties, which includes testimony from expert witnesses who testify as to the appropriate standard of care. After careful deliberation, the judge or jury will determine whether the practitioner violated the standard of care by performing his or her duties in a negligent or offensive way.

STANDARD OF CARE

Each profession or area in the health care delivery system has a standard of care. The standard for radiologic tech-

nology is not written in stone and is constantly changing because of the dynamic structure of the technology. Regardless of the changing nature of the discipline, guidelines must be established to help define the standard of care.

The general definition of the standard of care is the degree of skill (proficiency), knowledge, and care ordinarily possessed and employed by members in good standing within the profession. The test of whether the standard of care has been met by an individual under certain circumstances is to determine what a reasonable, prudent practitioner would have done under the same or similar circumstances.

The court looks to the profession as it tries to establish the standard of care for a particular practice. The determinative areas include federal and state regulations, job descriptions, curriculum guides, course goals and objectives, professional customs and standards of practice.

A document called the Practice Standards for Medical Imaging and Radiation Therapy has been developed by a group of medical imaging professionals and adopted by the American Society of Radiologic Technologists. These Standards outline the practice of medical imaging and radiation therapy professionals in clinical, quality, and professional performance. Each section offers standards for practice and helps direct the practitioner while allowing for variations in different localities and areas of practice. The Standards outline the standard of care for medical imaging and radiation therapy and will be used to determine whether an individual is compliant with a national standard. Expert witnesses, who are generally educators or long-term practitioners in the area under scrutiny, define these areas. Appendix A contains the Practice Standards for Radiography. The standard of care will change and grow as the profession grows; therefore all radiologic technologists must keep abreast of current trends in the profession because these standards are likely to be the ones to which they will be held. A governing body known as the Practice Standards Advisory Council has been established with the purpose of continually reviewing and updating the Practice Standards, as well as researching practice questions and rendering opinions as to the current standard as determined by literature, statute, regulation, and accepted practice.

CAUSES OF ACTION

Newspaper headlines often proclaim huge monetary awards given to an individual as a result of medical negligence. These headlines are followed by stories of horrendous injuries patients suffered at the hands of negligent physicians, nurses, or other health care professionals. These cases are quite disturbing, but they are generally found to be the exception instead of the rule. Even if these cases are the exception, the general public will clearly not tolerate actions by health care practitioners that are less than the generally accepted standard of care. An estimated 10% of all medical negligence claims are somehow related to diagnostic imaging, either by improper diagnosis or by injuries to patients suffered during diagnostic procedures. Therefore any radiographer may be called to testify at any time either as a defendant or as a witness to the practice of another.

TORTS

A patient's claim that he or she has been wronged or has suffered some injury, other than a breach of contract, for which he or she believes cause exists for an action for damages is known as a **tort**. This type of claim arises from a violation of a duty imposed by general law on all persons involved in a transaction or situation. For a patient to have a claim, some breach of duty must have occurred on the part of the health care practitioner.

In a case against a radiologic technologist, the patient contacts an attorney with the belief that an injury has occurred during a procedure or while present in the radiology department. The patient also may look for legal guidance if he or she believes that the care received has been less than optimal or that he or she has been threatened in any way. Although these legal inquiries may not lead to lawsuits, many of the complaints are based on legitimate concerns of negligent care or claims of assault, battery, false imprisonment, defamation, or fraud.

Assault

An **assault** claim may arise when a patient believes he or she has been threatened in such a way that reason to fear or to expect immediate bodily harm exists. This fear may arise from comments made by a technologist to the patient before or during the examination. For example, threatening to repeat a painful examination if the patient does not hold still may be construed as an assault. This type of threat may appear to be innocuous on the part of the technologist, but if the patient truly believes that he or she is threatened, the claim may be valid.

Battery

In a similar context, if a technologist performs an examination or touches a patient without that patient's per-

mission, a **battery** may occur even if no injury arises from such contact. Any unlawful touching may constitute a battery if the patient thinks that the technologist has touched him or her in an offensive way. Such a touch may occur if an examination is performed on the wrong patient or if a patient is moved roughly about the radiographic table while being positioned for an examination.

False Imprisonment

The common claim of **false imprisonment** arises when a person is restrained or believes that he or she is being restrained against his or her will. The individual must be aware of the confinement and have no reasonable means of escape. This phenomenon is most prevalent with patients who are unable to cooperate, such as inebriated, senile, or pediatric patients. Each of these types of patients poses an interesting and often confusing set of problems that must be handled without compromising the quality of medical care.

Inebriated patients pose a problem in that they are unable to consent to treatment and may oppose restraint. The general practice in such cases is to speak with the physician who has ordered the examination to determine whether the requested procedure is of the utmost importance and must be completed immediately or whether the examination may be delayed until the patient is coherent enough to make informed decisions. If the examination must be done immediately, or if the patient is in such a condition that he or she may bring harm to self or the technologist, appropriate restraints may be applied.

In the case of senile, pediatric, or other incompetent patients, obtaining consent to restrain or immobilize from someone authorized to give consent is important. This person may be a parent or guardian who has the legal right to make decisions about the treatment and care of the patient. This person must be informed as to the reasons for the restraint and the possible risks that may occur if restraints are not used before any such devices may be applied.

These principles may sometimes be in opposition to the paternalistic attitude of health care professionals. An important point to note, however, is that all health care professionals safeguard patient rights and autonomy.

Defamation

Health care professionals have an obligation to maintain patient confidentiality and are required to keep all information concerning the patient, the diagnosis, and the prognosis in strictest confidence. This information should be shared only with persons who need to know and who have a relationship with the patient in subsequent diagnosis and treatment. If information concerning a patient were leaked to individuals who did not need to know, and if the information were disseminated in such a way that the patient was subject to ridicule, scorn, or contempt or was injured in some other way as through loss of job or home, then an action for **defamation** might be brought against the individual responsible for the breach of patient confidence.

Two types of defamation are generally recognized: (1) slander, which involves the spoken word; and (2) libel, which involves written or published comments or pictures. In either case, the alleged injured party must prove that they have been defamed and that the defamation has caused an injury.

Fraud

Fraud in health care is on the rise and occurs in the areas of health care financing, as well as during attempts to cover up wrongdoing or errors on the part of the patient or provider. **Fraud** is generally defined as a wilful and intentional misrepresentation of facts that may cause harm to an individual or result in loss of an individual right or property. Cases of fraud may arise when a pathologic condition is missed on a radiograph or when a study is not completed with optimal images and a health care provider attempts to cover up the error by destroying or altering images or records. Other areas of fraud may include altering personnel records, changing patient's medical records, billing for procedures that were not performed, or altering other documentation in an attempt to mislead or cover up some wrongdoing. For a plaintiff to prevail in a claim of fraud, the alleged injury party must show that (1) an untrue statement, known to be untrue by the party making it, is made so as to mislead, (2) the injured party relied on the statement, and (3) damages were incurred as a result of the reliance.

PRIVACY OF RECORDS

Privacy of records and confidentiality are two principles clearly articulated in the American Hospital Association's Patient's Bill of Rights. Although the patient's health information belongs to the hospital, the information contained in the record belongs to the patient and therefore may not be distributed without the patient's consent. The records, which include radiographic films, should be kept in a secured area with access given only to persons who need to know what is contained in them. The patient

generally has a right to see what is contained in his or her records. In some limited cases, however, the physician may determine that the patient should not have access to the files. Such a case may arise when a physician believes that a patient may not be emotionally stable enough to understand or handle what has been written in the chart. A claim of invasion of privacy may be made if a person's records are released or used in a way contrary to the standard established by the health care community.

The issue of acquired immunodeficiency syndrome (AIDS) has brought to the attention of health care workers the sensitivity of the concept of confidentiality of records. Information disclosed from records of patients who are human immunodeficiency virus (HIV) positive or who have AIDS may cause them to lose their jobs or to incur discrimination. Such a breach of confidentiality may place a health care practitioner at legal risk for defamation or for negligence in the breach of the duty to hold information confidential.

The Health Insurance Portability and Accountability Act of 1996 (HIPAA) calls for the standardization of electronic data interchange, the protection of confidentiality, and the security of individually identifiable health information. The confidentiality standards establish guidelines for the storage, access, and transmission of individual health information. Under these guidelines, patients must authorize the release of health information, and a knowing misuse of health information by a health professional may result in fines and/or imprisonment. Every health provider must understand the rules for release of patient health information and follow the policies established by the employer for access and release. Any questions that arise about the appropriateness of the release of information should be directed to the facility's compliance officer.

NEGLIGENCE

"The existence of a medical injury shall not create any inference or presumption of negligence against the healthcare provider, and the claimant must provide the burden of proving that the injury was proximately caused by the breach in the prevailing professional standard of care." *McDonald vs. Medical Imaging Center of Boca Raton, 662So2d733 (Fla App 1995)*

Medical malpractice litigation is predominantly founded in the negligence theory of liability. **Negligence** is a failure to use such care as a reasonably prudent person would use under like or similar circumstances. Medical negligence uses this theory, but instead of the prudent person, the reasonably prudent health care professional or, in the case of radiologic technology, the reasonably prudent technologist is used as a model.

For a patient (plaintiff) to recover damages for injuries suffered because of alleged negligence, four elements must be proved: (1) a duty to the patient by the health care practitioner (in medical-related cases this is defined as the standard of care), (2) breach of this duty by an act or by failing to perform some act (deviation from the standard of care), (3) a compensable injury, and (4) a causal relationship between the injury and the breach of duty.

For example, a patient arrives in the radiology department on a cart. After the radiographer has completed the examination, the patient is transferred back to the cart, but the side rails are not raised. In moving about, the patient falls from the cart and fractures a hip. The radiographer has a duty to protect the patient from falls by raising the side rails on the cart, and this duty was breached by the radiographer's failure to lock the side rails in the raised position. The injury element is demonstrated by the fact that the patient has fractured a hip as a result of the fall. The causation factor is generally the most difficult to prove; however, the fractured hip was apparently a direct result of the fall from the cart, which, but for the failure of the radiographer to place the side rails in the raised position, would not have occurred.

Each of the four elements must be proved before the radiographer can be found to be negligent. The evidence requirements may vary from one jurisdiction to another, and other legal factors may affect the outcome. These same basic elements must be proved no matter where the case is filed.

OTHER LEGAL THEORIES

Whereas negligence is the primary theory of liability in medical malpractice claims, attorneys may use other legal theories to switch the burden of proof from the plaintiff to the defendant or to bring additional parties into the litigation. Such theories include *res ipsa loquitur,* respondeat superior, and corporate liability.

Res Ipsa Loquitur

The legal doctrine of *res ipsa loquitur* sometimes arises in cases of medical negligence and is used to switch the burden of proof from the plaintiff to the defendant. **Res ipsa loquitur** translates to *the thing speaks for itself* and describes how a patient is injured through no fault of his or her own while in the complete control of another. In these cases, the plaintiff must show that the action

causing the injury was in the exclusive control of the defendant and that the injury is a type that would not have occurred but for the negligent activity of the defendant. This type of case occurs most often in the surgical setting in which a patient is anesthetized and suffers an injury that would not have happened in the ordinary course of the operation. Radiology may be involved in such a case, for example, when a patient suffers a burn from a portable machine when the field light remains on while in contact with the patient's skin.

In a case in which the theory of *res ipsa loquitur* is raised, the burden of proof shifts from the patient's proving the negligence to the defendant health care practitioner's proving that he or she was not negligent.

Respondeat Superior

If the radiographer in the previous scenario were sued for negligence, then more often than not the hospital and surgeon would also be named as defendants. This legal theory is known as **respondeat superior** or *the master speaks for the servant.* In cases of medical negligence, the well-established theory asserts that the physician or the health care facility is responsible for the negligent acts of its employees. Many critics of this theory claim that this action is a *deep pocket* approach to legal recovery based primarily on the fact that a physician or health care facility has more money than an individual technologist. Although this circumstance may be true in many cases, other reasons and strategies are used when determining whom to name as defendants in a medical negligence complaint. Such a theory is that a lone technologist on the stand is a more sympathetic character than a wealthy physician or hospital corporation.

Corporate Liability

The theory of corporate liability requires the hospital or health care entity to be responsible for the quality of care delivered to consumers. This liability extends not only to actual employees of the corporation, but also to independent contractors, such as physicians who practice within the facility.

Courts have in recent years expanded the concept of corporate liability to include the following:

1. Duty of reasonable care in the selection and retention of employees and medical staff
2. Duty of reasonable care in the maintenance and use of equipment
3. Availability of equipment and services

Under these guidelines, the health care corporation has the responsibility to assess and evaluate the quality of care delivered and must be prepared to make changes as needed to protect the consumer of health care services. The corporation may be required to intervene if suboptimal care is being provided by one of its independent contractors.

INFORMED CONSENT

When patients enter a health care facility for examination or treatment, they place their trust in health care professionals. This trust includes an assumption that the correct procedures are being performed and that the professional is meeting the appropriate standard of care. This trust does not mean, however, that patients relinquish their right to make decisions about their own health care. They rely on the fact that health care professionals must give them all of the information necessary to make an informed decision.

Only when patients have all the information they need to make decisions about their health care will they be able to give an **informed consent** for examination and treatment. Informed consent is required when a patient is subjected to any type of invasive procedure. In radiology departments, this consent requirement runs the gamut from excretory urography to interventional vascular examinations.

When patients are informed that a particular procedure would assist the physician in making a diagnosis, they should also be informed of the techniques that will be used to complete the examination, the possible risks associated with it, the benefits, and any alternative procedures that might be performed. A good example may be the patient who is scheduled for a myelogram. The patient should receive a careful explanation of how the procedure is to be performed along with an enumeration of the benefits and risks that may be associated with it. The patient should also be informed of alternatives such as computed tomography or magnetic resonance imaging and should be informed of the risks and benefits of each alternative. All this information must be relayed to patients in language they can understand. Expecting a patient to understand the explanation of a procedure is impossible if the health care practitioner uses medical terminology that is foreign to the patient. This situation is similar to explaining something to a Spanish-speaking individual in English and expecting him or her to understand. Current guidelines recommend that consent be given in layperson's terms in the primary language of the patient. Hospitals are required to have interpreters who will be able to relay procedural and other health care information to patients.

After the patient has been given all the information necessary to make an informed decision, a consent form should be signed that documents the information that has been given. These forms are usually prepared by the health care facility. As a general rule, a consent form should contain (1) an authorization clause to permit the physician or other health care professional to perform the examination; (2) a disclosure clause to explain the procedure, its risks and benefits, and possible alternatives to the procedure; (3) an anesthesia clause if required; (4) a no-guarantee clause for therapeutic procedures; (5) a tissue-disposal clause if the removal of tissue may be necessary; (6) a patient understanding clause, which usually states that all the information contained in the consent form has been carefully explained to the patient; and (7) a signature clause, which calls for the signature of the patient, as well as that of a witness. The witness should be a disinterested third party who will not be involved in the actual performance of the procedure.

The amount of information given to the patient must be evaluated on a case-by-case basis. Because every individual is different, the need for information differs from patient to patient. The health care professional who is obtaining the consent must assess the patient as the information is received and base the disclosure of information on the responses and history of the patient. The circumstances surrounding the signing of consent forms are also important, and the department should establish a policy as to how consent forms are to be signed. The evaluation process in determining the policy should include when the consent should be signed, who will be available to answer questions from the patient, who will obtain the signature, and how it will be determined whether the patient is mentally and physically able to make an informed consent.

The patient's autonomy should always be considered when performing diagnostic or therapeutic procedures. If the patient consents to a procedure and then revokes the consent, the health care practitioner must then recognize the patient's right to revoke and must stop the procedure at a point at which the patient will not be injured in any way. Such a case may arise during a barium enema procedure when a patient with discomfort determines that he or she does not want to proceed with the examination. The radiologist and radiographer must comply with the patient's wishes by stopping the flow of barium and allowing any barium already administered to flow back into the enema bag. Simply stopping the procedure without allowing the barium to flow back may cause a subsequent injury to the patient because barium that is not evacuated in a timely fashion may cause a perforated colon or other injury.

SUMMARY

Radiologic technologists are legally liable for their actions in the daily performance of diagnostic procedures. They must follow the appropriate standard of care and should be well versed in current practice and procedure. They should also understand the civil liability of such actions as assault, battery, and false imprisonment. Any information the technologist acquires during the course of an examination must be kept in strictest confidence. The basic right to determine the course of diagnosis and treatment must always be recognized. Therefore the patient must be given information that allows for quality decision making and the ability to give informed consent.

Health care practitioners who do not remain current in the field or who do not follow the accepted standards may be liable under the legal theory of medical negligence. Similarly, the health care facility and the supervising physician may be liable under the theory of respondeat superior.

BIBLIOGRAPHY

Anderson GR, Glesnes-Anderson V: *Health care ethics: a guide for decision makers,* Rockville, Md, 1987, Aspen Publishers.

Berlin L: *Malpractice issues in radiology,* ed 2, Leesburg, Va, 2003, American Roentgen Ray Society.

Bundy AL: *Radiology and the law,* Rockville, Md, 1988, Aspen Publishers.

Capron A: Informed consent in catastrophic disease research and treatment, *PA Law Rev* 123:365, 1974.

Furrow BR et al: *Health law: cases, materials, and problems,* ed 4, St Paul, Minn, 2001, West Wadsworth Publishing.

Furrow BR: *Liability and quality issues in health care,* ed 3, St Paul, Minn, 1999, West Information Publishing Group.

Health Insurance Portability and Accountability Act of 1996. Available at: *http://www.hhs.gov.*

King JH: *The law of medical malpractice,* St Paul, Minn, 1977, West Publishing.

Miller RD: *Problems in hospital law,* ed 6, Rockville, Md, 1990, Aspen Publishers.

Pozgar GD: *Legal aspects of health care administration,* ed 9, Sudbury, Mass, 2004, Jones and Bartlett Publishers.

Practice Standards for Medical Imaging and Radiation Therapy, adopted by American Society of Radiologic Technology, 1998.

Sanbar SS, ed: *Legal medicine: American college of legal medicine,* ed 5, St Louis, 2001, Mosby.

Schloendorf v. Society of New York Hospital, 211 NY 125, 105 NE 92, 1914.

Review Questions and Patient Care Lab Activities
Patient Care Lab Activities

STUDENT NAME: _____ DATE: _____

LAB 13-1: PATIENT TRANSFER TECHNIQUES

Objective

- To demonstrate proper wheelchair and cart transfer techniques

Equipment

- Wheelchair and cart

Procedure

- On completion of this laboratory activity, the student will be able to:

STANDBY ASSIST WHEELCHAIR TRANSFER	YES	NO
1. Position the wheelchair at a 45-degree angle to the table.	☐	☐
2. Move the wheelchair footrests out of the way, and be sure that the wheelchair is locked.	☐	☐
3. Instruct the patient to sit on the edge of the wheelchair seat.	☐	☐
4. Instruct the patient to push down on the arms of the chair to assist in rising and then to stand up slowly.	☐	☐
5. Direct the patient to reach out and hold onto the table with the hand closest to the table and then to turn slowly until he or she feels the table behind him or her.	☐	☐
6. Instruct the patient to hold onto the table with both hands and then to sit down.	☐	☐

ASSISTED STANDING PIVOT WHEELCHAIR TRANSFER	YES	NO
1. Position the wheelchair at a 45-degree angle to the table with the patient's strongest side closest to the table. If the patient has loose-fitting clothes, then place a transfer belt around the patient's waist.	☐	☐
2. Move the wheelchair footrests out of the way, and be sure that the wheelchair is locked.	☐	☐

	YES	NO
3. Direct the patient to sit on the edge of the wheelchair seat, providing assistance as needed.	☐	☐
4. Instruct the patient to push down on the arms of the wheelchair to assist in rising.	☐	☐
5. Bend at the knees, keeping the back stationary, and grasp the transfer belt with both hands. Block the patient's feet and knees to provide stability, especially for patients who are paraplegic and hemiplegic.	☐	☐
6. Assist the patient in rising to a standing position.	☐	☐
7. Ask the patient whether he or she is feeling all right. If the patient reports any feelings of dizziness or exhibits any of the other signs of orthostatic hypotension, then let him or her stand for a moment until the feeling subsides.	☐	☐
8. Pivot the patient toward the table until the patient can feel the table against the back of the thighs.	☐	☐
9. Ask the patient to support himself or herself on the table with both hands and sit down, assisting as necessary.	☐	☐

TWO-PERSON WHEELCHAIR LIFT	YES	NO
1. Plan for the lift by locating an assistant who will lift the patient's feet as you lift the patient's torso.	☐	☐
2. Lock the wheelchair, remove the armrests, swing away or remove the leg rests, and direct the patient to cross his or her arms over the chest.	☐	☐
3. Stand behind the patient, reach under the patient's axillae, and grasp the patient's crossed forearms. Direct the assistant to squat in front of the patient and cradle the patient's thighs in one hand and the calves in the other hand.	☐	☐
4. On command, lift the patient to clear the wheelchair, and move the patient as a unit to the desired place.	☐	☐

CART TRANSFER WITH A MOVING DEVICE	YES	NO
1. Move the cart alongside the table, preferably on the patient's strong or less affected side. Place it as close to the table as possible, and then secure it by	☐	☐

depressing the wheel locks. In addition, place sandbags or other devices on the floor to block the wheels satisfactorily.

2. Place the patient at an oblique angle away from the table while the moving device is placed to the midpoint of the back. ☐ ☐

3. Return the patient to a supine position so that he or she is halfway onto the moving device. ☐ ☐

4. Grab the draw sheet, and use it to move the patient slowly onto the table. ☐ ☐

5. Remove the moving device, turning the patient obliquely if necessary. ☐ ☐

CART TRANSFER WITHOUT A MOVING DEVICE	YES	NO

1. Move the cart alongside the table, preferably on the patient's strong or less affected side. Place it as close to the table as possible, and then secure it by depressing the wheel locks. In addition, place sandbags or other devices on the floor to block wheels satisfactorily. ☐ ☐

2. Begin by rolling up the draw sheet on both sides of the patient. Be sure that the draw sheet is completely under the patient and straightened before the transfer. ☐ ☐

3. Support the patient's head and upper body from the far side of the radiographic table. Direct a second assistant to support the patient's pelvic girdle from the cart side and a third assistant to support the patient's legs from the table side. ☐ ☐

4. Cross the patient's arms over the chest to avoid injury or interfering with a smooth transfer. ☐ ☐

5. Direct the second assistant supporting the pelvic girdle to stand on the opposite side of the cart, and make sure that the cart does not move away from the table during the transfer. ☐ ☐

6. On command, grasp the rolled up draw sheet and slowly pull the patient to the edge of the cart. On a second command, slowly lift and pull the patient onto the table. ☐ ☐

COMMENTS: _____
_____
_____

EVALUATOR'S SIGNATURE: _____

STUDENT'S SIGNATURE: _____

STUDENT NAME: _____ DATE: _____

LAB 14-1: IMMOBILIZATION DEVICES

Objective

- To demonstrate proper technique for patient immobilization

Equipment

- Oblique sponge
- Finger sponge
- Strap
- Compression bands
- Sandbags
- Head clamp

Procedure

- On completion of this laboratory activity, the student will be able to:

IMMOBILIZATION DEVICES	YES	NO
1. Position a patient with a sponge for an oblique lumbar spine position.	☐	☐
2. Position a patient's hand in a fan lateral position on a sponge.	☐	☐
3. Position a patient for an axial calcaneus position using a strap.	☐	☐
4. Position a patient on a table in a semierect position using compression bands.	☐	☐
5. Position a patient in an erect lateral cervical position using sandbags.	☐	☐
6. Position a patient for an anteroposterior (AP) skull radiograph using head clamps.	☐	☐

COMMENTS: _____

_____

_____

EVALUATOR'S SIGNATURE: _____

STUDENT'S SIGNATURE: _____

STUDENT NAME: _____ DATE: _____

LAB 14-2: PEDIATRIC IMMOBILIZATION TECHNIQUES

Objective

- To demonstrate proper techniques for pediatric immobilization

Equipment

- Pediatric patient or doll
- Sheet
- Pigg-O-Stat
- Velcro restraint board
- Octostop

Procedure

- On completion of this laboratory activity, the student will be able to:

MUMMIFICATION TECHNIQUE	YES	NO
1. Position the child in the center of a triangularly folded sheet so that the shoulders are just above the top fold.	☐	☐
2. Bring the left corner of the sheet over the left arm and under the body so that approximately 2 feet of the sheet extends beyond the right side of the body. Make sure the child is not lying on the left arm.	☐	☐
3. Tuck the 2 feet of sheet over the right arm and under the body. Again, make sure the child is not lying on the arm.	☐	☐
4. Bring the remaining sheet over the body, tucking the sheet securely under the left side of the body. Secure the sheet in place with tape.	☐	☐

USING SPECIALIZED PEDIATRIC IMMOBILIZATION DEVICES	YES	NO
1. Position a pediatric patient in a Pigg-O-Stat for an AP chest radiograph.	☐	☐
2. Position a pediatric patient on a Velcro strap restraint board.	☐	☐
3. Position a pediatric patient on an Octostop restraint board.	☐	☐

COMMENTS: _____

_____

EVALUATOR'S SIGNATURE: _____

STUDENT'S SIGNATURE: _____

STUDENT NAME: _____ DATE: _____

LAB 15-1: MONITORING PATIENT VITAL SIGNS

Objective

- To measure a patient's vital signs of temperature, pulse, respiration, and blood pressure

Equipment

- Thermometer
- Blood pressure kit

Procedure

- On completion of this laboratory activity, the student will be able to:

TEMPERATURE—ORAL METHOD	YES	NO
1. Place the oral thermometer under the patient's tongue.	☐	☐
2. Ensure that the thermometer is kept in place until a stable reading is obtained.	☐	☐
3. Read the oral thermometer, and record the reading.	☐	☐

RESPIRATION	YES	NO
1. Measure a patient's respiration by observing the patient's chest or abdomen for a 60-second period.	☐	☐
2. Record the number of respirations per minute.	☐	☐

PULSE	YES	NO
1. Measure a patient's pulse rate at the radial artery near the wrist for a 60-second period.	☐	☐
2. Record the patient's pulse rate per minute.	☐	☐

BLOOD PRESSURE	YES	NO
1. Obtain a sphygmomanometer and stethoscope.	☐	☐
2. Place the cuff of the sphygmomanometer on the patient's upper arm midway between the elbow and shoulder.	☐	☐
3. Inflate the cuff above the systolic pressure to stop blood flow to the arm.	☐	☐
4. With the stethoscope placed over the brachial artery in the antecubital fossa of the elbow, slowly release the cuff of the sphygmomanometer.	☐	☐
5. When the first sound of blood flow is heard through the stethoscope, record the systolic pressure reading.	☐	☐
6. When the sound of blood flowing through the arm ceases, record the diastolic pressure reading.	☐	☐

COMMENTS: _____

_____

_____

EVALUATOR'S SIGNATURE: _____

STUDENT'S SIGNATURE: _____

STUDENT NAME: _____ DATE: _____

LAB 16-1: PROPER HAND-WASHING TECHNIQUE

Objective

- To demonstrate proper hand-washing technique

Equipment

- Sink
- Soap
- Toweling

Procedure

- On completion of this laboratory activity, the student will be able to:

HAND WASHING	YES	NO
1. Approach the sink. Consider it to be contaminated. Avoid contact with clothing. Use foot or knee levels when available. If not, use toweling to handle all controls. Adjust water flow to avoid splashing. Adjust water temperature to comfort.	☐	☐
2. Wet hands thoroughly with water, keeping the hands lower than the elbows.	☐	☐
3. Apply soap. Soap should be available in liquid form and can be applied by using foot or knee levers. Soap can also be dispensed from a pump.	☐	☐
4. Use a firm, vigorous, rotary motion, beginning at the wrist and working toward the fingertips. Rub the palms, back of the hands, between the fingers, and under the nails.	☐	☐
5. Rinse and allow water to run down over hands.	☐	☐
6. Repeat the entire process to cleanse from the elbow to the fingertips.	☐	☐
7. Turn off the water. Use toweling on handles if foot or knee levers are not available.	☐	☐
8. Dry from the elbow to the fingertips, never returning to an area.	☐	☐

COMMENTS: _____

_____

_____

EVALUATOR'S SIGNATURE: _____

STUDENT'S SIGNATURE: _____

STUDENT NAME: _____ DATE: _____

LAB 16-2: CONTACT PRECAUTIONS TECHNIQUE

Objective

- To demonstrate the proper method for performing a radiographic examination on a patient with contact precautions

Equipment

- Cassettes and cassette bags
- Gowns, gloves, caps, masks, goggles
- Portable machine
- Lead aprons

Procedure

- On completion of this laboratory activity, the student will be able to:

CONTACT PRECAUTIONS	YES	NO
1. Determine the correct number of cassettes needed for the examination, and place each cassette into a protective bag.	☐	☐
2. Move the portable machine to the isolated room.	☐	☐
3. Locate the isolation supplies for the room.	☐	☐
4. Remove all ornamentation, including watch, rings, earrings, and other such items, and place them in a pocket.	☐	☐
5. Put on a lead apron.	☐	☐
6. Wash hands as described previously.	☐	☐
7. Put on a clean gown, making sure it is sufficiently long to cover most of the uniform. Pick up the gown from the inside near the armhole openings and gently shake it open. Put one arm in and then the other. First tie the neck strings, then tie the waist strings.	☐	☐
8. Put on a mask, tying it securely, and then a cap. Goggles may also be worn, if available.	☐	☐
9. Put on the gloves. These gloves should be clean but need not be sterile.	☐	☐
10. Direct an assistant to put on a lead apron, gown, gloves, and a cap.	☐	☐
11. Enter the isolated area and explain to the patient who you are and what you are doing.	☐	☐
12. Position the patient and the cassette.	☐	☐
13. Direct the assistant to manipulate the machine and make the exposure.	☐	☐
14. Remove the cassette from behind the patient. Fold the edge of the protective bag back, never touching the inside.	☐	☐
15. Direct the assistant to remove the cassette, never touching the outside. Place the covering into an appropriate container. Instruct the assistant to remove the portable equipment from the room.	☐	☐
16. Untie the waist ties of the gown.	☐	☐
17. Remove the gloves. Remove the first glove with the other gloved hand, never touching the inside of the glove. Grasp the top of the glove and pull it inside out. Remove the other glove with the exposed hand, touching the inside only. Discard into an appropriate container.	☐	☐
18. Remove the cap and then untie the mask ties, touching the ties only, and remove the mask.	☐	☐
19. Untie the neckties of the gown and pull the gown forward and down from the shoulders. Pull the gown off so that the sleeves are inside out and the front of the gown is folded inward. Avoid touching the front of the gown. Discard into an appropriate container.	☐	☐
20. Wash hands.	☐	☐
21. Direct the assistant to follow the same protocol. Clean the portable equipment with an antiseptic.	☐	☐
22. Wash hands one last time.	☐	☐

COMMENTS: _____

_____

_____

EVALUATOR'S SIGNATURE: _____

STUDENT'S SIGNATURE: _____

STUDENT NAME: _____ DATE: _____

LAB 17-1: OPENING A STERILE PACKAGE

Objective

- To demonstrate the proper technique for opening a sterile package

Equipment

- Sterile package and table

Procedure

- On completion of this laboratory activity, the student will be able to:

OPENING A STERILE PACKAGE ON A TABLE	YES	NO
1. Place the package on the center of the surface with the top flap of the wrapper set to open away from you.	☐	☐
2. Pinch the first flap on the outside of the wrapper between the thumb and index finger by reaching around (not over) the package. Pull the flap open and lay it flat on the far surface.	☐	☐

	YES	NO
3. Use the right hand to open the right flap and the left hand to open the left flap.	☐	☐
4. Grasp the turned-down corner, and pull the fourth and final flap down, being sure not to touch the inner surface of any of the package with an unsterile object such as a sleeve.	☐	☐

OPENING A STERILE PACKAGE WHILE HOLDING IT	YES	NO
1. Hold the package in one hand with the top flap opening away from you.	☐	☐
2. Pull the top flap well back, and hold it away from both the contents of the package and the sterile field.	☐	☐
3. Drop the contents gently onto the sterile field from approximately 6 inches above the field and at a slight angle, making sure that the package wrapping does not touch the sterile field at any time.	☐	☐

COMMENTS: _____

_____

_____

EVALUATOR'S SIGNATURE: _____

STUDENT'S SIGNATURE: _____

STUDENT NAME: _____ DATE: _____

LAB 17-2: STERILE GOWNING TECHNIQUE

Objective

- To demonstrate the proper sterile technique for self-gowning and for gowning another person

Equipment

- Surgical gown

Procedure

- On completion of this laboratory activity, the student will be able to:

SELF-GOWNING	YES	NO
1. Stand approximately 12 inches from the sterile area, pick up the gown by the folded edges, and lift it directly up from the package. The gown is folded so that the outside faces away.	☐	☐
2. Step back from the table, making sure no objects are near the gown. Holding the gown at the shoulders, allow it to unfold gently. Do not shake the gown.	☐	☐
3. Place the hands inside the armholes, and guide each arm through the sleeves by raising and spreading the arms.	☐	☐
4. Direct an unsterile assistant to stand behind and reach inside the sleeves, grasp the sleeves, and pull them gently to adjust the gown.	☐	☐
5. For the open technique of gloving, the sleeves are pulled over the hands. For the closed technique of gloving, keep the hands and fingers covered by the sterile gown.	☐	☐
6. Direct an assistant to fasten the back and waistband of the gown.	☐	☐

GOWNING ANOTHER PERSON	YES	NO
1. After gowning and gloving using sterile technique, pick up the sterile gown by the neck band, hold it at arm's length, and allow it to unfold.	☐	☐
2. Hold the gown by the shoulder seams with the outside facing the sterile person.	☐	☐
3. Protect the sterile gloves by placing both hands under the back panel of the gown's shoulder.	☐	☐
4. Direct the person being gowned to slip the arms into the sleeves in a downward motion, sliding the gown up to the mid upper arms.	☐	☐
5. A nonsterile circulator pulls the gown up and fastens the back and waistband of the gown.	☐	☐
6. Gently pull the cuff back over the person's hands being careful that your gloved hands do not touch the bare hands.	☐	☐

COMMENTS: _____

_____

_____

EVALUATOR'S SIGNATURE: _____

STUDENT'S SIGNATURE: _____

STUDENT NAME: _____ DATE: _____

LAB 17-3: STERILE GLOVING TECHNIQUE

Objective

- To demonstrate proper sterile technique for the closed and open methods of self-gloving and for gloving another person

Equipment

- Surgical gloves
- Surgical gown

Procedure

- On completion of this laboratory activity, the student will be able to:

SELF-GLOVING: CLOSED TECHNIQUE	YES	NO
1. Have an assistant open the glove package so that the right glove is on his or her right side.	☐	☐
2. After donning a sterile gown with the fingers still inside the cuff of the gown, pick up the glove and lay it palm-down over the cuff of the gown. The fingers of the glove face toward you.	☐	☐
3. Working through the gown sleeve, grasp the cuff of the glove and bring it over the open cuff of the sleeve.	☐	☐
4. Unroll the glove cuff so that it covers the sleeve cuff.	☐	☐
5. Pull the glove on by grasping the glove cuff and advancing the hand into the glove.	☐	☐
6. Proceed with the opposite hand, using the same technique. Never allow the bare hand to contact the gown cuff edge or outside of glove.	☐	☐
7. Adjust the fingers until comfortable.	☐	☐

SELF-GLOVING: OPEN TECHNIQUE	YES	NO
1. Pick up the glove by its inside cuff with one hand. Do not touch the outside surface of the glove or the glove wrapper.	☐	☐
2. Slide the glove onto the opposite bare hand, leaving the cuff down.	☐	☐
3. With the gloved (and now sterile) hand, pick up the other glove by reaching under the cuff, being sure to touch only the outside surface of the glove with the sterile gloved hand.	☐	☐
4. Pull the glove onto the hand without touching the inside surface of the glove, which is actually the outside surface of the folded cuff.	☐	☐

GLOVING ANOTHER PERSON	YES	NO
1. After gloving using sterile technique, open the sterile package, and pick up the right gloves, placing the palm away from the person. Slide the fingers under the glove cuff and spread them so that a wide opening is created. Keep the thumbs under the cuff.	☐	☐
2. The person thrusts his or her hand into the glove. Be sure to have an extremely good grasp on the cuff because considerable force will be exerted when the hand is pushed down into the tight glove.	☐	☐
3. Gently release the cuff while rolling it over the wrist.	☐	☐
4. Proceed with the left glove using the same technique.	☐	☐

COMMENTS: _____
_____
_____

EVALUATOR'S SIGNATURE: _____

STUDENT'S SIGNATURE: _____

STUDENT NAME: _____ DATE: _____

LAB 18-1: ASSISTING PATIENTS WITH A URINAL AND A BEDPAN

Objective

- To demonstrate proper technique for assisting a patient with a urinal and a bedpan

Equipment

- Urinal
- Bedpan
- Gloves

Procedure

- On completion of this laboratory activity, the student will be able to:

ASSISTING A PATIENT WITH A URINAL	YES	NO
1. Put on clean, disposable gloves, and raise the cover sheet sufficiently to permit adequate visibility while being careful not to expose the patient excessively.	☐	☐
2. Spread the patient's legs, and place the urinal between them. Place the penis into the urinal far enough so that it does not slip out, and hold the urinal in place by the handle until the patient finishes voiding.	☐	☐
3. Remove the urinal, empty it, remove the gloves, and wash hands.	☐	☐

ASSISTING A PATIENT WITH A BEDPAN	YES	NO
1. Remove the bedpan cover and place it at the end of the table.	☐	☐
2. If the patient is able to move, then place one hand under the lower back and ask the patient to raise the hips. Place the pan under the hips, being sure the patient is covered with a sheet.	☐	☐
3. Direct the patient to sit up, if possible, so that the head is elevated approximately 60 degrees.	☐	☐
4. When the patient has finished using the bedpan, put on clean, disposable gloves. Direct the patient to lie back. Place one hand under the lumbar area, and instruct the patient to raise up at the hips.	☐	☐
5. Remove the pan, cover it, and empty it in the designated area. Rinse it thoroughly with cold water, and return it to the area where used equipment is placed.	☐	☐
6. Offer the patient a wet paper towel or washcloth to wash hands and a paper towel to dry them. Remove the gloves and wash hands.	☐	☐

COMMENTS: _____
_____
_____

EVALUATOR'S SIGNATURE: _____

STUDENT'S SIGNATURE: _____

STUDENT NAME: _____ DATE: _____

LAB 19-1: THE HEIMLICH MANEUVER

Objective

- To simulate the Heimlich maneuver on a conscious adult, an unconscious adult, a pregnant victim, and an infant

Equipment

- None

Procedure

- On completion of this laboratory activity, the student will be able to:

CONSCIOUS ADULT	YES	NO
1. Assess the victim to determine whether he or she is choking.	☐	☐
2. Stand behind the victim, and wrap both arms around him or her, clutching one fist with the other hand.	☐	☐
3. Place the thumb side of the fist at the midline of the victim's abdomen, above the navel and well below the sternum.	☐	☐
4. Hold the elbows out from the victim, and exert pressure inward and upward.	☐	☐
5. Administer each thrust separately, repeating the procedure quickly six to ten times or until the obstructing object is expelled.	☐	☐

UNCONSCIOUS ADULT	YES	NO
1. Place the unconscious patient in the supine position.	☐	☐
2. Kneel astride the victim, and place the heel of one hand in the midline of the abdomen, above the navel, and well below the sternum. Place the second hand directly on top of the first and apply pressure in a quick upward thrust.	☐	☐

	YES	NO
3. Repeat the procedure until the obstructing object is expelled.	☐	☐

PREGNANT VICTIM	YES	NO
1. Stand behind the pregnant victim, placing both arms under the victim's armpits and around the victim's chest. Place the thumb side of the fist in the center of the sternum and the second hand over the fist.	☐	☐
2. Apply backward thrusts until the obstructing object is expelled.	☐	☐

INFANT VICTIM	YES	NO
1. Hold the infant along your arm with the head lower than the trunk, and support the infant by holding the jaw.	☐	☐
2. Rest the arm holding the infant on your thigh, and, using the heel of the hand, deliver four back blows between the infant's scapulae.	☐	☐
3. Continue to support the head and neck, and turn the infant over.	☐	☐
4. Place the index finger on the sternum just below the intermammary line. Using two or three fingers, deliver four chest thrusts.	☐	☐
5. Alternately repeat back blows and chest thrusts until the obstructing object is expelled.	☐	☐

COMMENTS: _____

_____

_____

EVALUATOR'S SIGNATURE: _____

STUDENT'S SIGNATURE: _____

STUDENT NAME: _____ DATE: _____

LAB 20-1: FILLING A SYRINGE FROM AN AMPULE AND A VIAL

Objective

- To demonstrate proper technique for filling a syringe from an ampule and a vial

Equipment

- Glass ampule
- Vial
- Syringe
- Needle

Procedure

- On completion of this laboratory activity, the student will be able to:

FILLING A SYRINGE FROM A GLASS AMPULE	YES	NO
1. Direct an assistant to flick the top of the neck of the ampule until all the liquid is at the bottom of the container.	☐	☐
2. Direct the assistant to snap off the top of the ampule with a gauze pad.	☐	☐
3. Open a syringe package. Open a needle package and insert the needle on the end of the syringe without letting the end of the syringe or the end of the needle touch anything but each other.	☐	☐
4. Withdraw the contents of the ampule, being careful not to let the shaft of the needle touch the broken edge of the ampule.	☐	☐
5. After use, dispose of the ampule, syringe, and needle into an acceptable *sharps* biohazard container.	☐	☐

FILLING A SYRINGE FROM A VIAL	YES	NO
1. Break the seal, expose the rubber stopper, and wipe the stopper with an alcohol swab.	☐	☐
2. Open a syringe package, and pull back the syringe plunger to pull air into the syringe equal to the amount of drug that will be withdrawn from the vial.	☐	☐
3. Open a needle package, and insert the needle on the end of the syringe without letting the end of the syringe or the end of the needle touch anything but each other.	☐	☐
4. Invert the vial, and, with the dominant hand, insert the needle without letting the tip of the needle touch anything but the rubber stopper of the vial.	☐	☐
5. With the tip of the needle in the fluid, inject air equal to the volume of drug to be removed. Pull back on the plunger until the correct amount of drug has been drawn into the syringe.	☐	☐
6. Remove the needle, and hold the syringe with the needle pointing up while tapping it with a finger to move any air bubble toward the hub where it can be expelled by gently pushing on the plunger of the syringe.	☐	☐
7. After use, dispose of entire syringe and needle into an acceptable *sharps* biohazard container.	☐	☐

COMMENTS: _____
_____
_____

EVALUATOR'S SIGNATURE: _____

STUDENT'S SIGNATURE: _____

STUDENT NAME: _____ DATE: _____

LAB 20-2: PREPARING A DRIP INFUSION SETUP

Objective

- To demonstrate the proper technique for setting up a drip infusion set

Equipment

- Intravenous (IV) pole
- Drip infusion set
- Saline solution bag

Procedure

- On completion of this laboratory activity, the student will be able to:

PREPARING A DRIP INFUSION SETUP	YES	NO
1. Remove the administration set from the box, and straighten the tubing while checking for any cracks or holes.	☐	☐
2. Slide the clamp up to the drip chamber and close it.	☐	☐
3. Place the bag on a hard surface, remove the protective cap from the tubing insertion port on the bag, and wipe it with an alcohol sponge.	☐	☐
4. Remove the protective cap from the spike on the drip chamber of the tubing, and insert the spike into the port.	☐	☐
5. Check again to make certain the clamp is closed, hang the bag on the IV pole, and squeeze the drip chamber until it is one-half full.	☐	☐
6. Prime the IV setup by removing the protective cap from the end of the tubing and holding it over a sink or wastebasket.	☐	☐
7. Taking care to preserve the sterility of the cap and of the end of the tubing, release the clamp and allow the solution to run freely until all air bubbles are cleared from the tubing.	☐	☐
8. Reclamp the tubing to stop the flow, and replace the protective cap over the end of the tubing.	☐	☐

COMMENTS: _____

_____

_____

EVALUATOR'S SIGNATURE: _____

STUDENT'S SIGNATURE: _____

STUDENT NAME: _____ DATE: _____

LAB 20-3: VENIPUNCTURE AND INTRAVENOUS DRUG INJECTION

Objective

- To demonstrate the proper technique for venipuncture and intravenous drug injection

Equipment

- Disposable gloves
- Butterfly needle
- Syringe
- Venipuncture training arm kit

Procedure

- On completion of this laboratory activity, the student will be able to:

VENIPUNCTURE AND IV DRUG INJECTION	YES	NO
1. Wash hands thoroughly.	☐	☐
2. Check the patient's identification.	☐	☐
3. Explain the procedure to the patient.	☐	☐
4. Assemble all needed supplies, and prepare the drug for administration.	☐	☐
5. Put on disposable gloves.	☐	☐
6. Once an appropriate site for venipuncture has been selected, cleanse it with an alcohol swab, using a circular motion while moving from the center to the outside.	☐	☐
7. Apply a tourniquet above the site using sufficient tension to impede the flow of blood in the vein. Ask the patient to open and close the fist to distend the vein fully. When the vein has been identified, ask the patient to hold the fist in a clenched position.	☐	☐
8. To stabilize the vein, place the thumb on the tissue just below the site, and gently pull the skin and vein toward the hand.	☐	☐
9. Hold the needle with the bevel facing upward. Pinch the wings of the butterfly needle together tightly.	☐	☐
10. Insert the needle next to the vein at a 15-degree angle, and gently advance it into the vein. Blood will flow back into the tubing when the needle is correctly positioned.	☐	☐
11. If the tubing of the butterfly needle has not previously been filled with solution, then allow the blood to flow from the hub before attaching the syringe to ensure that no air bubbles are contained in the system.	☐	☐
12. Remove the tourniquet and inject the drug.	☐	☐
13. Unless otherwise instructed, remove the needle, and apply gentle pressure to the site with an alcohol swab.	☐	☐
14. Dispose of the syringe and needle properly.	☐	☐
15. Chart all relevant information.	☐	☐

COMMENTS: _____

_____

_____

EVALUATOR'S SIGNATURE: _____

STUDENT'S SIGNATURE: _____

Review Questions
and Patient Care
Lab Activities
Review Questions

CHAPTER 1

1. The term used to describe energy transmitted through matter is
   a. ionization
   b. physiology
   c. radiation
   d. therapy

2. Special protection should be taken to prevent excessive exposure to
   a. energy
   b. electromagnetic energy
   c. ionizing radiation
   d. radio waves

3. Which of the following specialties uses a nonionizing form of radiation?
   a. nuclear medicine technology
   b. radiation therapy
   c. radiography
   d. sonography

4. The discovery of x-rays occurred in
   a. 1858
   b. 1876
   c. 1895
   d. 1898

5. An individual who specializes in using x-rays to create images of the body is known as a
   a. diagnostic medical sonographer
   b. nuclear medicine technologist
   c. radiographer
   d. radiation therapist

6. An effective treatment of atherosclerosis that uses a special catheter with a balloon tip is termed
   a. angiography
   b. angioplasty
   c. arteriography
   d. cardiac catheterization

7. A discipline that visualizes sectional anatomy by the recording of a predetermined plane in the body is
   a. computed tomography
   b. cardiovascular interventional technology
   c. nuclear medicine technology
   d. radiation therapy

8. Radiography of the breast is termed
   a. angiography
   b. cytotechnology
   c. histology
   d. mammography

9. The study of diseases of muscles and bones is termed
   a. neurology
   b. orthopedics
   c. oncology
   d. urology

10. An individual who specializes in carrying out treatments designed to correct or improve the function of a particular body part or system is known as a
    a. diagnostician
    b. histologist
    c. technologist
    d. therapist

CHAPTER 2

1. Which of the following is a voluntary process through which an agency grants recognition to an individual on demonstration, usually by examination, of specialized professional skills?
   a. accreditation
   b. certification
   c. licensure
   d. registration

2. Which of the following is a listing of individuals holding certification in a particular profession?
   a. accreditation
   b. certification
   c. licensure
   d. registry

3. What organization certifies individuals in radiography?
   a. American Society of Radiologic Technologists
   b. American Registry of Radiologic Technologists
   c. Joint Review Committee on Education in Radiologic Technology
   d. Radiological Society of North America

4. Which of the following organizations represents the interests of radiologic technologists to the public and federal government?
   a. American Registry of Radiologic Technologists
   b. American Society of Radiologic Technologists
   c. International Society of Radiographers and Radiologic Technologists
   d. American Roentgen Ray Society

5. What purpose is served by the *Standards* document for a profession?
   a. It sets the legal and ethical standards for a profession.
   b. It determines the minimum standards for an individual to become certified by a registry organization.
   c. It establishes the sponsorship of a joint review committee.
   d. It specifies the requirements for accreditation of an educational program by a joint review committee.

6. Which of the following is the process by which a governmental agency (usually at the state level) grants permission to individuals to practice their profession?
   a. accreditation
   b. certification
   c. licensure
   d. registration

7. Which title is granted to a radiographer after successful completion of the American Registry of Radiologic Technologist's examination in radiography?
   a. radiologic technologist
   b. radiologic technologist, radiographer
   c. registered technologist
   d. registered technologist, radiographer

8. Which of the following organizations is a sponsor of the Joint Review Committee on Education in Radiologic Technology and the American Registry of Radiologic Technologists?
   a. Society of Nuclear Medicine
   b. American Society of Radiologic Technologists
   c. American Healthcare Radiology Administrators
   d. Radiological Society of North America

9. Which of the following is a voluntary peer process through which an agency grants recognition to an institution for a program of study that meets specified criteria?
   a. accreditation
   b. certification
   c. licensure
   d. registration

10. Approximately how many individuals are registered by the American Registry of Radiologic Technologists?
    a. 10,000
    b. 100,000
    c. 200,000
    d. 250,000

CHAPTER 3

1. Stress is defined as
   a. a feeling of anxiety and fear
   b. not having enough time to complete commitments
   c. a breaking point
   d. demand on time, energy, and resources with some threat included

2. Causes of stress include
   a. individual perception of wants
   b. poor physical health
   c. lack of time management
   d. all of the above

3. The best ways to reduce stress are by
   a. managing finances better and saving money
   b. controlling time, thinking positively, and buffering stressors
   c. choosing a nonmedical profession and vacationing often
   d. avoiding worry and practicing relaxation

4. When taking a test, always
   a. cram the night before.
   b. arrive early and review notes just before the test.
   c. answer all questions you know first, then go back and repeat, leaving the most difficult questions for last.
   d. review your test, but do not change answers.

5. In-control language
   a. is used when driving to class
   b. is positive and expresses choice
   c. identifies where others are wrong
   d. is critical and powerful

6. The biggest thief of time is
   a. indecision
   b. worry
   c. traffic
   d. mistakes

7. When managing time, practice self-management, which includes which of the following?
   a. setting your alarm and limiting telephone calls
   b. doing only the important tasks
   c. prioritizing, setting limits, and providing for self-care
   d. avoiding worry

8. Good study habits include
   a. reading out loud and writing down important facts
   b. planned group activity
   c. a regular plan for study and review
   d. all of the above

9. Stress buffers include
   a. exercise and good nutrition
   b. taking a personal day off work
   c. avoiding study the night before a test
   d. avoiding worry

10. Vitamins and minerals depleted as a result of stress are
    a. iron, B_{12}, and C
    b. B complex, C, and magnesium
    c. magnesium, E, and B complex
    d. A, E, and C

CHAPTER 4

1. Students in medical professions often learn to apply theories through the review of a real life situation or scenario. What is this activity called?
   a. code review
   b. case study
   c. role playing
   d. laboratory practice

2. What is the term for a new work or understanding that is created through the combination of multiple areas of knowledge?
   a. affective
   b. critique
   c. analysis
   d. synthesis

3. Which of the following is (are) characteristic of professional critical thinking?
   a. sound professional judgment
   b. uncomfortable and challenging decision making
   c. quick and inventive response
   d. action based on professional knowledge and experience
   e. all of the above

4. What is the first step involved in problem solving associated with critical thinking?
   a. Identify and clarify the problem.
   b. Remove yourself from the situation.
   c. Brainstorm all possible solutions.
   d. Analyze how the problem affects you personally.

5. The second step involved in problem solving associated with critical thinking is to undergo an objective examination of the problem. What element(s) of this step is (are) reflected below?
   a. implications of the problem
   b. safety risks and potential liability
   c. technical considerations
   d. number and type or types of solutions required
   e. all of the above

6. What is the primary factor in determining the solution to the problem in critical thinking?
   a. the solution that gives the most profit for the healthcare institution
   b. the solution that most closely resembles what the most experienced radiologic science profession in the department would do
   c. the solution that results in the least damage to your reputation
   d. the solution that provides the best outcome for the patient

7. In what aspect of the education program for a radiologic science professional is the student exposed to real-life experiences that allow him or her to transfer knowledge into action?
   a. cognitive
   b. classroom
   c. laboratory
   d. clinical

8. Which of the following statements is true regarding the clinical setting?
   a. All clinical sites operate in a nearly identical manner.
   b. Standard procedures taught in the classroom will match all experiences in the clinical setting.
   c. All patients will easily conform to the standards taught in the textbooks.
   d. Each radiologic science professional has his or her own style based on education and experience.

9. Analyzing personal values and feelings and managing uncomfortable ethical situations are components of what type of critical thinking?
   a. affective
   b. cognitive
   c. psychomotor
   d. technical

10. Which of the following describes a situation in which technical critical thinking skills are required?
    a. A patient arrives for a routine procedure and asks questions.
    b. A female patient responds that she is pregnant before a procedure.
    c. A male patient requests that he be permitted to go to the bathroom before the procedure.
    d. A trauma patient has a broken femur, and specialized hip radiographs are required.

CHAPTER 5

1. Clinical procedures and activities are performed in what setting?
   a. classroom
   b. hospital
   c. laboratory
   d. library

2. Cognitive learning includes
   a. attitudes, values, and beliefs
   b. physical actions, neuromuscular manipulations, and coordination
   c. assistance, observation, and performance
   d. knowledge, reason, and judgment

3. A qualified practitioner directly supervises a student radiographer by
   a. reviewing the request in relation to the student's achievement
   b. evaluating the condition of the patient in relation to the student's knowledge
   c. being present while the student conducts the examination
   d. reviewing and approving the procedure
   e. all of the above

4. A student's unsatisfactory radiographs must be repeated in the presence of a qualified practitioner because
   a. students are not instructed in how to repeat images.
   b. quality patient care and protection from radiation must be ensured and provided.
   c. the qualified practitioner is responsible for all unsatisfactory radiographs.
   d. patient preference mandates it.

5. Which program official often provides one-on-one instruction and evaluation of students?
   a. radiologist
   b. radiation safety officer
   c. clinical instructor
   d. didactic instructor

6. Which program official is responsible for the overall organization, administration, and assessment of the radiography program?
   a. program director
   b. clinical coordinator
   c. clinical instructor
   d. none of the above

7. Disciplinary action may be initiated if a student commits which serious infraction?
   a. disclosure of confidential information
   b. falsification of records
   c. cheating
   d. intoxication
   e. all of the above

8. An instructor may use which format to measure cognitive behaviors?
   a. rating scale
   b. critical incident form
   c. anecdotal note
   d. multiple-choice test
   e. none of the above

9. Affective behaviors influence a person's ability to
   a. comprehend
   b. analyze
   c. synthesize
   d. evaluate
   e. none of the above

10. If a radiography student is to perform radiologic procedures competently, he or she must always
    a. observe a qualified radiographer
    b. develop and refine the appropriate skills and behaviors
    c. help the radiologist as much as possible
    d. simulate as many radiographic procedures as possible

CHAPTER 6

1. The driving and guiding force that outlines the reason for the existence of a hospital is its
   a. chief executive officer
   b. medical director
   c. mission statement
   d. adherence to the Joint Commission on the Accreditation of Healthcare Organizations

2. The board of directors employs _____, who interacts with the medical staff to ensure coordination and quality of patient care and services.
   a. an insurance agent
   b. a radiology chairman
   c. a vice president of nursing
   d. a president or chief executive officer

3. Forces causing hospitals to reorganize include
   a. state regulators
   b. economic hardships
   c. total quality management
   d. the Joint Commission on the Accreditation of Healthcare Organizations

4. When an organization focuses on quality or patient safety, it
   a. undergoes a cultural revolution
   b. prohibits employees from participating in groups
   c. encourages employees to focus on one department to the exclusion of others
   d. lowers workers' perceptions of patient or physician expectations

5. The management function that charts a course of action for the future to enable coordinated and consistent fulfillment of goals and objectives is
   a. coordinating
   b. planning
   c. communicating
   d. setting goals

6. The management function that involves the development of a structure or framework that identifies how people do their work is
   a. staffing
   b. planning
   c. organizing
   d. coordinating

7. The management function that involves getting the right people to do the work and developing their abilities is
   a. staffing
   b. organizing
   c. directing
   d. describing

8. Performance standards or guidelines used to measure progress toward the goals of the organizations are defined as
   a. employee evaluations
   b. feedback
   c. controlling
   d. the Joint Commission on the Accreditation of Healthcare Organizations guidelines

9. The internal hospital committee that ensures safe operations for the facility for both patients and employers is the
   a. safety committee
   b. certificate of need
   c. hazardous chemicals group
   d. radiation safety committee

10. Besides acquiring a strong knowledge of technical skills, a radiologic technology student should develop
    a. a broad range of procedural abilities
    b. referrals of patients from physicians
    c. skills in magnetic resonance imaging, computed tomography, ultrasonography, and nuclear medicine
    d. superior skills in interactive relationships

CHAPTER 7

1. The process by which a beam of x-ray photons is altered as it passes through matter is known as
   a. density
   b. attenuation
   c. fog
   d. processing

2. The beam of radiation as it exits the x-ray tube and before it reaches the patient is
   a. primary radiation
   b. scatter
   c. remnant radiation
   d. potential difference

3. The chief controlling factor of radiographic contrast is
   a. milliampere seconds (mAs)
   b. source-to-image distance (SID)
   c. object-to-image distance (OID)
   d. kilovoltage peak

4. What mAs value would result using the 500 mA setting at 0.25 second?
   a. 12.5 mAs
   b. 20 mAs
   c. 125 mAs
   d. 2000 mAs

5. Which of the following sets of technical factors would produce the greatest radiographic density or image receptor exposure?
   a. 300 mA, $\frac{1}{10}$ sec, 36 inch SID
   b. 200 mA, $\frac{1}{10}$ sec, 40 inch SID
   c. 100 mA, $\frac{1}{10}$ sec, 40 inch SID
   d. 200 mA, $\frac{1}{10}$ sec, 72 inch SID

6. A radiograph is made using 40 mAs at a 40 inch SID. If the image must be repeated at a 72 inch SID, what mAs value is necessary to maintain the same exposure?
   a. 12 mAs
   b. 13 mAs
   c. 120 mAs
   d. 130 mAs

7. The 15% rule helps explain the effect of _____ on exposure.
   a. grids
   b. mAs
   c. SID
   d. kilovoltage peak

8. Which of the following is *not* a radiographic contrast medium?
   a. barium compounds
   b. air
   c. iodine compounds
   d. water

9. The most common cause of radiographic unsharpness is
   a. motion
   b. material unsharpness
   c. increased OID
   d. decreased SID

10. Which of the following uses *x-radiation* to produce a digital computer image?
    a. ultrasonography
    b. nuclear medicine
    c. computed tomography
    d. magnetic resonance imaging

CHAPTER 8

1. The device that produces radiation is the
   a. collimator
   b. Bucky tray
   c. x-ray tube
   d. cassette

2. The component that gives the operator control of the exposure factors (technique) is the
   a. control console
   b. fluoroscope
   c. spot image device
   d. x-ray tube

3. Milliamperage is usually selectable in increments of
   a. 10
   b. 100
   c. 250
   d. 500

4. The primary components of the x-ray tube are
   a. kilovoltage peak and milliamperage
   b. milliamperage and time
   c. diode and triode
   d. anode and cathode

5. The component that controls the size and shape of the x-ray field is the
   a. x-ray tube
   b. collimator
   c. anode
   d. spot image device

6. The device that holds the x-ray cassette in place under the x-ray table is the
   a. Bucky tray
   b. foot switch
   c. wall-mounted Bucky unit
   d. grid

7. The control that permits x-rays to be produced is
   a. kilovoltage peak
   b. milliamperage
   c. rotor-exposure
   d. timer

8. The component that supports and permits the x-ray tube to be moved in different directions is the
   a. tube stand
   b. Bucky mechanism
   c. spot image device
   d. collimator

9. Pivoting the x-ray tube at the point at which it is attached to its support is
   a. collimation
   b. vertical travel
   c. coning
   d. tube angulation

10. The component that allows the radiologist to take radiographs during a fluoroscopic procedure is the
    a. spot image device
    b. collimator
    c. cassette
    d. control console

CHAPTER 9

1. Which of the following is not necessary for x-rays to be produced?
   a. a source of electrons
   b. rapid particle acceleration
   c. a source of protons
   d. instantaneous deceleration

2. For pair production to occur, the energy of the incoming x-ray photon must be at least
   a. 10 keV
   b. 1.02 keV
   c. 10 MeV
   d. 1.02 MeV

3. The interaction of x-rays with matter that constitutes the greatest hazard to patients in diagnostic radiography is
   a. photoelectric interaction
   b. Compton interaction
   c. classic coherent scattering
   d. pair production

4. The unit used to measure the amount of energy absorbed in any medium is the
   a. radiation equivalent man (rem)
   b. radiation absorbed dose (rad)
   c. roentgen
   d. sievert

5. The maximum accumulated whole-body dose for a 35-year-old occupational worker is
   a. 85 rem
   b. 5 rem
   c. 35 rem
   d. 0.5 rem

6. According to the law of Bergonie and Tribondeau, the characteristics that determine the sensitivity of a cell to radiation are
   a. mitotic activity and metabolic function
   b. metabolic function and cell type
   c. mitotic activity and structure and function of the cell
   d. cell type and life span of the cell

7. The intensity of radiation from a radiographic tube was 35 mR at a distance of 2.5 m from the tube. What would the intensity be at a distance of 4 m from the tube, all other factors remaining the same?
   a. 5.5 mR
   b. 55 mR
   c. 14 mR
   d. 90 mR

8. Which of the following is not a component of an optically stimulated luminescence (OSL) dosimeter?
   a. exposure meter
   b. plastic blister pack
   c. aluminum oxide strip
   d. metal filters

9. The type of shielding device that is attached to the side of the collimator on a radiographic tube is a
   a. flat contact shield
   b. detachable shield
   c. shaped contact shield
   d. shadow shield

10. When ionizing radiation interacts with the suspending medium of the cell, it is termed a
    a. direct-hit interaction
    b. indirect-hit interaction
    c. target interaction
    d. random interaction

CHAPTER 10

1. Human diversity consists of characteristics associated with
   a. age
   b. ethnicity
   c. gender
   d. lifestyle
   e. all of the above

2. Individuals born between 1981 and 1995 are generally referred to as
   a. the baby boom generation
   b. generation X
   c. generation Y
   d. the lost generation

3. Over the next three decades, which of the following age groups is expected to be the fastest-growing segment of the population?
   a. 35+
   b. 55+
   c. 65+
   d. 75+
   e. 85+

4. Which one of the following does not relate to a person's ethnicity?
   a. dress
   b. language
   c. religion
   d. race

5. Which of the following is not one of the ways that culturally different individuals have interacted with the U.S. majority culture in the past?
   a. assimilation
   b. biculturalism
   c. multiculturalism
   d. a and b
   e. b and c

6. Government statutes to protect people from discrimination are based on
   a. ethnicity or race
   b. disability
   c. age
   d. all of the above
   e. none of the above

7. Sexual orientation regards an individual's designation as any of the following *except*
   a. asexuality
   b. bisexuality
   c. heterosexuality
   d. homosexuality

8. Approximately what percentage of world's population has some type of disability?
   a. 5
   b. 10
   c. 15
   d. 20

9. Which of the following is considered the most profound step that the United States has ever undertaken to prevent discrimination toward people with a disability?
   a. The Civil Rights Act of 1964
   b. The Rehabilitation Act of 1973
   c. The Americans with Disabilities Act of 1990
   d. The Human Rights Declaration of 1999

10. Of the following, which one is not considered an element that may contribute to the ability of an organization to become culturally competent?
    a. valuing diversity
    b. institutionalizing cultural knowledge
    c. possessing the capacity for cultural self-assessment
    d. ignoring cultural norms and values
    e. developing of adaptations for the delivery of services that reflect an understanding of a multicultural environment

CHAPTER 11

1. The highest level of Maslow's hierarchy of needs is
   a. self-actualization
   b. belonging
   c. physiologic
   d. self-esteem

2. The word *ambulatory* means that the patient
   a. must be confined to a wheelchair
   b. must be moved by ambulance
   c. can be moved by stretcher
   d. can walk

3. Which of the following would you not want to discuss with a patient?
   a. hobbies
   b. medical chart
   c. ability to walk
   d. weather

4. Questions about the diagnosis of an examination from a patient or visitor are best answered by
   a. explaining that only a radiologist can read radiographs
   b. providing the best diagnosis available
   c. explaining that the results are not available yet
   d. suggesting that the question is inappropriate

5. Which method is effective in communicating with a patient?
   1. professional appearance
   2. touch
   3. pantomime techniques
      a. 1 only
      b. 1 and 2 only
      c. 2 and 3 only
      d. 1, 2, and 3

6. When is touching a patient valuable?
   a. for emotional support
   b. for emphasis
   c. for palpation
   d. all of the above

7. Which of the following characterize the development of a toddler (1 to 3 years of age)?
   a. understands simple abstractions
   b. is unable to understand more than one word for something
   c. is unable to take the viewpoint of another
   d. all of the above

8. Of the changes that occur in geriatric patients that are especially important when patients are undergoing radiologic examinations, which of the following may produce patient paranoia about potential falls with potential for permanent loss of mobility?
   a. osteoporotic loss of bone mass
   b. arthritis
   c. decreased muscle strength
   d. atrophied muscle mass

9. Which of the following is considered to be the first stage of acceptance of dying for a terminally ill patient?
   a. anger
   b. frustration
   c. denial and isolation
   d. shock

10. Which of the following permits the patient to begin to work through the various stages that precede dying?
    a. suspicious awareness
    b. mutual pretense
    c. open awareness
    d. all of the above

CHAPTER 12

1. Which of the following is undesirable for conducting a clinical history interview?
   a. clarifying terminology
   b. asking open-ended questions
   c. asking vague questions
   d. repeating information

2. Which of the following includes a description of the color, quantity, and consistency of blood or other body substances?
   a. localization
   b. chronology
   c. quality
   d. occurrence

3. Which of the following is the determination of a precise area, usually through gentle palpation or careful wording of questions?
   a. localization
   b. chronology
   c. quality
   d. occurrence

4. Which of the following is (are) usually Included as part of the chronology of a clinical history?
   a. onset
   b. duration
   c. frequency
   d. all of the above

5. Which of the following includes the tone of voice, the speed of speech, and the position of the speaker's extremities and torso?
   a. nonverbal communication
   b. palpation
   c. quality
   d. facilitation

6. What term describes the primary medical problem as defined by the patient?
   a. chief complaint
   b. palpation
   c. onset
   d. nonverbal communication

7. Which of the following describes an undesirable method of questioning that provides information that may direct the answer toward a suspected symptom or complaint?
   a. facilitation
   b. palpation
   c. nonverbal communication
   d. leading question

8. Which of the following is (are) part of the *sacred seven* elements of the patient clinical history?
   a. localization
   b. aggravating factors
   c. quality
   d. all of the above

9. Which of the following is (are) desirable method(s) of conducting a clinical history interview?
   a. positive nonverbal communication
   b. defining and specifying terms
   c. subjectiveness
   d. a and b

10. Which term describes gentle touching to determine the precise location of a symptom or complaint?
    a. nonverbal communication
    b. palpation
    c. quality
    d. facilitation

CHAPTER 13

1. Which of the following is the foundation on which a body rests?
   a. center of gravity
   b. base of support
   c. orthostatic hypotension
   d. biomechanics

2. What term is used to describe the drop in blood pressure some patients experience when they stand up quickly?
   a. center of gravity
   b. base of support
   c. orthostatic hypotension
   d. a and b

3. Where is the human center of gravity located?
   a. at the center of the diaphragm
   b. within 1 to 2 inches of the umbilicus
   c. midway between the hip joints
   d. at approximately sacral level two

4. Which of the following transfers can be used to move a patient from a wheelchair to an examination table?
   a. pivot
   b. assisted standing
   c. standby assist
   d. all of the above

5. Toward which side should all transfers be initiated?
   a. left
   b. right
   c. patient's weak side
   d. patient's strong side

6. What causes patients to feel lightheaded, queasy, or faint when they stand up quickly from a sitting or supine position?
   a. increased respiration from the effort of standing
   b. decreased blood pressure
   c. increased body temperature
   d. increased pulse rate

7. What term describes the hypothetical point around which all mass appears to be concentrated?
   a. center of gravity
   b. base of support
   c. orthostatic hypotension
   d. a and b

8. If a patient arrives in a wheelchair and on a sling, which type of transfer is indicated?
   a. hydraulic lift
   b. pivot
   c. standby assist
   d. cart to table by means of a moving device

9. How can the base of support be increased?
   a. standing on one toe
   b. standing on one foot
   c. standing with the legs far apart
   d. bending the knees with the feet together

10. What is the minimum number of persons to use for a cart-to-table transfer when no moving devices are available?
    a. one
    b. two
    c. three
    d. four

CHAPTER 14

1. Voluntary motion is under the control of the
   a. technologist
   b. patient
   c. radiologist
   d. student

2. The most important communication that occurs in a radiology department takes place between the radiographer and the
   a. administrator
   b. patient
   c. radiologist
   d. student

3. A key component to effective communication with a patient is
   a. establishing rapport
   b. assessing the patient's physical condition
   c. introducing the patient to the radiologist
   d. giving a detailed, technical explanation of the examination

4. What is the most commonly used immobilization device?
   a. sheet restraint
   b. cervical collar
   c. positioning sponge
   d. Velcro straps

5. Which of the following might be used to immobilize a patient for an upright lateral chest radiograph?
   a. sandbags
   b. Velcro straps
   c. head clamps
   d. positioning sponge

6. Which of the following is an example of a spinal trauma immobilization device?
   a. air splint
   b. antishock garment
   c. traction splint
   d. backboard

7. When is removing a cervical collar permissible?
   a. before the initial radiographic examination
   b. after a radiographer makes the exposure
   c. at the conclusion of the entire examination
   d. after a paramedic reads the radiograph and approves removal

8. Which of the following devices might a radiographer encounter when hemorrhage is thought to exist as a result of pelvic trauma?
   a. air splint
   b. compression band
   c. antishock garment
   d. traction splint

9. The Pigg-O-Stat is an immobilization device used for which examination?
   a. upper extremity
   b. pelvis
   c. skull
   d. chest

10. One of the greatest fears of a geriatric patient is
    a. falling
    b. being unable to hear the radiographer
    c. having to lie on a radiolucent pad
    d. getting lost on the way to the radiology department

CHAPTER 15

1. A patient arrives to the emergency department with an oral temperature of 39.38°C. This finding is consistent with
   a. normal temperature
   b. hyperthermia
   c. hypothermia
   d. bradypnea

2. A patient is thought to have suffered cardiac arrest. The pulse should be checked at the
   a. radial artery
   b. brachial artery
   c. carotid artery
   d. femoral artery

3. In the healthy adult the normal range for blood pressure is
   a. systolic less than 95 mm Hg, diastolic less than 60 mm Hg
   b. systolic less than 60 mm Hg, diastolic greater than 95 mm Hg
   c. systolic less than 120 mm Hg, diastolic less than 80 mm Hg
   d. systolic less than 80 mm Hg, diastolic greater than 120 mm Hg

4. Hypoxia is
   a. a drug that must be prescribed by a physician
   b. necessary for cellular repair
   c. a state describing oxygen-deficient tissue
   d. necessary for cellular function

5. Which of the following devices can be classified as a high-flow oxygen delivery device?
   a. air-entrainment mask
   b. nasal cannula
   c. simple mask
   d. nonrebreathing mask

6. Regarding oxygen delivery, all of the following are true *except*
   a. Oxygen dose is ordered in liters per minute or in concentration as a fractional concentration of oxygen.
   b. The maximum dose should always be given to obtain the desired results.
   c. The oxygen flowmeter is green in color.
   d. The regulator attached to the oxygen tank consists of a flowmeter and pressure manometer.

7. Oxygen therapy is administered to
   a. minimize cardiopulmonary workload
   b. counteract hypoxemia
   c. treat tissue hypoxia
   d. all of the above

8. A properly placed endotracheal tube will be radiographically confirmed when the
   a. distal tip is positioned 1 inch inferior to the tracheal bifurcation
   b. distal tip is positioned 1 inch superior to the tracheal bifurcation
   c. distal tip is positioned adjacent to the vocal folds
   d. cuff is positioned between the vocal folds

9. Thoracostomy tubes are
   a. used to monitor pulmonary arterial pressures
   b. central venous lines used to administer parenteral nutrition
   c. chest tubes used to drain the intrapleural space
   d. used to administer oxygen with mechanical ventilators

10. Which of the following is a common complication associated with central venous line placement?
    a. pneumothorax
    b. pleural effusion
    c. atelectasis
    d. tracheal erosion

CHAPTER 16

1. Microorganisms that cause infectious diseases can be classified as
   a. lytic
   b. endogenous
   c. pathogenic
   d. nosocomial

2. The best method of preventing the spread of aerosol infections is by
   a. the patient's wearing a mask
   b. the health care worker's wearing a gown
   c. hand washing
   d. all of the above

3. All of the following are types of indirect transmission *except*
   a. fomite
   b. vector
   c. aerosol
   d. touching

4. The common cold Is an example of an infection by a
   a. bacterium
   b. virus
   c. fungus
   d. protozoan

5. The term that best describes the absolute removal of all life forms is
   a. antisepsis
   b. medical asepsis
   c. disinfection
   d. sterilization

6. A person is bitten by a mosquito and develops an infection. This type of transmission is known as
   a. vector
   b. fomite
   c. nosocomial
   d. iatrogenic

7. A health care worker is accidentally punctured with a contaminated needle. This type of transmission is known as
   a. vector
   b. fomite
   c. nosocomial
   d. iatrogenic

8. An outpatient develops a staphylococcal infection after a surgical procedure. This type of transmission is known as
   a. vector
   b. fomite
   c. nosocomial
   d. more than one of the above, but not all

9. An infectious microbe can gain entrance into the human body by
   a. ingression
   b. penetration
   c. both a and b
   d. neither a nor b

10. Hand washing employs which of the following methods of infection control?
    a. chemical
    b. physical
    c. sterile
    d. a and b

CHAPTER 17

1. A pacemaker prevents bradycardia by
   1. sensing the patient's heartbeats
   2. pacing the heart when it does not contract
   3. producing electrical impulses
      a. 1 and 2 only
      b. 1 and 3 only
      c. 2 and 3 only
      d. 1, 2, and 3

2. What type of catheter is the Foley?
   a. retention balloon
   b. straight
   c. coiled
   d. self-cleansing

3. When handling sterile gloves with a nonsterile hand, which of the following is not considered sterile?
   a. outside of the cuff
   b. inside of the cuff
   c. fingertips of the glove
   d. thumb of the glove

4. Outside air is prevented from entering the pleural cavity through the chest tube by the
   a. collection chamber
   b. water seal chamber
   c. suction control chamber
   d. first compartment

5. The number-one priority for good sterile technique is
   a. sterile drapes
   b. gowns
   c. hand washing
   d. saline solution

6. The first rule of caring for a tracheostomy patient is
   a. watch for secretions.
   b. establish communication.
   c. contact the nurse in charge of the patient.
   d. attempt to finish the procedure as quickly as possible.

7. The purpose of the surgical hand scrub is to
   1. Remove debris and transient microorganisms from the hands, nails, and forearms.
   2. Destroy infected material.
   3. Inhibit rapid rebound growth of microorganisms.
      a. 1 and 2 only
      b. 1 and 3 only
      c. 2 and 3 only
      d. 1, 2, and 3

8. Urine should flow in a female patient when the catheter has been inserted approximately
   a. $1\frac{1}{2}$ inches
   b. $2\frac{1}{2}$ inches
   c. $4\frac{1}{2}$ inches
   d. $8\frac{1}{2}$ inches

9. What parts of a gown are considered sterile?
   1. sleeves
   2. front from the waist up
   3. back below the waist
      a. 1 and 2 only
      b. 1 and 3 only
      c. 2 and 3 only
      d. 1, 2, and 3

10. Which of the following are types of intravenous lines?
    1. Swan-Ganz
    2. femoral
    3. Hickman
       a. 1 and 2 only
       b. 1 and 3 only
       c. 2 and 3 only
       d. 1, 2, and 3

CHAPTER 18

1. The two most common types of nasogastric tubes are
   1. Levin
   2. Salem-sump
   3. Miller-Abbott
   4. Cantor
      a. 1 and 2
      b. 2 and 3
      c. 2 and 4
      d. 1 and 4

2. How can leakage from a double-lumen tube be prevented?
   a. Clamp with a hemostat.
   b. Clamp with a regular clamping device.
   c. Use a piston-like syringe.
   d. Leakage is not a problem with a double-lumen tube.

3. Bedpans should be
   a. rinsed between uses
   b. sterilized between uses
   c. disposed of after use
   d. none of the above

4. Hypertonic solution is used when
   a. fluid must be of the same osmolarity as that of the interstitial spaces of the colon.
   b. stool must be softened.
   c. the patient cannot tolerate large amounts of fluid.
   d. infant safety is a primary concern.

5. The normal adult patient should be able to tolerate how much fluid from a cleansing enema?
   a. 200 ml
   b. 500 ml
   c. 1000 ml
   d. 1500 ml

6. What should be done if cramping occurs during a barium enema?
   a. The patient should be told to use deep oral breathing.
   b. The enema should be stopped.
   c. The bag should be raised.
   d. Both a and b should be done.

7. Desirable characteristics of a barium suspension include
   1. rapid flow
   2. good mucosal adhesion
   3. thick layering
      a. 1 only
      b. 1 and 2 only
      c. 1 and 3 only
      d. 1, 2, and 3

8. A postural drop in blood pressure can occur after a barium enema as a result of
   a. a reaction from the barium
   b. dehydration
   c. trapping of barium in the transverse colon
   d. none of the above

9. With a double-barrel colostomy, the proximal stoma delivers and the distal stoma delivers
   a. stool or mucus
   b. mucus or stool
   c. mucus or flatus
   d. solids or fluids

10. Approximately what percentage of colostomy patients have recurrences of cancer?
    a. 10%
    b. 20%
    c. 30%
    d. 40%

CHAPTER 19

1. In working with a patient, which of the following would be the first priority for attention?
   a. providing an open airway
   b. splinting a fractured extremity
   c. controlling bleeding
   d. treating shock

2. Which of the following signs or symptoms is typically associated with a deteriorating head injury?
   a. increasing pulse rate
   b. increasing respiratory rate
   c. lethargy
   d. thirst

3. Which of the following actions would help prevent a patient from going into shock?
   a. minimizing pain
   b. providing emotional support
   c. maintaining a normal body temperature
   d. all of the above

4. A patient suffering from hypoglycemia needs which of the following?
   a. rest
   b. insulin
   c. carbohydrates
   d. a and c

5. Where should the heel of the hand be placed when performing chest compressions during cardiopulmonary resuscitation on an adult?
   a. near the sternal angle
   b. at the xiphoid process
   c. two fingers above the xiphoid process
   d. anywhere along the length of the sternum

6. *Syncope* is a medical term for which of the following?
   a. dizziness
   b. fainting
   c. hemorrhage
   d. nosebleed

7. Which of the following is typically associated with shock?
   a. decreasing pulse rate
   b. decreasing blood pressure
   c. fever
   d. flushed face

8. The Heimlich maneuver is used in response to which of the following situations?
   a. asthmatic crisis
   b. cardiac arrest
   c. choking
   d. wound dehiscence

9. How long can the brain be deprived of oxygen before cerebral function impairment is likely?
   a. 30 seconds
   b. 60 seconds
   c. 2 minutes
   d. 4 to 6 minutes

10. Which of the following actions is the most appropriate in handling a patient who begins a violent seizure?
    a. Restrain the patient in any way possible.
    b. Ensure an open airway, putting your hands into the victim's mouth if necessary.
    c. Attempt to prevent the patient from injuring himself or herself.
    d. All of the above are true.

CHAPTER 20

1. Who is the person licensed to prepare and dispense drugs?
   a. nurse
   b. radiologist
   c. physician
   d. pharmacist

2. The name given to a drug manufactured by a specific company is the
   a. trade (brand) name
   b. chemical name
   c. generic name
   d. nonproprietary name

3. A drug that relieves pain without causing a loss of consciousness is a(an)
   a. sedative
   b. analgesic
   c. anesthetic
   d. hypnotic

4. A patient with an abnormal rhythm of the heart would most likely be receiving which of the following?
   a. corticosteroids
   b. anticholinergic agents
   c. nonsteroidal antiinflammatory drugs
   d. antiarrhythmics

5. What class of drug is Benadryl?
   a. diuretic
   b. antibiotic
   c. anticholinergic
   d. antihistamine

6. In case of emergency, a patient with chronic obstructive pulmonary disease would most likely receive which of the following?
   a. Zantac
   b. Proventil
   c. Prozac
   d. Levophed

7. Drugs placed under the tongue are said to be administered
   a. subcutaneously
   b. sublingually
   c. topically
   d. parenterally

8. Which of the following statements expresses the correct relation between lumen diameter and gauge number?
   a. As the diameter increases, the gauge number increases.
   b. As the diameter decreases, the gauge number decreases.
   c. As the diameter decreases, the gauge number increases.
   d. As the diameter increases, the gauge number stays the same.

9. Long bevel needles are generally used for
   1. subcutaneous injection
   2. intramuscular injection
   3. intravenous injection
      a. 1 only
      b. 3 only
      c. 1 and 2 only
      d. 1, 2, and 3

10. A severe life-threatening response to a drug is called
    a. idiosyncratic
    b. anaphylaxis
    c. palliative
    d. pharmacognosy

CHAPTER 21

1. Contrast media are used in radiographic imaging to
   a. increase the radiographic density of the area of interest
   b. enhance the subject contrast of the area of interest
   c. decrease the radiographic density of the area of interest
   d. lower the subject contrast of the area of interest

2. Radiographic images that demonstrate few density differences define
   a. low subject contrast
   b. high subject contrast
   c. low x-ray photon absorption
   d. high x-ray photon absorption

3. A negative contrast agent will
   a. increase density and is radiopaque
   b. decrease density and is radiopaque
   c. decrease density and is radiolucent
   d. increase density and is radiolucent

4. A radiopharmaceutical is a
   a. radioactive contrast agent
   b. molecular imaging contrast agent
   c. radiographic contrast agent
   d. radioactive organ specific pharmaceutical

5. Contrast media that dissociate into two molecular particles are known as
   a. ionic agents
   b. low osmolality agents
   c. nonionic agents
   d. oil-based agents

6. Hydroxyl groups on nonionic water-soluble iodinated contrast media act to increase
   a. osmotic effects
   b. solubility
   c. blood pressure
   d. bronchospasm

7. External contamination of a short-lived diagnostic radioisotope is a problem because it might
   a. cause major harm to the patient and the caregiver
   b. be misconstrued as pathology on an image
   c. burn a patient
   d. disable a gamma camera

8. Which one of the following drugs should be discontinued 48 hours before and 48 hours after administration of water-soluble iodine contrast media?
   a. insulin
   b. glucagons
   c. beta-blockers
   d. metformin

9. What can be done for a patient who will receive water-soluble iodine contrast media to reduce allergic-like effects?
   a. premedicate with steroids and antihistamines.
   b. give intravenous fluids.
   c. instruct the patient to drink warm salt water before the procedure.
   d. give a negative contrast agent with the iodinated medium.

10. Which of the following acute reactions to contrast media usually requires no medical treatment?
    a. bronchospasm
    b. laryngeal edema
    c. urticaria
    d. convulsions

CHAPTER 22

1. A personal value system can be defined in terms of
   a. virtues
   b. values
   c. ethical principles
   d. morals
   e. all of the above

2. Professional ethics can be best defined as
   a. reflective decision making
   b. rules of right living
   c. the science of rightness and wrongness of human conduct
   d. a common concern for collective self-discipline
   e. rules promulgated by professional societies

3. Which of the following statements is *not* true?
   a. Ethics apply to specific groups.
   b. Laws apply to political subdivisions.
   c. Morals apply to individuals.
   d. Morals control individuals within a group.
   e. Ethics control a group from within.

4. Which of the following statements is true?
   a. Codes of ethics are usually written by individuals.
   b. Religious writings form the basis for ethical control.
   c. Codes of ethics are a form of legislation.
   d. Conscience controls individual morality.
   e. Laws provide an internal control for society.

5. Which of the following statements is *not* true?
   a. Ethical dilemmas may have competing moral principles.
   b. Ethical dilemmas involve decisions based on human values.
   c. Ethical dilemmas are easily solved by codes of ethics.
   d. Ethical dilemmas can be resolved by problem solving.
   e. Ethical dilemmas invite a wide range of personal opinions.

6. Moral rules are best applied to ethical dilemmas when
   a. religious beliefs are strongly held
   b. religious beliefs are not strongly held
   c. the ethical dilemma is very narrow in scope
   d. the ethical dilemma is very wide in scope
   e. all individuals agree to use moral rules

7. Action to benefit others is defined as
   a. veracity
   b. fidelity
   c. beneficence
   d. justice
   e. autonomy

8. Which is *not* a step in the problem-solving process?
   a. identifying the problem
   b. developing alternative solutions
   c. selecting the best solution
   d. defending your selection
   e. determining ethical sanctions

9. The strict observance of promises or duties is defined as
   a. fidelity
   b. justice
   c. autonomy
   d. confidentiality
   e. veracity

10. Generally accepted customs of right living and conduct are
    a. codes
    b. morals
    c. laws
    d. ethics
    e. rules

CHAPTER 23

1. Which of the following is not a function of a hospital health information management department?
   a. coding of diagnoses and operative procedures and diagnosis-related group assignment
   b. documenting relevant patient information in the medical record
   c. quality management and performance improvement activities
   d. appropriate release of medical information

2. The prospective payment system is a payment system based on which of the following?
   a. the diagnosis-related group (DRG)
   b. the coding system based on the *International Classification of Diseases,* 9th edition, Clinical Modification (ICD-9-CM)
   c. the Current Procedural Terminology (CPT) coding system
   d. the resource-based relative value system (RBRVS)

3. Which of the following is an example of an organization that accredits hospitals and other health care institutions in the United States?
   a. American Hospital Association
   b. American Medical Association
   c. Joint Commission on the Accreditation of Healthcare Organizations
   d. American College of Radiology

4. The chief complaint, included in a patient's history, is a statement made by the
   a. physician
   b. patient
   c. admitting officer
   d. admitting nurse

5. The Health Insurance Portability and Accountability Act of 1996 (HIPAA) legislation affects radiology and other hospital departments by its focus on
   a. patient record confidentiality
   b. facility reimbursement
   c. quality management and performance improvement
   d. risk management

6. Which of the following is *not* required to be included in a patient's health record?
   a. medical history
   b. radiology reports
   c. patient's telephone number
   d. physical examination report

7. Criteria used in quality management activities must be all of the following *except*
   a. clinically valid
   b. diagnosis or procedure oriented
   c. generally acceptable to department staffs
   d. written

8. Assessment of problems in quality management activities must be
   a. ongoing
   b. physician directed
   c. subjective
   d. objective

9. In making a correction to an entry in the paper health record, the documenter should
   a. line out the error, authenticate, and insert correct information.
   b. erase the incorrect information, and insert correct information.
   c. leave the incorrect entry alone, and add the new correct information.
   d. remove the incorrect page from the record, and begin a new page of documentation.

10. The organization (chart order, forms) of a hospital patient record is determined by
    a. the accrediting body's suggested format
    b. Medicare regulations
    c. the American Hospital Association–suggested format
    d. the hospital's own preference

CHAPTER 24

1. If a technologist threatens a patient during the course of a procedure and has an apparent immediate ability to perform the threatened act, which of the following torts may be claimed?
   a. assault
   b. battery
   c. negligence
   d. false imprisonment

2. The legal theory of respondeat superior requires that
   a. the employee is responsible for the actions of the employee.
   b. each person is responsible for his or her superior.
   c. the employer is responsible for the employee's actions.
   d. the employee is responsible for the employer's actions.

3. A technologist who has completed a procedure on a patient leaves the area grumbling, "I hate to do AIDS patients because I am afraid of catching the disease." A member of the housekeeping staff hears the technologist and asks who has AIDS. The technologist responds by giving the patient's name and room number. After this incident, housekeeping personnel refuse to clean the room. One person from housekeeping tells the story to members of the housekeeper's church, where the patient is also a member. After learning of the patient's condition, the church asks the patient not to return. What type of complaint might be brought against the technologist?
   a. negligence
   b. defamation
   c. assault
   d. false imprisonment

4. The claim of false imprisonment requires the patient to show proof that the technologist restrained his or her freedom without consent. The defenses a technologist may raise include all of the following *except* the
   a. risk that the patient was going to hurt himself or herself
   b. risk that the patient was going to hurt the technologist
   c. life-threatening condition of the patient's health
   d. need for motionless images

5. In a case in which the legal theory of res ipsa loquitur is being raised, the evidence presented must show all the following elements *except* that the
   a. injury would not have occurred except for negligence
   b. patient contributed to his or her injury
   c. defendant was in complete control
   d. patient did not contribute to his or her injury in any way

6. A consent form has been signed by a patient who will be undergoing an excretory urogram. A witness should sign the form after the patient. Who is the best witness?
   a. a member of the patient's family
   b. the radiographer performing the procedure
   c. a ward clerk who has no relationship with the patient or the procedure
   d. the patient's physician

7. Informed consent requires that the patient be given enough information to make an educated decision about his or her health care. The information the patient needs to make this decision includes all of the following *except*
   a. how the procedure will be performed
   b. the benefits of the procedure
   c. the alternatives to the procedure
   d. the cost of the procedure

8. What complaint may be brought against a technologist if he or she touches a patient in any way without the patient's permission?
   a. assault
   b. battery
   c. false imprisonment
   d. harassment

9. A radiographer is performing an abdominal series on a patient from the emergency department. To complete the examination, the patient must be moved from a supine to an upright position using the remote control on the table. During this movement, the patient falls from the table and suffers a fractured hip. A complaint of negligence is brought against both the radiographer and the hospital. The elements that the patient (plaintiff) must prove include all the following *except*
   a. a breach of the duty to the patient
   b. an injury
   c. a direct causal relation between the breach of duty and the injury
   d. that the radiographer acted outside of his or her scope of practice

10. A patient consents to a procedure in the radiology department, but after it has started, he decides that he does not want the procedure completed. The technologist should
   a. stop immediately.
   b. complete the procedure because the patient may not revoke consent once it is given.
   c. stop the procedure as soon as it is safe to do so.
   d. none of the above should be done.

Practice Standards
for Radiography

INTRODUCTION TO RADIOGRAPHY PRACTICE STANDARDS

The complex nature of disease processes involves multiple imaging modalities. Although an interdisciplinary team of radiologists, radiographers, and support staff plays a critical role in the delivery of health services, it is the radiographer who performs the radiographic examination that creates the images needed for diagnosis. Radiography integrates scientific knowledge and technical skills with effective patient interaction to provide quality patient care and useful diagnostic information.

Radiographer

Radiographers must demonstrate an understanding of human anatomy, physiology, pathology, and medical terminology.

Radiographers must maintain a high degree of accuracy in radiographic positioning and exposure technique. They must maintain knowledge about radiation protection and safety. Radiographers prepare for and assist the radiologist in the completion of intricate radiographic examinations. They prepare and administer contrast media and medications in accordance with state and federal regulations.

Radiographers are the primary liaison between patients and radiologists and other members of the support team. They must remain sensitive to the physical and emotional needs of the patient through good communication, patient assessment, patient monitoring, and patient care skills.

Radiographers use professional and ethical judgment and critical thinking when performing their duties. Quality improvement and customer service allow the radiographer to be a responsible member of the health care team by continually assessing professional performance. Radiographers embrace continuing education for optimal patient care, public education, and enhanced knowledge and technical competence.

Education and Certification

Radiographers prepare for their role on the interdisciplinary team by satisfactorily completing an accredited educational program in radiologic technology. Two-year certificate, associate degree, and four-year baccalaureate degree programs exist throughout the United States.

Accredited programs must meet specific curricular and educational standards. The Joint Review Committee on Education in Radiologic Technology (JRCERT) is the accrediting agency for radiologic technology programs recognized by the U.S. Department of Education.

Upon completion of a course of study in radiologic technology, individuals may apply to take the national certification examination. The American Registry of Radiologic Technologists (ARRT) is the recognized certifying agency for radiographers and offers examinations three times per year. Those who successfully complete the certification examination in radiography may use the credential RT(R) following their name; the RT signifies registered technologist, and the (R) indicates radiography.

To maintain ARRT certification, a level of expertise, and awareness of changes and advances in practice, radiographers must complete 24 hours of appropriate continuing education every 2 years.

Practice Standards

The practice standards define the practice and establish general criteria to determine compliance. Practice standards are authoritative statements enunciated and promulgated by the profession for judging the quality of practice, service, and education. They include desired and achievable levels of performance against which actual performance can be measured.

Professional practice constantly changes, and actual practice varies from state to state as determined by local law and community custom. Recognizing this, the profession has adopted standards that are general in nature. The general format was favored over a *cookbook* style or *step-by-step* approach that would be difficult to maintain in a changing environment and confining for those practitioners with an expanded practice.

The standards focus on the dynamic nature of the health care delivery system. The standards are adaptable not only to the area of practice but also to the locality of practice and institutional needs. While a minimum standard of acceptable performance is appropriate and should be followed by all practitioners in a specific area, it is unrealistic and highly inappropriate to assume that professional practice is the same in all regions of the United

States.* State statute or regulation may dictate practice parameters. To conduct an appropriate review of the standards, one must look to the professional standard as well as local or state law that may impact the nature and scope of practice.

Format

The cohesive nature and inherent differences of medical imaging and radiation therapy are recognized in the general format of the standards. The standards are divided into three sections: clinical performance, quality performance, and professional performance.

CLINICAL PERFORMANCE STANDARDS. The clinical performance standards define the activities of the practitioner in the care of patients and delivery of diagnostic or therapeutic procedures and treatments. The section incorporates patient assessment and management with procedural analysis, performance, and evaluation.

QUALITY PERFORMANCE STANDARDS. The quality performance standards define the activities of the practitioner in the technical areas of performance, including equipment and material assessment, safety standards, and total quality management.

PROFESSIONAL PERFORMANCE STANDARDS. The professional performance standards define the activities of the practitioner in the areas of education, interpersonal relationships, personal and professional self-assessment, and ethical behavior.

Each section of the standards is subdivided into individual standards. The standards are numbered and followed by a term or set of terms that identify the standards, such as *"assessment"* or *"analysis/determination."* The next statement is the expected performance of the practitioner when performing the procedure or treatment. A rationale statement follows and explains why a practitioner should adhere to the particular standard of performance.

Criteria

Criteria are used in evaluating a practitioner's performance. Each set of criteria is divided into two parts: the general criteria and the specific criteria. Both the measurement and specific criteria should be used when evaluating performance.

GENERAL CRITERIA. General criteria are written in a general style that applies to either medical imaging or radiation therapy practitioners. These criteria are the same in all sections of the standards and should be used for the appropriate area of practice. For example, a radiographer should use good professional judgment to make decisions concerning the adaptation of equipment and technical variables for a diagnostic procedure. Under these circumstances, evaluation of the decision-making process concerning radiation therapy procedures would not be appropriate and should not be applied unless the procedure is diagnostic in nature, such as simulation.

SPECIFIC CRITERIA. Specific criteria meet the needs of the practitioners in the various areas of professional performance. While many areas of performance within medical imaging and radiation therapy are similar, others are not. The specific criteria are drafted with these differences in mind. For example, a criterion that calls for daily review of patient treatment records and doses to ensure that treatment does not exceed prescribed dose or normal tissue tolerance is imperative for those who practice in radiation therapy yet is not applicable to those who practice in the imaging professions.

A profession's practice standards serve as a guide for appropriate practice. Standards provide role definition for practitioners that can be used by individual facilities to develop job descriptions and practice parameters. Those outside the medical imaging and radiation therapy community can use the standards as an overview of the role and responsibilities of the practitioner as defined by the profession.

RADIOGRAPHY CLINICAL PERFORMANCE STANDARDS

Standard One: Assessment

The practitioner collects pertinent data about the patient and about the procedure.

RATIONALE. Information about the patient's health status is essential in providing appropriate imaging and therapeutic services.

GENERAL CRITERIA. The practitioner:

1. Uses consistent and appropriate techniques to gather relevant information from the medical record, significant others, and health care providers. The collection

---

*The term *practitioner* is used in all areas of the standards in place of the various names used in medical imaging and radiation therapy, such as radiologic technologist, sonographer, or radiation therapist. Practitioner is defined as any person practicing in a specific area or discipline. The profession believes that any person practicing in one of the defined disciplines or specialties should be held to a minimum standard of performance to protect the patients who receive professional services.

of information is determined by the patient's needs or condition.

2. Reconfirms patient identification and verifies the procedure requested or prescribed.
3. Verifies the patient's pregnancy status when appropriate.
4. Determines whether the patient has been appropriately prepared for the procedure.
5. Assesses factors that may contraindicate the procedure, such as medications, insufficient patient preparation, or artifacts.

SPECIFIC CRITERIA. The practitioner identifies artifact-producing objects, such as dentures, chest leads, jewelry, and hearing aids.

Standard Two: Analysis/Determination

The practitioner analyzes the information obtained during the assessment phase and develops an action plan for completing the procedure.

RATIONALE. Determining the most appropriate action plan enhances patient safety and comfort, optimizes diagnostic and therapeutic quality, and improves cost effectiveness.

GENERAL CRITERIA. The practitioner:

1. Selects the most appropriate and cost-effective action plan after reviewing all pertinent data and assessing the patient's abilities and condition.
2. Uses his or her professional judgment to adapt imaging and therapeutic procedures to improve diagnostic quality and therapeutic outcome.
3. Consults appropriate medical personnel to determine a modified action plan when necessary.
4. Determines the needs for accessory equipment.

SPECIFIC CRITERIA. The practitioner:

1. Evaluates laboratory values prior to administering contrast media and beginning interventional procedures.
2. Selects appropriate shielding devices.
3. Selects appropriate patient immobilization devices.
4. Determines appropriate type and dose of contrast agent to be administered, based on the patient's age, weight, and medical/physical status.
5. Reviews the patient's chart and the physician's request to determine optimal imaging procedure for suspected pathology.

Standard Three: Patient Education

The practitioner provides information about the procedure to the patient, significant others, and health care providers.

RATIONALE. Communication and education are necessary to establish a positive relationship with the patient, significant others, and health care providers.

GENERAL CRITERIA. The practitioner:

1. Verifies that the patient has consented to the procedure and fully understands its risks, benefits, alternatives, and follow-up; verifies that written consent has been obtained when appropriate.
2. Provides accurate explanations and instructions at an appropriate time and at a level the patient can understand; addresses and documents patient questions and concerns regarding the procedure when appropriate.
3. Refers questions about diagnosis, treatment, or prognosis to the patient's physician.
4. Provides appropriate information to any individual involved in the patient's care.

SPECIFIC CRITERIA. The practitioner:

1. Consults with other departments, such as patient transportation and anesthesia, for patient services.
2. Instructs patients regarding preparation prior to imaging procedures, including providing information about oral or bowel preparation and allergy preparation.
3. Ensures that all procedural requirements are in place to achieve a quality diagnostic examination.
4. Explains precautions regarding administration of contrast agents to nursing mothers.

Standard Four: Implementation

The practitioner implements the action plan.

RATIONALE. Quality patient services are provided through the safe and accurate implementation of a deliberate plan of action.

GENERAL CRITERIA. The practitioner:

1. Implements an action plan that falls within established protocols and guidelines.
2. Elicits the cooperation of the patient to carry out the action plan.
3. Uses an integrated team approach as needed.
4. Modifies the action plan according to changes in the clinical situation.

5. Administers first aid or provides life support in emergency situations.
6. Uses accessory equipment when appropriate.
7. Assesses and monitors the patient's physical and mental state.

SPECIFIC CRITERIA. The practitioner:

1. Performs venipuncture, IV patency, and maintenance procedures according to established guidelines.
2. Administers contrast agents according to established guidelines.
3. Monitors the patient for reactions to contrast agent.
4. Uses appropriate radiation safety devices.
5. Monitors the patient's physical condition during the procedure.
6. Applies appropriate patient immobilization devices when necessary.

Standard Five: Evaluation

The practitioner determines whether the goals of the action plan have been achieved.
RATIONALE. Careful examination of the procedure is necessary to determine that all goals have been met.
GENERAL CRITERIA. The practitioner:

1. Evaluates the patient and the procedure to identify variances that may affect patient outcome. The evaluation process should be timely, accurate, and comprehensive.
2. Measures the procedure against established protocols and guidelines.
3. Identifies any exceptions to the expected outcome.
4. Documents any exceptions clearly and completely.
5. Develops a revised action plan to achieve the intended outcome if necessary.
6. Disseminates reasons for revisions to all team members.

SPECIFIC CRITERIA. The practitioner reviews images to determine if additional images will enhance the diagnostic value of the procedure.

Standard Six: Implementation

The practitioner implements the revised action plan.
RATIONALE. It may be necessary to make changes to the action plan to achieve the intended outcome.
GENERAL CRITERIA. The practitioner:

1. Bases the revised action plan on the patient's condition and the most appropriate means of achieving the intended outcome.
2. Takes action based on patient and procedural variances.
3. Measures and evaluates the results of the revised action plan.
4. Notifies appropriate health provider when immediate clinical response is necessary based on procedural findings and patient's condition.

Specific Criteria. None added.

Standard Seven: Outcomes Measurement

The practitioner reviews and evaluates the outcome of the procedure.
RATIONALE. To evaluate the quality of care, the practitioner compares the actual outcome with the intended outcome.
GENERAL CRITERIA. The practitioner:

1. Reviews all diagnostic or therapeutic data for completeness and accuracy.
2. Determines whether the actual outcome is within the established criteria.
3. Evaluates the process and recognizes opportunities for future changes.
4. Assesses the patient's physical and mental status prior to discharge from the practitioner's care.

Specific Criteria. None added.

Standard Eight: Documentation

The practitioner documents information about patient care, the procedure, and the final outcome.
RATIONALE. Clear and precise documentation is essential for continuity of care, accuracy of care, and quality assurance.
GENERAL CRITERIA. The practitioner:

1. Documents diagnostic, treatment, and patient data in the appropriate record. Documentation must be timely, accurate, concise, and complete.
2. Documents any exceptions from the established criteria or procedures.
3. Records diagnostic or treatment data.

Specific Criteria. None added.

QUALITY PERFORMANCE STANDARDS

Assessment

The practitioner collects pertinent information regarding equipment, the procedures, and the work environment.

RATIONALE. The planning and provision of safe and effective medical services rely on the collection of pertinent information about equipment, procedures, and the work environment.

GENERAL CRITERIA. The practitioner:

1. Ensures that services are performed in a safe environment in accordance with established guidelines.
2. Ensures that equipment maintenance and operation comply with established guidelines.
3. Assesses equipment to determine acceptable performance based on established guidelines.
4. Ensures that protocol and procedure manuals include recommended criteria and are reviewed and revised on a regular basis.

SPECIFIC CRITERIA. The practitioner maintains controlled access to restricted area during radiation exposure to ensure the safety of patients, visitors, and hospital personnel.

Standard Two: Analysis/Determination

The practitioner analyzes information collected during the assessment phase and determines whether changes need to be made to equipment, procedures, or the work environment.

RATIONALE. Determination of acceptable performance is necessary for the provision of safe and effective services.

GENERAL CRITERIA. The practitioner:

1. Assesses whether services, procedures, and the work environment meet or exceed established guidelines. If not, the practitioner develops an action plan.
2. Evaluates equipment to determine if it meets or exceeds established standards. If not, the practitioner develops an action plan.
3. Analyzes information collected during the assessment phase to determine whether optimal services are being provided. If not, the practitioner develops an action plan.

Specific Criteria. None added.

Standard Three: Education

The practitioner informs patients, the public, and other health care providers about procedures, equipment, and facilities.

RATIONALE. Open communication promotes safe practices.

GENERAL CRITERIA. The practitioner:

1. Elicits confidence and cooperation from the patient, the public, and health care providers by providing timely communication and effective instruction.
2. Presents explanations and instructions at the learner's level of understanding and learning style.

SPECIFIC CRITERIA. The practitioner:

1. Instructs health care providers and students regarding radiographic procedures and radiation safety.
2. Educates the public about radiographic procedures and radiation safety.

Standard Four: Performance

The practitioner performs quality assurance activities or acquires information on equipment and materials.

RATIONALE. Quality assurance activities provide valid and reliable information regarding the performance of materials and equipment.

GENERAL CRITERIA. The practitioner:

1. Performs quality assurance activities based on established quality protocols.
2. Provides evidence of ongoing quality assurance activities.

SPECIFIC CRITERIA. The practitioner monitors image production to determine variance from established quality standards.

Standard Five: Evaluation

The practitioner evaluates quality assurance results and establishes an appropriate action plan.

RATIONALE. Materials, equipment, and procedure safety depend on ongoing quality assurance activities that evaluate performance based on established guidelines.

GENERAL CRITERIA. The practitioner:

1. Compares quality assurance results to established acceptable values.
2. Verifies quality assurance testing conditions and results.
3. Formulates an action plan following verification of testing.

Specific Criteria. None added.

Standard Six: Implementation

The practitioner implements the quality assurance action plan.

RATIONALE. Implementation of a quality assurance action plan is imperative for quality diagnostic and therapeutic procedures and patient care.

GENERAL CRITERIA. The practitioner:

1. Obtains assistance from appropriate personnel to implement the quality assurance action plan.
2. Implements the quality assurance action plan.

Specific Criteria. None added.

Standard Seven: Outcomes Measurement

The practitioner assesses the outcome of the quality assurance action plan in accordance with established guidelines.

RATIONALE. Outcomes assessment is an integral part of the ongoing quality assurance plan to enhance diagnostic and therapeutic services.

GENERAL CRITERIA. The practitioner:

1. Reviews the implementation process for accuracy and validity.
2. Determines whether the performance of equipment and materials is safe for practice based on outcomes assessment.
3. Develops and implements a modified action plan when testing results are not in compliance with guidelines.

Specific Criteria. None added.

Standard Eight: Documentation

The practitioner documents quality assurance activities and results.

RATIONALE. Documentation provides evidence of quality assurance activities designed to enhance the safety of patients, the public, and health care providers during diagnostic and therapeutic services.

GENERAL CRITERIA. The practitioner:

1. Maintains documentation of quality assurance activities, procedures, and results in accordance with established guidelines.
2. Provides timely, concise, accurate, and complete documentation.
3. Provides documentation that adheres to current protocol, policy, and procedures.

Specific Criteria. None added.

PROFESSIONAL PERFORMANCE STANDARDS

Quality

The practitioner strives to provide optimal care to all patients.

RATIONALE. All patients expect and deserve optimal care during diagnosis and treatment.

GENERAL CRITERIA. The practitioner:

1. Works with others to elevate the quality of care.
2. Participates in quality assurance programs.
3. Adheres to the accepted standards, policies, and procedures adopted by the profession and regulated by law.
4. Provides the best possible diagnostic study or therapeutic treatment for each patient by applying professional judgment and discretion.
5. Anticipates and responds to the needs of the patient.

Specific Criteria. None added.

Standard Two: Self-Assessment

The practitioner evaluates personal performance, knowledge, and skills.

RATIONALE. Self-assessment is an important tool in professional growth and development.

GENERAL CRITERIA. The practitioner:

1. Monitors personal work ethics, behaviors, and attitudes.
2. Monitors and evaluates orientation guidelines and recommends improvements or changes as needed.
3. Evaluates performance and recognizes opportunities for improvement.

4. Recognizes his or her strengths and uses them to benefit patients, co-workers, and the profession.
5. Performs procedures only after receiving appropriate education and training.
6. Recognizes and takes advantage of opportunities for educational growth and improvement in technical and problem-solving skills.
7. Actively participates in professional societies and organizations.

Specific Criteria. None added.

Standard Three: Education

The practitioner acquires and maintains current knowledge in clinical practice.
RATIONALE. Advancements in medical science require enhancement of knowledge and skills through education.
GENERAL CRITERIA. The practitioner:

1. Maintains appropriate credentials and certification related to clinical practice.
2. Demonstrates completion of the appropriate education related to clinical practice.
3. Participates in educational activities to enhance knowledge, skills, and performance.
4. Shares knowledge and expertise with others.

Specific Criteria. None added.

Standard Four: Collaboration and Collegiality

The practitioner promotes a positive, collaborative practice atmosphere with other members of the health care team.
RATIONALE. To provide quality patient care, all members of the health care team must communicate effectively and work together efficiently.
GENERAL CRITERIA. The practitioner:

1. Shares knowledge and expertise with colleagues, peers, students, and all members of the health care team.
2. Develops collaborative partnerships with other health care providers in the interest of diagnostic and therapeutic quality and cost effectiveness and safety.

Specific Criteria. None added.

Standard Five: Ethics

The practitioner adheres to the profession's accepted code of ethics.
RATIONALE. All decisions and actions made on behalf of the patient are based on a sound ethical foundation.
GENERAL CRITERIA. The practitioner:

1. Provides health care services with respect for the patient's dignity and age-specific needs.
2. Acts as a patient advocate to support patients' rights.
3. Takes responsibility for professional decisions.
4. Delivers patient care and service without bias based on personal attributes, nature of the disease, sex, race, creed, religion, or socioeconomic status.
5. Respects the patient's right to privacy and confidentiality.
6. Adheres to the established practice standards of the profession.

Specific Criteria. None added.

Standard Six: Exploration and Investigation

The practitioner participates in the acquisition, dissemination, and advancement of the professional knowledge base.
RATIONALE. Scholarly activities such as research, scientific investigation, presentation, and publication advance the profession and thereby improve the quality and efficiency of patient services.
GENERAL CRITERIA. The practitioner:

1. Reads and critically evaluates research in diagnostic and therapeutic services.
2. Investigates new, innovative methods and applies them in practice.
3. Shares information with colleagues through publication, presentation, and collaboration.
4. Pursues lifelong learning.
5. Participates in data collection.

Specific Criteria. None added.

RADIOGRAPHY GLOSSARY

Artifact: False feature in the image produced by patient instability or equipment deficiencies
Assess: To determine the significance, importance, or value

Clinical: Pertaining to or found on actual observation and treatment of patients

Competency: Having the ability to perform a task

Contrast medium: Substance administered to subject being imaged to alter selectively the image intensity of a particular anatomic or functional region

Contraindicate: To make the indicated or expected treatment or drug inadvisable

Disease: A disorder or abnormal condition having a characteristic train of symptoms that may affect the whole body or any of its parts. Its etiology, pathology, and prognosis may be known or unknown.

Ethical: Conforming to the standards of conduct of a given profession or group

Interpret: To understand and explain an image to provide a diagnostic report

Interventional procedure: Percutaneous catheterization for diagnostic and therapeutic purposes

Quality assurance: A comprehensive set of policies and procedures designed to optimize the performance of personnel and equipment

Radiation protection: Procedures followed to prevent inappropriate or accidental irradiation of patient, public, and health care professionals

Radiography: An image produced on a sensitized film by x-rays

Venipuncture: The puncture of a vein.

Professional Organizations

Contact information for most of the professional organizations discussed in this book is listed here to assist individuals who require more information or who wish to join or become involved in professional activities.

ACCREDITING AGENCIES

Joint Review Committee on Education in Diagnostic Medical Sonography
2025 Woodland Dr.
St. Paul, MN 55125
651-731-1582
http://www.jrcdms.org

Joint Review Committee on Education in Radiologic Technology
20 North Wacker Dr., Suite 2850
Chicago, IL 60606-2901
312-704-5300
http://www.jrcert.org

Joint Review Committee on Education Programs in Nuclear Medicine Technology
716 Black Point Rd.
PO Box 1149
Polson, MT 59860
406-883-0003
http://www.jrcnmt.org

REGISTRIES AND OTHER CERTIFICATION AGENCIES

American Registry of Diagnostic Medical Sonographers
15 Monroe St.
Plaza East One
Rockville, MD 20850
800-541-9754 or 301-738-8401
http://www.ardms.org

American Registry of Radiologic Technologists
1255 Northland Dr.
St. Paul, MN 55120-1155
612-687-0048
http://www.arrt.org

Nuclear Medicine Technology Certification Board
2970 Clairmont Rd., Suite 935
Atlanta, GA 30329
404-315-1739
http://www.nmtcb.org

STATE LICENSING AGENCIES

See Appendix C.

PROFESSIONAL SOCIETIES

American Healthcare Radiology Administrators
490B Boston Post Rd., Suite 101
PO Box 334
Sudbury, MA 01776
978-443-7591 or 800-334-2472
http://www.ahraonline.org

American Society of Radiologic Technologists
15000 Central Ave., SE
Albuquerque, NM 87123-3909
505-298-4500
http://www.asrt.org

Association of Educators in Imaging and Radiologic Sciences, Inc.
PO Box 90204
Albuquerque, NM 87199
505-823-4740
http://www.aers.org (soon to be *http://www.aeirs.org*)

Association of Vascular and Interventional Radiographers
10201 Lee Hwy., Suite 500
Fairfax, VA 22030
703-691-2350
http://www.avir.org

International Society for Clinical Densitometry
342 N. Main St.
West Hartford, CT 06117
860-586-7563
http://www.iscd.org

International Society of Radiographers and Radiologic Technologists
ISRRT Secretary-General
143 Bryn Pinwydden, Cardiff, CF23 7DG, Wales, United Kingdom
http://www.isrrt.org

Society of Breast Imaging
1891 Preston White Dr.
Reston, VA 20191
703-715-4390
http://www.sbi-online.org

The Society for Computer Applications in Radiology
10105 Cottesmore Ct.
Great Falls, VA 22066-3540
703-757-0054
e-mail: info@scarnet.org

Society of Diagnostic Medical Sonographers
2745 Dallas Pkwy, Suite 350
Plano, TX 75093
800-229-9506 or 214-473-8057
http://www.sdms.org

Society of Magnetic Resonance Technologists/ Society of Magnetic Resonance in Medicine/Society for Magnetic Resonance Imaging
2118 Milvia St., Suite 201
Berkeley, CA 94704
510-841-1899
http://www.ismrm.org/smrt

Society of Nuclear Medicine—Technologist Section
1850 Samuel Morse Dr.
Reston, VA 20190-5316
703-708-9000
http://www.snm.org

STATE AND LOCAL RADIOLOGIC TECHNOLOGY SOCIETIES

Because many state societies do not maintain an executive office, we suggest contacting the American Society of Radiologic Technologists for current addresses and telephone numbers. Local societies can usually be contacted through local radiologic technology educators or administrators or through the state society.

RADIOLOGIST ORGANIZATIONS

American Association of Physicists in Medicine
One Physics Ellipse
College Park, MD 20740
301-209-3350
http://www.aapm.org

American Board of Radiology
5441 E. Williams Blvd., Suite 200
Tucson, AZ 87511
520-790-2900
http://www.theabr.org

American College of Radiology
1891 Preston White Dr.
Reston, VA 22091
703-648-8900
http://www.acr.org

American Institute of Ultrasound in Medicine
14750 Sweitzer Ln., Suite 100
Laurel, MD 20707
301-498-4400 or 800-638-5352
http://www.aium.org

The American Medical Association
515 North State St.
Chicago, IL 60610
312-464-5000
http://www.ama-assn.org

American Roentgen Ray Society
44211 Slatestone Ct.
Leesburg, VA 20176
800-438-2777
http://www.arrs.org

American Society for Therapeutic Radiology and Oncology
12500 Fair Lakes Cir., Suite 375
Fairfax, VA 22033
800-962-7876
http://www.astro.org

Radiological Society of North America
820 Jorie Blvd.
Oak Brook, IL 60523
630-571-2670
http://www.rsna.org

APPENDIX

C

State Licensing
Agencies

Most states (including the territory of Puerto Rico and the District of Columbia) have licensing laws in effect or under development for radiographers. Although the laws and regulations vary widely from state to state, all states that require licenses accept the Examination in Radiography of the American Registry of Radiologic Technologists (ARRT) to obtain a license to practice.

Students or radiographers desiring information should contact the appropriate agency for the particular state. Although addresses and telephone numbers sometimes change, the most current for each are listed here. A current listing of contacts for state licensing agencies is maintained by the American Society of Radiologic Technologists on their website at *http://www.asrt.org* (check under Government Relations).

ALABAMA

Office of Radiation Control
State Department of Public Health
201 Monroe St./PO Box 303017
Montgomery, AL 36130-3017
334-206-5391, fax: 334-206-5387
kwhatley@adph.state.al.us
Brad Grinstead, X-ray Compliance & Registration
bgrinstead@adph.state.al.us
http://www.adph.org

ALASKA

Radiologic Health Program
4500 Boniface Pkwy.
Anchorage, AK 99507-1270
907-334-2107, fax: 907-334-2162
clyde_pearce@health.state.ak.us
http://www.hss.state.ak.us

ARIZONA

State of Arizona
Medical Radiologic Technology Board of Examiners
4814 South 40th St.
Phoenix, AZ 85040-2940
602-255-4845

ARKANSAS

Licensing Accreditation and Registration
Division of Radiation Control and Emergency Management
4815 W. Markham, Slot 30
Little Rock, AR 72205
501-661-2301

CALIFORNIA

Division of Food and Radiation Safety
Radiologic Health Branch
PO Box 997414
1500 Capitol
Sacramento, CA 95899-7414
916-440-7899, fax: 916-440-7900
ebailey@dhs.ca.gov
Victor Anderson, Certification Standards and Training
916-440-7931
vanderso@dhs.ca.gov
http://www.dhs.ca.gov/rhb

COLORADO

Radiation Control Division
Colorado Department of Health
4300 Cherry Creek Dr. South
Denver, CO 80222-1530
303-692-3441

CONNECTICUT

Applications, Examinations and Licensure
Department of Public Health
Radiographer Licensure
79 Elm St.
Hartford, CT 06106
860-424-3029

DELAWARE

State of Delaware
Office of Radiation Control
Robbins Building
PO Box 637
Dover, DE 19903
302-744-4944

DISTRICT OF COLUMBIA

Department of Health
51 N Street NE, Room 6025
Washington, DC 20002
202-535-2320

FLORIDA

State of Florida
Radiologic Technology Program
Department of Health/Bureau of Radiation Control
4052 Bald Cypress Way, Bin C21
Tallahassee, FL 32399-1741
850-245-4540

GEORGIA

Office of Regulatory Services—X-ray Unit
Department of Human Resources
2 Peachtree St., 19th Floor
Atlanta, GA 30303
404-657-5400

HAWAII

State of Hawaii
Radiologic Technology Board
Department of Health
Noise and Radiation Branch
591 Ala Moana Blvd.
Honolulu, HI 96801
808-586-4700

IDAHO

Idaho Department of Health and Welfare
Division of Health
Radiation Control
2220 Old Penitential Rd.
Boise, ID 83712
208-334-2235

ILLINOIS

State of Illinois
Division of Nuclear Safety
1035 Outer Park Dr.
Springfield, IL 62704
217-785-6982

INDIANA

State of Indiana
Department of Health
2 N. Meridian St.
Indianapolis, IN 46204
317-233-7146

IOWA

State of Iowa
Bureau of Radiological Health
401 SW 7th St., Suite D
Des Moines, IA 50309-4611
515-281-3478

KANSAS

State of Kansas
Radiation Section
1000 SW Jackson St., Suite 310
Topeka, KS 66612-1366
785-296-1565

KENTUCKY

State of Kentucky
Operator Certification Coordinator
Radiation Control Branch
275 East Main St.
Frankfort, KY 40621-0001
502-564-7818

LOUISIANA

Louisiana State Radiologic Technology
PO Box 4313
602 N. 5th
Baton Rouge, LA 70821
225-219-3366

MAINE

State of Maine
Radiologic Technology Board of Examiners
State House Station #35
Augusta, ME 04333-0035
207-624-8623

MARYLAND

Radiologic Health Program
1800 Washington Blvd., Suite 750
Baltimore, MD 21230-1724
410-537-3301

MASSACHUSETTS

Radiation Control Program
90 Washington St.
Dorchester, MA 02121
617-427-2944

MICHIGAN

Radiation Safety Section
Department of Community Health
PO Box 30664
Lansing, MI 48909
517-241-1989

MINNESOTA

Radiation Control Unit
Minnesota Department of Health
1645 Energy Park Dr., Suite 300
St. Paul, MN 55108
651-642-0492

MISSISSIPPI

Division of Radiological Health
PO Box 1700
3150 Lawson St.
Jackson, MS 39215-1700
601-987-6893

MISSOURI

Medical Radiation Control Program
PO Box 570
Jefferson City, MO 65102-0570
573-751-6083

MONTANA

Radiological Health Program
Department of Public Health and Human Services
Quality Assurance Division, Licensure Bureau
2401 Colonial Dr.
PO Box 202953
Helena, MT 59620-2951
406-444-2868

NEBRASKA

Nebraska Department of Health
Professional and Occupational Licensure Division
PO Box 94986
Lincoln, NE 68509-4986
402-471-0528

NEVADA

Radiological Health Section
1179 Fairview Dr., Suite 102
Carson City, NV 89701-5405
775-687-5394

NEW HAMPSHIRE

Bureau of Radiological Health
Health and Welfare Building
#29 Hazen Dr.
Concord, NH 03301
603-271-4588

NEW JERSEY

State of New Jersey
Department of Environmental Protection
Radiation Protection Programs
Box 415
Trenton, NJ 08625-0415
609-984-5636

NEW MEXICO

Radiologic Technologist Certification Program
New Mexico Environment Department
PO Box 26110
Santa Fe, NM 87502-6110
505-467-3264

NEW YORK

Bureau of Environment Radiation Protection
New York State Department of Health, Room 325
547 River St., Room 530
Troy, NY 12180-2216
518-402-7580

NORTH CAROLINA

Division of Radiation Protection
Electronic Production Radiation Section
3825 Barrett Dr.
Raleigh, NC 27609-7221
919-571-4141

NORTH DAKOTA

North Dakota State Department of Health
Division of Environmental Engineering
1200 Missouri Ave., Room 304
Box 5520
Bismarck, ND 58506-5520
701-328-5188

OHIO

Bureau of Radiation Protection
PO Box 118
Columbus, OH 43266-0118
614-644-2727

OKLAHOMA

Department of Environmental Quality
Radiation and Special Hazards
1000 NE 10th St.
Oklahoma City, OK 73117-1212
405-271-5243

OREGON

Board of Radiologic Technology
800 NE Oregon St., Suite 1160A
Portland, OR 97232-2187
503-731-4088

PENNSYLVANIA

Bureau of Radiation Protection
Department of Environmental Health
Health Licensing Division
PO Box 8469
Harrisburg, PA 17105-8469
717-783-5919

PUERTO RICO

Radiologic Health Division
Department of Environmental Health
PO Box 70184
San Juan, PR 00936-8184
787-274-7815

RHODE ISLAND

Professional Regulation
3 Capitol Hill, Room 104
Providence, RI 02908
401-277-2436

SOUTH CAROLINA

Bureau of Radiologic Health
2600 Bull St.
Columbia, SC 29201
803-545-4403

SOUTH DAKOTA

Licensure and Certification
Office of Health Care Facilities
615 East 4th St.
Pierre, SD 57501-1700
605-773-3356

TENNESSEE

Tennessee Board of Medical Examiners
Health Related Board
1st Floor, Cordell Hall Bldg.
426 Fifth Ave. North
Nashville, TN 37247-1010
1-800-778-4123

TEXAS

Texas Department of Health
Professional Licensing and Certification Division
1100 West 49th St.
Austin, TX 78756-3183
512-834-6617

UTAH

Division of Occupational and Professional Licensing
PO Box 144850
Salt Lake City, UT 84145
801-536-6403

VERMONT

Office of Radiological Health
PO Box 70
Burlington, VT 05402
802-865-7730

VIRGINIA

Board of Medicine for Radiologic Technology
6603 West Broad St., 5th Floor
Richmond, VA 23230-1712
804-662-9908

WASHINGTON

Washington State Department of Health
Radiologic Technologist/X-Ray Technician Program
PO Box 47869
Olympia, WA 98504-7869
360-236-4941

WEST VIRGINIA

WV Radiological Health Program
Bureau for Public Health, OEHS
815 Quarrier St., Suite 418
Charleston, WV 25301-2616
304-558-6772

WISCONSIN

Radiation Protection Section
Department of Health and Family Services
PO Box 2659
Madison, WI 53701-2659
608-267-4792

WYOMING

Wyoming Board of Radiologic
Technologist Examiners
First Bank Plaza, Suite 201
2020 Carey Ave.
Cheyenne, WY 82002
307-777-3507

The American Registry of Radiologic Technologists® Code of Ethics

The Code of Ethics forms the first part of the *Standards of Ethics*. The Code of Ethics shall serve as a guide by which Registered Technologists and Candidates may evaluate their professional conduct as it relates to patients, health care consumers, employers, colleagues, and other members of the health care team. The Code of Ethics is intended to assist Registered Technologists and Candidates in maintaining a high level of ethical conduct and in providing for the protection, safety, and comfort of patients. The Code of Ethics is aspirational.

1. The radiologic technologist conducts herself or himself in a professional manner, responds to patient needs, and supports colleagues and associates in providing quality patient care.

2. The radiologic technologist acts to advance the principal objective of the profession to provide services to humanity with full respect for the dignity of mankind.

3. The radiologic technologist delivers patient care and service unrestricted by the concerns of personal attributes or the nature of the disease or illness, and without discrimination, on the basis of sex, race, creed, religion, or socioeconomic status.

4. The radiologic technologist practices technology founded upon theoretical knowledge and concepts, uses equipment and accessories consistent with the purposes for which they were designed, and employs procedures and techniques appropriately.

5. The radiologic technologist assesses situations; exercises care, discretion, and judgment; assumes responsibility for professional decisions; and acts in the best interest of the patient.

6. The radiologic technologist acts as an agent through observation and communication to obtain pertinent information for the physician to aid in the diagnosis and treatment of the patient and recognizes that interpretation and diagnosis are outside the scope of practice for the profession.

7. The radiologic technologist uses equipment and accessories, employs techniques and procedures, performs services in accordance with an accepted standard of practice, and demonstrates expertise in minimizing the radiation exposure to the patient, self, and other members of the health care team.

8. The radiologic technologist practices ethical conduct appropriate to the profession and protects the patient's right to quality radiologic technology care.

9. The radiologic technologist respects confidences entrusted in the course of professional practice, respects the patient's right to privacy, and reveals confidential information only as required by law or to protect the welfare of the individual or the community.

10. The radiologic technologist continually strives to improve knowledge and skills by participating in continuing educational and professional activities, sharing knowledge with colleagues, and investigating new aspects of professional practice.

The Patient Care Partnership: Understanding Expectations, Rights, and Responsibilities

When you need hospital care, your doctor and the nurses and other professionals at our hospital are committed to working with you and your family to meet your health care needs. Our dedicated doctors and staff serve the community in all its ethnic, religious and economic diversity. Our goal is for you and your family to have the same care and attention we would want for our families and ourselves.

The sections explain some of the basics about how you can expect to be treated during your hospital stay. They also cover what we will need from you to care for you better. If you have questions at any time, please ask them. Unasked or unanswered questions can add to the stress of being in the hospital. Your comfort and confidence in your care are very important to us.

WHAT TO EXPECT DURING YOUR HOSPITAL STAY

- **High quality hospital care.** Our first priority is to provide you the care you need, when you need it, with skill, compassion, and respect. Tell your caregivers if you have concerns about your care or if you have pain. You have the right to know the identity of doctors, nurses and others involved in your care, and you have the right to know when they are students, residents or other trainees.
- **A clean and safe environment.** Our hospital works hard to keep you safe. We use special policies and procedures to avoid mistakes in your care and keep you free from abuse or neglect. If anything unexpected and significant happens during your hospital stay, you will be told what happened, and any resulting changes in your care will be discussed with you.
- **Involvement in your care.** You and your doctor often make decisions about your care before you go to the hospital. Other times, especially in emergencies, those decisions are made during your hospital stay. When decision-making takes place, it should include:

Discussing your medical condition and information about medically appropriate treatment choices. To make informed decisions with your doctor, you need to understand:

The benefits and risks of each treatment.
Whether your treatment is experimental or part of a research study.
What you can reasonably expect from your treatment and any long-term effects it might have on your quality of life.

What you and your family will need to do after you leave the hospital.
The financial consequences of using uncovered services or out-of-network providers.

Please tell your caregivers if you need more information about treatment choices.

Discussing your treatment plan. When you enter the hospital, you sign a general consent to treatment. In some cases, such as surgery or experimental treatment, you may be asked to confirm in writing that you understand what is planned and agree to it. This process protects your right to consent to or refuse a treatment. Your doctor will explain the medical consequences of refusing recommended treatment. It also protects your right to decide if you want to participate in a research study.

Getting information from you. Your caregivers need complete and correct information about your health and coverage so that they can make good decisions about your care. That includes:

Past illnesses, surgeries or hospital stays.
Past allergic reactions.
Any medicines or dietary supplements (such as vitamins and herbs) that you are taking.
Any network or admission requirements under your health plan.

Understanding your health care goals and values. You may have health care goals and values or spiritual beliefs that are important to your well-being. They will be taken into account as much as possible throughout your hospital stay. Make sure your doctor, your family and your care team know your wishes.

Understanding who should make decisions when you cannot. If you have signed a health care power of attorney stating who should speak for you if you become unable to make health care decisions for yourself, or a *"living will"* or *"advance directive"* that states your wishes about end-of-life care; give copies to your doctor, your family and your care team. If you or your family need help making difficult decisions, counselors, chaplains and others are available to help.

- **Protection of your privacy.** We respect the confidentiality of your relationship with your doctor and other caregivers, and the sensitive information about your health and health care that are part of that relationship. State and federal laws and hospital operating policies protect the privacy of your medical information. You will receive a *Notice of Privacy Practices* that describes the ways that we use, disclose and safeguard patient information and that explains how you can obtain a copy of information from our records about your care.

- **Preparing you and your family for when you leave the hospital.** Your doctor works with hospital staff and professionals in your community. You and your family also play an important role in your care. The success of your treatment often depends on your efforts to follow medication, diet and therapy plans. Your family may need to help care for you at home.

You can expect us to help you identify sources of follow-up care and to let you know if our hospital has a financial interest in any referrals. As long as you agree that we can share information about your care with them, we will coordinate our activities with your caregivers outside the hospital. You can also expect to receive information and, where possible, training about the self-care you will need when you go home.

Help with your bill and filing insurance claims. Our staff will file claims for you with health care insurers or other programs such as Medicare and Medicaid. They also will help your doctor with needed documentation. Hospital bills and insurance coverage are often confusing. If you have questions about your bill, contact our business office. If you need help understanding your insurance coverage or health plan, start with your insurance company or health benefits manager. If you do not have health coverage, we will try to help you and your family find financial help or make other arrangements. We need your help with collecting needed information and other requirements to obtain coverage or assistance.

While you are here, you will receive more detailed notices about some of the rights you have as a hospital patient and how to exercise them. We are always interested in improving.

Reprinted with permission of the American Hospital Association, copyright 2003.

Index